1,000 DIABETES RECIPES

JACKIE MILLS

WILEY

John Wiley & Sons, Inc.

To my loving husband, Nick. I would not be here without you.

This book is printed on acid-free paper. ♾

Copyright © 2011 by Jackie Mills. All rights reserved

Illustration Copyright © 2011 Gina Triplett

Published by John Wiley & Sons, Inc., Hoboken, New Jersey

Published simultaneously in Canada

For general information on our other products and services or for technical support, please contact our Customer Care Department within the United States at (877) 762–2974, outside the United States at (317) 572–3993 or fax (317) 572–4002.

Wiley also publishes its books in a variety of electronic formats. Some content that appears in print may not be available in electronic books. For more information about Wiley products, visit our web site at www.wiley.com.

Library of Congress Cataloging-in-Publication Data:

Mills, Jackie, 1961-

1,000 diabetes recipes / Jackie Mills.

    p. cm.

Includes index.

ISBN 978-0-470-40744-8 (cloth); ISBN 978-1-118-11041-6 (ebk); ISBN 978-1-118-11042-3 (ebk); ISBN 978-1-118-11043-0 (ebk)

1. Diabetes--Diet therapy--Recipes. I. Title. II. Title: One thousand diabetes recipes.

RC662.M54 2010

641.5'6314--dc22

            2010044591

All decorative spot art: © gettyimages/IMZ

Decorative borders & rules: ©istockphoto.com/dobric

Printed in the United States of America

10 9 8 7 6 5 4 3 2 1

Publisher: Natalie Chapman

Senior Editor: Linda Ingroia

Senior Production Editor: Amy Zarkos

Cover Designer: Jeffrey Faust

Interior Designer: Holly Wittenberg

Manufacturing Manager: Kevin Watt

Cover Illustrator: Gina Triplett

Contents

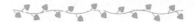

Acknowledgments

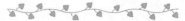

It takes a group of talented and passionate people to produce a book of this size and scope and luckily, the colleagues and friends who helped me create this one were rich in wisdom and more than generous with their time, expertise, and kindness.

I owe special gratitude to Betsy Bohannon, Lorena Drago, and Cindy Silver, all dietitians who work with people with diabetes in very different settings, and all of who graciously shared their expert knowledge with me. Bea Krinke and Madelyn Wheeler never lost patience with my endless questions on the intricacies of calculating diabetic exchanges.

I can never thank Molly Shuster enough. She spent tireless hours in my home kitchen testing and retesting recipes until they tasted too good to be healthy (but they are!). Her skill as a cook and her cheerful spirit were invaluable.

Thanks to my dear friends Judy Feagin, Julia Rutland, and Rebecca Reed for generously sharing their favorite healthy recipes. Thank you to my friend and word maven, Deborah Mintcheff, who read and commented on early drafts of the introduction of the book. I am grateful for the friendship of Eileen Runyan and for her unwavering support of my work. And thanks to Mark Fowler, my skillful advocate and advisor.

Linda Ingroia, my editor at Wiley, is professionalism personified. She made me believe that I was the person to write this book and her advice and knowledge kept me on track through the entire project. Thanks to Amy Zarkos for shepherding the book through production; Holly Wittenberg for creating the accessible, attractive design; and Jeff Faust for designing and Gina Triplett for illustrating such a fresh new cover. Thanks to copy editor Justine Gardener for making sure that the recipes were clear and consistent and that my words conveyed what I really meant to say.

Most of all, thank you to my husband, Nick, for his boundless love and encouragement and for grocery shopping almost daily for two years.

Introduction

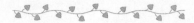

Sharing delicious food with friends and family is one of life's simplest and greatest pleasures. And when the food is chosen wisely, with good nutrition in mind, what we eat has lasting implications for good health and longevity. This is true for everyone, but is even more important for people who have a family history of diabetes.

Over the years I have watched several members of my family struggle with the challenges of living with diabetes—and you may have, too. As a registered dietitian, this made me determined to help others recognize the positive impact that a healthful diet has in preventing type 2 diabetes and in delaying complications for those who have the disease.

Preparing flavorful and nourishing meals is excellent advice for everyone, as it can prevent not just diabetes, but heart disease, high blood pressure, and some types of cancer. This book is an essential guide to eating healthfully, whether you have diabetes yourself, prepare meals for someone who does, or just want to cook delicious nourishing meals for your family. Let's start with a review of what diabetes is all about.

What is diabetes? Diabetes is a chronic condition where the body produces no insulin, produces too little insulin, or is unable to use the insulin it does produce efficiently. Insulin is a hormone produced in the pancreas. After eating a meal, the digestive juices in the body break down starches and sugars into glucose, a simple sugar. Glucose is the body's main source of fuel used for energy. Insulin is the "key" that unlocks the cells to allow glucose to enter.

When there is not enough insulin, or when the body cannot use the insulin it produces, the glucose remains in the bloodstream and ultimately passes out of the body unused in the urine. Over time, high levels of blood glucose can result in complications including heart disease, kidney damage, eye problems, and nerve damage.

Types of diabetes. There are two major types of diabetes: type 1 and type 2. As a general rule, though not always, type 1 diabetes is diagnosed in children and young adults. With this type of diabetes, the body doesn't produce any insulin and insulin must be injected several times a day. Only about 5 to 10 percent of people with diabetes have type 1.

Much more common is type 2 diabetes. Here the body does not produce enough insulin or the body isn't able to use the insulin it does produces (this is called insulin resistance). Type 2 diabetes used to be a disease of middle age. Now, because of obesity, it is being diagnosed in younger people.

What causes diabetes? There is a genetic factor in both type 1 and type 2 diabetes, but there is also a key environmental trigger that kick-starts the disease. In most cases of type 1, there has to be a family history of diabetes from both parents to get the disease. But family history alone does not mean the person will have diabetes. Something else—as of yet unknown—triggers the disease. Theories include a virus, early diet (those who were breastfed and those who ate solid food at a later age get type 1 less often), and cold weather (the disease is more commonly diagnosed in winter months and in people who live in cold climates).

A family history of diabetes is also a strong predictor of type 2 diabetes. But in almost all cases, the disease presents itself, no matter the family history, when a person is overweight and gets too little exercise.

What is pre-diabetes? There is also a condition called pre-diabetes. In this situation, blood glucose levels are not high enough to be diagnosed with diabetes, but they are higher than normal. The ADA estimates there are 57 million people who have pre-diabetes. Of those, an estimated 70 percent will eventually develop type 2 diabetes if they do not make lifestyle changes to lower their weight and increase their exercise.

Pre-diabetes is a serious condition, as permanent damage to the heart and circulatory system may occur when a person has it. With lifestyle changes such as a 5 to 10 percent weight loss and 30 minutes of physical activity a day, people with pre-diabetes can delay or even prevent the onset of type 2 diabetes.

Gestational diabetes. This occurs during pregnancy and requires treatment to prevent harm to the infant. Women who have a family history of diabetes and who are obese are more likely to develop gestational diabetes. After having it, women have a 35 to 65 percent greater chance of developing diabetes ten to twenty years after pregnancy.

Diabetes complications and care. People with type 1 and type 2 diabetes are at increased risk for serious health complications including eye disorders, high blood pressure, stroke, and kidney disease. Keeping blood glucose levels as close to normal as possible through medications, meal planning, and exercise will prevent or slow some of the complications.

If you have diabetes, it is crucial that you be under the regular care of a physician to get the health care advice and the medications you need. Your doctor will refer you to a health care provider, usually a diabetes educator, who will teach you about your diabetes medications and the daily aspects of living with diabetes. Visits to a registered dietitian, preferably one who specializes in diabetes, will be invaluable. A dietitian will help you reach your nutrition goals based on your diabetes medications, level of physical activity, food preferences, and cooking skills.

Treatment for diabetes must be individualized. Medications, foods, and exercise all affect each person differently and no single medication or eating or exercise plan will work the same for everyone.

Being overweight is without a doubt a strong predictor for developing type 2 diabetes: Fully 90 percent of people who have type 2 diabetes are overweight. Obesity and a sedentary lifestyle are fueling the diabetes epidemic in the United States. Between 1997 and 2007 the rate of diabetes doubled. The American Diabetes Association (ADA) estimates that there are 25.8 million people—8.3 percent of the population—who have diabetes. Of those, 18.8 million have been diagnosed, while the remaining 7 million people don't know they have diabetes.

The good news behind these discouraging statistics is that studies have shown that simple lifestyle changes such as eating a well-balanced diet and exercising moderately are the best way to prevent type 2 diabetes. Diet and exercise are also an essential part of the treatment plan when diagnosed with pre-diabetes or diabetes. In the early stages of type 2 diabetes, blood glucose may be kept under control through diet alone. In the later stages, however, insulin or other blood glucose–lowering medications will be recommended. But these medicines are not a substitute for a healthful diet. Unquestionably, a sensible diet plays a key role in good health, but for people who have a predisposition to developing type 2 diabetes, it can prevent or prolong the onset of the disease and delay its progression.

How to Eat Smart When You Have Diabetes

There's no such thing as a diabetic diet. There are no foods that a person with diabetes should or should not eat that any other person who is following a nutritious and healthy diet should or should not eat.

Eating smart when you have type 1 or type 2 diabetes means the same as it does for everyone else: consuming a level of calories that will maintain your weight or allow you to lose weight if you need to; enjoying a whole food–based diet that has a wide variety of whole grains, fruits, and vegetables; choosing lean protein sources and healthier fats and oils; and limiting salt intake. The only difference is that a person with diabetes must be aware of how many carbohydrates they consume. The goal is to be consistent with the amount consumed at each meal to keep blood glucose under control. People who take insulin or have an insulin pump can take a proscribed amount of insulin based on how many carbohydrates they eat at each meal.

The Role of Carbohydrates

Carbohydrates are essential in your diet. Carbohydrates are the main source of energy for every cell in your body, and in the case of the brain, carbohydrates are the only fuel it uses.

Carbohydrates aren't just in sugary foods. They're also in fiber-rich breads and grains, and in protein- and calcium-containing cheeses, yogurt, and milk. They're in vitamin- and mineral-rich fruits, and in vitamin A–packed vegetables like sweet potatoes and winter squash. Just like everyone else, people with diabetes need the energy and the nutrients from carbohydrate-containing foods in order to keep their bodies healthy.

Some carbohydrates are better than others. Different types of carbohydrates can affect blood sugar levels in different ways, but the total amount of carbohydrates eaten at each meal is what matters most. For example, if you eat three servings (or 3 Carb Choices, more about those later) of carbohydrates in a meal, whether those three servings are a slice of bread, a serving of peas, and a glass of milk, or if the three servings are mashed potatoes, an apple, and a chocolate brownie, your blood glucose will rise by about the same amount.

This doesn't mean you should have brownies at every meal. As a person with diabetes, you have an individualized eating plan you created with your health care team that distributes your daily carbohydrate intake over three meals and sometimes snacks. For most women, this ranges from 45 to 75 grams (3 to 5 servings or Carb Choices) per meal and from 60 to 90 grams (4 to 6 servings or Carb Choices) for most men.

Nutrient-rich carbohydrates such as whole wheat bread, oatmeal, whole grain cereal, fresh fruits, and low-fat milk and yogurt are always better options than sweets and desserts that contribute few nutrients other than empty calories. Everyone deserves—and absolutely should have—an occasional treat. Just not every day, and certainly not at every meal.

The benefits of fiber. Fiber is the indigestible part of fruits, vegetables, and grains. A high-fiber diet can improve long-term blood glucose control and lower blood lipids (fats) and cholesterol. Fiber gives a sense of fullness, which may help you eat less and feel satisfied longer, not to mention fiber's role in bowel regularity. The ADA recommends that people with diabetes should consume 25 to 30 grams of fiber per day, while the average American gets about 12 to 15 grams per day.

To improve your fiber intake, choose whole grains, such as bulgur, barley, oats, corn (including popcorn), quinoa, and brown and wild rice. Dried beans, lentils, split peas, artichokes, broccoli, raspberries, and unpeeled pears and apples are also excellent choices when you're trying to boost fiber. For help in choosing whole wheat bread that really does contain "whole" wheat, see Choosing Whole Wheat Bread (page 66). Many of the recipes in this book are good sources of fiber. Look for the symbol HIGH FIBER for dishes that contain 4 or more grams of fiber per serving.

What about the glycemic index? The glycemic index (GI) is the measure of how much your blood glucose rises after eating a 50-gram portion of a food compared to the rise after eating 50 grams of either white bread or glucose. The GI of a food can vary within an individual depending on a variety of factors, such as the time of day the food is consumed and what other foods were eaten at the same time. Aspects such as ripeness, cooking time, fat content, and fiber content also affect the GI measure. For these reasons, even though the GI measure does promote eating whole, fresh foods it is just one tool to consider when planning meals. Creating an eating plan using the GI is very complicated, and if you are interested in doing so, consult with a registered dietitian first.

A few words about sugar and artificial sweeteners. With good meal planning and sensible portion sizes, people with diabetes can enjoy desserts made with real sugar while staying within their carbohydrate goal for meals.

Sugar is essential to create desserts that have natural flavor, characteristic texture, and satisfying taste. Sugar provides more than sweetness in desserts. It gives cookies and muffins their distinguishing brown caramelized edge. It prevents dryness in cakes and loaf breads, giving them a moist, tender crumb. Sugar softens the protein in flour, so it expands easily to make cakes and muffins rise. In frozen desserts, sugar lowers the freezing point, making the ice crystals smaller and ice cream or sorbet creamier. The desserts in this book use a judicious amount of sugar and smart portion sizes to create sweet treats that are delicious, satisfying, and healthful.

There are many artificial sweeteners available and several are recommended for cooking. When substituting them for sugar in desserts, do not expect the characteristic flavors and textures of traditional baked goods. Artificial sweeteners are helpful in reducing the amount of carbohydrates and calories you consume, and when used to sweeten foods such as beverages, hot cereals, or yogurt, where the only property they provide is sweet taste, they offer a satisfactory substitute for sugar.

If you buy food products that are made with artificial sweeteners, read the label carefully. Just because it says "sugar-free" doesn't necessarily mean it's carbohydrate-free. A sugar-free cake contains carbohydrates from flour, while yogurt and ice cream have carbohydrates from naturally occurring milk sugars.

Always look at the "Total Carbohydrate" content on the label so that you will know how to budget the food into your meal plan.

Other Nutritional Considerations

How many calories do you need? It depends on whether you are male or female, how active you are, and whether you are trying to maintain the weight you are now or you are trying to lose weight. Only a registered dietitian or other diabetes care professional who knows your medical history, the medications you are taking, and your personal weight loss history can calculate exactly how many calories are right for you. Most people with diabetes are overweight, so weight reduction should be a goal when choosing a calorie level.

For a small woman with a sedentary lifestyle or for a woman trying to lose weight, 1,200 to 1,400 calories is a sensible goal. For a large active teenage boy or man, 2,400 to 2,800 would be the recommended range.

The menu examples on pages xxiv–xxvii provide you with models of 1,500-calorie and 1,800-calorie seven-day menus. Once you and your health care provider decide on a goal for you, use these sample menus as a starting point for planning meals for you and your family.

Limit—but don't eliminate—fat. Your body needs some fat, as it provides essential fatty acids and carries crucial fat-soluble vitamins, like vitamin A and D. Fat is essential in cooking, too. It helps foods brown when sautéing or baking, adds moisture to baked goods like cakes and muffins, gives a silky texture and rich flavor to sauces, and adds flavor on its own. But all fats are high in calories and should be used in moderation.

Choose healthy fats. Saturated fats, such as those in meats and butter, and trans fats, like those found in some fried foods, cookies, chips, and crackers can increase your risk for heart disease (they can raise your LDL or "bad" cholesterol). Fats that are monounsaturated, such as olive oil and canola oil and those that are polyunsaturated, such as corn, soybean, safflower, and sesame oils are better choices for heart-healthy eating. These oils help lower the cholesterol in your blood.

Eat saturated fat sensibly. You don't have to completely give up your favorite saturated fat–containing foods. Even if you follow healthy eating guidelines in the strictest sense, there are times throughout the year that you'll want to enjoy a juicy steak hot from the grill, a crisp buttery holiday cookie, a wedge of creamy cheese at a party, or some bacon with breakfast.

You can have all these foods as part of a healthful diet, as long as you limit the portion size and include them in the total amount of saturated fat that you should have in a day. See the chart at right for the recommended daily intakes of fat and saturated fat. As a point of reference, 2 strips of bacon have 2 grams of saturated fat, 2 teaspoons of butter have 8 grams, 3 ounces of lean sirloin steak have 5 grams, and a 1-ounce wedge of Brie has 8 grams.

In cooking, using small amounts of foods high in saturated fat to flavor an entire dish gives unparalleled taste. Using a couple of strips of bacon to flavor a large pot of vegetable soup, sprinkling a family-sized green salad with a few tablespoons of blue cheese, or making a butter sauce for a fish dish that serves four people using a tablespoon or two of butter is cooking in a way that makes nutritious food delicious.

RECOMMENDED DAILY FAT AND SATURATED FAT INTAKE

Calorie Level	Recommended Grams of Total Fat (30% of calories)	Recommend Grams of Saturated Fat (7% of calories)
1200	40	9
1500	50	12
1800	60	14
2000	67	16

Cholesterol. Cholesterol is a fatty substance that your body uses to make essential hormones and to make and repair cell membranes. Your body manufactures some cholesterol, and some enters the body through foods. Only animal products, such as meat, poultry, fish and shellfish, eggs, and butter contain cholesterol. Consuming saturated fat and trans fats can raise cholesterol levels, but eating cholesterol-rich foods can also raise blood cholesterol. The ADA recommends that people with diabetes consume 200 milligrams or less of cholesterol per day.

Protein. There are no special dietary recommendations for protein for people with diabetes. Most Americans get much more protein than they need. Protein should comprise about 15 to 20 percent of the calories in your diet, which translates to 56 to 75 grams of protein at the 1,500-calorie level.

To reduce fat, saturated fat, and calories, choose lean meats and poultry and trim away any visible fat before cooking. Fish is naturally lean and a good source of heart-healthy omega-3 fats. Meatless protein sources, like eggs, tofu, dried beans, lentils, and nuts, each have their own nutritional goodness and add flavor and variety to meals. Try to have at least two meals featuring fish and two meals containing a meatless protein every week.

Meal Planning

There are three different methods for keeping track of the carbohydrates you eat. It's important to choose a method you'll stick with that will fit your lifestyle. The goal in meal planning is to give you a tool to use so that you eat about the same amount of carbohydrates at each meal and/or snack every day in order to keep your blood glucose level in check.

Create your plate. If the thought of counting carbohydrates or keeping track of Exchanges seems overwhelming, then you should start with the "create your plate" method. The basic concept is that at lunch and dinner you fill half of your plate with non-starchy vegetables. Then, fill the other half with equal amounts of lean protein and starchy food.

At breakfast, with the "create your plate" method, choose small portions and have one or two servings of carbohydrate-containing food (cereal, a small muffin, a piece of toast, or a serving of fruit). If you like to have a dairy food at breakfast, such as milk, yogurt, or cottage cheese, take into account that a serving of these foods contains protein, but also contains carbohydrates. An egg is a carbohydrate-free protein source for breakfast.

There is no counting with this method, but you do have to observe portion control and utilize healthy cooking methods. See the discussion of portion control under "Measure and Weigh" and "When You Have to Estimate" on page xv–xvi.

Carb counting. Carb counting is just that—counting the number of carbohydrates you consume in each meal and/or snack. Your health care provider will set the number of grams of carbohydrate or the servings of carbohydrate, also known as Carb Choices that you should have based on your medications, weight, and activity level. Each Carb Choice has 15 grams of carbohydrate. Your health care provider may tell you to have 3 Carb Choices at each meal, or 45 grams of carbohydrate—both mean the same thing. People who take insulin or who have an insulin pump can use an advanced version of this method to take a proscribed amount of insulin depending on the amount of carbohydrate eaten at each meal or snack. It's also a simple way for people not taking insulin to keep track of carbohydrates.

Once you know the number of Carb Choices or the grams of carbohydrate you should have at each meal, you can figure out how many servings of carbohydrate-containing foods you should eat. When you need to figure the number of Carb Choices in a packaged food, from a listing in a carb-counter book, or from the nutrient analysis of a recipe in a magazine, use the chart on page xiii to find the number of Carb Choices. If a serving of crackers has 18 grams of carbohydrate, then that would be 1 Carb Choice, since 18 falls in the range of 11 to 20 grams. Using the chart, you can figure out the Carb Choices from any food if you know how many grams of carbohydrate it contains.

Even though all you're actually counting is carbohydrates, you have to make wise choices regarding the foods you eat in order to eat a balanced diet that has the right amount of nutrients. As with any of the methods of meal planning, portion control is vital, and healthy cooking methods are a must. Your health care provider or a registered dietitian will help you individualize your plan.

GRAMS OF CARBOHYDRATE IN CARB CHOICES (OR CARB SERVINGS)

Carb Choices or Carb Servings	Grams of Carbohydrate
0	0–5
½	6–10
1	11–20
1½	21–25
2	26–35
2½	36–40
3	41–50
3½	51–55
4	56–65

Exchange system. With this method, you track the starches, fruits, milk, non-starchy vegetables, proteins, and fats for each meal. All the foods in each group have about the same amount of carbohydrates, protein, and fat. Within each group is a list of the foods and the portion sizes.

For example, a serving or "Exchange" of fruit can be 1 small apple, half of a large pear, or 1 cup of raspberries. A protein or meat serving can be 1 ounce of fish, ¼ cup of cottage cheese, or 1 egg. If your health care provider recommends that you be very precise in the amounts of carbohydrate, fat, and calories that you consume, this is probably the best choice for you. Or, if you are the type of person who finds it easier when you have fewer decisions to make—you like to look at a list of foods and make your choices—then this might be the best way for you to plan your meals.

For all the recipes in this book, the Carb Choices, the number of grams of carbohydrate (as well as other nutrient data), and Exchanges are listed. Whichever method you choose, the recipes provided here will easily fit into your meal plan.

Eating Well for Life

Being diagnosed with diabetes can be overwhelming. There may be medications that you will have to take on a strict schedule, you will have to check your blood sugar level several times a day, and more than likely, you'll be asked by your health care provider to make changes in the way you eat in order to lose a few pounds. Managing your diabetes is a lifelong commitment, but the good news is you don't have to change everything at once. These tips will help get you started toward a healthier way of eating for life.

Set small goals. Making too many changes at once can make the whole process of improving your diet overwhelming. Work with a registered dietitian or a diabetes educator who will help you set small, attainable goals in achieving your ultimate healthy eating lifestyle. Switch from white bread to whole wheat, start eating one more serving of vegetables each day, or try one new healthful recipe each week. Before you know it, your blood sugars and lipid profiles will improve, you'll lose weight, and you'll feel better.

Train your taste buds. If you're accustomed to eating foods that are salty, very sweet, and laden with fat, eating healthfully will be a challenge at first. Give yourself time for your taste buds to adjust. After a month or so, you'll stop automatically reaching for the saltshaker; you'll find desserts you used to enjoy are now just too sweet and fried foods are simply too greasy. You'll now be enjoying the natural flavors of foods, not the salt, sugar, and fat.

Eat foods, not food products. The most satisfying meals start with fresh unprocessed foods you cook simply. Buying fresh fruits and vegetables to prepare for you and your family will guarantee you're eating healthfully. Processed foods may shave off a few minutes preparation time, but you get more calories, fat, additives, and preservatives, and less flavor.

Some people with diabetes have a tendency to eat packaged foods because the nutrition facts are listed on the label and they don't have to figure out how many carbohydrates they are having. You'll eat more healthfully and have meals with better flavor, however, if you avail yourself of online resources or books that list the amount of carbohydrates and other nutrient values of whole raw foods so you can create your own nutritious meals.

Double up on vegetables. The United States Department of Agriculture recommends that adults get 2½ to 3 cups of vegetables a day. Make it a goal to eat double that amount of non-starchy vegetables every day. These include asparagus, broccoli, cauliflower, celery, eggplant, green beans, leafy greens, mushrooms, peppers, radishes, tomatoes, yellow squash, and zucchini. These foods only have a small amount of carbohydrates and you can eat a lot of them with little effect on blood sugars. They fill you up without adding many calories, add fiber to your diet, and boost your nutrient intake. Three cups of non-starchy raw vegetables or 1½ cups of cooked count as 1 Carb Choice.

Plan ahead. Each day, you have a carbohydrate, calorie, and fat budget. Take a few minutes each morning to make some decisions about what you'll be eating that day. If you know you're going out to dinner with friends, maybe you'll want to have a light lunch. If it's a friend's birthday and you want to enjoy a slice of cake, you might want to limit the other carbohydrates in the same meal. If you think ahead and have a plan already in place at the start of each day, you'll make wise decisions at each meal. After a while, you'll make the smart choice without even thinking about it.

Shake the salt habit. Salt has nothing to do with blood sugar levels. An excess amount of salt raises blood pressure by causing your body to retain water, which makes your heart work harder and puts an extra burden on your blood vessels. Heart disease and stroke are the number one causes of death and disability in people with type 2 diabetes.

Your body only needs a miniscule amount of sodium—about 200 milligrams a day. Most Americans consume 3,000 to 3,600 milligrams. The American Heart Association recommends that healthy Americans eat less than 1,500 milligrams each day.

Work toward eliminating processed food and fast food. Seventy-five percent of sodium Americans consume comes not from the saltshaker at the table, but from processed foods such as prepared mixes, frozen meals, canned soups, and fast foods.

Use low-sodium or no-salt-added canned foods. Beans, tomatoes, tomato sauce, tomato paste, broths, and tuna are all available in lower-sodium versions. These ingredients are used in recipes in this book, and you'll note that almost all those recipes have added salt. The reason is that even with the added salt, the sodium levels are far below what they would be if you used regular versions of these foods. Sodium also lurks in some foods that you would never guess have a lot of salt, so always check the sodium on the label of items such as bread, breadcrumbs, salsas, cereals, pasta sauces, tomato juice, and cheeses.

Moderation is key. A small amount of added salt brings out the natural flavor of food. Without a tiny amount of salt, food can be bland and tasteless. Even dessert recipes contain just a little salt, as it rounds out the flavors and makes sweet foods taste sweeter. Foods such as broccoli, broccoli rabe, parsnips, and cauliflower have a mild bitter edge. Adding a little salt makes this almost disappear. Recipes that contain reduced-sodium soy sauce, fish sauce, or hoisin sauce, and recipes using cured ham, sausage, or bacon are naturally higher in sodium, so enjoy them only on occasion.

Use kosher salt for cooking. Most serious home cooks and professional chefs use kosher salt instead of table salt for cooking because of its clean natural flavor. But it can help you use less sodium in cooking, too. It's not because kosher salt contains less sodium—all salt has the same composition—but the crystals of kosher salt are large and irregularly shaped. When measured, kosher salt crystals

can't pack together, so you'll have less in the measuring spoon. Because you're adding salt in smaller increments, you will most likely realize that you don't need as much.

Add acidity or a fresh herb. If you think a dish needs a little something, instead of adding salt try adding a tiny bit of red or white wine vinegar, sherry vinegar, balsamic vinegar, cider vinegar, lemon juice, or lime juice, depending on the dish. Start by adding just ¼ teaspoon. It's amazing how just a touch of acidity really wakes up the flavors of soups, stews, sauces, salads, and vegetables.

Fresh herbs, even ones as ordinary as chopped parsley, also add a burst of freshness to foods. Try adding a tablespoon of chopped parsley, mint, basil, or cilantro to accentuate the flavor of a dish.

Measure and weigh. The serving sizes of foods in restaurants and in supermarkets just keep getting bigger. A sandwich roll can weigh 4 or 5 ounces and muffins can be large enough to make three servings. In restaurants, it's not unusual to be served a 1-pound steak or a baked potato large enough for four.

If you've never measured serving sizes, this is a good educational exercise to try for a couple weeks. Once you measure out ½ cup of a bean salad, or 3 ounces of cooked steak, or 1 tablespoon of dessert sauce, you'll develop an "eye" for estimating portion size and you can put the measuring tools away. It may be a good idea to bring them back out every couple of months just to refresh your memory and retrain your eye. Measuring and weighing food at home and taking note of what it looks like on a plate will keep you on track when you eat out or are at a party.

When you have to estimate. Here are some comparisons to help when eating away from home.

VISUAL CUES FOR FOOD MEASUREMENTS

Measure	Types of food	Visual
1 teaspoon	Butter	One dice
1 tablespoon	Mayonnaise, dips, spreads, sauces	Tip of a woman's thumb
¼ cup	Dried fruit	Golf ball
⅓ to ½ cup	Chopped fresh fruit, hot cereal, dried beans, cooked vegetables, rice and other grains	A small fist
1 cup	Salad greens, chopped raw vegetables, casserole, pasta entrée	A large fist
1-ounce portion	Nuts	A child's handful
1-ounce portion	Cheese	A woman's whole thumb
3-ounce portion	Cooked meats, poultry, and fish	A deck of cards

Be restaurant savvy. Most Americans eat out four to five times a week. And it's a fun and relaxing way to socialize with friends and family. Just because you have diabetes doesn't mean you have cut back on eating out: You simply have to be smarter about it.

Consider your carbohydrate budget based on your personal eating plan before you order. Will you choose a small piece of bread and a cup of pasta or rice, or will you have the crostini appetizer, no carbohydrates with your entrée, and treat yourself to dessert? If you start the meal with a budgeted amount of carbohydrates in mind, you're more likely to order a sensible meal.

Only eat in restaurants that have healthful menu options. If the entire menu is fried, steer clear. Don't be afraid to ask for sauces or dressings on the side, so you can decide how much to use.

Most restaurant meals are large enough for two meals. Eat only half of what you're served. If you know you can't resist finishing the meal, have the waiter wrap half of it up for you at once. Consider ordering an appetizer instead of an entrée. If you also have a soup or a salad along with it, most likely, it will be more than enough food.

Make your own treats. If triple-layer chocolate cake is what you consider a real indulgence, then bake the cake from scratch and share it with a dozen friends. This way, enjoying a treat becomes a special social occasion and there won't be any leftovers to tempt you later.

Try this homemade tactic no matter what you have a weakness for, be it French fries, fried chicken, lasagna, or cheese fondue. If you go to the effort of making it yourself and sharing it with a group of friends and family, in all likelihood, you'll eat the special high-calorie, high-fat food less often.

Eat together as a family. Whether you're preparing healthy meals for yourself or for someone who has diabetes, the wholesome foods that are recommended for people with diabetes—whole grains, fruits, and vegetables along with lean protein—are smart choices for everyone. If one person in your family has diabetes, that means others are at risk, so a healthy diet is a preventative measure against them developing type 2 diabetes.

Exercise on most days. Getting active is essential for being healthy—especially when you have diabetes. Exercise can help lower your blood glucose and improve your ability to use insulin. It can also lower blood pressure, improve blood lipids, reduce stress, and help you lose weight.

You don't have to join a gym or take up jogging. No matter what your physical abilities, there are ways to get your body moving. Start slowly and work your way up to about thirty minutes most days of the week. You can power walk, swim, ride a bike or a stationary bike, go dancing, or play tennis. Do what you enjoy and you'll be more likely to do it often. And don't overlook the exercise you get from typical daily activities like climbing stairs, gardening, strenuous housecleaning, and walking.

Consult with your health care provider before making any changes in your activity level. The health of your heart and nervous system need to be considered and adjustments may need to be made in your diabetes medications and your diet as you become more active.

Stocking the Healthy Pantry

Whether you chart out every meal for the week, make a list, and then head out for the supermarket, or you're more of a last-minute meal planner, having a basic well-stocked pantry of healthful foods will make it easier to make nourishing meals.

You've probably heard the advice to shop the perimeter of the grocery store for the healthiest foods, such as fresh produce, meats, poultry, fish, and dairy products. But don't skip the center aisles. For the savviest shopping, load up on the foods found around the perimeter and be choosy in the center aisles.

In the center of the supermarket are all kinds of foods that are not to be missed as part of a healthy diet: dried beans and lentils, oats, brown rice, barley, whole wheat pastas, low-sodium broths, canned tomatoes, canned tuna and salmon, healthy oils, mustards, vinegars, spices, nuts, natural peanut butter, honey, whole wheat breads, tortillas, crackers, and teas.

When you shop, avoid exposing yourself to irresistible temptations. Keep problem foods out of your shopping cart. If you feel guilty for denying family members treats and snacks, suggest that they have these foods when out with friends or other family members. Another trick is to individually portion foods. Place single muffins or cookies inside resealable plastic bags and allot yourself one bag per day. Store the others in the freezer so they are out of sight and out of mind.

Long-Lasting Pantry Staples

Oils. Use **canola oil** when cooking at high temperatures (such as stir-frying) or when you don't want to add any flavor (oiling pans for baking). Use **extra virgin olive oil** for almost everything else. It's a delicious all-purpose oil that is great for sautéing, roasting, salad dressings, and marinades. Colavita is a high-quality reasonably priced extra virgin oil found in most supermarkets. **Asian sesame oil** is a toasty oil that's indispensable for stir-fries and other Asian dishes. A tiny bit—just a teaspoon or less—will flavor a whole dish. **Walnut, hazelnut, and pecan oils** add an intense nutty flavor to salad dressings, sauces, and desserts. When you roast root vegetables, toss them with a teaspoon of nut oil just before serving to add another layer of flavor. Look for roasted nut oils, which have more concentrated flavor.

Salts. Diamond Crystal **kosher salt** and **table salt** have larger grains than other brands of salt and measure for measure will add less sodium to your food. Use kosher salt for cooking and table salt for baking and for making breads, since its finer grains mix better with dry ingredients such as flour. **Sea salt** is made from evaporated seawater, so it contains trace minerals that kosher salt and table salt do not. Because of how it is produced, sea salt is more expensive than other salts, but the flavor tends to be more concentrated so you can use less than you would of table salt. It is best used for sprinkling lightly over food at the table.

Flours. If you do a lot of baking, it's convenient to have whole wheat flour, white whole wheat flour, whole wheat pastry flour, and enriched white flour on hand. See Types of Flour (page 507) for a description of each of the flours and the types of recipes for which each one is best. Whole wheat flour goes rancid faster than white flour. If you buy more than you can use in three to four months, store the flour in an airtight container in the freezer.

Spices, herbs, and seasoning blends. These add lively flavor to all kinds of foods and you should have a diverse selection based on what you cook most. One note of caution: Always check the ingredient list when buying seasoning blends. Some are terrific-tasting blends of herbs and spices and some are mostly salt.

Pastas. If you don't like whole wheat pasta, here's how to retrain your taste buds. Start by combining half regular pasta and half whole wheat in recipes, or try pastas made with a blend of white and whole wheat flours. In time, you'll come to love the earthy, nutty flavor of whole wheat pasta while benefiting from its nutrients. Keep a good selection of short pastas (penne, macaroni, rigatoni) and long pastas (spaghetti, linguini, fettuccini) in your pantry. Pasta lasts almost indefinitely, so stock up when it's on sale.

Beans, rice, grains, and cornmeal. Buy dried beans and lentils in a store that has a lot of turnover. When old, they take longer to cook. Cooking dried beans is very easy and it takes less time than you might think. Check out Cooking Dried Beans (page 119) for no-soak instructions on cooking a variety of these protein and fiber powerhouses. Stock up on several kinds of whole grain rice—brown basmati, brown jasmine, Wehani, or wild rice—as a welcome change from ordinary brown rice. Have a few other grains on hand, too. Quinoa, bulgur, wheat berries, and barley make delicious salads and side dishes and healthful additions to soups. And with fine-grind cornmeal on hand, you can make a polenta side dish almost as fast as you can boil water.

Teas. If you drink sugary soft drinks or fruit-based beverages, brewing your own tea may be the best carb and calorie fighting change you can make in your diet. There are hundreds of teas, with and without caffeine, and they're easy to make (you don't even have to boil water). See 3 Ways to Brew Iced Tea (page 605).

Condiments, Seasonings, and Sweeteners

Mustards. Unless you're a mustard connoisseur, regular Dijon mustard and whole grain Dijon will suffice in most any recipe. Regular Dijon adds a tempting sharpness to salad dressings and sauces and both types of mustard add rich flavor to meat rubs and marinades. And they're great on sandwiches, too.

Mayonnaise. Because of its long list of ingredients and unnatural flavor, instead of using reduced-fat mayonnaise, try using regular mayonnaise mixed half and half with plain low-fat yogurt. It's a trick you'll see in a lot of the salad recipes in this book.

Vinegars. They are an essential ingredient in salad dressings, but they also lift the flavors of soups and stews when you add a few drops at the very end of the cooking time. Vinegars add a tang to dishes that makes you want less salt, too. At the least, have on hand red and white wine vinegar, balsamic vinegar, and cider vinegar. Sherry vinegar and rice vinegar are nice to have, but not essential.

Hot sauce and chipotles in adobo sauce. Whether used at the table or in cooking, a dash of your favorite hot sauce can wake up a meal. Chipotles in adobo are smoked jalapeños that are cooked in tomato sauce. They add heat (and a lot of it) and a smoky taste that gives oven-baked foods a barbecued flavor. Only a small amount of chipotles is used, so instead of mincing them every time you need a teaspoon or two, put the entire can of chipotles and the sauce in the food processor and puree it. Use it in equal measure whenever a recipe calls for minced chipotles in adobo sauce. The pureed chipotles will last for months in the refrigerator.

Asian sauces and flavorings. Hoisin sauce, oyster sauce, red and green curry paste, fish sauce, and reduced-sodium soy sauce are all must-haves if you enjoy cooking Asian dishes. Once opened, always store these items in the refrigerator. Asian sauces are all high in sodium, so when you do enjoy these, cut back on the sodium in other foods for the day.

Honey, maple syrup, and molasses. Used prudently in cooking, these sweeteners can round out the flavors of a dish while adding their own unique natural flavor. When you've budgeted your carbohydrates for a pancake breakfast, a few teaspoons of real maple syrup will add more flavor than a big splash of chemically sweetened artificial syrup.

Canned Foods

Tomato products. These are an absolute necessity for quick weeknight meals. Keep diced tomatoes, whole tomatoes, crushed tomatoes, tomato sauce, and tomato paste on hand. Tomatoes packaged in aseptic paper boxes are more expensive, but their flavor is fresher and more natural than canned. Look for Pomi brand diced tomatoes and strained tomatoes, which are like a thick tomato sauce.

Broths. Making your own is ideal and easier than you think (see Chicken Stock, page

149, and Leftover-Chicken Chicken Stock, page 150). When you do buy broth, always choose the low-sodium versions. You'll find lots of uses for chicken, beef, and vegetable broths, including soups, stews, chilis, sauces, and gravies. If you only have regular broth on hand for cooking in a recipe like soup or chili that uses several cups of broth, use half broth and half water to keep the sodium low.

Salmon and tuna. Don't overlook canned fish for making tasty salads and sandwiches. These pantry staples are a convenient way to eat more fish more often. Buy "dolphin-safe" tuna, which means the tuna was caught without using nets that sometimes ensnare dolphins and other sea life. Look for low-sodium canned tuna, which is widely available. Low-sodium salmon can be found, but not as easily, as it doesn't seem to be as popular as tuna.

Dried beans. Keep garbanzo, cannellini, black, red kidney, and pinto beans on hand to use in salads, soups, and chilis. They are an excellent source of low-fat protein and fiber. All varieties of canned dried beans come in no-salt-added versions, but they can be significantly more expensive than the regular ones. If you find that the regular beans fit best into your budget, rinsing the beans in a colander under cool running water will remove about 40 percent of the sodium.

Cheese and Dairy Products

Cheese. Mozzarella, Monterey Jack, sharp Cheddar, and ricotta are four cheeses that are available in good-quality reduced-fat versions. Parmesan, Pecorino Romano, blue cheese, feta, goat cheese, Gruyère, manchego, and provolone are best purchased in the full-fat versions. Just use small amounts.

Plain low-fat yogurt. Even if you don't like to eat yogurt on its own, you should keep it on hand for cooking and baking. It's great for mixing with mayonnaise to make a creamy salad dressing or vegetable dip, its acidity makes it a tenderizing marinade, and it adds tang and tenderness to cakes and muffins.

Reduced-fat sour cream and reduced-fat cream cheese. These lower-fat versions of their high-calorie counterparts taste natural and have a texture that's close to the original. Look for one-third less fat Neufchâtel when buying reduced-fat cream cheese.

Butter. There is no substitute for butter. It's high in saturated fat, but used in small amounts, it can be part of a healthful diet. Just ½ teaspoon of butter can give a serving of broccoli or green beans a delectably rich flavor. A pastry crust made with butter has a flaky, crisp texture with complex flavor. A tablespoon of butter whisked into a sauce to serve four people can mean the difference between a sharp-flavored one-note dish and a dinner with well-rounded nuanced flavors. Regardless of advertising slogans, nothing tastes like butter.

Fresh Fruits and Vegetables

Fresh fruit. Keep a few limes and lemons in the refrigerator at all times for adding to beverages. The juice and the grated rind are useful in all kinds of cooking, from soups and salads to seafood and desserts. Most food experts recommend storing fruit in the refrigerator. That's great advice for the fruit, but not for encouraging you to eat it. Buy a variety of fresh in-season fruit every time you shop, and unless it's something very perishable (like fresh berries), wash it when you get home and put it in a large bowl on the counter. Seeing the fruit will remind you and your family to eat it.

Vegetables. During the growing season shop at local farmers' markets for the freshest vegetables. They will taste better and stay fresher longer than produce that was picked and shipped from far away. If you have a Community Supported Agriculture (CSA) program in your area, consider joining it. They are community-based organizations where you pay a farmer a specific amount of money in early spring and receive vegetables from the farm throughout the summer and early fall. Because you get a large quantity of vegetables each week, you will be forced to incorporate them into your meals. When you do buy produce at the supermarket, shop at a busy store that has a lot of turnover so the produce is fresh, and base your meals on what looks best and what's on sale when you shop.

Herbs, garlic, and fresh ginger. Herbs can be expensive, especially in winter, but even a sprinkling of ordinary parsley can add a burst of fresh flavor to a pasta salad, a bowl of soup, or a sautéed chicken breast. Try to always have at least one fresh herb on hand (even if it's inexpensive parsley) and use that herb in different dishes over several days. If you find yourself with extra herbs, use them to make Herb Water (page 608). Garlic is a must-have ingredient that adds flavor to every kind of dish, and fresh ginger adds a punch to Asian dishes and desserts.

Frozen Foods

Vegetables. Frozen corn, baby lima beans, green peas, and shelled edamame are basic staples to have on hand for a quick side dish or to use in recipes.

Fruit. Keep a selection of frozen unsweetened fruits such as berries, peaches, cranberries, and cherries on hand to use in smoothies, for making flavored waters (see Berry Water, page 608), and for fruit desserts.

Shrimp. Buy frozen shrimp produced in the United States rather than abroad. The United States has environmental standards for farming seafood that other countries do not.

Essential Kitchen Equipment

Most people have basic kitchen equipment and tools, but there are a few things that make cooking healthy foods easier and more convenient. If you don't already have these tools, buy them one at a time until you have what you need.

Silicone pastry brush. Oil does not absorb into the bristles of these brushes, so you use less oil and can spread it thinner than when using a nylon or natural bristle pastry brush. Having one of these brushes enables you to eliminate your use of cooking spray (which tastes bad anyway). Just put a teaspoon (or two for a very large pan) of oil in a pan and spread it around on the bottom and sides with the silicone brush. It takes just seconds and the cleanup is easy—the brushes are dishwasher safe.

Microplane grater. Use this super-sharp tool for grating flavor-packed citrus zest, fresh ginger, hard cheese, chocolate, or nutmeg.

Large rimmed baking sheets. Serving roasted vegetables is the key to getting your family to love them. With two large (about 17 x 12-inch) rimmed baking sheets on hand, you can roast enough vegetables for two meals. Serve the leftovers on their own, or add them to salads, soups, and stews.

Salad spinner. You can save money and eat fresher greens if you wash your own. A salad spinner makes washing and drying greens really fast and easy. See Keeping Greens Fresh (page 85) for tips on washing and storing greens.

Very large salad bowl. Always serve a big leafy green salad at dinner and always toss the salad with the dressing before serving. By using a large bowl, you'll have plenty of room to toss the greens and coat them evenly with a miniscule amount of dressing. You'll use less dressing—and the salad will be more flavorful—than if you put the dressing on individual salads at the table.

Cast iron grill pan. This is a large skillet (they come round and square) with ridges that simulate cooking on an outdoor grill. There are nonstick versions, but cast iron pans heat more evenly and retain the heat when food is added, giving it a charred look and taste. The fat from whatever is cooked drips into the grooves away from the food. Use this pan to cook anything you would normally cook on a grill: chicken breasts or thighs, steaks, chops, shrimp, salmon, tuna, and vegetables.

Instant-read thermometer. These handy, inexpensive gadgets take the guesswork out of knowing when a beef or pork roast or a whole roasted chicken is done in a matter of seconds.

Techniques and Tips for Healthy Cooking

These techniques and tips are smart ways to help you use less fat, eat fewer calories, and add great flavor.

Heat the skillet first. When sautéing, pan-searing, or stir-frying, get the skillet hot *before* you add the oil. When oil is added to a hot pan, the pan heats the oil, making it thinner. Then when you tilt the pan to coat it with the oil, the oil skims the surface, coating the pan using less oil than you would use if the pan were cold. Food will not stick to a lightly oiled hot pan, even if the pan isn't nonstick, so cleanup is easier. Food added to a hot pan browns, caramelizing the natural sugars in foods, giving it better flavor.

Stir vegetables; let meat and fish set. When you sauté vegetables or make a stir-fry, begin stirring the food immediately to coat it with the small amount of oil you are using. For pan-searing steaks, chops, chicken breasts, or fish fillets, let the food cook on one side until it is well browned before turning it, usually 2 to 4 minutes. If you try to turn the food and it seems stuck, let it cook for another minute and it will release from the pan.

Salt and taste as you cook. Reducing sodium intake is a goal that almost everyone should have, but cooking without any added salt makes bland, boring meals that satisfy no one. Keep a small dish of Diamond Crystal kosher salt with a ⅛ teaspoon measure near the stove. Add salt to anything you cook—⅛ teaspoon at a time—and have a small taste after each addition. Adding salt little by little and tasting as you go will help you season food just right.

Crumble cheeses when they're cold. To distribute the fantastic flavor of feta, ricotta salata, blue cheese, and goat cheese while using as little as possible, crumble them when they are cold.

Serve meat in thin slices. Cut cooked steaks, boneless pork chops, pork tenderloin, and chicken breast into thin slices. It makes less look like more, and thin slices mean you take smaller bites and savor the meat more.

Nutrition Information

Nutrition information is provided for each recipe, including Carb Choices and Exchanges. The recipes are analyzed for carb (carbohydrate), cal (calories), fat, sat fat (saturated fat), chol (cholesterol), fib (fiber), pro (protein), and sod (sodium). Exchanges are given for starch, carb (carbohydrate), fruit, veg (non-starchy vegetables), fat-free milk, reduced-fat milk, high-fat protein, medium-fat protein, lean protein, plant-based protein, and fat. Every attempt has been made to provide accurate nutritional information. However, the information should be considered approximate as there may be variance in sizes of fruits and vegetables and different brands of foods contain different ingredients.

Nutrition information is for a single serving. Take note of the number of servings each dish makes when portioning your meals. When an ingredient is optional, it is not included in the analysis of the recipe. When there are two options listed for an ingredient, the analysis was done using the first ingredient. All recipes using kosher salt were analyzed using Diamond Crystal brand kosher salt.

When the fiber in a dish is more than 5 grams per serving, half the number of grams of fiber is subtracted from the number of grams of carbohydrate to calculate the Carb Choices and Exchanges. The reason for doing this is that fiber is not completely digested and the calories derived from fiber are only about half the amount from other carbohydrates.

In many recipes in this book, small amounts of high-fat cheeses are used to add flavor to a dish. In instances where the portion is so small that the protein in the cheese does not warrant being counted as a high-fat protein exchange, I have included the fat from the cheese in the Exchanges as "fat." Many people with diabetes strive to cut back on fat and the calories it contains, so I wanted to draw particular attention to the total fat in each dish.

Diabetes presents itself differently in each individual and it is a disease that requires personalized medical and dietary advice. Your health care provider may have given you special instructions regarding your diet. If there is any difference between this book and what your health care professional has advised, follow the instructions of your health care professional.

Note: The icon QUICK means the dish requires minimal prep and cooks in 30 minutes or less. The icon HIGH FIBER means the dish has 4 grams or more of fiber per serving.

Menus for Healthful Eating

7-DAY 1,500-CALORIE MENU

The average daily calorie level for these menus is 1,360 calories, leaving 140 discretionary calories for a snack during the day.

	Day 1	Day 2	Day 3
BREAKFAST	**Quick Overnight Steel-Cut Oatmeal** (page 3) topped with 1 small chopped apple 1 cup skim milk CARB CHOICES: 3 EXCHANGES: 1 starch, 1 fruit, 1 fat-free milk CALORIES: 249	**Tomato-Basil Frittata** (page 18) 1 slice whole wheat toast 1 cup skim milk 1¼ cups sliced fresh strawberries CARB CHOICES: 3 EXCHANGES: 1 starch, 1 fruit, 1 veg, 1 fat-free milk, 1 medium-fat protein, ½ fat CALORIES: 359	**Raspberry-Pear Smoothie** (page 606) 1 poached egg ½ whole wheat English muffin ⅔ cup plain fat-free yogurt CARB CHOICES: 3 EXCHANGES: 1 starch, 1 fruit, 1 fat-free milk, 1 medium-fat protein CALORIES: 289
LUNCH	**Muffuletta-Style Roast Beef Sandwiches** (page 72) **Marinated Cucumber and Sweet Onion Salad** (page 94) ⅔ cup plain fat-free yogurt with 1 sliced kiwi CARB CHOICES: 4 EXCHANGES: 2 starch, 1 fruit, 2 veg, 1 fat-free milk, 2 lean protein, 1 fat CALORIES: 491	**Italian Turkey Sausage and White Bean Soup** (page 181) 1 whole wheat roll 1 small orange CARB CHOICES: 4 EXCHANGES: 2½ starch, 1 fruit, 1 veg, 1 medium-fat protein, 1 plant-based protein CALORIES: 399	**Cilantro Chicken Salad Wraps** (page 65) **Chamomile-Ginger Summer Fruit Salad** (page 30) **Almond Biscotti** (page 579) CARB CHOICES: 4 EXCHANGES: 1½ starch, ½ carb, ½ fruit, 1 veg, 3 fat CALORIES: 532
DINNER	**Shrimp Summer Rolls** (page 49) **Peanut-Crusted Chicken with Honey-Sesame Sauce** (page 211) 1 cup steamed broccoli ¾ cup cooked brown rice CARB CHOICES: 4 EXCHANGES: 3 starch, 3 veg, 4 lean protein, 2 fat CALORIES: 631	**Wilted Spinach-Mushroom Salad** (page 86) **Pork Chops with Sautéed Apples** (page 300) **Roasted Butternut Squash with Goat Cheese** (page 495) 1 cup steamed cauliflower florets **Chocolate Mousse** (page 557) CARB CHOICES: 4 EXCHANGES: 1½ starch, 1 carb, 1 fruit, 2 veg, 1 high-fat protein, 3 lean protein, 2 fat CALORIES: 557	**Mixed Green Salad with Marinated Tomatoes** (page 87) **Lasagna with Greens and Ricotta** (page 379) 1 cup steamed yellow squash **Frozen Yogurt** (page 585) CARB CHOICES: 4 EXCHANGES: 1 starch, 1½ carb, 3 veg, 2 medium-fat protein, 1 fat CALORIES: 510

Day 4	Day 5	Day 6	Day 7
Everyday Granola (page 6) ¾ cup fresh blueberries ⅔ cup plain fat-free yogurt CARB CHOICES: 3 EXCHANGES: 1 starch, 1 carb, 1 fat, 1 fruit, 1 fat-free milk CALORIES: 309	**Moist Bran Muffin** (page 513) ½ cup plain fat-free yogurt ½ large grapefruit CARB CHOICES: 3 EXCHANGES: 1½ carb, 1 fruit, 1 fat-free milk, 1 fat CALORIES: 279	**Whole Wheat Pancakes with Orange Honey** (page 9) 2 slices bacon CARB CHOICES: 3 EXCHANGES: 2 starch, 1 carb, 2 fat CALORIES: 344	**Ham and Egg Breakfast Cups** (page 28) 1 slice whole wheat toast 1 cup cantaloupe cubes 1 cup skim milk CARB CHOICES: 3 EXCHANGES: 1 starch, 1 fruit, TK veg, 1 fat-free milk, 1½ medium-fat protein CALORIES: 345
Tuna Tabbouleh (page 107) **Mediterranean Bean Salad with Artichokes and Lemon** (page 118) 1 4-inch whole wheat pita bread CARB CHOICES: 4 EXCHANGES: 3 starch, 2 veg, 1 lean protein, 1 plant-based protein, 1½ fat CALORIES: 431	**Curried Lentil Soup** (page 174) **Yeast-Risen Cornmeal Loaf** (page 526) 2 cups salad greens with 2 teaspoons **Herbed Vinaigrette** (page 138) **Lemon Pound Cake** (page 568) CARB CHOICES: 4 EXCHANGES: 2 starch, 1½ carb, 1 veg, 2 plant-based protein, 3 fat CALORIES: 479	**Carrot-Ginger Soup** (page 164) **Barley Risotto with Asparagus and Peas** (page 382) 1 large sliced tomato with 2 teaspoons **Mustard Vinaigrette** (page 138) CARB CHOICES: 4 EXCHANGES: 2 starch, 4 veg, 2 fat CALORIES:441	**Grilled Fish Fillets with Citrus-Herb Gremolata** (page 334) **Grilled Fennel with Orange-Olive Vinaigrette** (page 463) ¾ cup **brown rice** (page 108) 1 cup **fresh raspberries** CARB CHOICES: 4 EXCHANGES: 2 starch, 1 fruit, 2 veg, 3 lean protein, 2 fat CALORIES: 477
Tomato and Roasted Red Pepper Soup (page 153) **Steak with Quick Mushroom-Rosemary Sauce** (page 266) **Buttermilk Mashed Potatoes** (page 482) ½ cup steamed Swiss chard **Banana Cream Pie** (page 552) CARB CHOICES: 4 EXCHANGES: 1½ starch, 1½ carb, 3 veg, 3 lean protein, 2 fat CALORIES: 597	**Caesar Salad** (page 84) **Fish Fillets, Potatoes, and Green Beans en Papillote** (page 332) **Fruit-Filled Meringues with Custard Sauce** (page 545) CARB CHOICES: 4 EXCHANGES: 1 starch, 2 carb, ½ fruit, 2 veg, 3 lean protein, 3 fat CALORIES: 606	**Chicken-Cheddar Quesadillas** (page 70) **Black Bean, Jicama, and Avocado Salad** (page 122) 1 cup fresh mango slices CARB CHOICES: 4 EXCHANGES: 2 starch, 2 fruit, 2 lean protein, ½ plant-based protein, 2½ fat CALORIES: 587	**Arugula and Melon Salad with Crispy Prosciutto** (page 89) **Herb-Crusted Sautéed Chicken** (page 207) **Roasted Fennel with Pernod** (page 464) **Asparagus with Sautéed Shiitake Mushrooms** (page 446) **Lemon Meringue Pie** (page 548) CARB CHOICES: 4 EXCHANGES: 2 carb, 1 fruit, 3 veg, 1 medium-fat protein, 3 lean protein, 3 fat CALORIES: 619

7-DAY 1,800-CALORIE MENU

The average daily calorie level for these menus is 1,550 calories, leaving 250 discretionary calories for two snacks during the day.

	Day 1	Day 2	Day 3
BREAKFAST	**Breakfast Barley with Honey and Walnuts** (page 5) 1 extra small banana 1 cup skim milk CARB CHOICES: 4 EXCHANGES: 2 starch, 1 fruit, 1 fat-free milk, ½ fat CALORIES: 325	**Fruit and Nut Muesli** (page 6) 1 poached egg 1 slice whole wheat toast 2 tablespoons **Fresh Strawberry Jam** (page 601) CARB CHOICES: 4 EXCHANGES: 2 starch, ½ carb, ½ fruit, 1 medium-fat protein, 1 fat CALORIES: 377	**Almond-Crusted French Toast with Berries** (page 13) ½ cup fresh orange juice ⅔ cup plain fat-free yogurt CARB CHOICES: 4 EXCHANGES: 1 starch, ½ carb, 1½ fruit, 1 fat-free milk, 1 fat, CALORIES: 375
LUNCH	**Open-Face Cheddar and Red Pepper Salad Sandwiches** (page 78) **Confetti Pasta Salad** (page 104) 2 cups mixed greens drizzled with 2 teaspoons **Lemon Vinaigrette** (page 139) **Pumpkin-Cranberry Bread** (page 506) CARB CHOICES: 4 EXCHANGES: 1½ starch, 1½ carb, 2 veg, 1 high-fat protein, 3 fat CALORIES: 583	**Avocado Dip** (page 38) with celery sticks **Homemade Tomato Soup** (page 153) 1 whole wheat roll **Tuna and White Bean Salad with Spinach** (page 135) 2 small fresh apricots CARB CHOICES: 4 EXCHANGES: 2 starch, ½ fruit, 5 veg, 2 lean protein, 2½ fat CALORIES: 524	**Grilled Vegetable and Goat Cheese Sandwiches** (page 77) **Tri-Color Salad** (page 86) **Orange and Pink Grapefruit Salad with Honey-Rosemary Syrup** (page 30) CARB CHOICES: 4 EXCHANGES: 2 starch, ½ carb, 1 fruit, 2 veg, 1 high-fat protein, 1½ fat CALORIES: 560
DINNER	**Creamy Onion Dip** (page 34) with cucumber slices **Falafel Burgers** (page 402) **Fattoush** (page 85) **Roasted Zucchini with Toasted Cumin and Basil** (page 488) **Walnut-Chocolate Chippers** (page 577) CARB CHOICES: 4 EXCHANGES: 3 starch, ½ carb, 2 veg, 1 plant-based protein, 3 fat CALORIES: 632	**Beef Saté with Peanut Sauce** (page 45) **Butternut Squash Soup with Red Curry and Coconut** (page 166) **Citrus Chicken and Snow Pea Stir-Fry** (page 212) ¾ cup brown rice CARB CHOICES: 4 EXCHANGES: 3 starch, ½ carb, 2 veg, 5 lean protein, 1 fat CALORIES: 654	**Roasted Beet and Green Bean Salad** (page 95) **Caper-Crusted Baked Fish** (page 338) **English Pea Puree** (page 481) 1 cup steamed yellow squash **Strawberry Shortcake** (page 541) CARB CHOICES: 4 EXCHANGES: ½ starch, 1½ carb, ½ fruit, 3 veg, 3 lean protein, 5 fat CALORIES: 585

Day 4	Day 5	Day 6	Day 7
Spiced Apple Cider Oatmeal (page 3)	**Spinach, Red Pepper, and Feta Quiche with Quinoa Crust** (page 20)	**Asparagus and Goat Cheese Omelet** (page 16)	**Blueberry Pancakes** (page 7)
¾ cup fresh pineapple	**Cranberry-Basted Baked Apple** (page 29)	1 whole wheat English muffin	½ extra small banana
1 cup skim milk	1 cup skim milk	1 cup cubed honeydew melon	1 cup skim milk
CARB CHOICES: 4	CARB CHOICES: 4	1 cup skim milk	CARB CHOICES: 4
EXCHANGES: 1½ starch, 2 fruit, 1 fat-free milk	EXCHANGES: 1 starch, 1 carb, 1 fruit, 1 fat-free milk, ½ medium-fat protein, 1 fat	CARB CHOICES: 4	EXCHANGES: 2 starch, ½ carb, ½ fruit, 1 fat-free milk, 1 fat
CALORIES: 306	CALORIES: 386	EXCHANGES: 2 starch, 1 fruit, 1 fat-free milk, 1 medium-fat protein, 1 fat	CALORIES: 356
		CALORIES: 456	
Avocado-Cucumber Salsa (page 42) with jicama spears	**Steak Sandwiches with Tomato Jam** (page 73)	**Artichoke, Feta, and Olive Pizza** (page 59)	**Lemony Lima Bean Spread** (page 38) with celery sticks
Chicken Tortilla Soup (page 180)	**Green Bean, Cherry Tomato, and Bacon Salad** (page 98)	**Mixed Green Salad with Marinated Tomatoes** (page 87)	**Oven-Fried Chicken Salad** (page 127)
Corn and Zucchini Muffin (page 515)	**Chiffon Cake** (page 567)	**Raspberry Granita** (page 584)	**Apricot-Almond Crostada** (page 555)
2 cups fresh baby spinach with 2 teaspoons **Cilantro-Lime Vinaigrette** (page 139)	CARB CHOICES: 4	CARB CHOICES: 4	CARB CHOICES: 4
Chocolate Brownie (page 581)	EXCHANGES: 1 starch, 2½ carb, 2 veg, 3 medium fat protein, 3½ fat	EXCHANGES: 2 starch, 2 veg, 2½ fat, 1 carb	EXCHANGES: 1 starch, 1½ carb, ½ fruit, 2 veg, 3 lean protein, 2 fat
CARB CHOICES: 4	CALORIES: 636	CALORIES: 387	CALORIES: 525
EXCHANGES: 2½ starch, 1 carb, 2 veg, 2½ lean protein, 3 fat			
CALORIES: 606			
Arugula and Pear Salad with Walnuts and Blue Cheese (page 89)	**Pumpkin and Roasted Red Pepper Soup** (page 160)	**Spinach Salad with Nut-Crusted Goat Cheese** (page 87)	**Egg Drop Soup** (page 169)
Pork Chops with White Beans and Sage (page 301)	**Parmesan-Crusted Oven-Baked Chicken Breasts** (page 233)	**Eye of Round with Roasted Garlic–Horseradish Sauce** (page 276)	**Miso-Orange Glazed Salmon** (page 345)
Broccoli Rabe with Garlic and Sun Dried Tomatoes (page 452)	**Polenta with Fresh Corn and Thyme** (page 422)	**Green Beans with Caramelized Onions and Cider Vinegar** (page 466)	**Asian Edamame and Radish Salad** (page 101)
Gingerbread Bundt Cake (page 569)	8 steamed asparagus spears	**Herb Mashed Potatoes** (page 482)	**Berry Rice Pudding** (page 560)
CARB CHOICES: 4	**Citrus Sugar Cookies** (page 576)	**Lemon Chiffon Pie** (page 550)	CARB CHOICES: 4
EXCHANGES: 1 starch, 2 carb, ½ fruit, 1 veg, 3 lean protein, 1 plant-based protein, 5½ fat	CARB CHOICES: 4	CARB CHOICES: 4	EXCHANGES: 4 carb, 5½ lean protein, 1 fat
CALORIES: 698	EXCHANGES: 2½ starch, 1 carb, 2 veg, 3 lean protein, 1½ fat	EXCHANGES: 1½ starch, 2 carb, 2 veg, 1 high-fat protein, 3 lean protein, 3 fat	CALORIES: 637
	CALORIES: 548	CALORIES: 696	

A Dozen Menus for Special Days

NEW YEAR'S DAY BRUNCH

Garden Vegetable Brunch Bundt "Cake" (page 25)

Orchard Fruit Salad (page 30)

Oatmeal-Raisin Bread (page 506)

CARB CHOICES: 3 EXCHANGES: 1½ carb, 1½ fruit, 1 veg, 1 high-fat protein, 1 medium-fat protein, 1½ fat, 435 calories

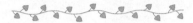

SPRING CELEBRATION

Crustless Asparagus and Feta Tart (page 411)

Pasta and Pea Salad (page 103)

Bibb and Whole Herb Salad (page 88)

Strawberry Shortcakes (page 541)

CARB CHOICES: 4 EXCHANGES: 1½ starch, 1½ carb, ½ fruit, 2 veg, 1 medium-fat protein, 564 calories

PICNIC IN THE PARK

Chunky Gazpacho (page 193)

Serrano Ham and Manchego Picnic Sandwich (page 79)

Roasted Vegetable and Pasta Salad (page 102)

Lemon Bars (page 582)

CARB CHOICES: 4 EXCHANGES: 2½ starch, ½ carb, 3 veg, 1 high-fat protein, 2 fat, 514 calories

CASUAL COOKOUT

Creamy Onion Dip (page 34) with fresh vegetables

Grilled BBQ Chicken (page 238)

Creamy Coleslaw (page 90)

Old-Fashioned Potato Salad (page 91)

Blueberry-Nectarine Crisp with Cornmeal-Pecan Topping (page 539)

CARB CHOICES: 4 EXCHANGES: 1 starch, 2 carb, ½ fruit, 1 veg, 3 lean protein, 4 fat, 583 calories

CHILDREN'S BIRTHDAY LUNCH

Peanut Sauce (page 594) with fresh vegetables

Panko-Crusted Chicken (page 234)

Steamed baby carrots

Chocolate Layer Cake with Fluffy White Frosting (page 564)

CARB CHOICES: 4 EXCHANGES: 1 starch, 2½ carb, 1 veg, 3 lean protein, 3½ fat, 543 calories

ADULT BIRTHDAY PARTY

Cured Salmon (Gravlax) (page 47)

Perfect-Every-Time Beef Tenderloin (page 275) with Romesco Sauce (page 593)

Green Beans with Caramelized Onions and Cider Vinegar (page 466)

Roasted Mushroom Salad (page 96)

Raspberry-Lemon Layer Cake (page 563)

CARB CHOICES: 3½ EXCHANGES: ½ starch, 2 carb, 3 veg, 4 lean protein, 4 fat, 742 calories

SUMMER'S BOUNTY LUNCH

Goat Cheese and Marinated Red Pepper
Bruschetta (page 50)

Broiled Salmon with Strawberry-Avocado
Salsa (page 345)

Tri-Color Salad (page 86)

Raspberry-Topped Cheesecake (page 573)

CARB CHOICES: 4 EXCHANGES: ½ starch, 2 carb,
½ fruit, 1 veg, 4 lean protein, 5 ½ fat, 717 calories

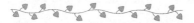

BRIDAL OR BABY SHOWER LUNCH

Creamy Smoked Salmon–Dill Spread
(page 48) with fresh vegetables

Spinach and Feta–Stuffed Chicken (page 234)

Wheat Berry, Fennel, and Parsley Salad
(page 109)

Angel Food Cake (page 568) with Raspberry
Sauce (page 588)

Citrus-Ginger Sparkler (page 606)

CARB CHOICES: 5 EXCHANGES: 1½ starch, 2 carb, 1 fruit,
1 medium-fat protein, 5 lean protein, 3 fat, 711 calories

VEGETARIAN DINNER

Tomatillo Salsa Verde (page 42) with
fresh vegetables

Black Bean Burritos with Creamy Avocado
Sauce (page 400)

Sautéed Zucchini with Cilantro and Lime
(page 486)

Flan (page 558)

CARB CHOICES: 4 EXCHANGES: 2 starch, 1½ carb,
3 veg, 1 plant-based protein, 1 fat, 575 calories

THANKSGIVING

Herb Roasted Turkey with Sage Gravy
(page 245)

Roasted Garlic Mashed Potatoes (page 482)

Brussels Sprouts with Apple Cider Glaze
(page 453)

Tangerine-Ginger Cranberry Sauce
(page 600)

Pumpkin Pie (page 548)

CARB CHOICES: 5 EXCHANGES: 1½ starch, 3 carb,
1 veg, 5 lean protein, 1½ fat, 574 calories

WINTER SOLSTICE CELEBRATION

Beer-Braised Beef Brisket (page 282)

Herb Mashed Potatoes (page 482)

Broccoli Rabe with Garlic and Sun-Dried
Tomatoes (page 452)

Apple-Cranberry Crisp (page 539)

CARB CHOICES: 3½ EXCHANGES: 1½ starch, 1 carb,
½ fruit, 1 veg, 3 lean protein, 3 fat, 556 calories

SUPER BOWL PARTY

Guacamole (page 38) with fresh vegetables

Buffalo Chicken Skewers (page 45)

Beef and Red Bean Chili (page 286)

Cornmeal Muffins with Chiles and Cheese
(page 516)

Classic Chocolate Chippers (page 576)

CARB CHOICES: 4½ EXCHANGES: 3 starch, 1 carb, 1 veg,
5 lean protein, 1 plant-based protein, 4 fat, 794 calories

Breakfasts and Brunches

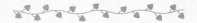

Cereals

Slow-Cooking Steel-Cut Oatmeal

Quick Overnight Steel-Cut Oatmeal

Spiced Apple Cider Oatmeal

Creamy Cherry-Almond Oatmeal

Breakfast Barley with Honey and Walnuts

Creamy Grits with Sharp Cheddar

Everyday Granola

Fruit and Nut Muesli

Pancakes, Waffles, and French Toast

Blueberry Pancakes

Cranberry-Orange Pancakes

Cornmeal-Cherry Pancakes

Whole Wheat Pancakes with Orange Honey

Ricotta Pancakes with Fresh Strawberries

Buckwheat Pancakes

Buttermilk Waffles

Chocolate-Chocolate Waffles

Pumpkin Waffles

Baked-Apple Pancake

Almond-Crusted French Toast with Berries

Maple-Raisin French Toast with Apples

Savory French Toast

Omelets, Frittatas, and Scrambles

Zucchini and Feta Omelet

Red Pepper and Manchego Omelet

Asparagus and Goat Cheese Omelet

Artichoke and Spinach Frittata

Asparagus and Mushroom Frittata

Tomato-Basil Frittata

Migas

Egg and Avocado Soft Tacos

Quiches, Breakfast Casseroles, and Other Egg Dishes

Asparagus Quiche with Couscous Crust

Spinach, Red Pepper, and Feta Quiche with Quinoa Crust

Crustless Broccoli and Cheddar Quiche

Crustless Sausage and Mushroom Quiche

Spinach and Mushroom Breakfast Casserole

Italian Vegetable Strata with Provolone

Sausage and Spinach Strata

Blueberry-Apricot Breakfast Casserole

Garden Vegetable Brunch Bundt "Cake"

Soufflé Roll with Asparagus, Mushrooms, and Mozzarella

Sausage and Cheddar Soufflé Roll

Ham and Egg Breakfast Cups

Huevos Rancheros

Compotes and Other Morning Fruits

Cranberry-Basted Baked Apples

Autumn Pear, Cranberry, and Pomegranate Compote

Orchard Fruit Salad

Orange and Pink Grapefruit Salad with Honey-Rosemary Syrup

Chamomile-Ginger Summer Fruit Salad

Basil-Lime Melon Compote

Yogurt-Berry Parfaits

Fresh Fruits with Yogurt-Maple Dip

Your mother was right—breakfast really is the most important meal of the day—and even more so if you have diabetes. People with diabetes need to eat at regular times throughout the day, starting with a nourishing breakfast, in order to control blood sugar levels.

Consuming fiber is fundamentally important for people with diabetes—the American Diabetes Association recommends 25 to 30 grams of fiber each day. And, for most people, breakfast is the easiest meal of the day to incorporate fiber. Eating fiber and whole grains is associated with a lowered risk of some cancers, lowered cholesterol, and better digestive regularity. Whole grains are good sources not only of fiber, but also of magnesium, vitamin E, and antioxidants.

Insoluble fiber adds bulk and volume to foods, but it is not digested, so it doesn't add calories. Foods that are high in fiber make you feel fuller longer, so if you're watching your weight, having a high-fiber breakfast helps keep you feeling full throughout the morning. It's no surprise that studies have shown that people who eat breakfast weigh less than those who skip the morning meal.

Typical breakfast foods such as oatmeal, bran muffins, high-fiber cereals, fresh fruits, or vegetable omelets are all good sources of fiber. If you think you don't have time for a fiber-rich breakfast, try Quick Overnight Steel-Cut Oatmeal (page 3)—it's ready in 10 minutes. If oatmeal seems like too much work in the morning, check out the muffin recipes on page 510–516. Most of these can be made ahead and frozen and you can reheat them

in a minute in the microwave. If you'd rather drink breakfast, try the smoothie recipes on page 606.

Even if what you eat isn't considered "breakfast food," that's okay, too. Some people don't like typical breakfast foods and certain people with diabetes have higher blood sugar levels in the mornings and need to restrict carbohydrates for the first part of the day. There are still options. Have some lean cold cuts or cheese, enjoy a handful of nuts, or even have a cup of soup to get your body going and ready to start the day.

You'll find recipes here for every kind of breakfast—from quick and easy ways to dress up your oatmeal, pancakes, and waffles for lazy mornings, to celebration dishes to enjoy when you host a weekend brunch.

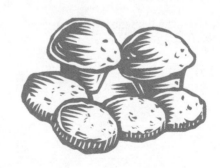

Cereals

Slow-Cooking Steel-Cut Oatmeal

makes 4 servings

Steel-cut oatmeal is a delicious creamy treat that tastes nothing like oatmeal made from regular rolled oats. Serve the oatmeal plain, or add a few raisins or currants during the last 5 minutes of cooking. You can add a pinch of cinnamon or nutmeg, too, if you wish.

3 cups water
Pinch of kosher salt
¾ cup steel-cut oats

1 Combine the water and salt in a medium saucepan and bring to a boil over medium-high heat. Slowly stir in the oats and return to a boil.

2 Reduce the heat to low, and simmer, uncovered, stirring occasionally, until the oats are tender, 20 to 25 minutes. Depending on how chewy you prefer your oats, you may need to add a little more water and cook them 5 to 10 minutes longer.

Each serving: 20 g carb, 111 cal, 2 g fat, 0 g sat fat, 0 mg chol, 3 g fib, 4 g pro, 18 mg sod • Carb Choices: 1; Exchanges: 1 starch

Quick Overnight Steel-Cut Oatmeal QUICK

makes 4 servings

If you love the hearty flavor and creamy texture of steel-cut oatmeal, but are too rushed in the mornings to make it, try this timesaving method. You'll have to do 5 minutes prep at night, but the oatmeal is ready in 10 minutes the next morning.

3 cups water
Pinch of kosher salt
¾ cup steel-cut oats

1 Combine the water and salt in a medium saucepan and bring to a boil over medium-high heat. Remove the pan from the heat and stir in the oats. Cover and let stand at room temperature overnight.

2 When ready to serve, set the saucepan over medium-high heat and bring to a boil over high heat. Reduce the heat, and simmer, covered, stirring occasionally, until the oats are tender, about 10 minutes.

Each serving: 20 g carb, 111 cal, 2 g fat, 0 g sat fat, 0 mg chol, 3 g fib, 4 g pro, 18 mg sod • Carb Choices: 1; Exchanges: 1 starch

Spiced Apple Cider Oatmeal QUICK

makes 4 servings

Shred the apple on a box grater just as you would shred a carrot for coleslaw. This comforting breakfast is good year-round, but especially so in the fall when fresh apples and apple cider are available.

1½ cups water
1 cup apple cider
1 small apple (any variety), peeled and coarsely shredded
¼ teaspoon ground cinnamon
Pinch of kosher salt
1½ cups old-fashioned rolled oats
1 tablespoon light brown sugar
½ teaspoon vanilla extract

1 Combine the water, apple cider, apple, cinnamon, and salt in a medium saucepan and bring to a boil over medium-high heat.

2 Stir in the oats, and cook, stirring constantly, until the liquid is absorbed and the oatmeal is thickened, 5 minutes. Stir in the sugar and the vanilla and serve at once.

Each serving: 35 g carb, 171 cal, 2 g fat, 0 g sat fat, 0 mg chol, 3 g fib, 4 g pro, 26 mg sod • Carb Choices: 2; Exchanges: 1½ starch, 1 fruit

Toasting Nuts

Since nuts are so high in calories, they are a special treat. Healthful recipes that call for nuts use only a small amount as a flavor accent. To get the most from a few nuts, it's worth the extra step to intensify their flavor by toasting them first.

It's best to toast whole shelled nuts or nut halves and then chop them. If you chop them before toasting, the pieces are so small that they can burn quickly. You can toast nuts in a dry skillet on the stovetop, but toasting them in the oven results in more even toasting and less chance of burning the nuts.

To toast nuts, place them in a single layer on a rimmed baking sheet and bake in a preheated 350°F oven. Most nuts take 8 to 10 minutes to toast. The exceptions are pine nuts, sunflower seeds, sesame seeds, and slivered or sliced almonds, which take 6 to 8 minutes. Stir the nuts once while they toast. Always set a timer when you're toasting nuts and once they get close to done, set the timer at 1-minute intervals to prevent them from burning. Once nuts are toasted, transfer them to a plate to cool.

Creamy Cherry-Almond Oatmeal QUICK

makes 4 servings

Customize this dressed-up oatmeal depending on what dried fruits you have on hand. Use cranberries, raisins, currants, or chopped apricots. It's a perfect quick-cooking breakfast to start your day in a flavorful and healthy way.

1½ cups water
1 cup skim milk
¼ cup dried tart cherries
Pinch of kosher salt
1½ cups old-fashioned rolled oats
2 tablespoons light brown sugar
⅛ teaspoon almond extract
2 tablespoons sliced almonds, toasted (left)

1 Combine the water, milk, cherries, and salt in a medium saucepan and bring to a boil over medium-high heat.

2 Stir in the oats, and cook, stirring constantly, until the liquid is absorbed and the oatmeal is thickened, 5 minutes. Stir in the sugar and the almond extract.

3 Spoon into 4 bowls, sprinkle evenly with the almonds, and serve at once.

Each serving: 37 g carb, 201 cal, 4 g fat, 0 g sat fat, 1 mg chol, 3 g fib, 7 g pro, 47 mg sod • Carb Choices: 2½; Exchanges: 2 starch, ½ fruit, ½ fat

Breakfast Barley with Honey and Walnuts

QUICK | HIGH FIBER

makes 4 servings

You don't think of barley as a breakfast food, but it's just as warm and comforting as a bowl of oatmeal. As with oatmeal, you can add any dried fruit that you have on hand instead of the currants. In summer, omit the dried fruit and top the cooked barley with fresh berries or chopped peaches.

⅔ cup pearl barley

2 cups water

2 tablespoons currants

Pinch of kosher salt

1 tablespoon honey

2 tablespoons walnuts, toasted and chopped (page 4)

1 Place the barley in a medium saucepan and set over medium heat. Toast, shaking the pan often, until the barley is lightly browned and fragrant, 5 minutes.

2 Add the water, currants, and salt and bring to a boil over high heat. Reduce the heat to low, cover, and simmer until the barley is tender, 20 to 25 minutes. Stir in the honey.

3 Spoon the barley into 4 bowls and sprinkle evenly with the walnuts. Serve at once.

Each serving: 34 g carb, 170 cal, 3 g fat, 0 g sat fat, 0 mg chol, 6 g fib, 4 g pro, 21 mg sod • Carb Choices: 2; Exchanges: 2 starch, ½ fat

Creamy Grits with Sharp Cheddar QUICK

makes 4 servings

Though I grew up in Kentucky and consider myself a Southerner, my mother never made grits. The first time I ever had them was in a restaurant where they were boiled with water and nothing else—not even salt. They were awful. Purists can have their plain cooked grits, but I need flavor. Cook grits in chicken broth or milk—or both—stir in almost any kind of cheese, and add roasted garlic, roasted red peppers, or thinly sliced prosciutto. Use this basic recipe to get started, then add whatever additions you enjoy. Do try this version first, though. They're so rich and creamy, they taste like they are made with whipping cream.

1 cup Chicken Stock (page 149) or low-sodium chicken broth

1 cup skim milk

½ cups uncooked quick-cooking grits

2 ounces shredded extra-sharp Cheddar cheese (about ½ cup)

Pinch of freshly ground pepper

1 Combine the stock and milk in a large saucepan and bring to a boil over medium-high heat.

2 Slowly stir in the grits, and cook, stirring constantly, until the grits are tender and the mixture is very thick, 5 minutes. Remove from the heat. Stir in the Cheddar and pepper and serve at once.

Each serving: 20 g carb, 158 cal, 5 g fat, 3 g sat fat, 17 mg chol, 0 g fib, 8 g pro, 153 mg sod • Carb Choices: 1; Exchanges: 1 starch, ½ high-fat protein

Everyday Granola

makes 12 cups

I store this granola in a big glass jar in my pantry and I have it with plain fat-free kefir for breakfast nearly every day. Sometimes I even take it with me if I'm traveling so I'm guaranteed a healthy breakfast. It's not a "gourmet" granola—it's not packed with sugar-coated nuts or chocolate chips. It's just a good solid breakfast that's a little bit sweet and has enough nuts to add some crunch. If you don't like kefir, serve the granola with yogurt or milk.

½ cup honey
4 tablespoons (½ stick) unsalted butter
1 tablespoon ground cinnamon
¼ teaspoon kosher salt
6 cups old-fashioned rolled oats
½ cup packed light brown sugar
¾ cup sliced almonds
½ cup dried cranberries

1 Preheat the oven to 350°F.

2 Combine the honey, butter, cinnamon, and salt in a medium saucepan. Bring to a boil over medium heat, stirring until the mixture is smooth.

3 Combine the oats and sugar in a large bowl. Using your fingers, evenly mix the sugar and oats. Stir in the almonds. Add the honey mixture in three additions, stirring well after each addition. Let the mixture stand until cool enough to handle, then mix thoroughly using your hands to evenly coat the oats and almonds with the honey mixture.

4 Transfer to an ungreased deep-sided roasting pan. Bake, stirring every 10 minutes, until the oats are lightly browned, 30 to 35 minutes.

5 Let stand to cool to room temperature (the granola will become crisp as it cools). Stir in the cranberries. Store the granola in an airtight container up to 1 month.

Each serving (generous ½ cup): 26 g carb, 155 cal, 5 g fat, 2 g sat fat, 5 mg chol, 2 g fib, 3 g pro, 15 mg sod • Carb Choices: 2; Exchanges: 1 starch, 1 carb, 1 fat

Fruit and Nut Muesli

QUICK | HIGH FIBER

makes 4 servings

As long as you keep the ratio of liquid to oats the same (1 part liquid, 1 part oats), you can vary this recipe according to the number of servings you need, to your taste, and to the season. Instead of the skim milk, use fat-free yogurt, buttermilk, or any kind of fruit juice. Instead of honey, use molasses, maple syrup, or brown sugar. And use whatever fresh fruit and nuts you have on hand. It's a simple, healthful breakfast that offers a delicious serving of fiber and fruit.

1 cup skim milk
1 tablespoon honey
1 cup old-fashioned rolled oats
1 cup fresh blueberries
¼ cup almonds, toasted and chopped (page 4)

1 Combine the milk and honey in a medium bowl and stir until well blended. Stir in the oats and blueberries.

2 Spoon into 4 bowls and sprinkle each serving with 1 tablespoon of the almonds. You can cover and refrigerate the muesli without the almonds for up to 4 days. Sprinkle with the remaining almonds just before serving.

Each serving: 28 g carb, 183 cal, 6 g fat, 1 g sat fat, 1 mg chol, 4 g fib, 7 g pro, 27 mg sod • Carb Choices: 2; Exchanges: 1 starch, ½ carb, ½ fruit, 1 fat

Pancakes, Waffles, and French Toast

Blueberry Pancakes QUICK

makes 6 servings

These light and tender pancakes are worth getting up early to make. They are packed with berries, but if you have extra on hand, sprinkle more on top of the pancakes, or serve them with Whole Blueberry Sauce (page 588).

¾ cup unbleached all-purpose flour
¾ cup whole wheat flour
1 tablespoon sugar
2 teaspoons baking powder
Pinch of salt
1¼ cups plain low-fat yogurt
½ cup skim milk
1 large egg
1 tablespoon plus 1½ teaspoons canola oil, divided
1 teaspoon vanilla extract
¾ cup fresh blueberries or unthawed frozen blueberries
3 tablespoons real maple syrup

1 Preheat the oven to 250°F. Place a large baking sheet in the oven.

2 Combine the flours, sugar, baking powder, and salt in a large bowl and stir to mix well. Combine the yogurt, milk, egg, 1 tablespoon of the oil, and the vanilla in a medium bowl and whisk until smooth. Add the yogurt mixture to the flour mixture and stir until a smooth batter forms.

3 Heat a large nonstick griddle or large nonstick skillet over medium heat. Brush with ½ teaspoon of the oil using a silicone brush. Spoon the batter by scant ¼ cup measures onto the griddle 4 at a time. Sprinkle about 1 tablespoon of the blueberries onto each pancake. Turn the pancakes when the tops are covered with bubbles and the edges look cooked. Place the pancakes on the baking sheet in the oven to keep warm. Repeat the procedure with the remaining oil, batter, and blueberries to make 12 pancakes.

4 Place 2 pancakes on each serving plate. Drizzle ½ tablespoon of the maple syrup over each serving.

Each serving: 39 g carb, 237 cal, 5 g fat, 1 g sat fat, 39 mg chol, 3 g fib, 9 g pro, 287 mg sod • Carb Choices: 2½; Exchanges: 2 starch, ½ carb, 1 fat

PEACHY PANCAKES QUICK : Follow the Blueberry Pancakes recipe, at left, but substitute 1 large fresh peach, peeled, pitted, and chopped for the blueberries in step 3 and proceed as directed.

Each serving: 38 g carb, 236 cal, 5 g fat, 1 g sat fat, 39 mg chol, 3 g fib, 9 g pro, 214 mg sod • Carb Choices: 2½; Exchanges: 2 starch, ½ carb, 1 fat

10 PANCAKE AND WAFFLE TOPPINGS UNDER 10 GRAMS OF CARBS

Topping	Carbs (grams)	Calories
Unsweetened applesauce (¼ cup)	7 (½ Carb Choice)	26
Low-sugar fruit spread (1 tablespoon)	6 (½ Carb Choice)	25
Apple butter (1 tablespoon)	8 (½ Carb Choice)	31
Plain low-fat yogurt (¼ cup)	4 (0 Carb Choice)	40
¼ cup mashed fresh strawberries mixed with ¼ cup plain low-fat yogurt (2-tablespoon serving)	3 (0 Carb Choice)	17
Fresh raspberries (½ cup)	7 (½ Carb Choice)	32
Fresh blueberries (½ cup)	7 (½ Carb Choice)	28
Fresh strawberries (½ cup)	6 (½ Carb Choice)	27
Confectioners' sugar (1 teaspoon)	2 (0 Carb Choice)	10
Maple syrup (½ tablespoon)	7 (½ Carb Choice)	26

Cranberry-Orange Pancakes QUICK | HIGH FIBER

makes 6 servings

These pancakes will put you in a festive mood during the winter holidays. In-season cranberries and bright orange segments make them a healthful and colorful breakfast to enjoy before heading out for holiday shopping or errands.

2 navel oranges

¾ cup unbleached all-purpose flour

¾ cup whole wheat flour

1 tablespoon sugar

2 teaspoons baking powder

¼ teaspoon ground cinnamon

Pinch of salt

1¼ cups plain low-fat yogurt

1 large egg

1 tablespoon plus 1½ teaspoons canola oil, divided

1 teaspoon vanilla extract

¾ cup fresh cranberries or unthawed frozen cranberries

1 Preheat the oven to 250°F. Place a large baking sheet in the oven.

2 Remove ½ teaspoon of the zest from 1 of the oranges and reserve. Cut a thin slice from the top and bottom of the orange, exposing the flesh. Stand the orange upright, and using a sharp knife, thickly cut off the peel, following the contour of the fruit and removing all the white pith and membrane. Holding the orange over a bowl, carefully cut along both sides of each section to free it from the membrane. Discard any seeds and let the sections fall into the bowl. Drain the orange segments, reserving ½ cup of the juice. Reserve any remaining juice for another use. Repeat with the remaining orange.

3 Combine the flours, sugar, baking powder, cinnamon, and salt in a large bowl and stir to mix well. Combine the yogurt, orange juice and zest,

egg, 1 tablespoon of the oil, and the vanilla in a medium bowl and whisk until smooth. Add the yogurt mixture to the flour mixture and stir until a smooth batter forms.

4 Heat a large nonstick griddle or large nonstick skillet over medium heat. Brush with ½ teaspoon of the oil using a silicone brush. Spoon the batter by scant ¼ cup measures onto the griddle 4 at a time. Sprinkle about 1 tablespoon of the cranberries onto each pancake. Turn the pancakes when the tops are covered with bubbles and the edges look cooked. Place the pancakes on the baking sheet in the oven to keep warm. Repeat the procedure with the remaining oil, batter, and cranberries to make 12 pancakes.

5 Place 2 pancakes on each plate. Using a slotted spoon, top each serving of the pancakes with about ⅓ cup of the orange segments.

Each serving: 45 g carb, 258 cal, 5 g fat, 1 g sat fat, 39 mg chol, 4 g fib, 8 g pro, 215 mg sod • Carb Choices: 3; Exchanges: 2 starch, ½ carb, ½ fruit, 1 fat

Cornmeal-Cherry Pancakes QUICK

makes 6 servings

These are a special treat if you're able to use fresh ripe summer cherries, but they're almost as good with the frozen variety. Be sure to wear an apron when you cut up the cherries to prevent a permanent stain on your clothes. Instead of syrup, these are also great topped with a dollop of low-fat Greek yogurt.

1 cup fine-grind yellow cornmeal

½ cup unbleached all-purpose flour

1 tablespoon sugar

2 teaspoons baking powder

Pinch of salt

1½ cups low-fat buttermilk

1 large egg

1 tablespoon plus 1½ teaspoons canola oil, divided

1 teaspoon vanilla extract

¾ cup fresh pitted cherries or partially thawed frozen cherries, quartered

3 tablespoons real maple syrup

1 Preheat the oven to 250°F. Place a large baking sheet in the oven.

2 Combine the cornmeal, flour, sugar, baking powder, and salt in a large bowl and stir to mix well. Combine the buttermilk, egg, 1 tablespoon of the oil, and the vanilla in a medium bowl and whisk until smooth. Add the buttermilk mixture to the cornmeal mixture and stir until a smooth batter forms.

3 Heat a large nonstick griddle or large nonstick skillet over medium heat. Brush with ½ teaspoon of the oil using a silicone brush. Spoon the batter by scant ¼ cup measures onto the griddle 4 at a time. Sprinkle about 1 tablespoon of the cherries onto each pancake. Turn the pancakes when the tops are covered with bubbles and the edges look cooked. Place the pancakes on the baking sheet in the oven to keep warm. Repeat the procedure with the remaining oil, batter, and cherries.

4 Place 2 pancakes on each plate. Drizzle ½ tablespoon of the maple syrup over each serving.

Each serving: 44 g carb, 255 cal, 6 g fat, 1 g sat fat, 38 mg chol, 2 g fib, 7 g pro, 243 mg sod • Carb Choices: 3; Exchanges: 2 starch, 1 carb, 1 fat

Whole Wheat Pancakes with Orange Honey

QUICK | HIGH FIBER

makes 6 servings

Adding beaten egg whites to the batter makes these so light and fluffy it's hard to believe they are made with whole wheat flour. The mixture of honey and orange juice lets you enjoy the sweetness of honey but in a less concentrated form of carbohydrates. For no-carb and low-carb pancake toppings, see 10 Pancake and Waffle Toppings Under 10 Grams of Carbs (page 7).

2 cups whole wheat flour

1 tablespoon sugar

2 teaspoons baking powder

Pinch of salt

2 cups low-fat buttermilk

1 large egg

1 tablespoon plus 1½ teaspoons canola oil, divided

1 teaspoon vanilla extract

3 large egg whites

3 tablespoons honey

3 tablespoons orange juice

1 Preheat the oven to 250°F. Place a large baking sheet in the oven.

2 Combine the flour, sugar, baking powder, and salt in a large bowl and stir to mix well. Combine the buttermilk, egg, 1 tablespoon of the oil, and the vanilla in a medium bowl and whisk until smooth. Add the buttermilk mixture to the flour mixture and stir until a smooth batter forms.

3 Place the egg whites in a large bowl and beat at high speed with an electric mixer until soft peaks form. Fold the egg whites into the batter in 3 additions, stirring until no white streaks appear.

4 Heat a large nonstick griddle or large nonstick skillet over medium heat. Brush with ½ teaspoon of the oil using a silicone brush. Spoon the batter by scant ¼ cup measures onto the griddle 4 at a time. Turn the pancakes when the tops are covered with bubbles and the edges look cooked. Place the pancakes on the baking sheet in the oven to keep warm. Repeat the procedure with the remaining oil and batter.

5 Combine the honey and orange juice in a small saucepan. Set over medium heat until hot.

6 Place 2 pancakes on each plate. Drizzle 1 tablespoon of the orange honey over each serving.

Each serving: 44 g carb, 284 cal, 6 g fat, 1 g sat fat, 38 mg chol, 5 g fib, 12 g pro, 139 mg sod • Carb Choices: 3; Exchanges: 2 starch, 1 carb, 1 fat

Ricotta Pancakes with Fresh Strawberries QUICK

makes 6 servings

Syrup would overwhelm the delicate flavor and texture of these airy pancakes. Serve them with a light dusting of confectioners' sugar and fresh berries, sliced peaches, or orange segments.

1 cup part-skim ricotta
⅓ cup skim milk
2 large eggs, separated
⅓ cup unbleached all-purpose flour
1 tablespoon granulated sugar
2 teaspoons grated orange zest
Pinch of salt
1½ teaspoons canola oil, divided
2 teaspoons confectioners' sugar
3 cups sliced fresh strawberries

1 Preheat the oven to 250°F. Place a large baking sheet in the oven.

2 Combine the ricotta, milk, egg yolks, flour, granulated sugar, orange zest, and salt in a large bowl and whisk until smooth.

3 Place the egg whites in a large bowl and beat at high speed with an electric mixer until stiff peaks form. Fold the egg whites into the ricotta mixture in 3 additions, stirring until no white streaks appear.

4 Heat a large nonstick griddle or large nonstick skillet over medium heat. Brush with ½ teaspoon of the oil using a silicone brush. Spoon the batter by scant ¼-cup measures onto the griddle 4 at a time. Turn the pancakes when the tops are covered with bubbles and the edges look cooked. Place the pancakes on the baking sheet in the oven to keep warm. Repeat the procedure with the remaining oil and batter to make 12 pancakes.

5 Place 2 pancakes on each plate. Sprinkle the pancakes evenly with the confectioners' sugar. Accompany each serving with ½ cup of the strawberries.

Each serving: 17 g carb, 156 cal, 6 g fat, 3 g sat fat, 84 mg chol, 2 g fib, 8 g pro, 106 mg sod • Carb Choices: 1; Exchanges: 1 starch, 1 fat

Buckwheat Pancakes

HIGH FIBER

makes 6 servings

If you love the flavor of buckwheat, these pancakes are a perfect make-ahead breakfast. Be sure to use a large bowl for the batter when you refrigerate it overnight to allow for expansion. Serve the pancakes topped with any fruit from berries to bananas.

1 cup warm 1% low-fat milk
1 package active dry yeast
1 cup buckwheat flour
½ cup unbleached all-purpose flour
1 tablespoon granulated sugar
¼ teaspoon salt
1 large egg, separated
⅓ cup plain low-fat Greek yogurt or strained yogurt (page 11)
½ teaspoon baking soda
1½ teaspoons canola oil, divided
2 teaspoons confectioners' sugar

1 Combine the milk and yeast in a large bowl and stir until the yeast dissolves. Let stand 5 minutes. Add the flours, granulated sugar, and salt and stir until a smooth batter forms. Cover and refrigerate overnight.

2 Preheat the oven to 250°F. Place a large baking sheet in the oven.

3 Add the egg yolk, yogurt, and baking soda to the batter and stir until smooth. Place the egg white in a medium mixing bowl and beat at high speed with an electric mixer until stiff peaks form. Fold the egg white into the pancake batter in 2 additions, stirring until no white streaks remain.

4 Heat a large nonstick griddle or large nonstick skillet over medium heat. Brush with ½ teaspoon of the oil using a silicone brush. Spoon the batter by scant ¼-cup measures onto the griddle 4 at a time. Turn the pancakes when the tops are covered with bubbles and the edges look cooked. Place the pancakes on the baking sheet in the oven to keep warm. Repeat the procedure with the remaining oil and batter to make 12 pancakes.

5 Place 2 pancakes on each plate. Sprinkle the pancakes evenly with the confectioners' sugar.

Each serving: 24 g carb, 157 cal, 3 g fat, 1 g sat fat, 38 mg chol, 4 g fib, 7 g pro, 139 mg sod • Carb Choices: 1½; Exchanges: 1½ starch, ½ fat

Making Strained Yogurt

Straining the liquid whey from yogurt makes an extra-thick tangy yogurt that is delicious to enjoy on its own, for use in baking, and for dips and spreads. To make it, line a strainer or a colander with several thicknesses of cheesecloth or coffee filters and set the strainer over a bowl. Spoon 2 cups plain low-fat yogurt into the strainer, cover, and refrigerate overnight. Discard the liquid. Two cups of yogurt makes 1 cup of strained yogurt. The yogurt can be refrigerated, covered, for up to a week. If you want to skip the straining, look for plain low-fat Greek yogurt near the regular yogurt in most large supermarkets.

Buttermilk Waffles QUICK

makes 6 servings

This is a terrific basic waffle recipe with a light wheat flavor. It's good year-round for serving with fresh strawberries in the spring or sautéed apples in the fall and winter.

¾ cup unbleached all-purpose flour
⅓ cup whole wheat flour
2 tablespoons granulated sugar
1 teaspoon baking powder
Pinch of salt
½ cup low-fat buttermilk
1 large egg
2 large egg whites
1 tablespoon plus 2 teaspoons canola oil, divided
1 teaspoon vanilla extract
2 teaspoons confectioners' sugar
1½ cups fresh sliced strawberries

1 Preheat the oven to 250°F. Place a large baking sheet in the oven.

2 Combine the flours, granulated sugar, baking powder, and salt in a medium bowl and stir to mix well. Combine the buttermilk, egg, egg whites, 1 tablespoon of the oil, and the vanilla in a separate medium bowl and stir to mix well. Add the buttermilk mixture to the flour mixture and stir just until moistened.

3 Preheat the waffle iron and lightly brush with part of the remaining 2 teaspoons canola oil using a silicone brush. Spoon about ¼ cup of batter onto the hot waffle iron, spreading the batter to the edges. Cook for 4 to 5 minutes or until the steaming stops. Place the waffles on the baking sheet in the oven to keep warm. Repeat with the remaining batter to make 6 waffles.

4 Place 1 waffle on each plate. Sprinkle the waffles evenly with the confectioners' sugar. Accompany each serving with ½ cup of the strawberries.

Each serving: 24 g carb, 163 cal, 5 g fat, 1 g sat fat, 35 mg chol, 2 g fib, 5 g pro, 198 mg sod • Carb Choices: 1½; Exchanges: 1½ starch, 1 fat

Chocolate-Chocolate Waffles QUICK | HIGH FIBER

makes 6 servings

When you want to start someone's day in a special way, make these double chocolate waffles for breakfast. Whether it's a birthday, a graduation, anniversary, or other milestone, begin the celebration early with a surprise treat for breakfast.

½ cup unbleached all-purpose flour
⅓ cup whole wheat flour
¼ cup unsweetened cocoa
2 tablespoons sugar
1 teaspoon baking powder
Pinch of salt
½ cup low-fat buttermilk
1 large egg
2 large egg whites
1 tablespoon plus 2 teaspoons canola oil, divided
1 teaspoon vanilla extract
2 ounces semisweet chocolate, chopped

1 Preheat the oven to 250°F. Place a large baking sheet in the oven.

2 Combine the flours, cocoa, sugar, baking powder, and salt in a medium bowl and stir to mix well. Combine the buttermilk, egg, egg whites, 1 tablespoon of the oil, and the vanilla in a separate medium bowl and stir to mix well. Add the buttermilk mixture to the flour mixture and stir just until moistened.

3 Preheat the waffle iron and lightly brush with part of the remaining 2 teaspoons oil using a silicone brush. Spoon about ¼ cup of batter onto the hot waffle iron, spreading the batter to the edges. Cook for 4 to 5 minutes or until the steaming stops. Place the waffles on the baking sheet in the oven to keep warm. Repeat with the remaining batter to make 6 waffles.

4 Meanwhile, bring a small saucepan of water to a boil over high heat. Place the chocolate in a small resealable plastic bag. Remove the saucepan from the heat; place the bag in the saucepan and let stand until the chocolate melts, about 3 minutes.

5 Place 1 waffle on each plate. Snip a tiny corner off the plastic bag; drizzle the melted chocolate evenly over the waffles.

Each serving: 29 g carb, 197 cal, 8 g fat, 3 g sat fat, 35 mg chol, 4 g fib, 6 g pro, 199 mg sod • Carb Choices: 2; Exchanges: 1½ starch, ½ carb, 1½ fat

Pumpkin Waffles QUICK

makes 8 servings

Serve these waffles with the Autumn Pear, Cranberry, and Pomegranate Compote on page 29. They make a festive Halloween or Thanksgiving breakfast.

¾ cup unbleached all-purpose flour
½ cup whole wheat flour
1 tablespoon sugar
1 teaspoon baking powder
¾ teaspoon pumpkin pie spice
Pinch of salt
¾ cup 1% low-fat milk
½ cup canned pumpkin (not pumpkin pie filling)
1 large egg
1 tablespoon plus 2 teaspoons canola oil, divided
1 teaspoon vanilla extract
4 tablespoons real maple syrup

1 Preheat the oven to 250°F. Place a large baking sheet in the oven.

2 Combine the flours, sugar, baking powder, pumpkin pie spice, and salt in a large bowl; stir to mix well.

3 Combine the milk, pumpkin, egg, 1 tablespoon of the oil, and the vanilla in a medium bowl; whisk until smooth. Add the buttermilk mixture to the flour mixture; stir until a moist batter forms.

4 Preheat the waffle iron and lightly brush with part of the remaining 2 teaspoons oil using a silicone brush. Spoon about ¼ cup of batter

for each 4-inch waffle onto the hot waffle iron, spreading the batter to the edges. Cook for 4 to 5 minutes or until the steaming stops. Repeat with the remaining batter. Place the waffles on the baking sheet in the oven to keep warm. Repeat the procedure with the remaining oil and batter to make 8 waffles.

5 Place 1 waffle on each plate. Drizzle ½ tablespoon of the maple syrup over each serving.

Each serving: 25 g carb, 151 cal, 4 g fat, 1 g sat fat, 28 mg chol, 2 g fib, 4 g pro, 71 mg sod • Carb Choices: 1½; Exchanges: 1 starch, ½ carb, ½ fat

Baked-Apple Pancake

makes 8 servings

Also known as a Dutch baby, this rustic-looking pancake is too delicate to remove to a serving platter. Serve it at the table in the skillet to show off the contrast of the lofty crisp edge to the flat and custardy center. When you need something simple and fast, it makes a great dessert, too. Don't substitute whole wheat flour in this recipe—the pancake won't rise.

4 tablespoons granulated sugar, divided

¼ teaspoon ground cinnamon

1 large Granny Smith, Gala, or Golden Delicious apple, peeled, cored, and thinly sliced

2 teaspoons plus 1 tablespoon canola oil, divided

¾ cup 1% low-fat milk

½ cup unbleached all-purpose flour

2 large eggs

2 large egg whites

½ teaspoon vanilla extract

Pinch of salt

1 teaspoon confectioners' sugar

1 Preheat the oven to 425°F.

2 Combine 1 tablespoon of the granulated sugar and the cinnamon in a medium bowl and stir to mix well. Add the apple and toss to coat. Brush the bottom and sides of a 10-inch ovenproof nonstick skillet with 2 teaspoons of the oil. Arrange the apples in concentric circles in the skillet and set over medium heat. Cook, without stirring or turning the apples, until they begin to soften and brown lightly, 6 to 8 minutes.

3 Meanwhile, combine the milk, flour, eggs, egg whites, vanilla, salt, the remaining 3 tablespoons granulated sugar, and the remaining 1 tablespoon oil in a medium bowl and whisk until smooth.

4 Pour the batter over the apple slices and bake until the edge is puffed and lightly browned, 12 to 15 minutes. Sprinkle with the confectioners' sugar and serve at once.

Each serving: 17 g carb, 122 cal, 4 g fat, 1 g sat fat, 54 mg chol, 1 g fib, 4 g pro, 60 mg sod • Carb Choices: 1; Exchanges: 1 carb, ½ fat

Almond-Crusted French Toast with Berries

QUICK | HIGH FIBER

makes 4 servings

Be careful not to let the almonds burn when you make this French toast. Cook the toast over medium heat and watch it closely, adjusting the heat if necessary.

2 large eggs

1 large egg white

2 tablespoons 1% low-fat milk

2 tablespoons sugar

½ teaspoon vanilla extract

⅛ teaspoon ground cinnamon

4 slices 100% whole wheat bread

¼ cup sliced almonds

1 teaspoon canola oil, divided

2 cups fresh blueberries or raspberries

1 Combine the eggs, egg white, milk, sugar, vanilla, and cinnamon in a large shallow dish and whisk until the sugar dissolves. Place the bread in the dish and let stand, turning the bread often, until the egg mixture is absorbed, about 5 minutes. Sprinkle both sides of each slice of bread evenly with the almonds, pressing to adhere.

continues on next page

2 Heat a large nonstick griddle or large nonstick skillet over medium heat. Brush with ½ teaspoon of the oil using a silicone brush. Place 2 bread slices on the griddle and cook, turning once, until lightly browned, about 2 minutes per side. Set aside to keep warm. Repeat the procedure with the remaining oil and bread.

3 Place 1 slice of French toast on each plate. Accompany each serving with ½ cup of the berries.

Each serving: 35 g carb, 228 cal, 7 g fat, 1 g sat fat, 53 mg chol, 4 g fib, 9 g pro, 171 mg sod • Carb Choices: 2; Exchanges: 1 starch, ½ carb, ½ fruit, 1 fat

Maple-Raisin French Toast with Apples QUICK

makes 4 servings

This French toast tastes like an apple pie—without all the work. Choose a good-quality whole wheat or multigrain raisin bread for this recipe.

2 large eggs
1 large egg white
2 tablespoons 1% low-fat milk
2 tablespoons real maple syrup
½ teaspoon vanilla extract
Pinch of ground nutmeg
Pinch of salt
4 slices whole wheat raisin bread
1 teaspoon canola oil, divided
2 small apples, peeled, cored, and diced

1 Combine the eggs, egg white, milk, maple syrup, vanilla, nutmeg, and salt in a large shallow dish and whisk until smooth. Place the bread in the dish and let stand, turning the bread often, until the egg mixture is absorbed, about 5 minutes.

2 Heat a large nonstick griddle or large nonstick skillet over medium heat. Brush with ½ teaspoon of the oil using a silicone brush. Place 2 bread slices on the griddle and cook, turning once until

lightly browned, about 2 minutes per side. Set aside to keep warm. Repeat the procedure with the remaining oil and bread.

3 Place 1 slice of French toast on each plate. Sprinkle each serving with about ¼ cup of the diced apple.

Each serving: 30 g carb, 184 cal, 5 g fat, 1 g sat fat, 106 mg chol, 3 g fib, 7 g pro, 195 mg sod • Carb Choices: 2; Exchanges: 1½ starch, ½ carb, 1 fat

Savory French Toast QUICK

makes 4 servings

I grew up eating savory French toast—it was simply bread dipped in beaten eggs, seasoned with salt and pepper, and cooked in a skillet. I've dressed this version up with a touch of Dijon and a little freshly grated cheese. Serve it with sliced tomatoes or with Fresh Tomato Salsa (page 41) for a satisfying summer breakfast.

2 large eggs
1 large egg white
2 tablespoons 1% low-fat milk
1 ounce freshly grated Parmesan (about ¼ cup)
¼ teaspoon Dijon mustard
¼ teaspoon kosher salt
⅛ teaspoon freshly ground pepper
4 slices 100% whole wheat bread or rye bread
1 teaspoon extra virgin olive oil, divided

1 Combine the eggs, egg white, milk, Parmesan, mustard, salt, and pepper in a large shallow dish and whisk until smooth. Place the bread in the dish and let stand, turning the bread often, until the egg mixture is absorbed, about 5 minutes.

2 Heat a large nonstick griddle or large nonstick skillet over medium heat. Brush with ½ teaspoon of the oil using a silicone brush. Place 2 bread slices on the griddle and cook, turning once, until lightly browned, about 2 minutes per side. Set aside to keep warm. Repeat the procedure with the remaining oil and bread. Serve immediately.

Each serving: 17 g carb, 166 cal, 6 g fat, 2 g sat fat, 110 mg chol, 2 g fib, 10 g pro, 342 mg sod • Carb Choices: 1; Exchanges: 1 starch, ½ fat

Omelets, Frittatas, and Scrambles

Zucchini and Feta Omelet QUICK

makes 2 servings

Omelets are a great way to enjoy a serving of vegetables early in the day. I love to make them filled with plenty of vegetables and a modest amount of cheese for a healthful start to a busy weekend morning.

2 large eggs
2 large egg whites
2 teaspoons chopped fresh dill
1/8 teaspoon kosher salt
1/8 teaspoon freshly ground pepper
2 teaspoons extra virgin olive oil, divided
1 medium zucchini, diced (about 1 1/2 cups)
2 tablespoons finely crumbled feta cheese

1 Whisk together the eggs, egg whites, dill, salt, and pepper in a medium bowl. Set aside.

2 Heat a medium nonstick skillet over medium-high heat. Add 1 teaspoon of the oil and tilt the pan to coat. Add the zucchini and cook, stirring often, until crisp-tender, about 3 minutes. Spoon into a bowl and set aside.

3 Add the remaining 1 teaspoon oil to the skillet and tilt to coat the pan. Pour the egg mixture into the skillet. Reduce the heat to medium and cook, lifting the edge of the egg with a spatula to allow the uncooked portion to flow underneath until the bottom is set, about 2 minutes. Reduce the heat to medium-low. Cover and cook until the top of the egg is set, about 2 minutes more.

4 Gently slide the cooked egg onto a large plate; spoon the cooked zucchini and the feta down the center of the egg. Carefully fold two opposite sides of the egg over the zucchini mixture to cover. Cut the omelet in half and arrange each half on a plate. Serve immediately.

Each serving: 5 g carb, 168 cal, 11 g fat, 3 g sat fat, 218 mg chol, 1 g fib, 12 g pro, 286 mg sod • Carb Choices: 0; Exchanges: 1 medium-fat protein, 1 fat

Red Pepper and Manchego Omelet QUICK

makes 2 servings

Manchego is a Spanish sheep's milk cheese that lends a mild nutty flavor to any dish. It melts to a creamy consistency, making it perfect for omelets and pasta dishes. If you have smoked or hot paprika on hand, sprinkle the top of the omelet with just a pinch to give your breakfast a kick.

2 large eggs
2 large egg whites
2 teaspoons chopped fresh Italian parsley
⅛ teaspoon kosher salt
⅛ teaspoon freshly ground pepper
2 teaspoons extra virgin olive oil, divided
1 medium red or yellow bell pepper, thinly sliced
2 tablespoons shredded manchego

1 Whisk together the eggs, egg whites, parsley, salt, and ground pepper in a medium bowl. Set aside.

2 Heat a medium nonstick skillet over medium-high heat. Add 1 teaspoon of the oil and tilt the pan to coat. Add the bell pepper and cook, stirring often, until crisp-tender, about 3 minutes. Spoon into a bowl and set aside.

3 Add the remaining 1 teaspoon oil to the skillet and tilt to coat the pan. Pour the egg mixture into the skillet. Reduce the heat to medium and cook, lifting the edge of the egg with a spatula to allow the uncooked portion to flow underneath until the bottom is set, about 2 minutes. Reduce the heat to medium-low. Cover until the top of the egg is set, about 2 minutes more.

continues on next page

4 Gently slide the cooked egg onto a large plate; spoon the cooked bell pepper and the manchego down the center of the egg. Carefully fold two opposite sides of the egg over the bell pepper mixture to cover. Cut the omelet in half and arrange each half on a plate. Serve immediately.

Each serving: 4 g carb, 179 cal, 13 g fat, 4 g sat fat, 221 mg chol, 1 g fib, 13 g pro, 226 mg sod • Carb Choices: 0; Exchanges: 1 medium-fat protein, 1 fat

Asparagus and Goat Cheese Omelet QUICK

makes 2 servings

This omelet is a delicious celebration of spring that's ready to eat in just a few minutes. If your asparagus spears are thick, cut them in half lengthwise before cutting into 2-inch pieces so they will cook quickly. Serve the omelet with rustic wheat toast and sliced melon.

2 large eggs
2 egg whites
2 teaspoons chopped fresh basil or dill
1/8 teaspoon kosher salt
1/8 teaspoon freshly ground pepper
2 teaspoons extra virgin olive oil, divided
1 1/2 cups 2-inch pieces asparagus
2 tablespoons crumbled goat cheese

1 Whisk together the eggs, egg whites, basil, salt, and pepper in a medium bowl. Set aside.

2 Heat a medium nonstick skillet over medium-high heat. Add 1 teaspoon of the oil and tilt the pan to coat. Add the asparagus and cook, stirring often, until crisp-tender, about 5 minutes. Spoon into a bowl and set aside.

3 Add the remaining 1 teaspoon oil to the skillet and tilt to coat the pan. Pour the egg mixture into

skillet. Reduce the heat to medium and cook, lifting the edge of the egg with a spatula to allow the uncooked portion to flow underneath until the bottom is set, about 2 minutes. Reduce heat to medium-low. Cover and cook until the top of the egg is set, about 2 minutes more.

4 Gently slide the cooked egg onto a large plate; spoon the cooked asparagus and the goat cheese down the center of the egg. Carefully fold two opposite sides of the egg over the asparagus mixture to cover. Cut the omelet in half and arrange each half on a plate. Serve immediately.

Each serving: 4 g carb, 178 cal, 12 g fat, 4 g sat fat, 217 mg chol, 2 g fib, 13 g pro, 234 mg sod • Carb Choices: 0; Exchanges: 1 medium-fat protein, 1 fat

Artichoke and Spinach Frittata QUICK

makes 4 servings

Frittatas are like pasta—you can add almost anything to them and they'll taste good. Plus, they are quick and easy to make. This recipe doesn't have any added salt because of the salty canned artichokes. Serve the frittata with toasted whole wheat English muffins.

4 large eggs
4 large egg whites
1/4 cup skim milk
1/8 teaspoon freshly ground pepper
2 teaspoons extra virgin olive oil
1 small onion, halved and thinly sliced
1 garlic clove, minced
2 cups chopped fresh spinach or baby spinach leaves
1 cup canned artichokes, drained, quartered, and blotted dry
2 tablespoons freshly grated Parmesan

1 Combine the eggs, egg whites, milk, and pepper in a medium bowl and whisk until smooth. Set aside.

2 Heat a medium ovenproof nonstick skillet over medium heat. Add the oil and tilt the pan to coat the bottom evenly. Add the onion and cook, stirring often, until softened, 5 minutes. Add the garlic and cook, stirring constantly, until fragrant, 30 seconds. Stir in the spinach and artichokes, and cook, stirring constantly, until the spinach is wilted and the liquid has evaporated, 3 minutes.

3 Preheat the broiler.

4 Pour the egg mixture evenly over the vegetables. Allow to cook 30 seconds, then use a spatula to move the edges of the egg toward the center, allowing the uncooked egg to seep to the bottom of the pan. Repeat until the bottom of the frittata is set, about 3 minutes. Place the skillet under the broiler and broil until the top is set, about 1 minute.

5 Sprinkle the frittata with the Parmesan, return to the broiler, and broil until the frittata is lightly browned and completely set, about 2 minutes. Cut into 4 wedges and serve at once.

Each serving: 7 g carb, 156 cal, 8 g fat, 2 g sat fat, 214 mg chol, 1 g fib, 13 g pro, 308 mg sod • Carb Choices: ½; Exchanges: 1 veg, 1 medium-fat protein, ½ fat

Asparagus and Mushroom Frittata QUICK

makes 4 servings

The classic combination of asparagus, mushrooms, and goat cheese makes this omelet special enough for guests for brunch or a light supper. If you have fresh dill or basil on hand, stir in a couple tablespoons along with the egg mixture.

4 large eggs
4 large egg whites
¼ cup skim milk
¼ teaspoon kosher salt
⅛ teaspoon freshly ground pepper
2 teaspoons extra virgin olive oil
1 small onion, halved and thinly sliced
1 cup 2-inch asparagus pieces
1 cup sliced white or cremini mushrooms
1 garlic clove, minced
¼ cup crumbled goat cheese

1 Combine the eggs, egg whites, milk, salt, and pepper in a medium bowl and whisk until smooth. Set aside.

2 Heat a medium ovenproof nonstick skillet over medium heat. Add the oil and tilt the pan to coat the bottom evenly. Add the onion, asparagus, and mushrooms and cook, stirring often, until the vegetables are tender, about 5 minutes. Add the garlic and cook, stirring constantly, until fragrant, 30 seconds.

3 Preheat the broiler.

4 Pour the egg mixture evenly over the vegetables. Allow to cook 30 seconds, then use a spatula to move the edges of the egg toward the center, allowing the uncooked egg to seep to the bottom of the pan. Repeat until the bottom of the frittata is set, about 3 minutes. Place the skillet under the broiler and broil until the top is set, about 1 minute.

5 Sprinkle the frittata with the goat cheese, return to the broiler, and broil until the frittata is lightly browned and completely set, about 2 minutes. Cut into 4 wedges and serve at once.

Each serving: 5 g carb, 153 cal, 10 g fat, 3 g sat fat, 217 mg chol, 1 g fib, 12 g pro, 240 mg sod • Carb Choices: 0; Exchanges: 1 veg, 1 medium-fat protein, 1 fat

Tomato-Basil Frittata QUICK

makes 4 servings

Keep this recipe in mind to make for brunch, lunch, or dinner when you think you've got nothing in the house to eat. You can substitute ½ teaspoon dried basil for the fresh and you can even use diced canned tomatoes if you drain them well first. Serve it with toasted slices of whole wheat baguette for a simple satisfying meal any time of day.

4 large eggs
4 large egg whites
¼ cup skim milk
¼ teaspoon kosher salt
⅛ teaspoon freshly ground pepper
2 plum tomatoes, chopped
2 tablespoons chopped fresh basil
2 teaspoons extra virgin olive oil
1 small onion, halved and thinly sliced
1 garlic clove, minced
¼ cup shredded part-skim mozzarella

1 Combine the eggs, egg whites, milk, salt, and pepper in a medium bowl and whisk until smooth. Stir in the tomatoes and basil. Set aside.

2 Heat a medium ovenproof nonstick skillet over medium heat. Add the oil and tilt the pan to coat the bottom evenly. Add the onion and cook, stirring often, until softened, about 5 minutes. Add the garlic and cook, stirring constantly, until fragrant, 30 seconds.

3 Preheat the broiler.

4 Pour the egg mixture evenly over the onion. Allow to cook 30 seconds, then use a spatula to move the edges of the egg toward the center, allowing the uncooked egg to seep to the bottom of the pan. Repeat until the bottom of the frittata is set, about 3 minutes. Place the skillet under the broiler and broil until the top is set, about 1 minute.

5 Sprinkle the frittata with the mozzarella, return to the broiler, and broil until the frittata is lightly browned and completely set, about 2 minutes. Cut into 4 wedges and serve at once.

Each serving: 5 g carb, 140 cal, 8 g fat, 2 g sat fat, 214 mg chol, 1 g fib, 12 g pro, 172 mg sod • Carb Choices: 0; Exchanges: 1 veg, 1 medium-fat protein, ½ fat

Migas QUICK

makes 4 servings

Migas in Tex-Mex cooking is scrambled eggs mixed with tortilla strips. They are usually prepared with fried corn tortillas, making them an addictively delicious—though unhealthy—breakfast. I've discovered that they're just as good made with baked tortillas. It takes extra time for baking, but you can prepare the jalapeño, cheese, and cilantro for the recipe while the tortillas bake. Try them with Fresh Tomato Salsa (page 41) or Tomatillo Salsa Verde (page 42).

2 (6-inch) corn tortillas, cut into thin strips
4 large eggs
4 large egg whites
2 tablespoons cold water
2 teaspoons canola oil
1 small onion, diced
1 jalapeño, seeded and minced
2 ounces finely shredded reduced-fat sharp Cheddar or Monterey Jack cheese (about ¼ cup)
4 tablespoons chopped fresh cilantro
½ cup salsa

1 Preheat the oven to 350°F. Place the tortilla strips on a medium baking sheet and bake, stirring once, until lightly toasted, 8 to 10 minutes. Set aside.

2 Combine the eggs, egg whites, and water in a medium bowl and whisk until smooth.

3 Heat a large nonstick skillet over medium-high heat. Add the oil and tilt the pan to coat the bottom evenly. Add the onion and jalapeño and cook, stirring often, until softened, 5 minutes.

4 Add the egg mixture to the onion mixture. Cook, stirring constantly, until soft-scrambled, about 3 minutes. Stir in the baked tortillas.

5 Spoon the migas onto 4 plates. Sprinkle each serving with 1 tablespoon of the Cheddar and 1 tablespoon of the cilantro. Accompany each serving with 2 tablespoons of the salsa.

Each serving: 10 g carb, 156 cal, 8 g fat, 2 g sat fat, 212 mg chol, 1 g fib, 11 g pro, 257 mg sod • Carb Choices: ½; Exchanges: ½ starch, 1 medium-fat protein, ½ fat

BACON MIGAS QUICK : Follow the Migas recipe, at left, but crumble 2 strips of center-cut crisp-cooked bacon and sprinkle evenly over the migas with the cheese in step 5.

Each serving: 10 g carb, 170 cal, 9 g fat, 2 g sat fat, 215 mg chol, 1 g fib, 12 g pro, 321 mg sod • Carb Choices: ½; Exchanges: ½ starch, 1 medium-fat protein, 1 fat

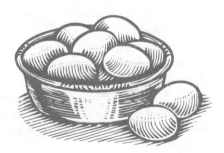

Egg and Avocado Soft Tacos QUICK | HIGH FIBER

makes 4 servings

Silky rich avocados get their creamy texture from a high content of monounsaturated fat, which is good for your heart. Canola and olive oils and nuts are other good sources of monounsaturated fat. Accompany the tacos with homemade salsa, such as Winter Tomato Salsa (page 41) or Tomato, Black Bean, and Corn Salsa (page 41), and serve them for a weekend family brunch.

4 large eggs
4 large egg whites
2 tablespoons 1% low-fat milk
2 teaspoons canola oil
¼ cup diced onion
¼ cup diced green bell pepper
1 jalapeño, seeded and minced
½ medium avocado, pitted, peeled, and diced
4 (6-inch) whole wheat flour tortillas, warmed
½ cup salsa

1 Combine the eggs, egg whites, and milk in a medium bowl and whisk until smooth. Set aside.

2 Heat a large nonstick skillet over medium-high heat. Add the oil and tilt the pan to coat the bottom evenly. Add the onion, bell pepper, and jalapeño and cook, stirring often, until softened, 5 minutes.

3 Add the egg mixture to the onion mixture. Cook, stirring constantly, until soft-scrambled, about 3 minutes. Stir in the avocado.

4 To assemble the tacos, spoon about ½ cup of the egg mixture down the center of each tortilla and top the egg mixture with 2 tablespoons of the salsa.

Each serving: 27 g carb, 245 cal, 12 g fat, 2 g sat fat, 212 mg chol, 4 g fib, 14 g pro, 427 mg sod • Carb Choices: 2; Exchanges: 2 starch, 1 medium-fat protein, 1 fat

Quiches, Breakfast Casseroles, and Other Egg Dishes

Asparagus Quiche with Couscous Crust

makes 8 servings

This light and delicate quiche is a delicious way to serve the first asparagus of spring. Serve it with fresh strawberries and pink grapefruit juice for a simple seasonal menu. This recipe uses couscous for the crust, which is a great technique to add flavor, fiber, and texture without adding a lot of carbohydrates.

2½ teaspoons extra virgin olive oil, divided
¾ cup low-sodium vegetable or chicken broth
½ cup whole wheat couscous
1 pound asparagus, tough ends removed, cut into 1-inch pieces
1 medium onion, chopped
2 garlic cloves, minced
¾ teaspoon kosher salt, divided
4 large eggs
4 large egg whites
½ cup 1% low-fat milk
2 ounces freshly grated Parmesan (about ½ cup)
⅛ teaspoon freshly ground pepper

1 Preheat the oven to 350°F. Brush a 10-inch ceramic quiche pan or a 10-inch glass or ceramic pie plate with ½ teaspoon of the oil.

2 Bring the broth to a boil in a small saucepan over high heat. Stir in the couscous, remove from the heat, cover, and let stand 5 minutes. Spoon the couscous into the prepared pan. Using a spatula, form a "crust" around the side and bottom of the pan. Set aside.

3 Meanwhile, heat a large nonstick skillet over medium heat. Add the remaining 2 teaspoons

oil and tilt the pan to coat. Add the asparagus, onion, garlic, and ½ teaspoon of the salt and cook, stirring often, until the asparagus is crisp-tender, 5 minutes. Spoon the vegetable mixture evenly into the prepared "crust."

4 Whisk together the eggs, egg whites, milk, Parmesan, remaining ¼ teaspoon salt, and the pepper in a medium bowl. Pour the egg mixture evenly over the vegetable mixture. Place the quiche pan on a large baking sheet. Bake until the edges are lightly browned and the center is set, 30 to 35 minutes. Let stand 5 minutes. Cut the quiche into wedges using a serrated knife.

Each serving: 10 g carb, 134 cal, 6 g fat, 2 g sat fat, 111 mg chol, 2 g fib, 10 g pro, 326 mg sod • Carb Choices: ½; Exchanges: ½ starch, ½ medium-fat protein, 1 fat

Spinach, Red Pepper, and Feta Quiche with Quinoa Crust

makes 8 servings

Colorful peppers and spinach make this quiche as vibrant as it is delicious. When you cook with quinoa, rinse it before cooking. It contains a harmless but bitter-tasting residue that naturally develops on the grain.

1⅓ cups low-sodium vegetable or chicken broth
⅔ cup quinoa, rinsed
2½ teaspoons extra virgin olive oil, divided
1 ounce freshly grated Parmesan (about ¼ cup)
1 medium onion, chopped
12 ounces fresh spinach, trimmed and chopped
¾ cup red Roasted Bell Peppers (page 21) or roasted red peppers from a jar, cut into short, thin strips
2 garlic cloves, minced
½ teaspoon kosher salt
4 large eggs
4 large egg whites
½ cup 1% low-fat milk
2 ounces finely crumbled feta cheese (about ½ cup)
⅛ teaspoon freshly ground pepper

1 Combine the broth and quinoa in a medium saucepan and bring to a boil over high heat. Reduce the heat to low, cover, and simmer until tender, about 20 minutes. Drain and transfer to a bowl and cool.

2 Preheat the oven to 375°F. Brush a 10-inch ceramic quiche pan or a 10-inch glass or ceramic pie plate with ½ teaspoon of the oil. Stir the Parmesan into the cooked quinoa. Spoon the quinoa mixture into the prepared pan. Using a spatula, form a "crust" around the side and bottom of the pan. Place the quiche pan on a baking sheet; bake 10 minutes. Maintain oven temperature.

3 Meanwhile, heat a large nonstick skillet over medium heat. Add the remaining 2 teaspoons of the oil and tilt the pan to coat. Add the onion and cook, stirring until softened, 5 minutes. Add the spinach, peppers, garlic, and salt and cook, stirring until the spinach is wilted, about 2 minutes. Spoon the vegetable mixture into the prepared "crust."

4 Whisk together the eggs, egg whites, milk, feta, and pepper in a medium bowl. Pour the egg mixture evenly over the vegetable mixture. Place the quiche pan on a baking sheet. Bake until the center is set, 30 to 35 minutes. Let stand 5 minutes. Cut into wedges using a serrated knife.

Each serving: 16 g carb, 174 cal, 8 g fat, 3 g sat fat, 116 mg chol, 2 g fib, 11 g pro, 367 mg sod • Carb Choices: 1; Exchanges: 1 starch, ½ medium-fat protein, 1 fat

Roasted Bell Peppers

To roast bell peppers, preheat the broiler and line a rimmed baking sheet with foil. Place the peppers in the pan. Broil, turning them occasionally, until the skins are blackened and blistered, 8 to 10 minutes. Place the peppers in a bowl, cover, and let stand until cool enough to handle. Discard the seeds and peel away the skins. The roasted peppers can be covered in an airtight container and refrigerated for up to a week.

Crustless Broccoli and Cheddar Quiche

makes 8 servings

If there are leftovers, you can enjoy this quiche cold or at room temperature for lunch the next day. When you bake it in a quiche pan, this quiche will rise above the sides of the pan as it bakes. It won't spill out of the pan, though, and as soon as it begins to cool, the quiche will deflate.

1½ teaspoons extra virgin olive oil, divided
1 small red onion, chopped
2 garlic cloves, minced
3 cups broccoli florets, cut into 1-inch pieces
4 large eggs
4 large egg whites
1 cup 1% low-fat milk
2 tablespoons unbleached all-purpose flour
½ teaspoon kosher salt
¼ teaspoon freshly ground pepper
4 ounces shredded reduced-fat extra-sharp
   Cheddar cheese (about 1 cup)

1 Preheat the oven to 350°F. Brush a 10-inch ceramic quiche pan or a 10-inch glass or ceramic pie plate with ½ teaspoon of the oil.

2 Heat a large skillet over medium-high heat. Add the remaining 1 teaspoon oil and tilt the pan to coat. Add the onion and cook, stirring often, until softened, 5 minutes. Add the garlic and cook, stirring constantly, until fragrant, 30 seconds.

3 Meanwhile, place the broccoli florets in a medium bowl. Cover with plastic wrap and microwave on high until crisp-tender, about 1 minute. Drain, cool slightly, and blot dry with paper towels.

4 Combine the eggs, egg whites, milk, flour, salt, and pepper in a large bowl and whisk until smooth. Add the broccoli, the onion mixture, and

continues on next page

the Cheddar and stir to combine. Pour into the prepared pan and arrange the broccoli evenly.

5 Place the quiche on a large baking sheet. Bake until the top is golden and the center is set, 40 to 45 minutes. Let stand 5 minutes. Cut the quiche into wedges using a serrated knife.

Each serving: 5 g carb, 124 cal, 6 g fat, 3 g sat fat, 102 mg chol, 0 g fib, 10 g pro, 238 mg sod • Carb Choices: 0; Exchanges: 1 veg, ½ medium-fat protein, ½ high-fat protein

Crustless Sausage and Mushroom Quiche

makes 8 servings

Hearty and filling, this is a quiche for big appetites. At breakfast or brunch, just add a fruit salad. It makes an easy and satisfying lunch or dinner when served with steamed broccoli or green beans and a tossed green salad.

1½ teaspoons extra virgin olive oil, divided
4 ounces turkey breakfast sausage
8 ounces white or cremini mushrooms, sliced
1 small onion, chopped
2 garlic cloves, minced
4 large eggs
4 large egg whites
1 cup 1% low-fat milk
2 tablespoons unbleached all-purpose flour
2 tablespoons minced fresh Italian parsley
½ teaspoon kosher salt
¼ teaspoon freshly ground pepper
 4 ounces shredded part-skim mozzarella (about 1 cup)

1 Preheat the oven to 350°F. Brush a 10-inch ceramic quiche pan or a 10-inch glass or ceramic pie plate with ½ teaspoon of the oil.

2 Heat a large nonstick skillet over medium-high heat. Add the remaining 1 teaspoon oil and tilt the pan to coat. Remove and discard the sausage casings, crumble the sausage, and add to the skillet. Add the mushrooms and onion and cook, stirring often, until the mushrooms are tender and

most of the liquid evaporates, 6 to 8 minutes. Add the garlic and cook, stirring constantly, until fragrant, 30 seconds. Transfer to a large plate to cool slightly.

3 Combine the eggs, egg whites, milk, flour, parsley, salt, and pepper in a large bowl and whisk until smooth. Add the sausage mixture and the mozzarella and stir to combine. Pour into the prepared pan.

4 Place the quiche on a large baking sheet. Bake until the top is golden and the center is set, 40 to 45 minutes. Let stand 5 minutes. Cut the quiche into wedges using a serrated knife.

Each serving: 8 g carb, 174 cal, 10 g fat, 4 g sat fat, 116 mg chol, 0 g fib, 14 g pro, 308 mg sod • Carb Choices: ½; Exchanges: 1 veg, ½ medium-fat protein, ½ high-fat protein

Spinach and Mushroom Breakfast Casserole

makes 8 servings

You can substitute a chopped red bell pepper for the mushrooms if you wish. Cook the bell pepper along with the onion and garlic. Chopped roasted red bell peppers also make a good switch from the mushrooms; add those when you add the cheese.

2½ teaspoons extra virgin olive oil, divided
1 medium onion, chopped
8 ounces cremini or white mushrooms, sliced
2 garlic cloves, minced
1 pound fresh spinach, trimmed and chopped
4 large eggs
4 large egg whites
½ teaspoon kosher salt
⅛ teaspoon freshly ground pepper
4 ounces shredded Gruyère or extra-sharp Cheddar cheese (about 1 cup)

1 Preheat the oven to 350°F. Brush a shallow 2-quart baking dish with ½ teaspoon of the oil.

2 Heat a large nonstick skillet over medium-high heat. Add the remaining 2 teaspoons oil and tilt

the pan to coat. Add the onion, mushrooms, and garlic, and cook, stirring often, until the vegetables are softened, about 5 minutes. Add the spinach in batches and cook, stirring constantly, until the spinach is wilted and most of the liquid has evaporated, 2 minutes. Spoon the vegetable mixture into a large bowl and let cool slightly.

3 Combine the eggs, egg whites, salt, and pepper in a medium bowl and whisk until smooth. Stir in the Gruyère. Add the egg mixture to the vegetable mixture and stir to mix well. Spoon into the prepared baking dish. Bake until the center is set, 25 to 30 minutes. Let stand 5 minutes before slicing.

Each serving: 4 g carb, 140 cal, 9 g fat, 4 g sat fat, 121 mg chol, 1 g fib, 11 g pro, 215 mg sod • Carb Choices: 0; Exchanges: 1 veg, ½ medium-fat protein, ½ high-fat protein

SPINACH, MUSHROOM, AND BACON BREAKFAST CASSEROLE: Follow the Spinach and Mushroom Breakfast Casserole recipe, at left, but stir in 4 strips of center-cut crisp-cooked bacon with the cheese in step 3.

Each serving: 4 g carb, 153 cal, 10 g fat, 4 g sat fat, 124 mg chol, 1 g fib, 12 g pro, 279 mg sod • Carb Choices: 0; Exchanges: 1 veg, ½ medium-fat protein, ½ high-fat protein

Italian Vegetable Strata with Provolone

makes 12 servings

You can assemble this casserole a day ahead. Cover it and refrigerate overnight, leaving off the ½ cup of cheese on the top until just before baking. If you do make it ahead of time, let the casserole stand at room temperature 15 minutes before baking and add 5 minutes to the baking time. Serve this with a fresh fruit salad and you've got a delicious and easy brunch menu.

3 teaspoons extra virgin olive oil, divided

2 medium leeks, halved lengthwise, and thinly sliced

2 cups 1% low-fat milk

4 large eggs

4 large egg whites

1 teaspoon kosher salt, divided

¼ teaspoon freshly ground pepper

10 slices day-old 100% whole wheat bread, cut into ½-inch cubes (about 8 cups)

2 medium zucchini, halved lengthwise and thinly sliced

1 red bell pepper, cut into short, thin strips

2 garlic cloves, minced

1 teaspoon dried oregano

½ teaspoon dried basil

6 ounces shredded sharp provolone (about 1½ cups), divided

1 Preheat the oven to 350°F. Brush a shallow 3-quart baking dish with 1 teaspoon of the oil.

2 Submerge the sliced leeks in a large bowl of water, lift them out, and drain in a colander. Repeat, using fresh water, until no grit remains in the bottom of the bowl. Drain the leeks well.

3 Whisk together the milk, eggs, egg whites, ½ teaspoon of the salt, and the ground pepper in a large bowl. Add the bread cubes and toss to combine. Let stand while you prepare the vegetables, stirring occasionally.

4 Heat a large nonstick skillet over medium heat. Add the remaining 2 teaspoons oil and tilt the pan to coat. Add the leeks and cook, stirring often, until softened, about 5 minutes. Add the zucchini, bell pepper, garlic, oregano, basil, and the remaining ½ teaspoon salt and cook, stirring often, until the vegetables are crisp-tender, 6 to 8 minutes. Spoon the vegetable mixture into a bowl and let cool slightly.

5 Stir the vegetable mixture and 1 cup of the provolone into the bread mixture. Spoon into the prepared baking dish. Sprinkle the top of the strata with the remaining ½ cup of provolone. Bake, uncovered, until the strata is bubbly and the top is lightly browned, 30 to 35 minutes. Let stand 5 minutes before serving.

Each serving: 17 g carb, 192 cal, 8 g fat, 3 g sat fat, 88 mg chol, 2 g fib, 12 g pro, 417 mg sod • Carb Choices: 1; Exchanges: 1 starch, 1 veg, ½ high-fat protein

Sausage and Spinach Strata

makes 12 servings

Hearty sausage and healthful spinach make this a satisfying casserole for chilly fall and winter mornings when appetites are heartier. Have it for breakfast or a late-morning brunch with a bowl of orange and pink grapefruit segments served alongside.

3 teaspoons extra virgin olive oil, divided

2 cups 1% low-fat milk

4 large eggs

4 large egg whites

¼ teaspoon freshly ground pepper

10 slices day-old 100% whole wheat bread, cut into ½-inch cubes (about 8 cups)

6 ounces turkey breakfast sausage

1 medium onion, diced

1 red bell pepper, diced

2 cloves garlic, minced

1 (10-ounce) package frozen chopped spinach, thawed and squeezed dry

4 ounces shredded part-skim mozzarella (about 1 cup)

2 tablespoons freshly grated Parmesan

1 Preheat the oven to 350°F. Brush a shallow 3-quart baking dish with 1 teaspoon of the oil.

2 Whisk together the milk, eggs, egg whites, and ground pepper in a large bowl. Add the bread cubes and toss to combine. Let stand while you prepare the sausage and vegetables, stirring occasionally.

3 Heat a large nonstick skillet over medium heat. Add the remaining 2 teaspoons oil and tilt the pan to coat the bottom evenly. Remove and discard the sausage casings, crumble the sausage, and add to the skillet. Add the onion and bell pepper and cook, stirring often, until the sausage is browned and the vegetables are softened, 5 minutes. Add the garlic and cook, stirring constantly, until fragrant, 30 seconds. Spoon the sausage mixture into a bowl and let cool slightly.

4 Stir the sausage mixture, the spinach, and the mozzarella into the bread mixture. Spoon into the prepared baking dish. Sprinkle the top of the strata with the Parmesan. Bake, uncovered, until the strata is bubbly and the top is lightly browned, 30 to 35 minutes. Let stand 5 minutes before serving.

Each serving: 19 g carb, 189 cal, 7 g fat, 3 g sat fat, 86 mg chol, 3 g fib, 14 g pro, 408 mg sod • Carb Choices: 1; Exchanges: 1 starch, 2 medium-fat protein, ½ fat

Blueberry-Apricot Breakfast Casserole

makes 6 servings

Similar to bread pudding, this lightly sweetened custardy casserole makes a great weekend breakfast treat. Serve it in shallow bowls and sprinkle a handful of additional berries on top of each serving. Try sliced strawberries, fresh raspberries, or even more blueberries. One word of caution: Make this only with fresh blueberries; the frozen ones are too soft to use here.

1 teaspoon canola oil

2 large eggs

4 large egg whites

½ cup 1% low-fat milk

⅓ cup apricot preserves

½ teaspoon vanilla extract

6 slices day-old 100% whole wheat bread, cut into ½-inch cubes (about 5 cups)

1 cup fresh blueberries

1 Preheat the oven to 350°F. Preheat the oven to 350°F. Brush an 8-inch square baking pan with the oil.

2 Whisk together the eggs, egg whites, milk, preserves, and vanilla in a large bowl. Add the bread cubes and toss to combine. Let stand 5 minutes, tossing occasionally. Add the blueberries and toss to combine.

3 Spoon into the prepared baking dish. Bake, uncovered, until the top is lightly browned and the center is almost set, 30 to 35 minutes. Let stand 5 minutes before serving.

Each serving: 32 g carb, 190 cal, 4 g fat, 1 g sat fat, 73 mg chol, 3 g fib, 9 g pro, 227 mg sod • Carb Choices: 2; Exchanges: 1 starch, 1 carb, 1 lean protein

Garden Vegetable Brunch Bundt "Cake"

makes 12 servings

I got the idea of baking a quiche filling in a Bundt cake pan from *Food to Live By—The Earthbound Farm Organic Cookbook* by Myra Goodman. I've used low-carb vegetables (the original recipe had potatoes) and used a judicious amount of eggs in this version. The result is healthy and delicious.

3 teaspoons extra virgin olive oil, divided
Unbleached all-purpose flour for dusting the pan
1 large red bell pepper, chopped
1 medium red onion, chopped
2 garlic cloves, minced
½ teaspoon kosher salt, divided

1 pound fresh spinach, trimmed and chopped
8 large eggs
8 large egg whites
⅛ teaspoon freshly ground pepper
8 ounces shredded Gruyère or extra-sharp Cheddar cheese (about 2 cups)
1 (14-ounce) can artichoke hearts, well drained and coarsely chopped

1 Preheat the oven to 350°F. Brush a 10- or 12-cup Bundt pan with 1 teaspoon of the oil. Dust the pan lightly with flour, shaking the pan to remove the excess.

2 Heat a large nonstick skillet over medium-high heat. Add the remaining 2 teaspoons oil and tilt the pan to coat. Add the bell pepper, onion, garlic, and ¼ teaspoon of the salt and cook, stirring often, until the vegetables are softened, about 5 minutes. Add the spinach in batches and cook, stirring constantly, until the spinach is wilted and most of the liquid has evaporated, 2 minutes. Spoon the vegetable mixture into a large bowl and let cool slightly.

3 Combine the eggs, egg whites, remaining ¼ teaspoon salt, and the ground pepper in a medium bowl and whisk until smooth. Stir in the Gruyère and artichokes. Add the egg mixture to the vegetable mixture and stir to mix well. Pour into the prepared pan. Bake until the "cake" is set, 35 to 40 minutes. Let stand 5 minutes. Cut the "cake" into slices using a serrated knife.

Each serving: 5 g carb, 173 cal, 11 g fat, 5 g sat fat, 162 mg chol, 1 g fib, 14 g pro, 279 mg sod • Carb Choices: 0; Exchanges: 1 veg, 1 medium-fat protein, 1 high-fat protein

Soufflé Roll with Asparagus, Mushrooms, and Mozzarella

makes 12 servings

This recipe is not difficult, but it is time consuming. It's worth the work for the stunning presentation and wonderful flavor. For a buffet, cut the roll into slices and arrange on a platter garnished with fresh herbs.

8 large eggs
4 large egg whites
1 tablespoon unsalted butter
2 tablespoons unbleached all-purpose flour
1 cup 1% low-fat milk
¾ teaspoon kosher salt, divided
⅛ teaspoon freshly ground pepper
2½ teaspoons extra virgin olive oil, divided
1 pound asparagus, tough ends removed and spears cut into ¾-inch pieces
8 ounces cremini or white mushrooms, sliced
1 small onion, chopped
6 ounces shredded part-skim mozzarella (about 1½ cups)

1 Separate the eggs, placing the egg yolks in a medium bowl and the egg whites, including the 4 additional egg whites for a total of 12, in a large bowl. Set aside.

2 Melt the butter in a large saucepan over medium heat. Add the flour and whisk until smooth. Gradually whisk in the milk. Cook, whisking constantly, until the mixture comes to a boil and thickens, about 3 minutes. Whisk in ¼ teaspoon of the salt and the pepper. Remove from the heat.

3 Whisk the egg yolks until smooth. Slowly whisk about ¼ cup of the milk mixture into the egg yolks. Slowly whisk the egg yolk mixture into the milk mixture remaining in the saucepan. Return the mixture to medium heat and cook, whisking constantly until the mixture thickens and coats the back of a spoon. Strain through a fine wire mesh strainer into a clean bowl. Place a sheet of plastic wrap on the surface to prevent a skin from forming. Let stand to cool to room temperature.

4 Meanwhile, heat a large nonstick skillet over medium heat. Add 2 teaspoons of the oil and tilt the pan to coat the bottom evenly. Add the asparagus, mushrooms, onion, and the remaining ½ teaspoon salt. Cook, stirring often, until the asparagus is crisp-tender, about 6 minutes. Transfer to a bowl and set aside.

5 Preheat the oven to 400°F. Line a 15 x 10-inch jellyroll pan or large rimmed baking sheet with parchment paper and brush the paper with the remaining ½ teaspoon oil.

6 Beat the egg whites at high speed with an electric mixer until stiff peaks form. Fold the egg whites into the cooled milk mixture in 3 additions, stirring until no white streaks remain. Spread the batter evenly into the prepared pan. Bake until the top is lightly browned and the center is set, 12 to 15 minutes. Reduce the oven temperature to 350°F. Cool the soufflé in the pan on a wire rack for 5 minutes.

7 Turn the soufflé upside down onto a clean sheet of parchment paper. Peel off the top layer of parchment and return the parchment to the pan. Spoon the asparagus mixture evenly over the soufflé and sprinkle evenly with the mozzarella. Starting with the long end, roll the soufflé up jellyroll-style. Place the roll seam side down on the parchment paper in the baking pan. Bake until heated through, 10 to 15 minutes. Cut the roll into slices using a serrated knife. Serve hot or warm.

Each serving: 5 g carb, 136 cal, 8 g fat, 4 g sat fat, 152 mg chol, 1 g fib, 10 g pro, 251 mg sod • Carb Choices: 0; Exchanges: 1 medium-fat protein, ½ fat

Sausage and Cheddar Soufflé Roll

makes 12 servings

Filled with flavorful breakfast sausage and sharp Cheddar cheese, this soufflé roll is a delicious contrast of light textured egg stuffed with hearty ingredients. Serve it in the fall or winter with Orchard Fruit Salad (page 30) and assemble friends and family for a special brunch.

8 large eggs
4 large egg whites
1 tablespoon unsalted butter
2 tablespoons unbleached all-purpose flour
1 cup 1% low-fat milk
¼ teaspoon kosher salt
⅛ teaspoon freshly ground pepper
2½ teaspoons extra virgin olive oil, divided
4 ounces turkey breakfast sausage
8 ounces cremini or white mushrooms, sliced
1 small onion, chopped
2 teaspoons minced fresh rosemary or ½ teaspoon crumbled dried rosemary
6 ounces shredded reduced-fat extra-sharp Cheddar cheese (about 1½ cups)

1 Separate the eggs, placing the egg yolks in a medium bowl and the egg whites, including the 4 additonal egg whites for a total of 12, in a large bowl. Set aside.

2 Melt the butter in a large saucepan over medium heat. Add the flour and whisk until smooth. Gradually whisk in the milk. Cook, whisking constantly, until the mixture comes to a boil and thickens, about 3 minutes. Whisk in the salt and pepper. Remove from the heat.

3 Whisk the egg yolks until smooth. Slowly whisk about ¼ cup of the milk mixture into the egg yolks. Slowly whisk the egg yolk mixture into the milk mixture remaining in the saucepan. Return the mixture to medium heat and cook, whisking constantly until the mixture thickens and coats the back of a spoon. Strain through a fine wire mesh strainer into a clean bowl. Place a sheet of plastic wrap on the surface to prevent a skin from forming. Let stand to cool to room temperature.

4 Meanwhile, heat a large nonstick skillet over medium heat. Add 2 teaspoons of the oil and tilt the pan to coat the bottom evenly. Remove and discard the sausage casings, crumble the sausage, and add to the skillet. Add the mushrooms and onion and cook, stirring often, until the mushrooms are tender and most of the liquid evaporates, 6 to 8 minutes. Transfer to a bowl and set aside.

5 Preheat the oven to 400°F. Line a 15 x 10-inch jellyroll pan or large rimmed baking sheet with parchment paper and brush the paper with the remaining ½ teaspoon oil.

6 Beat the egg whites at high speed with an electric mixer until stiff peaks form. Fold the egg whites into the cooled milk mixture in three additions, stirring until no white streaks remain. Stir in the rosemary. Spread the batter evenly into the prepared pan. Bake until the top is lightly browned and the center is set, 12 to 15 minutes. Reduce the oven temperature to 350°F. Cool the soufflé in the pan on a wire rack for 5 minutes.

7 Turn the soufflé upside down onto a clean sheet of parchment paper. Peel off the top layer of parchment and return the parchment to the pan. Spoon the sausage mixture evenly over the soufflé and sprinkle evenly with the Cheddar. Starting with the long end, roll the soufflé up jellyroll-style. Place the roll seam side down on the parchment paper in the pan. Bake until heated through, 10 to 15 minutes. Cut the roll into slices using a serrated knife. Serve hot or warm.

Each serving: 4 g carb, 179 cal, 12 g fat, 5 g sat fat, 170 mg chol, 0 g fib, 14 g pro, 346 mg sod • Carb Choices: 0; Exchanges: 1 high-fat protein, 1 medium-fat protein, ½ fat

Ham and Egg Breakfast Cups QUICK

makes 4 servings

Roasted red peppers and prosciutto turn ordinary eggs into an extravagant breakfast. Serve these with thin slices of rustic multigrain toast. To make this dish kid-friendly, substitute thin slices of deli ham for the prosciutto.

1 teaspoon extra virgin olive oil
1 cup red Roasted Bell Peppers (page 21) or roasted red peppers from a jar, finely chopped
2 ounces prosciutto, trimmed and finely chopped
4 large eggs
2 tablespoons freshly grated Parmesan
⅛ teaspoon freshly ground pepper

1 Preheat the oven to 325°F. Brush 4 (6-ounce) baking dishes with the oil.

2 Divide the roasted peppers and prosciutto evenly among the baking dishes. Carefully break 1 egg into each dish.

3 Place the dishes on a small rimmed baking sheet and bake just until the eggs begin to set, about 15 minutes. Sprinkle each egg evenly with the Parmesan and the ground pepper. Bake until the egg whites are opaque and the yolks are set, about 4 minutes longer. Serve at once.

Each serving: 4 g carb, 138 cal, 9 g fat, 3 g sat fat, 226 mg chol, 1 g fib, 12 g pro, 382 mg sod • Carb Choices: 0; Exchanges: 1½ medium-fat protein

Huevos Rancheros

QUICK | HIGH FIBER

makes 4 servings

This flavorful Mexican egg dish is a special treat for weekend entertaining or a special family meal. To save time, you can make the sauce up to two days ahead and reheat it just before serving. When you make it ahead, leave out the cilantro and stir it in just before serving the dish. Sliced mangoes tossed with grated lime zest are a colorful accompaniment.

2 teaspoons canola oil
1 poblano chile, seeded and chopped
1 small onion, chopped
2 garlic cloves, minced
½ teaspoon ground cumin
1 (14-ounce) can no-salt-added whole tomatoes, undrained and chopped
¼ teaspoon kosher salt
⅛ teaspoon freshly ground pepper
2 tablespoons chopped fresh cilantro
4 large eggs
1 tablespoon white vinegar
4 (6-inch) whole wheat flour tortillas, warmed
1 ounce shredded reduced-fat sharp Cheddar cheese (about ¼ cup)

1 Heat a large nonstick skillet over medium heat. Add the oil and tilt the pan to coat the bottom evenly. Add the chile and onion, and cook, stirring often, until softened, 5 minutes. Add the garlic and cumin and cook, stirring constantly, until fragrant, 30 seconds.

2 Stir in the tomatoes and their juices, the salt, and pepper and bring to a boil over high heat. Reduce the heat to low, cover, and simmer 10 minutes. Uncover and simmer until the sauce is slightly thickened, 5 minutes longer. Stir in the cilantro.

3 When the sauce is almost done, prepare the eggs. Fill a large deep skillet or broad saucepan with 3 inches of water. Add the vinegar and bring to a boil. Reduce the heat until the water is just at a simmer and break the eggs into the water. Turn off the heat, cover, and let stand 2 to 3 minutes.

4 Place 1 tortilla on each plate. Using a slotted spoon, top each tortilla with a poached egg. Spoon the sauce evenly over the eggs and sprinkle evenly with the Cheddar. Serve at once.

Each serving: 20 g carb, 225 cal, 11 g fat, 3 g sat fat, 217 mg chol, 10 g fib, 12 g pro, 395 mg sod • Carb Choices: 1; Exchanges: ½ starch, 1 veg, 1 medium-fat protein, ½ fat

Compotes and Other Morning Fruits

Cranberry-Basted Baked Apples

makes 4 servings

Baked apples are a comforting addition to a cold weather breakfast. Serve them with a quiche or a strata for a filling meal. Watch the apples carefully during the last 10 minutes of baking so they don't overcook and burst.

½ teaspoon canola oil
4 medium Granny Smith or Rome apples
1 cup cranberry juice
2 tablespoons sugar
2 teaspoons unbleached all-purpose flour
2 teaspoons grated orange zest

1 Preheat the oven to 350° F. Brush an 8-inch square glass baking dish with the oil.

2 Core the apples, cutting to, but not through, the bottoms. Cut away 1 inch of the peel from the tops of the apples and arrange them upright in the prepared baking dish.

3 Combine the cranberry juice, sugar, flour, and orange zest in a medium bowl and whisk until smooth. Pour over the apples, filling the cavities.

4 Bake, uncovered, 40 to 45 minutes or until the apples are tender, basting twice with the sauce.

5 To serve, place the apples in shallow bowls and drizzle evenly with the sauce. Serve hot, warm, or at room temperature. Cover and refrigerate leftover apples and bring to room temperature before serving.

Each serving: 33 g carb, 129 cal, 1 g fat, 0 g sat fat, 0 mg chol, 3 g fib, 1 g pro, 10 mg sod • Carb Choices: 2; Exchanges: 1 carb, 1 fruit

Autumn Pear, Cranberry, and Pomegranate Compote [HIGH FIBER]

makes 6 servings

Serve this compote on its own or pair it with waffles, pancakes, or oatmeal for breakfast or brunch. It's also a delicious dessert served with biscotti alongside.

2 cups pomegranate juice
2 tablespoons sugar
3 barely ripe Bartlett or Anjou pears, peeled, cored, and cut into 8 wedges
6 dried apricots
½ cup fresh cranberries
2 teaspoons grated orange zest

1 Combine the pomegranate juice and sugar in a medium saucepan. Bring to a boil over medium heat.

2 Add the pears and apricots and return to a boil. Reduce the heat to low and simmer, uncovered, until the pears are barely tender, about 5 minutes. Stir in the cranberries and simmer just until the cranberries begin to pop, 3 to 4 minutes.

3 Remove from the heat and stir in the orange zest. Cool to room temperature. Serve at once or cover and refrigerate up to 2 days. Bring to room temperature before serving.

Each serving: 34 g carb, 135 cal, 0 g fat, 0 g sat fat, 0 mg chol, 4 g fib, 1 g pro, 11 mg sod • Carb Choices: 2; Exchanges: 2 fruit

Orchard Fruit Salad QUICK

makes 6 servings

Tangy yogurt and a combination of sweet fruits make a refreshing version of the old-fashioned Waldorf salad. It's a great partner to a quiche or a breakfast casserole, but it's also a good dish to take to a potluck or a fall picnic.

2 barely ripe Bartlett pears, halved, cored, and cut into ¾-inch pieces

2 Granny Smith apples, halved, cored, and cut into ¾-inch pieces

1 stalk celery, thinly sliced

½ cup red seedless grapes, halved

2 tablespoons dried currants

½ cup plain low-fat Greek or regular plain low-fat yogurt

¼ cup walnuts, toasted and chopped (page 4)

Combine the pears, apples, celery, grapes, and currants in a large bowl. Add the yogurt and toss to coat. Serve at once or cover and refrigerate up to 6 hours. Sprinkle with the walnuts just before serving.

Each serving: 22 g carb, 115 cal, 3 g fat, 1 g sat fat, 1 mg chol, 3 g fib, 3 g pro, 13 mg sod • Carb Choices: 1½; Exchanges: 1½ fruit, ½ fat

Orange and Pink Grapefruit Salad with Honey-Rosemary Syrup

makes 4 servings

This salad makes a gorgeous addition to any winter brunch menu. To make it even more festive, sprinkle the citrus slices with fresh pomegranate seeds and garnish with rosemary sprigs.

2 tablespoons honey

2 tablespoons orange juice

2 teaspoons fresh rosemary leaves

2 large navel oranges

1 large pink grapefruit

1 Combine the honey, orange juice, and rosemary in a small saucepan. Bring to a boil over medium heat. Let stand 30 minutes to cool. Pour through a fine wire mesh strainer into a small bowl. Discard the rosemary.

2 Meanwhile, cut a thin slice from the top and bottom of the oranges and the grapefruit, exposing the flesh. Stand each fruit upright, and using a sharp knife, thickly cut off the peel, following the contour of the fruit and removing all the white pith and membrane. Thinly slice the fruit into rounds.

3 To serve, layer the grapefruit and orange slices alternately on a serving platter and drizzle with the syrup.

Each serving: 25 g carb, 96 cal, 0 g fat, 0 g sat fat, 0 mg chol, 2 g fib, 1 g pro, 1 mg sod • Carb Choices: 1½; Exchanges: ½ carb, 1 fruit

Chamomile-Ginger Summer Fruit Salad

makes 6 servings

This salad makes a beautiful display for a brunch buffet, but when summer fruit is at its peak, it's delicious with any meal. Chamomile tea bags are a convenient way to add heady floral flavor to a fresh fruit salad. Use the chamomile-infused syrup on any fresh summer fruits or berries.

¼ cup sugar

¼ cup water

4 chamomile tea bags

1 cup 1-inch cantaloupe or honeydew melon balls

1 cup 1-inch watermelon balls

1 medium peach, peeled, pitted, and sliced

½ cup fresh blueberries

2 tablespoons chopped crystallized ginger

1 Combine the sugar and water in a small saucepan and bring to a boil over medium heat, stirring until the sugar dissolves. Remove from the heat, add the tea bags, and let stand 30 minutes to cool. Remove and discard the tea bags, squeezing out the liquid.

2 Combine the melon balls, peach slices, and blueberries in a large glass serving bowl. Drizzle with the syrup and toss gently to coat. Sprinkle with the ginger and serve.

Each serving: 16 g carb, 64 cal, 0 g fat, 0 g sat fat, 0 mg chol, 1 g fib, 1 g pro, 5 mg sod • Carb Choices: 1; Exchanges: ½ carb, ½ fruit

Basil-Lime Melon Compote

makes 6 servings

On a hot summer day, melon, basil, and lime make the perfect cooling salad. This chilly combination is as delicious for brunch as it is for dinner. You can substitute mint for the basil, if you wish.

¼ cup water
¼ cup sugar
6 whole basil leaves
2 teaspoons grated lime zest
1 cup cubed seedless watermelon
1 cup cubed honeydew melon
1 cup cubed cantaloupe
1 tablespoon lime juice
1 tablespoon thinly sliced basil leaves

1 Combine the water and sugar in a medium saucepan. Bring to a boil over medium heat, stirring until the sugar dissolves. Remove from the heat and stir in the whole basil leaves and the lime zest. Let stand 30 minutes to cool. Pour the mixture through a fine wire mesh strainer and discard the basil and lime zest.

2 Combine the watermelon, honeydew, and cantaloupe in a large glass serving bowl. Drizzle with the syrup and the lime juice and toss gently to coat. Serve at once or cover and refrigerate up to 6 hours. Sprinkle with the sliced basil leaves just before serving.

Each serving: 16 g carb, 61 cal, 0 g fat, 0 g sat fat, 0 mg chol, 1 g fib, 1 g pro, 10 mg sod • Carb Choices: 1; Exchanges: ½ carb, ½ fruit

Yogurt-Berry Parfaits

QUICK | HIGH FIBER

makes 4 servings

Making your own fruit-flavored yogurt is as simple as stirring mashed or finely chopped fruit into plain yogurt. It tastes better than the purchased variety and there's no added sugar. This recipe uses raspberries, but try it with strawberries, mangoes, peaches, or bananas.

1 cup fresh raspberries
1 cup plain fat-free yogurt
2 cups fresh strawberries, halved if large
1 cup fresh blueberries

1 Place the raspberries in a medium bowl and mash with a fork or a potato masher until lightly crushed. Add the yogurt and stir until blended.

2 To make the parfaits, layer ½ cup of the yogurt mixture, ½ cup of the strawberries, and ¼ cup of the blueberries into each of four parfait glasses or glass bowls. Serve at once.

Each serving: 19 g carb, 94 cal, 1 g fat, 1 g sat fat, 1 mg chol, 4 g fib, 5 g pro, 49 mg sod • Carb Choices: 1; Exchanges: 1 fruit

Fresh Fruits with Yogurt-Maple Dip QUICK

makes 8 servings

Assemble seasonal fruits on a tray with the dip for an attractive, healthy, crowd-pleasing dessert for any breakfast or brunch get together.

½ cup plain fat-free Greek yogurt or strained
    yogurt (page 11)
1 tablespoon real maple syrup
½ teaspoon grated fresh ginger
4 cups any variety fresh fruits, cut into bite-size
    pieces

Stir together the yogurt, maple syrup, and ginger in a small bowl. Serve alongside the fruits for dipping.

Each serving: 11 g carb, 45 cal, 0 g fat, 0 g sat fat, 0 mg chol, 2 g fib, 1 g pro, 4 mg sod • Carb Choices: 1; Exchanges: 1 fruit

Starters and Snacks

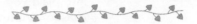

Dips and Spreads

Creamy Onion Dip

Hot Spinach Dip

Hot Black Bean Dip

Hummus

Lemon-Herb White Bean Dip

Rosemary White Bean Dip with Artichokes

Herbed Edamame Dip

Edamame Guacamole

Roasted Garlic Eggplant Dip

Avocado Dip

Guacamole

Lemony Lima Bean Spread

Cranberry-Olive Tapenade

Eggplant Caponata

Feta Cheese Spread

Broccoli Pesto

Tzatziki

Salsas

Fresh Tomato Salsa

Winter Tomato Salsa

Tomato, Black Bean, and Corn Salsa

Avocado-Cucumber Salsa

Mango-Jicama Salsa

Melon Salsa

Tomatillo Salsa Verde

Small Bites

Stuffed Eggs with Horseradish

Curried Stuffed Eggs

Smoky Spiced Stuffed Eggs

Buffalo Chicken Skewers

Beef Saté with Peanut Sauce

Baked Egg Rolls

Shrimp Pot Stickers with Sweet Soy Dipping Sauce

Cured Salmon (Gravlax)

Creamy Smoked Salmon–Dill Spread

Shrimp Summer Rolls

Spanakopita

Goat Cheese and Marinated Red Pepper Bruschetta

Shrimp Bruschetta

Crunchy Nibbles

Lemon-Garlic Pita Chips

Sugar-and-Spice Pita Chips

Baked Wonton Chips

Crispy Baked Root Vegetable Chips

Crispy Baked Garbanzos

Parmesan Popcorn

Romano–Black Pepper Biscotti

Portable Fruit and Nut Snack Mix

Serving bite size starters before a meal is probably not something you've thought about doing for your family on a weeknight. But maybe it's not a bad idea. If you and your family are more likely to eat vegetables when they are raw—and especially when dunked into a flavorful dip—then try serving one of the dishes from the Dips and Spreads section of this chapter before dinner starts.

A lot of these recipes are make-ahead and will keep for several days in the refrigerator, so all you have to do to serve them is uncover the plastic container. Rather than serving high-carb crackers and chips alongside, serve fresh vegetables instead. Take a look at Better Than Sliced Bread (at right) for inspiration. It's an easy and delicious way for you to encourage everyone in the family to eat their vegetables.

When you do entertain or want to serve something out of the ordinary, you'll find options here for plain and fancy versions of stuffed eggs and a quick Spanakopita recipe (page 49) that looks like it took hours to make. If you want something more exotic, serve a platter of Beef Saté with Peanut Sauce (page 45) or Shrimp Pot Stickers with Sweet Soy Dipping Sauce (page 46). There's even a healthy version of chicken wings to serve while watching the game. Buffalo Chicken Skewers (page 45) are made with boneless skinless chicken breast, but they're seasoned with a fiery yogurt marinade, so they're moist and flavorful.

All the salsas in this chapter can be served as a starter or a snack with tortilla chips, but they can do double duty as accompaniments to simply prepared chicken breasts, fish, or shrimp.

You'll find recipes here for making your own pita chips, wonton chips, and root vegetable chips, so you can easily create your favorite snacks with less fat and less sodium than commercial brands. With these recipes, snacking is good for you.

Better Than Sliced Bread

Instead of serving hors d'oeuvres and dips on crackers, chips, sliced baguettes, or other high-carbohydrate options, try these low-carb choices.

Celery sticks

Baby carrots

Large carrots, thinly sliced on the diagonal

Bell pepper spears

Thin slices of large radishes

Thin slices of cucumber

Thin slices of turnip or rutabaga

Broccoli or cauliflower florets

Cherry tomatoes

Trimmed snow peas

Fresh fennel spears

Belgian endive leaves

Jicama spears

Small mushroom caps

Baby zucchini or summer squash

Cooked and chilled asparagus or green beans

Cooked and chilled artichoke leaves

Dips and Spreads

Creamy Onion Dip

makes 1 cup

Classic onion dip is great with anything from carrots to crackers. Try it with Crispy Baked Root Vegetable Chips (page 52) or Lemon-Garlic Pita Chips (page 51). This is a chunky dip, but if you prefer it smooth, put the dip in a food processor and pulse it a few times before chilling.

2 teaspoons extra virgin olive oil
1 medium sweet onion, chopped
¼ teaspoon kosher salt
¼ cup mayonnaise
¼ cup plain low-fat yogurt
1 teaspoon lemon juice
¼ teaspoon Worcestershire sauce
Pinch of ground cayenne

1 Heat a medium nonstick skillet over medium heat. Add the oil and tilt the pan to coat the bottom evenly. Add the onion and salt and cook, covered, stirring occasionally, until the onion is very tender, about 30 minutes. Increase the heat to medium-high, uncover, and cook, stirring often, until the onion is golden brown and most of the liquid has evaporated, 8 to 10 minutes longer. Transfer the onion to a medium bowl to cool.

2 Add the mayonnaise, yogurt, lemon juice, Worcestershire sauce, and cayenne to the onions and stir to mix well. Cover and refrigerate until chilled, at least 2 hours and up to 2 days.

Each serving (2 tablespoons): 4 g carb, 84 cal, 7 g fat, 1 g sat fat, 3 mg chol, 0 g fib, 1 g pro, 88 mg sod • Carb Choices: 0; Exchanges: 1 fat

Hot Spinach Dip

makes 3¾ cups

A perennial favorite, this lightened up spinach dip uses reduced-fat cream cheese and low-fat yogurt to give it creamy texture without all the calories of the traditional version. It's pretty and perfect to serve with a tray of colorful raw vegetables.

3 teaspoons extra virgin olive oil, divided
1 medium onion, chopped
1 garlic clove, minced
3 ounces reduced-fat cream cheese, at room temperature
¼ cup plain low-fat yogurt
¼ teaspoon freshly ground pepper
2 (10-ounce) packages frozen chopped spinach, thawed and squeezed dry
1 (14-ounce) can artichoke hearts, well drained and coarsely chopped
4 ounces freshly grated Parmesan (about 1 cup)
3 ounces shredded part-skim mozzarella (about ¾ cup)
½ teaspoon hot sauce

1 Preheat the oven to 400°F. Brush a shallow 2-quart baking dish with 1 teaspoon of the oil.

2 Heat a large nonstick skillet over medium-high heat. Add the remaining 2 teaspoons oil and tilt the pan to coat the bottom evenly. Add the onion and cook, stirring often, until softened, 5 minutes. Add the garlic and cook, stirring constantly, until fragrant, 30 seconds. Set aside.

3 Combine the cream cheese, yogurt, and pepper in a large bowl and whisk until smooth. Add the onion mixture, the spinach, artichoke hearts, Parmesan, mozzarella, and hot sauce and stir to mix well. Spoon the mixture into the prepared baking dish, cover, and bake until the dip is bubbly, 25 to 30 minutes. Serve hot or warm with baked whole wheat pita chips, baked tortilla chips, or fresh raw vegetables.

Each serving (¼ cup): 5 g carb, 88 cal, 5 g fat, 3 g sat fat, 11 mg chol, 1 g fib, 7 g pro, 222 mg sod • Carb Choices: ½; Exchanges: 1 veg, 1 fat

Hot Black Bean Dip

makes 3¾ cups

If you're serving this to adults only, add ½ to 1 teaspoon minced chipotle in adobo sauce for more spice and a touch of smoky flavor. You can assemble the dip through step 5 and cover and refrigerate it for up to a day. Let the dip stand at room temperature for 15 minutes before baking and add 6 to 8 minutes to the baking time.

3 teaspoons canola oil, divided

1 (14½-ounce) can no-salt-added diced tomatoes, undrained

2 (15-ounce) cans no-salt-added black beans, rinsed and drained, divided

1 small onion, diced

½ cup diced red bell pepper

1 jalapeño, seeded and minced

2 garlic cloves, minced

2 teaspoons chili powder

1 teaspoon ground cumin

½ teaspoon kosher salt

¼ cup chopped fresh cilantro

1 tablespoon lime juice

¼ cup thinly sliced scallions

2 ounces shredded reduced-fat sharp Cheddar cheese (about ½ cup)

1 Preheat the oven to 350°F. Brush a shallow 2-quart baking dish with 1 teaspoon of the oil.

2 Place a colander inside a bowl and place the tomatoes in the colander to drain. Reserve the liquid.

3 Place 1 can of the beans in a medium bowl. Using a potato masher, mash the beans until chunky. Stir in the remaining 1 can of beans and the reserved tomato liquid. Set the bean mixture and the drained tomatoes aside.

4 Heat a large nonstick skillet over medium heat. Add the remaining 2 teaspoons oil and tilt the pan to coat the bottom evenly. Add the onion, bell pepper, and jalapeño and cook, stirring often, until the vegetables are softened, 5 minutes. Add the garlic, chili powder, cumin, and salt and cook, stirring constantly, until fragrant, 30 seconds.

5 Add the bean mixture and cook, stirring often, until heated through, about 3 minutes. Remove from the heat and stir in the cilantro and lime juice. Spoon the bean mixture into the prepared baking dish. Sprinkle with the drained tomatoes, the scallions, and Cheddar.

6 Bake, uncovered, until the dip is bubbly and the cheese melts, about 20 minutes. Serve hot or warm with fresh raw vegetables, baked tortilla chips, or baked whole wheat pita chips.

Each serving (¼ cup): 11 g carb, 76 cal, 2 g fat, 1 g sat fat, 3 mg chol, 3 g fib, 4 g pro, 96 mg sod • Carb Choices: 1; Exchanges: 1 starch, 1 plant-based protein, ½ fat

Hummus QUICK

makes 1½ cups

Hummus is so easy to make at home and it's a perfect healthy afternoon snack to have with raw vegetables. It has just enough fat and protein to fend off hunger until dinnertime. Use this basic recipe as a stepping-off point and add flavorings that you enjoy. Try a couple tablespoons of cilantro or basil, ¼ teaspoon minced chipotle in adobo, a couple drained and chopped sun-dried tomatoes, or ¼ cup chopped roasted red bell pepper.

1 (15-ounce) can no-salt-added garbanzo beans, rinsed and drained

¼ cup tahini (sesame paste)

¼ cup cold water

¼ cup lemon juice

1 garlic clove, chopped

½ teaspoon ground cumin

½ teaspoon kosher salt

Pinch of ground cayenne

Combine all the ingredients in a food processor and process until smooth. Cover and refrigerate until chilled, at least 2 hours and up to 5 days.

Each serving (¼ cup): 13 g carb, 123 cal, 6 g fat, 1 g sat fat, 0 mg chol, 3 g fib, 5 g pro, 174 mg sod • Carb Choices: 1; Exchanges: 1 starch, 1 plant-based protein, 1 fat

Lemon-Herb White Bean Dip QUICK

makes 1½ cups

This flavorful dip is not only great for snacks, but great for delicious sandwiches, too. To make a portable lunch, pack the dip separately, then at lunchtime, spoon it into whole wheat pita bread and top with sliced cucumbers and radishes.

1 (15-ounce) can no-salt-added cannellini
    beans, rinsed and drained
2 tablespoons lemon juice
1 tablespoon extra virgin olive oil
1 garlic clove, chopped
½ teaspoon kosher salt
Pinch of freshly ground pepper
2 tablespoons chopped fresh dill, basil, Italian
    parsley, or mint
1 teaspoon grated lemon zest

1 Combine the beans, lemon juice, oil, garlic, salt, and pepper in a food processor and process until smooth.

2 Transfer to a serving bowl and stir in the dill and lemon zest. Serve at once, or refrigerate, covered, for up to 3 days.

Each serving (scant ¼ cup): 10 g carb, 78 cal, 3 g fat, 0 g sat fat, 0 mg chol, 3 g fib, 3 g pro, 115 mg sod • Carb Choices: ½; Exchanges: ½ starch, ½ fat

Rosemary White Bean Dip with Artichokes QUICK | HIGH FIBER

makes 2 cups

To make a sophisticated presentation with this dip, spread it onto small whole grain crackers, and then top each one with a pitted niçoise olive. The dip tastes better if you have time to let it chill and allow the flavors to develop, but it's perfectly delicious straight from the food processor.

1 (14-ounce) can artichoke hearts
1 (15-ounce) can no-salt-added cannellini
    beans, rinsed and drained
1 small garlic clove, chopped
2 tablespoons extra virgin olive oil
2 tablespoons lemon juice
2 teaspoons minced fresh rosemary
⅛ teaspoon freshly ground pepper

1 Drain the artichoke hearts and cut into halves. Place the artichokes on several thicknesses of paper towels and gently blot dry.

2 Combine the artichoke hearts and the remaining ingredients in a food processor and process until smooth.

3 Transfer to a serving bowl and serve at once, or refrigerate, covered, for up to 3 days.

Each serving (¼ cup): Each serving: 13 g carb, 104 cal, 4 g fat, 1 g sat fat, 0 mg chol, 4 g fib, 4 g pro, 319 mg sod • Carb Choices: 1; Exchanges: ½ starch, 1 veg, 1 fat

Herbed Edamame Dip QUICK

makes 1½ cups

You can easily turn this dip into colorful crostini. Toast thin slices of whole wheat baguette, spread with the dip, then top with diced tomatoes, diced cucumber, colorful diced bell peppers, crumbled feta cheese, or minced fresh herbs. Choose several different toppings and arrange the crostini on a platter for the centerpiece of a cocktail party.

1½ cups frozen shelled edamame, thawed
⅓ cup Chicken Stock (page 149) or low-sodium
    chicken broth
¼ cup chopped fresh basil, dill, mint, or Italian
    parsley
1 teaspoon grated lemon zest
2 tablespoons lemon juice
1 tablespoon extra virgin olive oil
½ teaspoon kosher salt
Pinch of freshly ground pepper

1 Bring a medium saucepan of water to a boil over high heat. Add the edamame and cook until tender, about 5 minutes. Drain in a colander and rinse with cold running water until cool.

2 Combine the edamame and the remaining ingredients in a food processor and process until smooth. Serve at once, or refrigerate, covered, for up to 3 days.

Each serving (¼ cup): 5 g carb, 74 cal, 4 g fat, 0 g sat fat, 0 mg chol, 2 g fib, 4 g pro, 116 mg sod • Carb Choices: 0; Exchanges: 1 plant-based protein, ½ fat

Edamame Guacamole QUICK

makes 2 cups

This chile-spiked dip has just enough avocado to give it creamy texture and rich flavor. Serve it with anything you'd serve with ordinary guacamole: baked tortilla chips, fresh vegetables, or even tacos.

1¾ cups frozen shelled edamame, thawed
½ avocado, pitted, peeled, and chopped
1 small scallion, chopped
1 small jalapeño, seeded and chopped
1 garlic clove, minced
½ teaspoon ground cumin
3 tablespoons lime juice
¼ cup fresh cilantro leaves
¾ cup cold water
½ teaspoon kosher salt
1 plum tomato, diced

1 Bring a medium saucepan of water to a boil over high heat. Add the edamame and cook until tender, about 5 minutes. Drain in a colander and rinse with cold running water until cool.

2 Combine the edamame and the remaining ingredients except the tomato in a food processor and process until smooth. Serve at once, or refrigerate, covered, for up to 3 days. To serve, spoon the guacamole into a shallow serving bowl and sprinkle with the tomato.

Each serving (¼ cup): 6 g carb, 69 cal, 3 g fat, 0 g sat fat, 0 mg chol, 3 g fib, 4 g pro, 86 mg sod • Carb Choices: ½; Exchanges: ½ starch, 1 plant-based protein, ½ fat

Roasted Garlic Eggplant Dip HIGH FIBER

makes 1½ cups

Lemon-Garlic Pita Chips (page 51) or warmed whole wheat pita bread, cut into wedges, are perfect accompaniments for this silky dip. Cutting the eggplant in half and roasting it cut side down allows the surface to caramelize, lending a smoky nuance to the flavor.

1 large eggplant (about 1½ pounds)
1 teaspoon extra virgin olive oil
1 head of garlic
3 tablespoons lemon juice
2 tablespoons tahini (sesame paste)
2 tablespoons chopped fresh Italian parsley or basil
¾ teaspoon kosher salt

1 Preheat the oven to 375°F.

2 Cut the eggplant in half lengthwise and brush the cut side with the oil. Place the eggplant cut side down on a medium rimmed baking sheet. Wrap the garlic in a sheet of foil and place on the baking sheet.

3 Bake until the eggplant and the garlic are very tender, about 1 hour. Let stand to cool to room temperature.

4 Scoop out the eggplant flesh and squeeze the pulp from each garlic clove. Combine the eggplant, garlic, lemon juice, tahini, parsley, and salt in a food processor and process until smooth. The dip can be refrigerated, covered, for up to 3 days. Bring to room temperature before serving.

Each serving (generous ¼ cup): 9 g carb, 68 cal, 4 g fat, 1 g sat fat, 0 mg chol, 4 g fib, 2 g pro, 145 mg sod • Carb Choices: ½; Exchanges: 1 veg, ½ fat

Avocado Dip QUICK

makes 1½ cups

Serve this light and refreshing dip with fresh raw vegetables, baked tortilla chips, or chilled shrimp.

1 avocado, pitted and peeled
½ cup low-fat buttermilk
¼ cup plain low-fat yogurt
1 tablespoon lime juice
2 tablespoons thinly sliced scallions
½ teaspoon ground cumin
⅛ teaspoon ground cayenne
¼ teaspoon kosher salt

Combine all the ingredients in a food processor and process until smooth. Cover and refrigerate until chilled, at least 2 hours and up to 1 day.

Each serving (¼ cup): 5 g carb, 70 cal, 5 g fat, 1 g sat fat, 1 mg chol, 2 g fib, 2 g pro, 78 mg sod • Carb Choices: 0; Exchanges: 1 fat

Guacamole QUICK HIGH FIBER

makes 1½ cups

Hass avocados have bumpy purplish-black skin. They are preferred for guacamole because of their soft creamy texture. Squeeze the fruit with the palm of your hand. If it yields to light pressure, it is ready to eat. Guacamole is great with baked tortilla chips, but you can also serve this flavorful accompaniment alongside grilled tuna, shrimp, or chicken breasts.

1 ripe Hass avocado, pitted, peeled, and chopped
1 large plum tomato, chopped
2 tablespoons minced red onion
2 tablespoons chopped fresh cilantro
1 tablespoon lime juice
1 garlic clove, crushed through a press
½ jalapeño, seeded and minced
½ teaspoon kosher salt

Place the avocado in a medium bowl and gently mash with a spatula or fork until the avocado is creamy, but still chunky. Add the tomato, onion, cilantro, lime juice, garlic, jalapeño, and salt and stir to combine. Serve at once, or cover the surface of the guacamole with wax paper to prevent browning and refrigerate up to 4 hours.

Each serving (¼ cup): 6 g carb, 88 cal, 7 g fat, 1 g sat fat, 0 mg chol, 4 g fib, 1 g pro, 145 mg sod • Carb Choices: ½; Exchanges: ½ carb, 1½ fat

Lemony Lima Bean Spread QUICK

makes 2 cups

Baby lima beans make a creamy bright green dip that pairs perfectly with baked whole wheat pita chips, baked tortilla chips, or raw vegetables. Don't tell the kids it's made from lima beans—they will love the flavor and will never guess they are eating their vegetables.

1 (10-ounce) package frozen baby lima beans
½ teaspoon grated lemon zest
3 tablespoons lemon juice
3 tablespoons Chicken Stock (page 149) or low-sodium chicken broth
3 tablespoons chopped fresh basil, dill, mint, or Italian parsley
1 tablespoon extra virgin olive oil
1 garlic clove, chopped
½ teaspoon kosher salt
⅛ teaspoon freshly ground pepper

1 Bring a medium saucepan of water to a boil over high heat. Add the lima beans and cook 2 minutes. Drain in a colander and rinse with cold running water until cool.

2 Transfer the lima beans to a food processor. Add the remaining ingredients and process until the mixture is smooth. Serve at once, or refrigerate, covered for up to 3 days.

Each serving (scant ¼ cup): 10 g carb, 65 cal, 2 g fat, 0 g sat fat, 0 mg chol, 2 g fib, 3 g pro, 92 mg sod • Carb Choices: ½; Exchanges: ½ starch

Cranberry-Olive Tapenade QUICK

makes 1¼ cups

This flavor-packed tapenade is delicious any time of year, but it's festive red and green color make it especially appealing during the holidays. Spread a thin layer of it on thin slices of toasted whole wheat baguette, then top with crumbled goat cheese for an instant appetizer or serve it with fresh vegetables and whole wheat crackers.

½ cup cranberry juice
¾ cup dried cranberries
¼ cup green olives, pitted (such as manzanilla or picholine)
¼ cup loosely packed fresh Italian parsley leaves
2 tablespoons extra virgin olive oil
1 tablespoon capers, rinsed and drained
1 tablespoon lemon juice
1 teaspoon honey
1 small clove garlic, crushed through a press
½ teaspoon lemon zest

1 Place the cranberry juice in a small saucepan and bring to a boil over medium heat. Remove from the heat and add the cranberries. Cover and let stand to cool to room temperature. Drain.

2 Combine the cranberries and the remaining ingredients in a food processor and pulse until the mixture is coarsely chopped. The tapenade can be refrigerated, covered, for up to a week.

Each serving (1 tablespoon): 5 g carb, 35 cal, 2 g fat, 1 g sat fat, 0 mg chol, 0 g fib, 0 g pro, 58 mg sod • Carb Choices: 0; Exchanges: ½ fat

Eggplant Caponata

makes 4 cups

Serve the caponata in a bowl, surrounded with toasted whole grain baguette slices. Offer different toppings for guests to use for garnishes. Try crumbled goat cheese or feta cheese, freshly grated Parmesan, toasted pine nuts or slivered almonds, or thin strips of prosciutto. The caponata makes a delicious pasta sauce, too.

2 teaspoons extra virgin olive oil
1 medium onion, diced
2 garlic cloves, minced
1 large eggplant (about 1½ pounds), peeled and chopped
2 large tomatoes, peeled and chopped
½ cup water
⅓ cup Kalamata olives, pitted and chopped
¼ cup chopped fresh basil or Italian parsley
1 tablespoon capers, rinsed and drained
2 teaspoons red wine vinegar
½ teaspoon kosher salt
⅛ teaspoon freshly ground pepper

1 Heat a large nonstick skillet over medium heat. Add the oil and tilt the pan to coat the bottom evenly. Add the onion and cook, stirring often, until softened, 5 minutes. Add the garlic and cook, stirring constantly, until fragrant, 30 seconds.

2 Add the eggplant, tomatoes, and water and bring to a boil over high heat. Cover, reduce the heat to low, and simmer, stirring occasionally, until the eggplant is very tender, 30 to 35 minutes. Remove from the heat and stir in the olives, basil, capers, vinegar, salt, and pepper. Serve the caponata thick and chunky, or mash the mixture with a potato masher for a smoother texture. The caponata can be refrigerated, covered, for up to 4 days. Bring to room temperature before serving.

Each serving (¼ cup): 4 g carb, 29 cal, 1 g fat, 0 g sat fat, 0 mg chol, 2 g fib, 1 g pro, 92 mg sod • Carb Choices: 0; Exchanges: 1 veg

Feta Cheese Spread QUICK

makes 1 cup

Smear this spread on baked pita chips and sprinkle with diced tomatoes, cucumber, Kalamata olives, or red bell pepper. You can serve it as a dip, too. Just add 1% low-fat milk a tablespoon at a time until you reach the consistency you want.

  2 ounces crumbled feta cheese, at room
     temperature (about ½ cup)
½ cup reduced-fat cream cheese, cut into small
     pieces, at room temperature
2 tablespoons minced scallion
2 tablespoons chopped fresh Italian parsley
2 teaspoons grated lemon zest
1 tablespoon lemon juice

Combine all the ingredients in a food processor and process until the mixture is smooth. The spread can be refrigerated, covered, for up to 3 days.

Each serving (2 tablespoons): 2 g carb, 61 cal, 5 g fat, 3 g sat fat, 17 mg chol, 0 g fib, 3 g pro, 150 mg sod • Carb Choices: 0; Exchanges: 1 fat

Broccoli Pesto QUICK

makes 1½ cups

Using the traditional ingredients of pesto—Parmesan, pine nuts, garlic, and olive oil—turns broccoli into a delicious appetizer to serve with any kind of chips, toasted bread, or fresh vegetables. Use the leftovers to fill a pita for lunch or toss with hot pasta for dinner.

5 cups broccoli florets
2 garlic cloves, minced
Pinch of ground cayenne
1 ounce freshly grated Parmesan (about ¼ cup)
¼ cup pine nuts, toasted (page 4)
¼ cup water
1 teaspoon grated lemon zest
1 tablespoon lemon juice
1 tablespoon extra virgin olive oil
½ teaspoon kosher salt

1 Place the broccoli in a microwave-safe dish and cover with plastic wrap. Microwave on high until the broccoli is tender, yet still bright green, about 5 minutes.

2 Carefully uncover the broccoli and drain in a colander. Let cool slightly and pat dry with paper towels. Transfer the broccoli to a food processor. Add the remaining ingredients and process until the mixture is smooth. Serve at once, or refrigerate, covered, for up to 1 day. Bring to room temperature before serving.

Each serving (generous ¼ cup): 4 g carb, 92 cal, 7 g fat, 1 g sat fat, 3 mg chol, 2 g fib, 4 g pro, 161 mg sod • Carb Choices: 0; Exchanges: 1 veg, 1½ fat

Tzatziki QUICK

makes ¾ cup

You can make this with plain yogurt, but when made with Greek yogurt it's extra thick and rich tasting. Tzatziki is perfect to serve as a dip with whole wheat pita chips, wedges of grilled whole wheat pita bread, or any fresh vegetables. Stir in a tablespoon of chopped fresh dill or basil if you wish. You can also serve it as a sauce to accompany broiled or grilled fish.

½ cup plain low-fat Greek yogurt or strained
     yogurt (page 11)
½ cup peeled, seeded, shredded hothouse
     (English) cucumber
1 teaspoon grated lemon zest
⅛ teaspoon kosher salt

Stir together all the ingredients in a small bowl. Serve at once, or refrigerate, covered, for up to 3 days.

Each serving (2 tablespoons): 1 g carb, 14 cal, 0 g fat, 0 g sat fat, 1 mg chol, 0 g fib, 2 g pro, 30 mg sod • Carb Choices: 0

Salsas

Fresh Tomato Salsa [QUICK]

makes 1½ cups

Serve this classic salsa with tortilla chips, of course, but it's also good on any Tex-Mex dish from tacos to burritos. You can also serve it on top of grilled chicken breasts or salmon fillets to add instant flavor to an otherwise ho-hum dinner.

2 medium tomatoes, chopped
¼ cup chopped fresh cilantro
3 tablespoons diced red onion
2 tablespoons lime juice
1 jalapeño, seeded and minced
1 garlic clove, crushed through a press
½ teaspoon kosher salt

Combine all the ingredients in a medium bowl and stir to mix well. Serve at once or cover and refrigerate up to 6 hours.

Each serving (¼ cup): 3 g carb, 14 cal, 0 g fat, 0 g sat fat, 0 mg chol, 1 g fib, 1 g pro, 96 mg sod • Carb Choices: 0; Exchanges: 1 veg

Winter Tomato Salsa [QUICK]

makes 2½ cups

A generous splash of lime juice and a handful of cilantro give this canned tomato salsa amazing flavor. It's not as good as fresh salsa made with summer tomatoes, but it beats anything you'll find premade at the supermarket. This makes a big batch, but it keeps for several days in the refrigerator.

2 (14½-ounce) cans no-salt-added diced
    tomatoes, undrained
¼ cup minced red onion
¼ cup chopped fresh cilantro
3 tablespoons lime juice
1 jalapeño, seeded and minced
½ teaspoon kosher salt
Pinch of ground cayenne

1 Drain 1 can of the tomatoes and discard the liquid. Place the drained tomatoes and the remaining can of tomatoes with its juices in a food processor and pulse 4 or 5 times or until the tomatoes are finely chopped.

2 Transfer the tomatoes to a bowl and stir in the onion, cilantro, lime juice, jalapeño, salt, and cayenne. Serve at once, or refrigerate, covered, for up to 4 days.

Each serving (¼ cup): 5 g carb, 20 cal, 0 g fat, 0 g sat fat, 0 mg chol, 1 g fib, 1 g pro, 89 mg sod • Carb Choices: 0; Exchanges: 1 veg

Tomato, Black Bean, and Corn Salsa [QUICK]

makes 2 cups

This versatile salsa can be scooped up with any kind of chip you have on hand. You can serve it to top almost any main dish, too—try shrimp, salmon, chicken, or pork chops.

1 cup canned no-salt-added black beans, rinsed
    and drained
1 small ear corn, kernels cut from the cob,
    or ½ cup frozen corn kernels, thawed
1 medium tomato, chopped
1 jalapeño, seeded and minced
¼ cup diced green bell pepper
2 tablespoons chopped fresh cilantro
2 tablespoons lime juice
2 teaspoons canola oil
½ teaspoon kosher salt

Combine all the ingredients in a medium bowl and stir to mix well. Serve at room temperature within 2 hours.

Each serving (¼ cup): 8 g carb, 49 cal, 1 g fat, 0 g sat fat, 0 mg chol, 2 g fib, 2 g pro, 76 mg sod • Carb Choices: ½; Exchanges: ½ starch

Avocado-Cucumber Salsa QUICK

makes 2 cups

Spoon a little of this salsa alongside a few grilled shrimp or a couple slices of rare grilled tuna to make an elegant appetizer.

1 avocado, pitted, peeled, and chopped
½ hothouse (English) cucumber, chopped
¼ cup diced red onion
¼ cup diced yellow or red bell pepper
1 jalapeño, seeded and minced
2 tablespoons chopped fresh cilantro
2 tablespoons lime juice
½ teaspoon kosher salt

Combine all the ingredients in a medium bowl and stir to mix well. Serve at once, or refrigerate, covered, for up to 4 hours.

Each serving (¼ cup): 4 g carb, 47 cal, 4 g fat, 1 g sat fat, 0 mg chol, 2 g fib, 1 g pro, 72 mg sod • Carb Choices: 0; Exchanges: ½ fat

Mango-Jicama Salsa QUICK

makes 2 cups

The textures and colors of crunchy white jicama and creamy sweet mango play off each other in this sweet and spicy salsa. Serve it with baked tortilla chips, pita chips, or wonton chips.

1 large mango, peeled, pitted, and diced
1 cup diced jicama
1 scallion, thinly sliced
¼ cup diced red bell pepper
2 tablespoons chopped fresh cilantro
1 tablespoon lime juice
1 jalapeño, seeded and minced
¼ teaspoon kosher salt

Combine all the ingredients in a medium bowl and stir to mix well. Serve at once, or refrigerate, covered, for up to 4 hours.

Each serving (¼ cup): 7 g carb, 26 cal, 0 g fat, 0 g sat fat, 0 mg chol, 1 g fib, 0 g pro, 37 mg sod • Carb Choices: ½; Exchanges: ½ fruit

Melon Salsa QUICK

makes 2 cups

Serve this salsa with pita chips or salmon.

2 cups diced watermelon
2 cups diced honeydew melon
2 tablespoons minced red onion
1 jalapeño, seeded and minced
2 tablespoons chopped fresh cilantro
1 tablespoon lime juice
¼ teaspoon kosher salt

Combine all the ingredients in a medium bowl and stir to mix well. Serve at once, or refrigerate, covered, for up to 1 hour.

Each serving (¼ cup): 7 g carb, 29 cal, 0 g fat, 0 g sat fat, 0 mg chol, 1 g fib, 1 g pro, 43 mg sod • Carb Choices: ½; Exchanges: ½ fruit

Tomatillo Salsa Verde QUICK

makes 2 cups

Serve this vivid sauce with tortilla chips or shrimp.

1 pound tomatillos, husks removed and halved
2 jalapeños, halved and seeded
1 small onion, cut into 8 wedges
2 garlic cloves, halved
2 teaspoons canola oil
½ cup loosely packed fresh cilantro leaves
1 tablespoon lime juice
½ teaspoon kosher salt
¼ teaspoon sugar

1 Preheat the broiler.

2 Place the tomatillos, jalapeños, onion, and garlic on a medium rimmed baking sheet. Drizzle with the oil and toss to coat. Arrange the vegetables in a single layer. Broil, stirring twice, until the vegetables are softened, 12 to 15 minutes.

3 Transfer the vegetables to a food processor. Add the cilantro, lime juice, salt, and sugar and process until smooth. Cover and refrigerate until chilled, at least 2 hours and up to 2 days.

Each serving (¼ cup): 5 g carb, 35 cal, 2 g fat, 0 g sat fat, 0 mg chol, 1 g fib, 1 g pro, 72 mg sod • Carb Choices: 0; Exchanges: 1 veg

Small Bites

Stuffed Eggs with Horseradish

makes 8 servings

No matter if it's a black-tie affair or a backyard barbecue, stuffed eggs are always welcome. All the stuffed egg recipes here use part of the egg white to stuff the eggs. This trick cuts back on fat, cholesterol, and calories, but all these eggs are excellent and packed with flavor. If you don't tell your guests, they will never know.

12 large eggs
2 tablespoons mayonnaise
2 tablespoons plain low-fat yogurt
1 tablespoon prepared horseradish, drained
1 teaspoon white wine vinegar
1 teaspoon Dijon mustard
¼ teaspoon kosher salt
2 tablespoons minced red onion
2 tablespoons minced celery
1 tablespoon chopped fresh Italian parsley
Paprika

1 Place the eggs in a large saucepan and cover with cold water. Cover and bring to a boil over medium heat. Turn off the heat and let the eggs stand 12 minutes. Drain and peel under cold running water.

2 Cut the eggs in half lengthwise. Remove and discard 6 of the egg yolks. Combine the remaining egg yolks, the mayonnaise, yogurt, horseradish, vinegar, mustard, and salt and stir until smooth, breaking up the egg yolks with a spatula or fork.

3 Finely chop 8 of the egg white halves and add to the egg yolk mixture. Stir in the onion, celery, and parsley. Spoon the egg yolk mixture evenly into the remaining 16 egg white halves. Arrange on a serving plate. Cover and refrigerate until chilled, at least 2 hours and up to 1 day. Sprinkle with paprika just before serving.

Each serving: 2 g carb, 97 cal, 6 g fat, 2 g sat fat, 155 mg chol, 0 g fib, 8 g pro, 168 mg sod • Carb Choices: 0; Exchanges: 1 lean protein, ½ fat

Perfect Hard-Cooked Eggs

The cooking method for these stuffed eggs will ensure that your hard-cooked eggs are perfect every time. Place the eggs in a saucepan, then cover with cold water. Cover the saucepan and bring the water to a boil over medium heat. When the water comes to a boil, immediately turn off the heat and let the eggs stand, covered, for 12 minutes. Drain the eggs and cool them under cold running water. You can store hard-cooked eggs in the refrigerator for up to a week.

Curried Stuffed Eggs

makes 8 servings

A bit of mango chutney adds a sweet tang to this classic version of stuffed eggs. You can use chopped fresh cilantro instead of the parsley in this recipe if you wish.

12 large eggs
2 tablespoons mayonnaise
2 tablespoons plain low-fat yogurt
2 tablespoons finely minced mango chutney
1 teaspoon white wine vinegar
1 teaspoon curry powder
¼ teaspoon kosher salt
2 tablespoons minced red onion
2 tablespoons minced celery
1 tablespoon chopped fresh Italian parsley

1 Place the eggs in a large saucepan and cover with cold water. Cover and bring to a boil over medium heat. Turn off the heat and let the eggs stand 12 minutes. Drain and peel under cold running water.

2 Cut the eggs in half lengthwise. Remove and discard 6 of the egg yolks. Combine the remaining egg yolks, the mayonnaise, yogurt, chutney, vinegar, curry powder, and salt and stir until smooth, breaking up the egg yolks with a spatula or fork.

3 Finely chop 8 of the egg white halves and add to the egg yolk mixture. Stir in the onion, celery, and parsley. Spoon the egg yolk mixture evenly into the remaining 16 egg white halves. Arrange on a serving plate. Cover and refrigerate until chilled, at least 2 hours and up to 1 day.

Each serving: 4 g carb, 104 cal, 6 g fat, 2 g sat fat, 155 mg chol, 0 g fib, 8 g pro, 157 mg sod • Carb Cholces: 0; Exchanges: 1 lean protein, ½ fat

Smoky Spiced Stuffed Eggs

makes 8 servings

Once you try the unexpected smoky flavor of these eggs, they may become your favorite. Serve them as a starter at a Tex-Mex–themed party—they're great with beer or margaritas.

12 large eggs
2 tablespoons mayonnaise
2 tablespoons plain low-fat yogurt
1 teaspoon lime juice
½ teaspoon minced chipotle in adobo sauce
¼ teaspoon kosher salt
2 tablespoons minced red onion
2 tablespoons minced celery
2 tablespoons chopped fresh cilantro
Chili powder

1 Place the eggs in a large saucepan and cover with cold water. Cover and bring to a boil over medium heat. Turn off the heat and let the eggs stand 12 minutes. Drain and peel under cold running water.

2 Cut the eggs in half lengthwise. Remove and discard 6 of the egg yolks. Combine the remaining egg yolks, the mayonnaise, yogurt, lime juice, chipotle, and salt and stir until smooth, breaking up the egg yolks with a spatula or fork.

3 Finely chop 8 of the egg white halves and add to the egg yolk mixture. Stir in the onion, celery, and cilantro. Spoon the egg yolk mixture evenly into the remaining 16 egg white halves. Arrange on a serving plate. Cover and refrigerate until chilled, at least 2 hours and up to 1 day. Sprinkle with chili powder just before serving.

Each serving: 2 g carb, 98 cal, 6 g fat, 2 g sat fat, 155 mg chol, 0 g fib, 8 g pro, 167 mg sod • Carb Choices: 0; Exchanges: 1 lean protein, ½ fat

Buffalo Chicken Skewers

makes 8 servings

Look, Mom, no bones! This healthful dish has all the spicy flavor of Buffalo chicken wings, but it uses broiled boneless skinless chicken breast instead. It's a healthful and satisfying alternative to everyone's favorite fried chicken snack. Kids will love these, but remember to adjust the hot sauce to your family's liking.

¼ **cup plain low-fat yogurt**
1 **tablespoon hot sauce**
2 **garlic cloves, crushed through a press**
1 **pound boneless skinless chicken breasts**
1 **teaspoon canola oil**
½ **teaspoon kosher salt**
4 **stalks celery, halved lengthwise and cut into 3-inch pieces**
1 **recipe Creamy Blue Cheese–Peppercorn Dressing (page 141)**

1 Combine the yogurt, hot sauce, and garlic in a large resealable plastic bag. Slice the chicken into 24 thin strips. Add the chicken to the bag, seal, and refrigerate 2 to 4 hours.

2 Place 24 (6-inch) wooden skewers in a bowl of water to soak at least 30 minutes.

3 Remove the chicken from the marinade and discard the marinade. Thread 1 slice of chicken onto each of the soaked skewers.

4 Preheat the broiler. Brush a broiler pan with the oil.

5 Place the skewers on the broiler pan, sprinkle with the salt, and broil, turning once, until the chicken is cooked through, about 3 minutes on each side. Serve hot or at room temperature with the celery and the dressing.

Each serving: 3 g carb, 117 cal, 6 g fat, 1 g sat fat, 35 mg chol, 1 g fib, 13 g pro, 243 mg sod • Carb Choices: 0; Exchanges: 2 lean protein, ½ fat

Beef Saté with Peanut Sauce

makes 8 servings

To serve the beef, arrange the skewers on a platter with the sauce in the center. Intersperse colorful wedges of bell pepper, celery sticks, and whole radishes with the beef skewers. The vegetables will make a vibrant presentation and taste great with the Peanut Sauce, too.

2 **tablespoons reduced-sodium soy sauce**
1 **tablespoon light brown sugar**
2 **teaspoons grated fresh ginger**
1 **garlic clove, crushed through a press**
½ **teaspoon Asian sesame oil**
1 **pound flank steak, trimmed of all visible fat**
1 **teaspoon canola oil**
1 **recipe Peanut Sauce (page 594)**

1 Place 24 (6-inch) wooden skewers in a bowl of water to soak at least 30 minutes.

2 Whisk together the soy sauce, sugar, ginger, garlic, and sesame oil in a medium bowl. Slice the steak across the grain into 24 slices. Add to the soy sauce mixture and toss to coat. Cover and refrigerate 30 minutes. Remove the steak from the marinade and discard the marinade. Thread 1 slice of steak onto each of the soaked skewers.

3 Preheat the broiler. Brush a broiler pan with the canola oil.

4 Place the skewers on the broiler pan and broil, turning once, about 2 minutes on each side. Serve hot or at room temperature with the sauce.

Each serving: 5 g carb, 155 cal, 9 g fat, 2 g sat fat, 22 mg chol, 1 g fib, 14 g pro, 205 mg sod • Carb Choices: 0; Exchanges: 2 lean protein, 1 fat

Baked Egg Rolls

makes 8 servings

Sweet hoisin sauce in the egg roll filling plays off the salty dipping sauce. Asian appetizers are almost always high in sodium, so make lower-sodium food choices on a day when you enjoy these.

8 ounces boneless center-cut pork chops, trimmed and cubed
4 teaspoons canola oil, divided
1 cup finely chopped white mushrooms
½ cup diced onion
1 tablespoon minced fresh ginger
2 garlic cloves, minced
1 cup finely chopped green cabbage
½ cup coarsely shredded carrot
2 tablespoons hoisin sauce
8 egg roll wrappers
1 recipe Asian Dipping Sauce (page 595)

1 Place the pork in a food processor in 2 batches and pulse until the meat is finely minced but not ground, 4 to 5 times.

2 Heat a large nonstick skillet over medium-high heat. Add 2 teaspoons of the oil and tilt the pan to coat the bottom evenly. Add the ground pork, mushrooms, onion, ginger, and garlic and cook, stirring often, until the mushrooms are tender and most of the liquid has evaporated, 6 to 8 minutes. Add the cabbage and carrot and cook, stirring often, until the cabbage is softened, about 3 minutes. Remove from the heat and stir in the hoisin sauce. Transfer to a plate to cool.

3 Preheat the oven to 425°F. Brush a medium baking sheet with 1 teaspoon of the remaining oil.

4 Working with 1 egg roll wrapper at a time (keep the remaining wrappers covered to prevent drying), place the wrapper on a work surface with one corner pointing toward you. Spoon about ¼ cup of the pork mixture in the center of the wrapper. Fold the bottom corner of the wrapper over the filling. Fold in the sides. Brush the top corner of the wrapper lightly with water and roll up. Place the egg rolls on a plate and cover with damp paper towels to prevent drying. Repeat with the remaining wrappers and filling.

5 Brush the egg rolls lightly on all sides with the remaining 1 teaspoon oil. Arrange the egg rolls seam side down on the prepared baking sheet. Bake until the bottoms are browned, 10 to 12 minutes. Turn the egg rolls and bake 5 minutes longer. Serve hot or warm with the sauce.

Each serving: 25 g carb, 182 cal, 5 g fat, 1 g sat fat, 20 mg chol, 1 g fib, 10 g pro, 616 mg sod • Carb Choices: 1½; Exchanges: 1 starch, 1 veg, 1 lean protein, ½ fat

Shrimp Pot Stickers with Sweet Soy Dipping Sauce

makes 6 servings

Mirin, a Japanese cooking wine with added sugar, lends a touch of sweetness to the sauce. If you don't have it available, use any white wine that you have on hand and add ½ teaspoon of sugar to the sauce. For a party, you can assemble the pot stickers, cover them with a damp paper towel, and refrigerate for up to 4 hours before cooking them.

POT STICKERS
1 cup Chicken Stock (page 149) or low-sodium chicken broth
4 teaspoons reduced-sodium soy sauce, divided
8 ounces medium cooked peeled deveined shrimp, finely chopped
2 tablespoons minced scallion
2 tablespoons chopped fresh cilantro
2 teaspoons grated fresh ginger
1 large egg white
1 garlic clove, crushed through a press
½ teaspoon Asian sesame oil
18 wonton wrappers
4 teaspoons canola oil, divided

SAUCE

2 tablespoons reduced-sodium soy sauce

1 tablespoon cold water

4 teaspoons mirin

4 teaspoons rice vinegar

¼ teaspoon Asian sesame oil

1 tablespoon thinly sliced scallion, green tops only

1 To make the pot stickers, combine the stock and 2 teaspoons of the soy sauce in a measuring cup. Set aside.

2 Stir together the shrimp, scallion, cilantro, ginger, egg white, garlic, sesame oil, and the remaining 2 teaspoons soy sauce in a medium bowl. Working with 1 wonton wrapper at a time (keep the remaining wrappers covered to prevent drying), place the wonton wrapper on a work surface. Place 1 rounded teaspoon of the shrimp mixture in the center. Moisten the edge of the wrapper with water, bring the opposite corners together, and pinch the edges together to seal. Place the shaped pot stickers on a plate and cover with damp paper towels to prevent drying. Repeat with the remaining wrappers and filling.

3 Heat a large nonstick skillet over medium-high heat. Add 2 teaspoons of the canola oil and tilt the pan to coat the bottom evenly. Add half of the pot stickers and cook until the bottoms are browned, 2 to 3 minutes. Add half of the stock mixture and bring to a boil. Cover and cook until the stock is absorbed, about 3 minutes. Transfer the pot stickers to a large plate and cover to keep warm. Repeat with the remaining 2 teaspoons canola oil, the remaining pot stickers, and the remaining broth mixture. Serve at once with the sauce.

4 To make the sauce, whisk together the soy sauce, water, mirin, vinegar, and oil in a small bowl. Stir in the scallions.

Each serving: 16 g carb, 170 cal, 5 g fat, 0 g sat fat, 79 mg chol, 1 g fib, 14 g pro, 619 mg sod • Carb Choices: 1; Exchanges: 1 starch, 1 lean protein, ½ fat

Cured Salmon (Gravlax)

makes 12 servings

Make a double recipe of the salmon and check out 10 More Ways to Use Cured Salmon (page 48) for ideas on how to use the leftovers.

1 (1-pound) salmon fillet (about 1-inch thick)

¾ cup fresh dill sprigs

¼ cup kosher salt

¼ cup sugar

2 teaspoons grated lemon zest

12 thin slices pumpernickel bread

½ cup reduced-fat cream cheese, softened

¼ cup finely diced red onion

3 tablespoons capers, rinsed and drained

1 Place the salmon skin side down, in a glass baking dish. Top the salmon with the dill. Stir together the salt, sugar, and lemon zest in a small bowl and sprinkle evenly over the salmon.

2 Place a sheet of plastic wrap over the salmon. Place a plate on top of the salmon, then place a heavy can or other weighted object on the plate. Refrigerate 24 hours. Turn the salmon over, replace the plastic wrap, plate, and can and refrigerate 24 hours longer.

3 Remove the salmon from the dish and discard the accumulated liquid. Rub off all but a smattering of the curing mixture. At this point, the salmon can be refrigerated, covered, for up to 4 days.

4 To serve, place the salmon on a cutting board and cut into paper thin slices, turning the knife up after each cut to separate the salmon from the skin.

5 Trim the crusts from the bread and toast the bread. Cut each slice of bread into 4 triangles. Spread each triangle with ½ teaspoon of the cream cheese. Sprinkle the triangles evenly with the red onion and capers. Top evenly with the sliced salmon and serve at once.

Each serving: 10 g carb, 132 cal, 5 g fat, 2 g sat fat, 29 mg chol, 1 g fib, 11 g pro, 504 mg sod • Carb Choices: ½; Exchanges: ½ starch, 1 lean protein

10 More Ways to Use Cured Salmon

1. Place sliced cured salmon on small squares of pumpernickel toast and top with a bit of whole grain mustard.

2. Spread cucumber rounds with a smear of softened reduced-fat cream cheese, top with sliced cured salmon, and garnish with fresh dill.

3. Spread fresh fennel spears with softened goat cheese, top with sliced cured salmon, and garnish with fresh fennel fronds.

4. Toss chopped cured salmon with diced cucumber, avocado, red onion, and lemon juice. Serve in purchased phyllo shells or Belgian endive leaves.

5. Cook baby potatoes until just tender, then drain and let cool. Cut the potatoes in half and scoop out the centers. Stir together sour cream and minced scallions and spoon into the potato shells. Top with sliced cured salmon.

6. Serve thinly sliced cured salmon with cooked chilled asparagus spears as a first course. Top with plain low-fat yogurt, or for a special treat, serve with Yogurt Tartar Sauce (page 594).

7. Stir together equal parts mayonnaise and reduced-fat sour cream, then add drained prepared horseradish to taste. Spread the mayonnaise mixture on small squares of pumpernickel toast and top with sliced cured salmon. Garnish with minced chives.

8. Add chopped cured salmon and minced chives to eggs before scrambling them and serve with thin slices of rye toast.

9. Replace the canned tuna in Niçoise Salad (page 134) with sliced cured salmon. It is especially good drizzled with Mustard Vinaigrette (page 138).

10. Turn summer salads into special treats. Add short, thin strips of cured salmon to Cucumber-Dill Potato Salad (page 92), Pasta and Pea Salad (page 103), Marinated Cucumber and Sweet Onion Salad (page 94), or Asian Edamame and Radish Salad (page 101).

Creamy Smoked Salmon–Dill Spread QUICK

makes 8 servings

When you're in a rush, but need to serve something delicious, this dip fits the bill. Not only is it a perfect spread for toasted whole wheat bagels, but it turns any kind of cracker or vegetable into an extra-special treat.

8 ounces reduced-fat cream cheese, at room temperature

4 ounces smoked salmon

2 tablespoons thinly sliced scallion, white parts only

2 tablespoons chopped fresh dill

1 teaspoon grated lemon zest

1 tablespoon lemon juice

Pinch of freshly ground pepper

Combine all the ingredients in a food processor and process until smooth. Cover and refrigerate until chilled, at least 2 hours and up to 2 days.

Each serving (generous 2 tablespoons): 2 g carb, 92 cal, 7 g fat, 4 g sat fat, 16 mg chol, 0 g fib, 6 g pro, 186 mg sod • Carb Choices: 0; Exchanges: 1 medium-fat protein, 1 fat

Shrimp Summer Rolls

makes 4 servings

These rolls make an attractive and refreshing start to any Asian-themed get-together. You can also serve them with Peanut Sauce (page 594).

6 ounces cooked peeled deveined shrimp, halved lengthwise
½ hothouse (English) cucumber, cut into short, thin strips
½ cup coarsely shredded carrots
¼ cup thinly sliced scallions
¼ cup fresh mint leaves
¼ cup fresh cilantro leaves
8 (8-inch) rice paper wrappers
8 small leaf lettuce or Bibb lettuce leaves, ribs removed
1 recipe Asian Dipping Sauce (page 595)

1 Toss together the shrimp, cucumber, carrots, scallions, mint, and cilantro in a medium bowl.

2 Pour hot water into a large shallow dish. Dip each rice paper wrapper into the hot water until softened, about 30 seconds. Place the wrapper on a flat surface and top with a lettuce leaf, tearing the leaf to be slightly smaller than the wrapper.

3 Spoon about ¼ cup of the shrimp mixture onto the lettuce leaf. Fold in two sides of the wrapper and roll up. Place on a serving platter and top with damp paper towels to prevent drying. Repeat with the remaining wrappers, lettuce leaves, and shrimp mixture. Serve at once, or refrigerate, topped with damp paper towels and wrapped in plastic wrap, up to 4 hours. Serve with the sauce.

Each serving: 23 g carb, 152 cal, 1 g fat, 0 g sat fat, 86 mg chol, 1 g fib, 13 g pro, 836 mg sod • Carb Choices: 1½; Exchanges: 1 starch, 1 veg, 1 lean protein

Spanakopita

makes 12 servings

These classic Greek phyllo pastries made with spinach and cheese are not as difficult to make as it may seem. Keep the phyllo covered with a damp towel to keep it from drying out as you assemble the dish. Spanakopita makes a wonderful vegetarian entrée, too.

4 teaspoons plus 2 tablespoons extra virgin olive oil, divided
1 cup thinly sliced scallions
2 garlic cloves, minced
6 ounces finely crumbled feta cheese (about 1½ cups)
2 (10-ounce) packages frozen chopped spinach, thawed and squeezed dry
1 (16-ounce) container low-fat cottage cheese (about 1¾ cups)
2 large eggs
2 tablespoons chopped fresh dill or 1 teaspoon dried dill
¼ teaspoon freshly ground pepper
8 (14 x 9-inch) sheets frozen phyllo dough, thawed

1 Preheat the oven to 375°F. Brush a 13 x 9-inch baking pan with 2 teaspoons of the oil.

2 Heat a medium nonstick skillet over medium heat. Add 2 teaspoons of the remaining oil and tilt the pan to coat the bottom evenly. Add the scallions and garlic and cook, stirring often, until the scallions are softened, about 3 minutes. Transfer to a large bowl.

3 Add the feta, spinach, cottage cheese, eggs, dill, and pepper to the scallion mixture and stir to mix well.

4 Unroll the phyllo and place one sheet in the bottom of the prepared pan. Brush the phyllo lightly with some of the remaining 2 tablespoons oil. Repeat with 3 more layers of phyllo. Spread the

continues on next page

spinach mixture evenly over the phyllo. Top with a sheet of phyllo and brush with oil. Repeat the layering with the remaining 3 sheets of phyllo and the remaining oil. Brush the top sheet of phyllo with oil.

5 Bake until the top of the phyllo is well browned, about 35 minutes. Let cool in the pan on a wire rack for 10 minutes. Cut into 12 squares. Serve warm or at room temperature.

Each serving: 11 g carb, 169 cal, 9 g fat, 3 g sat fat, 55 mg chol, 1 g fib, 10 g pro, 477 mg sod • Carb Choices: 1; Exchanges: 1 carb, 1 medium-fat protein, 1 fat

Goat Cheese and Marinated Red Pepper Bruschetta

makes 8 servings

You can make countless toppings for bruschetta, but this goat cheese and pepper version is a popular favorite and easy to make. Try your own combinations. The peppers will keep for up to a week in the refrigerator. You can add them to green salads, pasta salads, or sandwiches. If you're storing the peppers for several days, use ½ teaspoon dried oregano or basil instead of a fresh herb. The dried herbs will last longer.

1 tablespoon balsamic vinegar

1 tablespoon extra virgin olive oil

1 garlic clove, crushed through a press

¼ teaspoon kosher salt

⅛ teaspoon freshly ground pepper

1 cup red Roasted Bell Peppers (page 21) or roasted red peppers from a jar, thinly sliced

1 tablespoon capers, rinsed and drained

2 tablespoons chopped fresh basil or Italian parsley

2 ounces goat cheese (about ½ cup), at room temperature

16 (¼-inch) slices 100% whole wheat baguette, toasted

1 Whisk together the vinegar, oil, garlic, salt, and ground pepper in a medium bowl. Add the roasted peppers and capers and stir to combine. Cover and refrigerate at least 8 hours and up to 4 days. Stir in the basil just before serving.

2 To assemble, spread ½ tablespoon of the goat cheese on each of the baguette slices. Top the cheese with about 1 tablespoon of the bell pepper mixture. Serve at once.

Each serving: 8 g carb, 84 cal, 4 g fat, 2 g sat fat, 6 mg chol, 2 g fib, 4 g pro, 164 mg sod • Carb Choices: ½; Exchanges: ½ starch, 1 fat

Shrimp Bruschetta QUICK

makes 8 servings

This is my go-to recipe when I need an appetizer that looks as good as it tastes and is ready to serve in about 15 minutes. The coriander and lemon give the shrimp remarkable flavor and the bell pepper and scallion add plenty of color. You can make the shrimp mixture ahead of time and refrigerate, covered, up to 4 hours before serving.

1 tablespoon mayonnaise

1 tablespoon plain low-fat yogurt

1 teaspoon grated lemon zest

1 tablespoon lemon juice

½ teaspoon ground coriander

¼ teaspoon kosher salt

6 ounces cooked peeled deveined shrimp, chopped

2 tablespoons minced red or yellow bell pepper

2 tablespoons chopped fresh Italian parsley

1 tablespoon minced scallions, green tops only

16 (¼-inch) slices whole wheat baguette, toasted

1 Stir together the mayonnaise, yogurt, lemon zest, lemon juice, coriander, and salt in a medium bowl. Add the shrimp, bell pepper, parsley, and scallions.

2 To assemble, spoon about 1 tablespoon of the shrimp mixture on each of the baguette slices. Arrange on a platter and serve at once.

Each serving: 13 g carb, 117 cal, 3 g fat, 0 g sat fat, 44 mg chol, 2 g fib, 10 g pro, 253 mg sod • Carb Choices: 1; Exchanges: 1 starch, 1 lean protein, ½ fat

Crunchy Nibbles

Lemon-Garlic Pita Chips QUICK

makes 8 servings

Addictively crunchy, these chips are handy to have on hand. They're perfect for dipping or just for snacking.

1 tablespoon extra virgin olive oil
1 garlic clove, crushed through a press
1 teaspoon grated lemon zest
2 (6-inch) whole wheat pita breads
⅛ teaspoon kosher salt

1 Preheat the oven to 350°F.

2 Combine the oil and garlic in a small saucepan and set over medium heat just until hot, about 2 minutes. Stir in the lemon zest.

3 Split each pita in half to make 4 rounds. Brush the rough side of the rounds with the oil mixture. Cut each round into 12 wedges. Place the pita wedges in a single layer rough side up on a large baking sheet and sprinkle with the salt.

4 Bake until the pita wedges are crisp and lightly toasted, 10 to 12 minutes. Cool the chips in the pan on a wire rack. The chips can be covered in an airtight container and stored at room temperature for up to 5 days.

Each serving: 9 g carb, 59 cal, 2 g fat, 0 g sat fat, 0 mg chol, 1 g fib, 2 g pro, 103 mg sod • Carb Choices: ½; Exchanges: ½ starch, ½ fat

CUMIN-LIME PITA CHIPS QUICK: Follow the Lemon-Garlic Pita Chips recipe, above, adding ¼ teaspoon ground cumin with the garlic in step 2. Substitute grated lime zest for the lemon zest and proceed with the recipe.

Each serving: 9 g carb, 59 cal, 2 g fat, 0 g sat fat, 0 mg chol, 1 g fib, 2 g pro, 103 mg sod • Carb Choices: ½; Exchanges: ½ starch, ½ fat

Sugar-and-Spice Pita Chips QUICK

makes 8 servings

These chips are a great afternoon treat for kids. Serve them with Melon Salsa (page 42), omitting the jalapeño if you wish. They're also great spread with a little natural peanut butter.

2 (6-inch) whole wheat pita breads
2 tablespoons sugar
¼ teaspoon ground cinnamon
Pinch kosher salt

1 Preheat the oven to 350°F. Line a large baking sheet with parchment paper.

2 Split each pita in half to make 4 rounds. Cut each round into 12 wedges. Place the pita wedges in a single layer on the prepared pan, rough side up.

3 Stir together the sugar, cinnamon, and salt in a small bowl. Sprinkle the pita wedges evenly with the sugar mixture.

4 Bake until the pita wedges are crisp and lightly toasted, 10 to 12 minutes. Cool the chips in the pan on a wire rack. The chips can be covered in an airtight container and stored at room temperature for up to 5 days.

Each serving: 12 g carb, 55 cal, 0 g fat, 0 g sat fat, 0 mg chol, 1 g fib, 2 g pro, 94 mg sod • Carb Choices: 1; Exchanges: 1 starch

Baked Wonton Chips QUICK

makes 4 servings

You can make a double (or triple) batch of these chips and store them in an airtight container at room temperature for up to 2 weeks. Experiment with seasonings, too. You can use chili powder, cumin, coriander, five-spice powder, or garam masala. Use them to serve with any kind of dip or spread.

12 wonton wrappers
2 teaspoons extra virgin olive oil
⅛ teaspoon fennel seeds
⅛ teaspoon kosher salt
Pinch of freshly ground pepper

1 Preheat the oven to 375°F.

2 Brush both sides of each wonton wrapper with the oil. Cut each wrapper in half to form 2 triangles. Arrange the triangles in a single layer on a large baking sheet.

3 Sprinkle the fennel seeds, salt, and pepper evenly over the wonton wrappers. Bake until golden brown, 7 to 9 minutes. Transfer the chips to a wire rack to cool.

Each serving: 14 g carb, 91 cal, 3 g fat, 0 g sat fat, 2 mg chol, 0 g fib, 2 g pro, 172 mg sod • Carb Choices: 1; Exchanges: 1 starch, ½ fat

Crispy Baked Root Vegetable Chips

makes 4 servings

These baked chips are time-consuming to make, but they are addictively delicious. Children love them—especially if they get to help with the prep. Once the slicing is done and the vegetables are tossed with oil, enlist small hands to help arrange them on the baking sheets. You can also make these with rutabagas, turnips, or beets (keep the beets separate from the other vegetables or use golden beets to prevent staining).

2 large carrots, peeled
1 small sweet potato, peeled
1 small baking potato, well scrubbed
2 teaspoons extra virgin olive oil
⅛ teaspoon salt

1 Preheat the oven to 375°F.

2 Using the thin slicing blade on a food processor or a mandolin, cut the carrots and potatoes into ¹/₁₆-inch slices. Place the vegetables in a large bowl, drizzle with the oil, and toss to coat evenly.

3 Arrange the vegetables in a single layer on two large rimmed baking sheets. Bake until the chips are browned, 30 to 35 minutes, checking the chips often during the last 10 minutes of baking. Transfer the chips to a large bowl as they are done. Sprinkle the chips with the salt and toss to coat. The chips are best on the day they are made. If you do store them, they will likely lose their crispness. You can bake them on a baking sheet in a 250°F oven for 6 to 8 minutes to restore their crunch.

Each serving (½ cup): 14 g carb, 81 cal, 2 g fat, 0 g sat fat, 0 mg chol, 2 g fib, 2 g pro, 106 mg sod • Carb Choices: 1; Exchanges: 1 starch, ½ fat

Crispy Baked Garbanzos

HIGH FIBER

makes 8 servings

Keep a close watch on these during the last 10 minutes of baking. They should look dry and some of the garbanzos will begin to split. If they aren't crisp once they've cooled, return the garbanzos to the oven for 5 minutes longer.

3 teaspoons canola oil
2 (15-ounce) cans no-salt-added garbanzos, rinsed and drained
1 teaspoon ground cumin
1 teaspoon ground coriander
¾ teaspoon kosher salt
⅛ teaspoon ground cayenne

1 Preheat the oven to 400°F. Brush a large rimmed baking sheet with 1 teaspoon of the oil.

2 Place the garbanzos between several layers of paper towels and blot dry, discarding any skins that rub off. Transfer the garbanzos to a medium bowl. Add the remaining 2 teaspoons oil, the cumin, coriander, salt, and cayenne and toss to coat.

3 Transfer the garbanzos to the baking sheet and bake, shaking the pan occasionally, until the garbanzos are browned and beginning to split, 45 to 50 minutes. The garbanzos will crisp as they cool. The garbanzos can be stored in an airtight container at room temperature for up to 1 week.

Each serving (¼ cup): 19 g carb, 123 cal, 3 g fat, 0 g sat fat, 0 mg chol, 4 g fib, 6 g pro, 130 mg sod • Carb Choices: 1; Exchanges: 1 starch, 1 plant-based protein

Parmesan Popcorn   QUICK

makes 4 servings

Popcorn is a fun, easy, and inexpensive snack to make at home with plain popcorn kernels. You don't need a microwave, a popcorn popper, or even melted butter to make mouthwatering popcorn. This version uses freshly grated Parmesan to embellish the popped corn, but it's just as delicious without it.

2 teaspoons canola oil
¼ cup popcorn kernels
3 tablespoons freshly grated Parmesan
⅛ teaspoon salt

1 Heat a large saucepan over medium heat. Add the oil and tilt the pan to coat the bottom evenly. Add 4 or 5 popcorn kernels and cover the pan. When the kernels pop, add the remaining popcorn kernels and tilt the pan to coat the kernels. Cover the pan and cook until the popping stops, about 3 minutes.

2 Transfer the popcorn to a large serving bowl. Immediately sprinkle with the Parmesan and the salt and toss to coat. Serve at once.

Each serving (generous 1 cup): 10 g carb, 87 cal, 4 g fat, 1 g sat fat, 3 mg chol, 2 g fib, 3 g pro, 131 mg sod • Carb Choices: ½; Exchanges: ½ starch, ½ fat

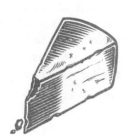

Romano–Black Pepper Biscotti

makes 24 biscotti

This savory version of biscotti will be a hit at your next cocktail party. The best part of this recipe (other than the decadent Pecorino Romano cheese) is that you can make it days ahead.

1½ cups white whole wheat flour or unbleached all-purpose flour

1 ounce freshly grated Pecorino Romano (about ¼ cup)

1 teaspoon baking powder

½ teaspoon salt

¼ teaspoon freshly ground pepper

¼ cup extra virgin olive oil

¼ cup 1% low-fat milk

1 large egg

1 garlic clove, crushed through a press

1 Preheat the oven to 350°F. Line a large baking sheet with parchment paper.

2 Combine the flour, Pecorino Romano, baking powder, salt, and pepper in a large bowl and whisk to mix well. Combine the oil, milk, egg, and garlic in a medium bowl and whisk until smooth.

3 Add the oil mixture to the flour mixture and stir just until the dough is moistened and holds together. Place the dough on the prepared baking sheet, press into a 12-inch log, and press on the log to flatten it slightly.

4 Bake until the top is lightly browned, 25 to 30 minutes. Remove from the baking sheet and transfer to a wire rack. Let cool until just slightly warm, about 20 minutes.

5 Reduce the oven temperature to 325°F.

6 Cut the log diagonally into 24 (½-inch) slices using a serrated knife. Place on a parchment-lined baking sheet and bake 20 minutes. Turn the biscotti and bake until lightly browned, 10 to 15 minutes longer. Remove from the baking sheet and transfer to a wire rack to cool completely. The biscotti can be stored in an airtight container at room temperature for up to 3 days.

Each serving (2 biscotti): 12 g carb, 118 cal, 6 g fat, 1 g sat fat, 21 mg chol, 2 g fib, 4 g pro, 182 mg sod • Carb Choices: 1; Exchanges: 1 starch, 1 fat

Portable Fruit and Nut Snack Mix   QUICK | HIGH FIBER

makes 10 servings

Little bits of dark chocolate make this snack mix taste like a special treat. Be sure to store it in a cool place to keep the chocolate from melting.

1 cup whole raw almonds

1 cup dry-roasted soy nuts

2 ounces excellent quality dark chocolate, coarsely chopped

½ cup dried tart cherries

Combine all the ingredients in a small resealable plastic bag. Store at cool room temperature for up to a month.

Each serving (¼ cup): 14 g carb, 176 cal, 11 g fat, 1 g sat fat, 0 mg chol, 4 g fib, 7 g pro, 0 mg sod • Carb Choices: 1; Exchanges: 1 carb, 2 fat

Pizzas and Sandwiches

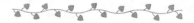

Pizzas

Whole Wheat Pizza Crust

Pizza Sauce

Roasted Red Pepper Pizza Sauce

Pizza with Fresh Tomatoes and Mozzarella

Asparagus and Asiago Pizza with Red Pepper Sauce

Artichoke, Feta, and Olive Pizza

BBQ Chicken Pizza

Sausage and Red Onion Pizza

Prosciutto and Arugula Salad Pizza

Greek Beef and Feta Pizza

Taco Salad Pizza

Caramelized Onion, Apple, and Blue Cheese Pizza

Eggplant and Provolone Pizza with Pesto Sauce

Shrimp and Spinach Pizza

Tomato and Roasted Pepper Phyllo Pizza

Salad-Topped Goat Cheese Lavash Pizza

Quick Tortilla Vegetable Pizzas

Sandwiches

Cilantro Chicken Salad Wraps

Chicken Sandwiches with Mango-Yogurt Sauce

Grilled Chicken, Pear, and Arugula Panini

Peanut-Chicken Pitas

Chicken and Vegetable Wraps with Sun-Dried Tomato-Basil Spread

Chicken Souvlaki Sandwiches

Black Bean and Roasted Red Pepper Quesadillas

Chicken-Cheddar Quesadillas

Middle Eastern Quesadillas

Zucchini and Tomato Quesadillas

Open-Face Turkey Sandwiches with Avocado Butter

Muffuletta-Style Roast Beef Sandwiches

Roast Beef and Apple Pitas with Blue Cheese–Honey Dressing

Steak Sandwiches with Tomato Jam

Greek Steak Sandwiches

Pulled Pork Sandwiches with Apple Slaw

Vietnamese Banh Mi

Lobster Rolls

Catfish Po Boys

Tuna Tartines

Grilled Vegetable and Goat Cheese Sandwiches

Portobello Mushroom, Feta, and Arugula Sandwiches

Open-Face Cheddar and Red Pepper Salad Sandwiches

Grilled Broccoli Rabe, Provolone, and Prosciutto Sandwiches

Serrano Ham and Manchego Picnic Sandwich

Most people think of pizzas and sand-wiches as junk food. They're what you order in when you're too tired to cook, or what you have for lunch when you only have time for a drive-through meal. And since they're both high in carbs, they must certainly be bad news for people with diabetes. Right?

Wrong. Pizzas and sandwiches that you make at home are actually some of the healthiest, most nutritious—and quickest—meals that you can enjoy. Even when you have to watch your carb intake, pizzas and sandwiches are not off limits.

The pizzas you'll find here start with a home-made crust that's so easy it almost makes itself (or you can use a purchased whole wheat crust to save time) and the toppings are combina-tions of lean meats, vegetables, and modest amounts of cheese. There are also pizza reci-pes that use nontraditional crusts like phyllo, whole wheat lavash, and whole wheat tortillas. If they're not already part of your repertoire, tortilla pizzas are a brilliant idea. They make a quick and nutritious snack that your kids will actually eat. Or you can serve them with soup or a salad for a light lunch that you'll love just as much as the little ones do.

When it comes to sandwiches, it's all about the fillings. Or is it all about the bread? No matter which camp you're in, there are deli-cious—and best of all—quick options for healthful lunches and dinners in this chapter. Check out Choosing Whole Wheat Bread (page 66) for tips on buying bread that truly is *whole* wheat. Read Smart-Sizing Rolls, Buns, and Sandwich Breads on page 68 for tips on reining in portion sizes and carb counts when you're making sandwiches. And, if there aren't enough ideas here for you, scan Salads to Make into Sandwiches (page 75) for other recipes in this book that you can use to make sandwiches.

As long as you make smart choices with top-pings and fillings and enjoy a sensible por-tion, pizzas and sandwiches are genuinely healthy fast food.

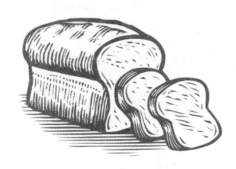

Pizzas

Whole Wheat Pizza Crust

HIGH FIBER

makes 1 (12-inch) crust

This no-fuss crust is simple to make even if you've never made homemade pizza crust. You dump the ingredients in a bowl and stir, then let the dough rise. After an hour, you press the dough into a pizza pan (no kneading) and let it rise again. Then you add the toppings and bake. Most of the work is in the waiting—and this crisp and delicious whole wheat crust is worth the wait.

½ cup lukewarm water
1 package active dry yeast
3 teaspoons extra virgin olive oil, divided
1 teaspoon sugar
1 cup whole wheat flour
¼ cup unbleached all-purpose flour
¼ teaspoon salt
1½ teaspoons fine-grind yellow cornmeal

1 Combine the water, yeast, 1 teaspoon of the oil, and the sugar in a medium bowl and stir until the yeast and sugar dissolve. Let stand 5 minutes. Add the whole wheat flour, all-purpose flour, and salt and stir until a soft dough forms.

2 Brush a medium bowl with 1 teaspoon of the remaining oil. Place the dough in the bowl and turn to coat the top. Cover and let rise in a warm place (85°F), free from drafts, until doubled in size, about 1 hour.

3 Brush a 12-inch pizza pan with the remaining 1 teaspoon oil. Sprinkle the pan with the cornmeal. Shape the dough into a flat disc and place on the prepared pan. Pat the dough to evenly cover the pan. If you have trouble stretching the dough, let it rest 5 minutes, then try again.

4 Cover the dough loosely with lightly oiled plastic wrap and let rise in a warm place (85°F), free from drafts, until doubled in size, about 45 minutes. Follow each recipe to top and bake the pizza.

Each serving (⅛th of crust): 30 g carb, 163 cal, 4 g fat, 1 g sat fat, 0 mg chol, 4 g fib, 6 g pro, 292 mg sod • Carb Choices: 2; Exchanges: 2 starch, ½ fat

Pizza Sauce QUICK

makes ¾ cup

You can easily double or triple this recipe if you make pizza often. It will keep in the refrigerator for a week. Compared to purchased pizza sauce, this one has less than one-quarter of the sodium and none of the added sugar.

2 teaspoons extra virgin olive oil
½ cup diced onion
1 garlic clove, minced
1 (8-ounce) can no-salt-added tomato sauce
⅛ teaspoon dried basil
⅛ teaspoon dried oregano
⅛ teaspoon kosher salt
Pinch of freshly ground pepper

1 Heat a medium skillet over medium heat. Add the oil and tilt the pan to coat the bottom evenly. Add the onion and cook, stirring occasionally, until softened, 5 minutes. Add the garlic and cook, stirring constantly, until fragrant, 30 seconds.

2 Stir in the tomato sauce, basil, oregano, salt, and pepper and bring to a boil over high heat. Reduce the heat to low and simmer until the sauce is slightly thickened, about 8 minutes.

Each serving (3 tablespoons): 6 g carb, 51 cal, 2 g fat, 0 g sat fat, 0 mg chol, 1 g fib, 1 g pro, 42 mg sod • Carb Choices: ½; Exchanges: 1 veg, ½ fat

Roasted Red Pepper Pizza Sauce QUICK

makes ¾ cup

You don't even have to cook to make this fresh vibrant sauce. Prepare a double batch when you make it and keep it in the refrigerator for up to 5 days—it's good on pasta, salmon, shrimp, or chicken breasts. If you have fresh herbs on hand, add 2 tablespoons chopped fresh basil or use 1 teaspoon fresh chopped oregano instead of the dried.

1 cup chopped plum tomatoes
½ cup red Roasted Bell Peppers (page 21) or roasted red peppers from a jar, chopped
1 tablespoon no-salt-added tomato paste
1 small garlic clove, chopped
¼ teaspoon kosher salt
⅛ teaspoon dried oregano
Pinch of freshly ground pepper

Combine all the ingredients in a food processor and process until smooth.

Each serving (3 tablespoons): 3 g carb, 14 cal, 0 g fat, 0 g sat fat, 0 mg chol, 1 g fib, 1 g pro, 73 mg sod • Carb Choices: 0; Exchanges: none

Pizza with Fresh Tomatoes and Mozzarella HIGH FIBER

makes 4 servings

The simplest foods are often the most satisfying and this basic pizza is a perfect example. Even when the only toppings are tomatoes and cheese, pizza is paradise!

1 prepared Whole Wheat Pizza Crust (page 57) or 1 (12-inch) purchased prebaked whole wheat thin pizza crust
1 recipe Pizza Sauce (page 57)
2 plum tomatoes, thinly sliced
3 ounces fresh mozzarella, cut into small cubes, or ¾ cup shredded part-skim mozzarella
4 basil leaves, thinly sliced

1 Position an oven rack on the lowest rung of the oven. Preheat the oven to 450°F.

2 Place the crust on the bottom rack of the oven and bake 5 minutes. Remove the crust from the oven and spread the sauce evenly over the crust, leaving a ½-inch border. Arrange the tomato slices evenly over the sauce in a single layer. Sprinkle with the mozzarella. Bake on the bottom rack until the crust is browned and the cheese melts, about 8 minutes. Sprinkle with the basil, cut into 8 wedges, and serve at once.

Each serving: 37 g carb, 273 cal, 11 g fat, 2 g sat fat, 8 mg chol, 5 g fib, 11 g pro, 205 mg sod • Carb Choices: 2½; Exchanges: 2 starch, 1 veg, 2 fat

Asparagus and Asiago Pizza with Red Pepper Sauce HIGH FIBER

makes 4 servings

Stunning to look at and delectable to eat, this pizza is a delight for the senses. If you are using very thin asparagus spears you don't have to cut them in half lengthwise. You can top the pizza with a few halved cherry tomatoes in addition to the asparagus if you wish.

8 asparagus spears, tough ends trimmed, spears halved lengthwise, and cut into 2-inch pieces
1 prepared Whole Wheat Pizza Crust (page 57) or 1 (12-inch) purchased prebaked whole wheat thin pizza crust
1 recipe Roasted Red Pepper Pizza Sauce (at left)
3 ounces shredded Asiago cheese (about ¾ cup)

1 Position an oven rack on the lowest rung of the oven. Preheat the oven to 450°F.

2 Bring a small pot of water to a boil over high heat. Add the asparagus and cook until crisp-tender, 2 minutes. Drain and pat dry with paper towels.

3 Place the crust on the bottom rack of the oven and bake 5 minutes.

4 Remove the crust from the oven and spread the sauce evenly over the crust, leaving a ½-inch border. Arrange the asparagus evenly over the sauce. Sprinkle with the Asiago. Bake on the bottom rack until the crust is browned and the cheese melts, about 8 minutes. Cut into 8 wedges and serve at once.

Each serving: 35 g carb, 268 cal, 11 g fat, 4 g sat fat, 19 mg chol, 6 g fib, 11 g pro, 425 mg sod • Carb Choices: 2; Exchanges: 2 starch, 1 high-fat protein, 1 fat

Artichoke, Feta, and Olive Pizza HIGH FIBER

makes 4 servings

This pizza grew out of my insistence on keeping the pantry stocked with my favorite ingredients—artichokes and olives. You've probably got all the ingredients you need to make this simple pizza in your pantry, too.

1 cup canned artichoke hearts, drained
1 prepared Whole Wheat Pizza Crust (page 57) or 1 (12-inch) purchased pre-baked whole wheat thin pizza crust
1 recipe Roasted Red Pepper Pizza Sauce (page 58)
2 tablespoons thinly sliced pitted Kalamata olives
2 ounces finely crumbled feta cheese (about ½ cup)

1 Position an oven rack on the lowest rung of the oven. Preheat the oven to 450°F.

2 Cut the artichokes into quarters. Place on several thicknesses of paper towels and gently blot dry. Set aside.

3 Place the crust on the bottom rack of the oven and bake 5 minutes.

4 Remove the crust from the oven and spread the sauce evenly over the crust, leaving a ½-inch border. Arrange the artichokes evenly over the sauce. Sprinkle with the olives, then with the feta. Bake on the bottom rack until the crust is browned and the cheese melts, about 8 minutes. Cut into 8 wedges and serve at once.

Each serving: 37 g carb, 248 cal, 9 g fat, 3 g sat fat, 13 mg chol, 5 g fib, 9 g pro, 579 mg sod • Carb Choices: 2½; Exchanges: 2 starch, 1 veg, 1½ fat

BBQ Chicken Pizza HIGH FIBER

makes 4 servings

This kid-pleasing pizza is only mildly spicy, so if you're serving it to adults only, you might want to double the chipotles. The crisp crust, a slightly sweet sauce, and extra-sharp Cheddar combine to make this one of my favorite pizzas.

2 tablespoons light brown sugar
1 teaspoon white wine vinegar
½ teaspoon minced chipotle in adobo sauce
1 recipe Roasted Red Pepper Pizza Sauce (page 58)
1½ cups shredded cooked chicken breast
1 prepared Whole Wheat Pizza Crust (page 57) or 1 (12-inch) purchased prebaked whole wheat thin pizza crust
¼ cup thinly sliced scallions
3 ounces shredded reduced-fat extra-sharp Cheddar cheese (about ¾ cup)

1 Position an oven rack on the lowest rung of the oven. Preheat the oven to 450°F.

2 Add the sugar, vinegar, and chipotle to the pizza sauce and pulse to combine. Transfer ¼ cup of the sauce to a medium bowl. Add the chicken and toss to coat. Set aside.

3 Place the crust on the bottom rack of the oven and bake 5 minutes.

4 Remove the crust from the oven and spread the remaining sauce evenly over the crust, leaving a ½-inch border. Arrange the chicken mixture evenly over the sauce. Sprinkle with the scallions, then with the Cheddar. Bake on the bottom rack until the crust is browned and the cheese melts, about 8 minutes. Cut into 8 wedges and serve at once.

Each serving: 39 g carb, 365 cal, 11 g fat, 4 g sat fat, 60 mg chol, 5 g fib, 28 g pro, 482 mg sod • Carb Choices: 2½; Exchanges: 2 starch, ½ carb, 1 medium-fat protein, 2 lean protein, 1 fat

Sausage and Red Onion Pizza [HIGH FIBER]

makes 4 servings

Creamy Gouda cheese elevates this pizza to a real treat. Its nutty flavor and smooth texture make it a natural for using on pizza. It's also great with plain old mozzarella.

2 teaspoons extra virgin olive oil
4 ounces Italian turkey sausage
1 small red onion, halved lengthwise and thinly sliced
1 garlic clove, minced
1 prepared Whole Wheat Pizza Crust (page 57) or 1 (12-inch) purchased prebaked whole wheat thin pizza crust
1 recipe Pizza Sauce (page 57)
2 ounces shredded Gouda (about ½ cup)

1 Position an oven rack on the lowest rung of the oven. Preheat the oven to 450°F.

2 Heat a large nonstick skillet over medium heat. Add the oil and tilt the pan to coat the bottom evenly. Remove and discard the sausage casings, crumble the sausage, and add to the skillet. Add the onion and cook, stirring often, until the sausage is browned and the onion is softened, 5 minutes. Add the garlic and cook, stirring constantly, until fragrant, 30 seconds.

3 Place the crust on the bottom rack of the oven and bake 5 minutes.

4 Remove the crust from the oven and spread the sauce evenly over the crust, leaving a ½-inch border. Spoon the sausage mixture evenly over the sauce. Sprinkle with the Gouda. Bake on the bottom rack until the crust is browned and the cheese melts, about 8 minutes. Cut into 8 wedges and serve at once.

Each serving: 37 g carb, 343 cal, 16 g fat, 4 g sat fat, 33 mg chol, 5 g fib, 16 g pro, 485 mg sod • Carb Choices: 2½; Exchanges: 2 starch, 1 veg, 1 high-fat protein, 1 medium-fat protein, 1½ fat

Prosciutto and Arugula Salad Pizza [HIGH FIBER]

makes 4 servings

This pizza is so flavorful from the sharp provolone, the salty ham, and the peppery greens that you can leave off the Pizza Sauce if you want to save a few minutes prep time. Either way, it's a great-tasting play on flavors.

1 prepared Whole Wheat Pizza Crust (page 57) or 1 (12-inch) purchased prebaked whole wheat thin pizza crust
1 recipe Pizza Sauce (page 57)
2 ounces shredded provolone (about ½ cup)
2 ounces prosciutto, cut into thin strips
½ cup grape tomatoes, halved
1½ cups loosely packed baby arugula or mixed baby greens
1 teaspoon red wine vinegar

1 Position an oven rack on the lowest rung of the oven. Preheat the oven to 450°F.

2 Place the crust on the bottom rack of the oven and bake 5 minutes.

3 Remove the crust from the oven and spread the sauce evenly over the crust, leaving a ½-inch border. Sprinkle the provolone evenly over the sauce. Arrange the prosciutto and tomatoes evenly over the cheese. Bake on the bottom rack until the crust is browned and the cheese melts, about 8 minutes.

4 Meanwhile, place the arugula in a medium bowl. Sprinkle with the vinegar and toss to coat.

5 Place the arugula on top of the pizza. Cut into 8 wedges and serve at once.

Each serving: 35 g carb, 300 cal, 12 g fat, 4 g sat fat, 22 mg chol, 5 g fib, 14 g pro, 589 mg sod • Carb Choices: 2; Exchanges: 2 starch, 1 veg, 1 high-fat protein, 1 lean protein, 1 fat

Greek Beef and Feta Pizza

HIGH FIBER

makes 4 servings

Kids will love this pizza—maybe minus the pepperoncini, depending on how adventurous your little ones are. Inexpensive to make, loaded with flavor, and faster and healthier than delivery—this pizza is guaranteed to be a hit.

6 ounces 95% lean ground beef
½ cup diced red onion
1 garlic clove, minced
½ teaspoon ground cumin
½ teaspoon dried oregano
½ cup no-salt-added tomato sauce
1 prepared Whole Wheat Pizza Crust (page 57) or 1 (12-inch) purchased prebaked whole wheat thin pizza crust
1 plum tomato, thinly sliced
2 pepperoncini peppers, thinly sliced
2 ounces finely crumbled feta cheese (about ½ cup)

1 Position an oven rack on the lowest rung of the oven. Preheat the oven to 450°F.

2 Combine the beef, onion, garlic, cumin, and oregano in a medium nonstick skillet. Place over medium-high heat and cook, stirring occasionally, until the beef is browned, about 8 minutes. Add the tomato sauce and bring to a boil. Cook, stirring often, until the mixture is thickened, about 3 minutes.

3 Place the crust on the bottom rack of the oven and bake 5 minutes.

4 Remove the crust from the oven and top evenly with the beef mixture. Arrange the tomato slices evenly on the pizza in a single layer. Sprinkle with the pepperoncini and the feta. Bake until the crust is browned and the cheese melts, about 8 minutes. Cut into 8 wedges and serve at once.

Each serving: 36 g carb, 280 cal, 9 g fat, 4 g sat fat, 37 mg chol, 5 g fib, 17 g pro, 483 mg sod • Carb Choices: 2½; Exchanges: 2 starch, 1 veg, 1 lean protein, 1½ fat

Taco Salad Pizza HIGH FIBER

makes 4 servings

6 ounces 95% lean ground beef
½ cup diced red onion
1 jalapeño, seeded and minced
1 garlic clove, minced
2 teaspoons chili powder
½ teaspoon ground cumin
¼ teaspoon kosher salt
½ cup no-salt-added tomato sauce
1 prepared Whole Wheat Pizza Crust (page 57) or 1 (12-inch) purchased prebaked whole wheat thin pizza crust
1 plum tomato, thinly sliced
3 ounces shredded reduced-fat Monterey Jack cheese (about ¾ cup)
1½ cups thinly sliced romaine lettuce
¼ cup loosely packed fresh cilantro leaves
2 teaspoons lime juice

1 Position an oven rack on the lowest rung of the oven. Preheat the oven to 450°F.

2 Combine the beef, onion, jalapeño, garlic, chili powder, cumin, and salt in a medium nonstick skillet. Place over medium-high heat and cook, stirring until the beef is browned, 8 minutes. Add the tomato sauce and bring to a boil. Cook until thickened, 3 minutes. Set aside.

3 Place the crust on the bottom rack of the oven and bake 5 minutes.

4 Remove the crust from the oven and top with the beef mixture. Arrange the tomato slices on the pizza in a single layer. Sprinkle with the cheese. Bake until the crust is browned, about 8 minutes.

5 Meanwhile, combine the romaine, cilantro, and lime juice in a medium bowl and toss to coat.

6 Place the salad on top of the pizza. Cut into 8 wedges and serve at once.

Each serving: 37 g carb, 319 cal, 11 g fat, 4 g sat fat, 38 mg chol, 6 g fib, 21 g pro, 396 mg sod • Carb Choices: 2; Exchanges: 2 starch, 1 veg, 1 medium-fat protein, 1 lean protein, 1 fat

Caramelized Onion, Apple, and Blue Cheese Pizza HIGH FIBER

makes 4 servings

This grown-up pizza is delicious with a salad of sharp-tasting greens like arugula or watercress. Or cut it into thin wedges and serve it with cocktails or wine. It's fine to serve it at room temperature.

2 teaspoons extra virgin olive oil
1 medium sweet onion, halved lengthwise and thinly sliced
⅛ teaspoon kosher salt
1 prepared Whole Wheat Pizza Crust (page 57) or 1 (12-inch) purchased prebaked whole wheat thin pizza crust
1 medium Granny Smith apple, cored and thinly sliced
1 ounce finely crumbled blue cheese (about ¼ cup)
Pinch of freshly ground pepper
2 tablespoons walnuts, toasted and chopped (page 4)

1 Position an oven rack on the lowest rung of the oven. Preheat the oven to 450°F.

2 Heat a medium nonstick skillet over medium-high heat. Add the oil and tilt the pan to coat the bottom evenly. Add the onion and salt, cover, and cook, stirring often, until the onion begins to soften, about 3 minutes. Uncover and cook, stirring occasionally, until the onion is tender and golden brown, about 10 minutes.

3 Place the crust on the bottom rack of the oven and bake 5 minutes.

4 Remove the crust from the oven and top evenly with the onion. Arrange the apple slices in a single layer over the onion. Sprinkle with the blue cheese and the pepper. Bake on the bottom rack until the crust is browned and the cheese melts, about 8 minutes. Sprinkle with the walnuts. Cut into 8 wedges and serve hot, warm, or at room temperature.

Each serving: 39 g carb, 278 cal, 11 g fat, 2 g sat fat, 5 mg chol, 5 g fib, 8 g pro, 287 mg sod • Carb Choices: 2½; Exchanges: 2 starch, ½ carb, 2 fat

Eggplant and Provolone Pizza with Pesto Sauce

HIGH FIBER

makes 4 servings

This pizza is an explosion of flavors and textures. A crisp crust with earthy wheat flavor, fresh basil pesto sauce, smoky roasted eggplant, and sharp creamy provolone cheese makes this a pizza lover's masterpiece.

3 teaspoons extra virgin olive oil, divided
3 small Japanese (Asian) eggplants
1 prepared Whole Wheat Pizza Crust (page 57) or 1 (12-inch) purchased prebaked whole wheat thin pizza crust
3 tablespoons Basil Pesto (page 597), or purchased pesto
2 ounces shredded provolone (about ½ cup)

1 Position an oven rack on the lowest rung of the oven. Preheat the broiler.

2 Brush a large rimmed baking sheet with 1 teaspoon of the oil. Cut each eggplant lengthwise into ¼-inch slices, discarding the end slices, which have too much skin. Brush the eggplant slices with the remaining 2 teaspoons oil. Arrange the eggplant in a single layer on the prepared baking sheet and broil, turning once, until the eggplant is tender and browned, about 3 minutes on each side. Preheat the oven to 450°F.

3 Place the crust on the bottom rack of the oven and bake 5 minutes.

4 Remove the crust from the oven and spread the sauce evenly over the crust, leaving a ½-inch border. Arrange the eggplant slices in a single

layer over the sauce. Sprinkle with the provolone. Bake on the bottom rack until the crust is browned and the cheese melts, about 8 minutes. Cut into 8 wedges and serve at once.

Each serving: 34 g carb, 314 cal, 17 g fat, 4 g sat fat, 14 mg chol, 6 g fib, 11 g pro, 272 mg sod • Carb Choices: 2; Exchanges: 2 starch, 1 veg, 3 fat

Shrimp and Spinach Pizza

HIGH FIBER

makes 4 servings

You could call this shrimp scampi pizza because of the loads of garlicky shrimp in the topping. Serve it with Bibb and Whole Herb Salad (page 88) for a simple, yet sophisticated supper.

2 teaspoons extra virgin olive oil
2 garlic cloves, minced
6 ounces medium peeled deveined shrimp
¼ teaspoon kosher salt, divided
12 ounces fresh spinach, trimmed and chopped
1 prepared Whole Wheat Pizza Crust (page 57) or 1 (12-inch) purchased prebaked whole wheat thin pizza crust
3 ounces shredded part-skim mozzarella (about ¾ cup)
¼ cup thinly sliced scallions

1 Position an oven rack on the lowest rung of the oven. Preheat the oven to 450°F.

2 Heat a large nonstick skillet over medium-high heat. Add the oil and tilt the pan to coat the bottom evenly. Add the garlic and cook, stirring constantly, until fragrant, 30 seconds. Add the shrimp and ⅛ teaspoon of the salt, and cook, stirring often, just until the shrimp turn pink, about 2 minutes. Transfer to a plate.

3 Add the spinach in batches and the remaining ⅛ teaspoon salt to the skillet and cook, stirring constantly, until the spinach is wilted and most of the liquid has evaporated, about 2 minutes. Drain the spinach.

4 Place the crust on the bottom rack of the oven and bake 5 minutes.

5 Remove the crust from the oven and arrange the shrimp and the spinach evenly over the crust. Sprinkle with the mozzarella and the scallions. Bake on the bottom rack until the crust is browned and the cheese melts, about 8 minutes. Cut into 8 wedges and serve at once.

Each serving: 31 g carb, 298 cal, 11 g fat, 4 g sat fat, 75 mg chol, 5 g fib, 20 g pro, 451 mg sod • Carb Choices: 2; Exchanges: 2 starch, 1 veg, 1 high-fat protein, 1 lean protein, 1 fat

Tomato and Roasted Pepper Phyllo Pizza

makes 4 servings

Keep the pizza in the pan for slicing because the crust makes it very delicate. You can cut the pizza into smaller pieces and serve it as an appetizer. It's almost as good at room temperature as it is hot.

2 teaspoons plus 1 tablespoon extra virgin olive oil, divided
8 (14 x 9-inch) sheets frozen phyllo dough, thawed
⅓ cup freshly grated Parmesan
¾ cup chopped plum tomatoes
¾ cup red Roasted Bell Peppers (page 21) or roasted red peppers from a jar, cut into short, thin strips
3 ounces shredded part-skim mozzarella (about ¾ cup)
¼ cup thinly sliced scallions
¼ cup chopped fresh basil

1 Preheat the oven to 375°F. Brush a large rimmed baking sheet with 2 teaspoons of the oil.

2 Unroll the phyllo and place one sheet in the prepared pan. Brush the phyllo lightly with some of the remaining 1 tablespoon of oil. Sprinkle the phyllo with about 2 teaspoons of the Parmesan. Repeat

continues on next page

the layering with the remaining phyllo, oil, and Parmesan. Brush the top layer of the phyllo with oil.

3 Sprinkle the phyllo evenly with the tomatoes and roasted pepper, then with the mozzarella and scallions. Bake until the crust is well browned and the cheese melts, 18 to 20 minutes. Sprinkle with the basil. Cut into 12 pieces and serve hot, warm, or at room temperature.

Each serving: 25 g carb, 276 cal, 14 g fat, 5 g sat fat, 17 mg chol, 2 g fib, 11 g pro, 402 mg sod • Carb Choices: 1½; Exchanges: 1 starch, 1 veg, 1 high-fat protein, 1½ fat

Salad-Topped Goat Cheese Lavash Pizza QUICK

makes 4 servings

If you can't find lavash bread, you can make this recipe using four 6-inch whole wheat tortillas (be sure to take the extra carbs into account). This makes a fresh light lunch or dinner in the middle of summer.

1 whole wheat lavash bread (about 18 x 14 inches)
2 teaspoons extra virgin olive oil
3 ounces crumbled goat cheese (about ¾ cup)
1 cup grape tomatoes, halved
¼ cup green olives, pitted and coarsely chopped
4 cups loosely packed mixed baby greens, baby spinach, or baby arugula
2 teaspoons white wine vinegar
Pinch of freshly ground pepper

1 Position an oven rack on the lowest rung of the oven for baking the pizza. Preheat the broiler.

2 Brush the lavash on both sides with the oil and place the lavash on a large baking sheet. Broil until the lavash is just barely beginning to brown and crisp, 45 seconds to 1 minute per side. Preheat the oven to 450°F.

3 Sprinkle the lavash evenly with the goat cheese, tomatoes, and olives. Bake on the

lowest oven rack until the lavash is crisp and the cheese just begins to melt, 5 to 7 minutes.

4 Toss together the greens, vinegar, and pepper in a medium bowl. Arrange on top of the baked pizza and serve at once.

Each serving: 20 g carb, 199 cal, 10 g fat, 5 g sat fat, 17 mg chol, 2 g fib, 8 g pro, 355 mg sod • Carb Choices: 1; Exchanges: 1 starch, 1 veg, 1 high-fat protein, 2 fat

Quick Tortilla Vegetable Pizzas QUICK HIGH FIBER

makes 2 servings

This recipe is more of an idea than a strict recipe. It's quick and easy to make with whatever ingredients you have on hand. Use any quick-cooking vegetables (try thinly sliced zucchini or yellow squash, bell peppers, or scallions), add leftover shredded chicken or turkey, or spread the tortillas with a thin layer of hummus or fat-free refried beans. The possibilities are endless.

2 (6-inch) whole wheat tortillas
1 ounce shredded part-skim mozzarella (about ¼ cup)
½ cup thinly sliced white mushrooms
½ cup chopped plum tomatoes
2 tablespoons diced red onion
Pinch of freshly ground pepper

1 Preheat the broiler.

2 Place the tortillas on a baking sheet and broil just until beginning to brown and crisp, about 1 minute on each side. Preheat the oven to 450°F.

3 Sprinkle the tortillas evenly with the mozzarella, then sprinkle with the mushrooms, tomatoes, and onion. Sprinkle with the pepper. Bake until the tortillas are crisp and the cheese melts, 4 to 5 minutes. Serve at once.

Each serving: 17 g carb, 142 cal, 5 g fat, 2 g sat fat, 8 mg chol, 9 g fib, 8 g pro, 321 mg sod • Carb Choices: 1; Exchanges: 1 starch, 1 fat

Sandwiches

Cilantro Chicken Salad Wraps QUICK | HIGH FIBER

makes 4 servings

You can use this technique to turn any kind of chunky salad—egg salad, tuna salad, or ham salad—into a sandwich wrap. Place leaf lettuce (you can use Bibb or romaine, too) on top of the tortillas, then top with thinly sliced tomatoes. Top the tomatoes with the salad of your choice and roll it up. These sturdy sandwiches are perfect to pack for lunch.

2 tablespoons mayonnaise
2 tablespoons plain low-fat yogurt
½ teaspoon grated lime zest
1 tablespoon lime juice
1 jalapeño, seeded and minced
1 small garlic clove, minced
⅛ teaspoon ground cumin
½ teaspoon kosher salt
12 ounces chopped cooked chicken breast (about 2 cups)
2 tablespoons minced red onion
2 tablespoons chopped fresh cilantro
4 (8-inch) whole wheat flour tortillas
4 large leaves leaf lettuce
2 plum tomatoes, thinly sliced

1 Stir together the mayonnaise, yogurt, lime zest, lime juice, jalapeño, garlic, cumin, and salt in a medium bowl. Add the chicken, onion, and cilantro and stir to mix well.

2 Top each of the tortillas with a lettuce leaf, then top the lettuce evenly with the tomato slices. Top evenly with the chicken mixture and roll up. Cut each roll in half.

Each serving: 26 g carb, 359 cal, 13 g fat, 3 g sat fat, 75 mg chol, 6 g fib, 32 g pro, 607 mg sod • Carb Choices: 2; Exchanges: 1½ starch, 1 veg, 2 fat

Chicken Sandwiches with Mango-Yogurt Sauce QUICK | HIGH FIBER

makes 4 servings

You could have an ordinary chicken sandwich, or with a couple extra minutes spent to make an Indian-inspired spice mix and a fruity yogurt sauce, you can have an exotic meal.

1 teaspoon ground cumin
½ teaspoon ground turmeric
½ teaspoon kosher salt
¼ teaspoon ground cinnamon
¼ teaspoon freshly ground pepper
4 (4-ounce) boneless skinless chicken breasts
2 teaspoons canola oil
2 tablespoons plain low-fat Greek yogurt or strained yogurt (page 11)
2 tablespoons mango chutney, finely minced
½ teaspoon grated orange zest
½ teaspoon hot sauce
4 whole wheat kaiser rolls
½ hothouse (English) cucumber, thinly sliced
¼ cup thinly sliced red onion

1 Stir together the cumin, turmeric, salt, cinnamon, and pepper in a small dish. Transfer ½ teaspoon of the spice mixture to a separate small bowl. Sprinkle the chicken with the remaining spice mixture.

2 Heat a large skillet over medium heat. Add the oil and tilt the pan to coat the bottom evenly. Add the chicken and cook, turning once, until the juices run clear, about 4 minutes on each side.

3 Meanwhile, stir the yogurt, chutney, orange zest, and hot sauce into the reserved spice mixture.

4 Spread the cut sides of the rolls evenly with the yogurt mixture. Place the chicken breasts cucumber, and onion on bottoms of rolls. Cover with the top half of each roll and serve at once.

Each serving: 30 g carb, 293 cal, 7 g fat, 1 g sat fat, 63 mg chol, 4 g fib, 28 g pro, 440 mg sod • Carb Choices: 2; Exchanges: 1½ starch, ½ carb, 3 lean protein, ½ fat

Choosing Whole Wheat Bread

One-hundred-percent whole wheat bread is made with flour that contains the bran, germ, and endosperm of the wheat grains. White flour, also known as enriched flour or all-purpose flour, has had these stripped away from the grains before they are ground into flour. Because 100% whole wheat bread still contains the whole grains of wheat, it is a good source of healthful fiber, vitamins, minerals, and antioxidants.

For many people, bread and breakfast cereals are the easiest way to incorporate whole grains into meals. These two food items do not require cooking, whereas other whole grains such as brown rice, corn, oats, barley, or quinoa require time spent in the kitchen.

Making the choice between white bread and whole wheat bread is a nutritional no-brainer. But how do you make the best selection of whole wheat bread when you're faced with an aisle of options at the supermarket?

Look at the ingredient list when you buy bread, not the splashy wording on the front of the label. The front of the package might say "6-grain wheat bread," "100% natural," "high-fiber," or "organic." The bread may be all those things, but none of those words means that the bread is made with 100% whole wheat flour.

The first ingredient in the ingredient list, and the only flour ingredient listed, should be "whole wheat flour" or "100% whole wheat flour." The word "whole" must be there if the bread is made from whole grain wheat.

If the bread is labeled "whole grain," it can be made with some whole wheat flour and some white flour, as well as other whole grains, such as oats, rye, millet, or buckwheat. As long as there is a small amount of whole grain in the bread, it can be labeled "whole grain." If the words "enriched flour" are in the ingredient list, this means that there is white flour in the bread. Ideally, the only other ingredients in the list other than whole wheat flour should be yeast, salt, and water. Any other ingredients are there to act as dough stabilizers, conditioners, or preservatives.

Something else to look at while you're checking the bread label is sodium. Most people are shocked to find that many breads are high in sodium. Try to buy bread that has less than 150 milligrams of sodium per slice. This amount allows for bread that tastes good (because salt-free bread tastes awful), yet it's still easy to enjoy the bread as part of a moderate sodium diet. (The American Heart Association recommends less than 1,500 milligrams of sodium each day.) Of course, you can make your own whole wheat bread (page 522).

Grilled Chicken, Pear, and Arugula Panini QUICK | HIGH FIBER

makes 4 servings

Gruyère cheese elevates anything to a gourmet meal—even a sandwich. And it's so flavorful, you only need a tiny amount to get a big punch of flavor. If you prefer not to make these as panini, simply put the ingredients on any sturdy toasted wheat bread.

4 (4-ounce) boneless skinless chicken breasts
2 tablespoons Dijon mustard, divided
¼ teaspoon freshly ground pepper
1 teaspoon canola oil, divided
1 (8-ounce) loaf whole wheat ciabatta
1 pear, cored and thinly sliced
2 ounces shredded Gruyère (about ½ cup)
1 cup baby arugula

1 Brush the chicken with 1 tablespoon of the mustard and sprinkle with the pepper. Heat a large grill pan over medium-high heat. Brush the pan with ½ teaspoon of the oil.

2 Place the chicken in the grill pan and grill, turning often, until the juices of the chicken run clear, 8 to 10 minutes. Transfer the chicken to a cutting board and cut into thin slices.

3 Cut the ciabatta in half crosswise, then cut each piece in half lengthwise. Remove and discard the soft inner crumbs from each piece of bread. Spread the cut sides of the bread evenly with the remaining 1 tablespoon mustard. Arrange the chicken evenly on the bottom halves of the bread. Top evenly with the pear slices, then with the Gruyère. Cover with the top half of each piece of bread.

4 Wipe out the grill pan with paper towels and set over medium heat. Brush the pan with the remaining ½ teaspoon oil. Place the sandwiches in the pan and top with a heavy skillet. Cook, turning once, until well browned on each side, 4 to 5 minutes. Remove the top halves of the bread and top evenly with the arugula. Replace the top halves of the bread. Cut each sandwich in half and serve at once.

Each serving: 28 g carb, 337 cal, 10 g fat, 4 g sat fat, 78 mg chol, 4 g fib, 32 g pro, 452 mg sod • Carb Choices: 2; Exchanges: 1½ starch, ½ fruit, 1 high-fat protein, 3 lean protein

Peanut-Chicken Pitas

QUICK | HIGH FIBER

makes 4 servings

The addictive Peanut Sauce (page 594) and gingery chicken makes this a sandwich that will appeal to everyone. If you have small children, they will find these sandwiches delightful if you serve them in mini whole wheat pita breads.

4 (4-ounce) boneless skinless chicken breasts
2 teaspoons minced fresh ginger
1 garlic clove, minced
¼ teaspoon kosher salt
2 teaspoons canola oil
4 (6-inch) whole wheat pita breads, warmed and halved
1 cup alfalfa sprouts
4 radishes, thinly sliced
½ hothouse (English) cucumber, thinly sliced
1 recipe Peanut Sauce (page 594)
2 tablespoons unsalted dry-roasted peanuts, chopped

1 Sprinkle the chicken with the ginger, garlic, and salt.

2 Heat a large skillet over medium heat. Add the oil and tilt the pan to coat the bottom evenly. Add the chicken and cook until the juices run clear, about 4 minutes on each side. Transfer the chicken to a cutting board and thinly slice.

3 Fill the pita bread halves evenly with the alfalfa sprouts, then with the sliced chicken. Top evenly with the radishes and cucumbers. Drizzle each half evenly with the sauce and sprinkle with the peanuts. Serve at once.

Each serving: 32 g carb, 413 cal, 16 g fat, 2 g sat fat, 63 mg chol, 5 g fib, 33 g pro, 578 mg sod • Carb Choices: 2; Exchanges: 2 starch, 3 lean protein, 2 fat

Smart-Sizing Rolls, Buns, and Sandwich Breads

In case you hadn't noticed, sandwich rolls and buns have been supersized along with most other foods in the supermarket. Like everything else, you become accustomed to them being big, and think that's the norm. Just because a roll or a bun weighs almost 4 ounces and is the size of a salad plate does not mean that it's a wise choice to eat the entire thing.

You have options to turn these carb overloads into smart-size portions. The easiest thing to do is simply cut the roll or bun in half and turn it into two servings. You can also cut a thin slice from the top using a serrated knife, then turn it over and cut a thin slice from the bottom. Discard the middle, turn it into breadcrumbs to use in a recipe, or feed it to the birds. Even if a bun or roll is a sensible size, you can cut the carbs by pulling out the soft inner crumbs of the bread. You'll still be left with plenty of sturdy bread to hold your sandwich fillings together.

When choosing sliced bread for a sandwich, buy thin-sliced whole wheat bread. If you buy from a bakery that slices bread to order, ask them to slice the bread as thinly as possible. And, if you buy unsliced loaves of bread, you can cut thin slices yourself using a sharp serrated knife.

Chicken and Vegetable Wraps with Sun-Dried Tomato-Basil Spread

QUICK | HIGH FIBER

makes 4 servings

Flavor-packed tomato spread makes these sandwiches truly special. You can use the spread on any sandwich or serve it as a vegetable dip.

¼ cup dry-packed sun-dried tomatoes, minced
¼ cup water
4 ounces reduced-fat cream cheese, softened
¼ teaspoon kosher salt, divided
¼ teaspoon freshly ground pepper, divided
2 tablespoons chopped fresh basil
2 teaspoons extra virgin olive oil
3 (4-ounce) boneless skinless chicken breasts
4 (8-inch) whole wheat flour tortillas
8 leaves Bibb lettuce
½ hothouse (English) cucumber, very thinly sliced

1 Combine the tomatoes and water in a small saucepan. Set over medium heat and bring to a boil over high heat. Remove from the heat, cover, and let stand 15 minutes. Drain the tomatoes.

2 Combine the tomatoes, cream cheese, ⅛ teaspoon of the salt, and ⅛ teaspoon of the pepper in a small bowl and stir until smooth. Stir in the basil.

3 Meanwhile, sprinkle the chicken with the remaining ⅛ teaspoon salt and remaining ⅛ teaspoon pepper. Heat a large nonstick skillet over medium-high heat. Add the oil and tilt the pan to coat the bottom evenly.

4 Add the chicken and cook until the juices run clear, 4 minutes on each side. Cut into thin slices.

5 Spread each tortilla with a generous tablespoon of cream cheese mixture. Top with the lettuce leaves, cucumber slices, and chicken. Roll up and cut each roll in half.

Each serving: 28 g carb, 343 cal, 14 g fat, 6 g sat fat, 63 mg chol, 6 g fib, 26 g pro, 727 mg sod • Carb Choices: 1½; Exchanges: 1½ starch, 2 lean protein, 2 fat

Chicken Souvlaki Sandwiches QUICK | HIGH FIBER

makes 4 servings

4 (4-ounce) boneless skinless chicken breasts, thinly sliced
2 garlic cloves, minced
½ teaspoon dried oregano
½ teaspoon kosher salt
¼ teaspoon freshly ground pepper
3 teaspoons extra virgin olive oil, divided
1 yellow or red bell pepper, thinly sliced
1 sweet onion, halved lengthwise and sliced
2 teaspoons grated lemon zest
1 tablespoon lemon juice
4 (6-inch) whole wheat pita breads, warmed and halved
2 plum tomatoes, sliced
8 Bibb lettuce leaves
1 recipe Tzatziki (page 40)

1 Toss together the chicken, garlic, oregano, salt, and pepper in a medium bowl.

2 Heat a large skillet over medium heat. Add 2 teaspoons of the oil and tilt the pan to coat the bottom evenly. Add the chicken and cook, stirring often, until the juices run clear, about 8 minutes. Transfer to a plate.

3 Add the remaining 1 teaspoon oil to the skillet and tilt the pan to coat the bottom evenly. Add the bell pepper and onion and cook, stirring often, until just crisp-tender, about 3 minutes. Return the chicken to the skillet and cook until heated through, 2 minutes. Remove from the heat and stir in the lemon zest and lemon juice.

4 Fill the pita bread halves with the lettuce, then with the chicken mixture and the tomatoes. Serve the tzatziki on the side for drizzling.

Each serving: 31 g carb, 324 cal, 8 g fat, 2 g sat fat, 65 mg chol, 5 g fib, 31 g pro, 485 mg sod • Carb Choices: 2; Exchanges: 1½ starch, 2 veg, 3 lean protein, 1 fat

Black Bean and Roasted Red Pepper Quesadillas

QUICK | HIGH FIBER

makes 2 servings

These quesadillas make a great-tasting "emergency meal" from basic pantry staples. Serve them with a green salad and a cup of soup or chili and you've got a satisfying supper in no time flat.

½ cup canned no-salt-added black beans, rinsed and drained
¼ cup red Roasted Bell Peppers (page 21) or roasted red peppers from a jar, chopped
1 ounce shredded reduced-fat Monterey Jack cheese (about ¼ cup)
2 tablespoons thinly sliced scallion
2 tablespoons chopped fresh cilantro
4 (6-inch) whole wheat flour tortillas
1 teaspoon canola oil
½ cup Fresh Tomato Salsa (page 41) or purchased salsa

1 Combine the beans, roasted peppers, Monterey Jack, scallion, and cilantro in a medium bowl and stir to mix well.

2 Brush one side of each of the tortillas with the oil. Place two of the tortillas oiled side down on a work surface. Top the tortillas evenly with the bean mixture. Cover with the remaining two tortillas, oiled side up.

3 Heat a large nonstick skillet over medium-high heat. Add one of the quesadillas and cook until the tortillas are lightly browned and the cheese melts, about 2 minutes on each side. Repeat with the remaining quesadilla. Cut the quesadillas into wedges and serve each one with ¼ cup of the salsa.

Each serving: 35 g carb, 317 cal, 12 g fat, 5 g sat fat, 13 mg chol, 20 g fib, 14 g pro, 701 mg sod • Carb Choices: 2; Exchanges: 2 starch, 1 veg, 2 fat

Chicken-Cheddar Quesadillas QUICK | HIGH FIBER

makes 2 servings

Quesadillas are a go-to dish for quick lunches and dinners. And just because they are quick doesn't mean they're not healthy or tasty. Using whole wheat tortillas, lean meats, canned or dried beans, and reduced-fat cheeses makes them healthful, filling, and delicious.

3 ounces chopped cooked chicken breast (about ½ cup)
1 ounce shredded reduced-fat sharp Cheddar cheese (about ¼ cup)
2 tablespoons thinly sliced scallion
2 tablespoons chopped fresh cilantro
½ teaspoon chili powder
4 (6-inch) whole wheat flour tortillas
1 teaspoon canola oil
1 cup loosely packed fresh baby spinach
½ cup Fresh Tomato Salsa (page 41) or purchased salsa

1 Combine the chicken, Cheddar, scallion, cilantro, and chili powder in a medium bowl and stir to mix well.

2 Brush one side of each of the tortillas with the oil. Place 2 of the tortillas oiled side down on a work surface. Top the tortillas evenly with the chicken mixture, then top evenly with the spinach. Cover with the remaining 2 tortillas, oiled side up.

3 Heat a large nonstick skillet over medium-high heat. Add 1 of the quesadillas and cook until the tortillas are lightly browned and the cheese melts, about 2 minutes on each side. Repeat with the remaining quesadilla. Cut the quesadillas into wedges and serve each one with ¼ cup of the salsa.

Each serving: 26 g carb, 319 cal, 13 g fat, 4 g sat fat, 49 mg chol, 17 g fib, 23 g pro, 640 mg sod • Carb Choices: 1; Exchanges: 1 starch, 2 lean protein, 2 fat

Middle Eastern Quesadillas

QUICK | HIGH FIBER

makes 2 servings

Who says quesadillas have to have Tex-Mex flavors and Middle Eastern food must be served with pita? Here cultures blend beautifully—tortillas are filled with hummus, roasted peppers, and feta—and it tastes fantastic. A sprinkle of chopped tomato and cucumber adds a colorful and crunchy touch to the finished quesadillas.

4 (6-inch) whole wheat flour tortillas
1 teaspoon canola oil
½ cup Hummus (page 35) or purchased hummus
¼ cup red Roasted Bell Peppers (page 21) or roasted red peppers from a jar, chopped
1 ounce finely crumbled feta cheese (about ¼ cup)
2 tablespoons thinly sliced scallion

1 Brush one side of each of the tortillas with the oil. Place 2 of the tortillas oiled side down on a work surface. Spread the tortillas evenly with the hummus, then top evenly with the roasted peppers, feta, and scallion. Cover with the remaining two tortillas, oiled side up.

2 Heat a large nonstick skillet over medium-high heat. Add 1 of the quesadillas and cook until the tortillas are lightly browned and the filling is heated through, about 2 minutes on each side. Repeat with the remaining quesadilla. Cut the quesadillas into wedges and serve at once.

Each serving: 35 g carb, 337 cal, 16 g fat, 6 g sat fat, 17 mg chol, 20 g fib, 14 g pro, 879 mg sod • Carb Choices: 1½; Exchanges: 1½ starch, ½ plant-based protein, 2 fat

Zucchini and Tomato Quesadillas QUICK HIGH FIBER

makes 2 servings

When you've run out of ideas for using zucchini in the summer, try these unusual and delicious quesadillas for lunch. They cook in just a few minutes so making them won't heat up the kitchen on a hot summer day.

2 teaspoons extra virgin olive oil, divided
2 cups shredded zucchini
1 garlic clove, minced
¼ teaspoon kosher salt
2 tablespoons chopped fresh basil
4 (6-inch) whole wheat flour tortillas
½ cup chopped plum tomatoes
1 ounce shredded part-skim mozzarella
    (about ¼ cup)

1 Heat a large nonstick skillet over medium-high heat. Add 1 teaspoon of the oil and tilt the pan to coat the bottom evenly. Add the zucchini, garlic, and salt and cook, stirring often, just until the zucchini begins to brown, about 5 minutes. Remove from the heat and stir in the basil.

2 Brush one side of each of the tortillas with the remaining 1 teaspoon oil. Place 2 of the tortillas oiled side down on a work surface. Spread the tortillas evenly with the zucchini mixture, then top evenly with the tomatoes and cheese. Cover with the remaining 2 tortillas, oiled side up.

3 Wipe out the skillet with paper towels. Heat the skillet over medium-high heat. Add 1 of the quesadillas and cook until the tortillas are lightly browned and the filling is heated through, about 2 minutes on each side. Repeat with the remaining quesadilla. Cut the quesadillas into wedges and serve at once.

Each serving: 29 g carb, 267 cal, 12 g fat, 5 g sat fat, 8 mg chol, 18 g fib, 11 g pro, 666 mg sod • Carb Choices: 1; Exchanges: 1 starch, 1½ fat

Open-Face Turkey Sandwiches with Avocado Butter QUICK HIGH FIBER

makes 4 servings

Turn leftover turkey into something unrecognizable with these sandwiches. Topped with creamy avocado butter, sweet red peppers, and crisp greens, this is an impressive turkey sandwich. Keep the avocado butter in mind and serve it as an accompaniment when you need to dress up plain grilled fish or chicken in a hurry.

½ avocado, pitted, peeled, and
    chopped
2 teaspoons lemon juice
⅛ teaspoon kosher salt
Pinch of freshly ground pepper
1 tablespoon chopped fresh basil
4 thin slices whole wheat bread, toasted
1½ cups mixed baby greens, baby spinach, or
    baby arugula
12 ounces thinly sliced cooked skinless turkey
    breast
¾ cup red Roasted Bell Peppers (page 21)
    or roasted red peppers from a jar, thinly
    sliced

1 Place the avocado in a shallow bowl and mash with a fork until smooth. Add the lemon juice, salt, and ground pepper and stir until blended. Stir in the basil.

2 Spread the avocado mixture evenly over one side of each slice of the bread. Place the bread on 4 plates. Top with the greens, then with the turkey. Top evenly with the roasted peppers and serve at once.

Each serving: 21 g carb, 256 cal, 5 g fat, 1 g sat fat, 71 mg chol, 5 g fib, 31 g pro, 222 mg sod • Carb Choices: 1½; Exchanges: 1 starch, ½ carb, 4 lean protein, ½ fat

Muffuletta-Style Roast Beef Sandwiches QUICK

makes 4 servings

The olive relish in this sandwich is what is served on traditional New Orleans cold cuts and cheese sandwiches. It can turn any ordinary sandwich into a masterpiece. Serve these sandwiches with a simple slaw such as Lemon–Poppy Seed Slaw (page 90).

¼ cup pimento-stuffed green olives, finely chopped

¼ cup red Roasted Bell Peppers (page 21) or roasted red peppers from a jar, finely chopped

¼ cup diced celery

1 tablespoon chopped fresh Italian parsley

1 teaspoon red wine vinegar

1 teaspoon extra virgin olive oil

1 small garlic clove, minced

¼ teaspoon dried oregano

1 (8-ounce) loaf whole wheat ciabatta

8 ounces thinly sliced rare roast beef

4 (½-ounce) slices Swiss cheese

2 plum tomatoes, thinly sliced

1½ cups thinly sliced romaine lettuce or fresh spinach

1 Stir together the olives, roasted peppers, celery, parsley, vinegar, oil, garlic, and oregano in a small bowl.

2 Cut the ciabatta in half crosswise, then cut each piece in half lengthwise. Remove and discard the soft inner crumbs from each piece of bread. Spread half of the olive mixture on the bottom halves of the bread. Top evenly with the beef and Swiss cheese, then with the remaining half of the olive mixture. Top with the tomatoes and lettuce. Cover with the top half of each piece of bread. Cut each sandwich in half and serve at once.

Each serving: 28 g carb, 314 cal, 11 g fat, 4 g sat fat, 44 mg chol, 2 g fib, 25 g pro, 452 mg sod • Carb Choices: 2; Exchanges: 2 starch, 1 veg, 2 lean protein, 1 fat

Roast Beef and Apple Pitas with Blue Cheese–Honey Dressing QUICK HIGH FIBER

makes 4 servings

From the ordinary list of ingredients, you wouldn't think this is a great sandwich—but it is. Salty blue cheese, sweet honey, crunchy tart apple, and hearty slices of roast beef come together to make a unique and flavorful sandwich.

1 tablespoon honey

1 tablespoon white wine vinegar

1 tablespoon apple juice or orange juice

1 tablespoon extra virgin olive oil

⅛ teaspoon kosher salt

⅛ teaspoon freshly ground pepper

2 tablespoons finely crumbled blue cheese

4 (6-inch) whole wheat pita breads, warmed and halved

2 cups loosely packed arugula or 4 large leaves Bibb lettuce

12 ounces thinly sliced rare roast beef

1 large Granny Smith apple, cored and thinly sliced

1 To make the dressing, whisk together the honey, vinegar, apple juice, oil, salt, and pepper in a small bowl. Stir in the blue cheese.

2 Fill the pita bread halves evenly with the arugula, then with the beef and apple slices. Drizzle each half evenly with the dressing and serve at once.

Each serving: 37 g carb, 346 cal, 11 g fat, 3 g sat fat, 78 mg chol, 11 g fib, 32 g pro, 388 mg sod • Carb Choices: 2; Exchanges: 1½ starch, ½ fruit, 3 lean protein, 1 fat

Steak Sandwiches with Tomato Jam HIGH FIBER

makes 4 servings

Fancy greens and a homemade jam smarten up an ordinary steak sandwich. If you don't have time to prepare the Tomato Jam, you can make Fresh Tomato Vinaigrette (page 138) for a quicker alternative.

1 teaspoon grated lemon zest
2 tablespoons lemon juice
3 teaspoons extra virgin olive oil, divided
1 garlic clove, minced
1 (1-pound) flank steak, trimmed of all visible fat
½ teaspoon kosher salt
⅛ teaspoon freshly ground pepper
4 (½-inch) diagonally cut slices whole wheat
    Italian bread, toasted
2 cups loosely packed arugula
½ cup Tomato Jam (page 599)

1 Stir together the lemon zest, lemon juice, 1 teaspoon of the oil, and the garlic in a large shallow dish. Add the steak and turn to coat. Cover and refrigerate at least 6 hours or up to 12 hours.

2 Sprinkle the steak with the salt and pepper. Heat a large heavy-bottomed skillet over medium-high heat. Add the remaining 2 teaspoons oil and tilt the pan to coat the bottom evenly. Add the steak and cook, turning once, 4 minutes on each side for medium-rare, or to the desired degree of doneness.

3 Transfer the steak to a cutting board, cover loosely with foil, and let stand 5 minutes. Cut across the grain into thin slices.

4 Place the bread on each of 4 plates. Top each slice with ½ cup of the arugula. Top evenly with the steak. Top the steak evenly with the jam and serve at once.

Each serving: 27 g carb, 337 cal, 13 g fat, 4 g sat fat, 43 mg chol, 4 g fib, 29 g pro, 348 mg sod • Carb Choices: 2; Exchanges: 1 starch, 1 carb, 3 medium-fat protein, ½ fat

Greek Steak Sandwiches

QUICK

makes 4 servings

These open-face sandwiches are a filling and substantial low-carb option. Piled high with flavorful steak and drizzled with creamy yogurt sauce, these sandwiches won't have you missing that extra slice of bread.

1 (1-pound) flank steak, trimmed of all visible fat
¼ teaspoon kosher salt
⅛ teaspoon freshly ground pepper
2 teaspoons canola oil
½ cup plain low-fat yogurt
2 teaspoons grated lemon zest
4 (½-inch) diagonally cut slices whole wheat
    Italian bread, toasted
2 cups thinly sliced romaine lettuce
2 plum tomatoes, sliced
½ hothouse (English) cucumber, thinly sliced
4 pepperoncini peppers, drained and thinly sliced
1 ounce finely crumbled feta cheese
    (about ¼ cup)

1 Sprinkle the steak with the salt and pepper. Heat a large heavy-bottomed skillet over medium-high heat. Add the oil and tilt the pan to coat the bottom evenly. Add the steak and cook, turning once, 4 minutes on each side for medium-rare, or to the desired degree of doneness.

2 Transfer the steak to a cutting board, cover loosely with foil, and let stand 5 minutes. Cut across the grain into thin slices.

3 Meanwhile, stir together the yogurt and lemon zest in a small bowl.

4 Place the bread on each of 4 plates. Top each slice evenly with the lettuce, tomatoes, cucumber, and pepperoncini. Top evenly with the steak, drizzle with the yogurt mixture, and sprinkle with the feta. Serve at once.

Each serving: 13 g carb, 281 cal, 13 g fat, 5 g sat fat, 57 mg chol, 2 g fib, 29 g pro, 398 mg sod • Carb Choices: 1; Exchanges: 1 starch, 3 lean protein, 1 fat

Pulled Pork Sandwiches with Apple Slaw [HIGH FIBER]

makes 6 servings

Using lean pork tenderloin to make these sandwiches means they are low in fat and they are quick to make, since the tenderloin does not have to simmer for hours to become tender. The apple slaw is a tart counterpoint to the sweet sauce on the pork.

PULLED PORK

1 (8-ounce) can no-salt-added tomato sauce

¼ cup apple cider vinegar

¼ cup water

3 tablespoons light brown sugar

1 garlic clove, crushed through a press

½ teaspoon kosher salt

1 teaspoon chili powder

⅛ teaspoon ground cayenne

1 pound pork tenderloin, trimmed of all visible fat

SLAW

1½ cups thinly sliced green cabbage

1 small Granny Smith apple, peeled, cored, and coarsely grated

1 tablespoon mayonnaise

½ teaspoon apple cider vinegar

¼ teaspoon kosher salt

Pinch freshly ground pepper

6 whole wheat buns, toasted

1 To make the sandwiches, combine the tomato sauce, vinegar, water, sugar, garlic, salt, chili powder, and cayenne in a large saucepan and stir to mix well. Cut the pork into quarters lengthwise, then cut into 1-inch pieces. Add the pork to the tomato sauce mixture. Set over medium-high heat and bring to a boil over high heat. Cover, reduce the heat to low, and simmer until the pork is very tender, about 45 minutes. Transfer the pork to a medium bowl using a slotted spoon.

2 Increase the heat to medium-high and bring the tomato sauce mixture to a boil. Cook, stirring occasionally, until the sauce is reduced to about ½ cup, 10 to 12 minutes.

3 Shred the pork into small pieces using your fingers. Return the pork to the saucepan and stir to coat with the sauce. Cook just until heated through, about 2 minutes.

4 Meanwhile, to make the slaw, combine the cabbage, apple, mayonnaise, vinegar, salt, and pepper in a medium bowl and stir to mix well. Cover and refrigerate until ready to serve.

5 Fill the buns evenly with the pork mixture, top evenly with the slaw, and serve at once.

Each serving: 37 g carb, 285 cal, 7 g fat, 2 g sat fat, 50 mg chol, 5 g fib, 21 g pro, 417 mg sod • Carb Choices: 2½; Exchanges: 1½ starch, ½ carb, 1 veg, 2 lean protein, ½ fat

Vietnamese Banh Mi

makes 4 servings

Banh mi are traditional Vietnamese sandwiches, typically served on a baguette, and filled with pork or chicken and pickled vegetables. You can use boneless skinless chicken breast or a flank steak instead of the pork in this recipe.

3 tablespoons sugar, divided

2 tablespoons lime juice

2 tablespoons Asian fish sauce

2 garlic cloves, chopped

1 scallion, chopped

1 tablespoon chopped fresh ginger

1 (1-pound) pork tenderloin, trimmed of all visible fat

½ cup rice vinegar

¼ teaspoon kosher salt

1 carrot, peeled and cut into thin matchstick strips

1 daikon radish or 1 small jicama, peeled and cut into thin matchstick strips

1 jalapeño, halved lengthwise, seeded, and thinly sliced

2 teaspoons canola oil

4 (6-inch) whole wheat baguettes, split and toasted

2 tablespoons mayonnaise

½ cup loosely packed cilantro leaves

1 Combine the 1 tablespoon of the sugar, the lime juice, fish sauce, garlic, scallion, and ginger in a large resealable plastic bag. Add the pork and turn to coat. Seal the bag and refrigerate 4 hours and up to 8 hours, turning the bag occasionally.

2 Combine the vinegar, remaining 2 tablespoons sugar, and salt in a small saucepan and bring to a boil over high heat, stirring to dissolve the sugar. Place the carrot, daikon, and jalapeño in a medium bowl. Add the vinegar mixture and toss to coat. Cover and refrigerate until ready to serve.

3 Preheat the oven to 400°F.

4 Remove the pork from the bag and discard the marinade. Pat the pork dry with paper towels.

5 Heat a large ovenproof skillet over medium-high heat until hot. Add the oil and tilt the pan to coat the bottom evenly. Add the tenderloin and cook, until browned on all sides, about 5 minutes. Transfer to the oven and bake, turning once, until an instant-read thermometer inserted into the center reads 145°F, 15 to 20 minutes. Cover with foil and let stand 10 minutes. Cut into thin slices.

6 To serve, spread the cut sides of the baguettes evenly with the mayonnaise. Drain the daikon mixture. Divide the pork among the baguettes and top evenly with the daikon mixture and cilantro leaves. Serve at once.

Each serving: 22 g carb, 316 cal, 14 g fat, 2 g sat fat, 66 mg chol, 3 g fib, 27 g pro, 638 mg sod • Carb Choices: 1½; Exchanges: 1½ starch, 3 lean protein, 2½ fat

Salads to Make into Sandwiches

In the Salads chapter of this book, you'll find lots of other recipes to turn into sandwiches. Here are some to try using rolls, buns, sandwich breads, or whole wheat tortillas:

Classic Chicken Salad (page 126)
Curried Chicken Salad (page 126)
Artichoke-Lemon Chicken Salad (page 126)
Cranberry-Pecan Chicken Salad (page 126)

Egg Salad (page 130)
Tuna Salad (page 133)
Curried Tuna Salad with Apple (page 133)
Pesto–Red Pepper Tuna Salad (page 133)
No-Mayo Tuna Salad (page 134)

Turn these into sandwiches using whole wheat pita bread:

Lima Bean, Corn, and Tomato Salad (page 100)
Edamame and Grape Tomato Salad (page 101)
Asian Edamame and Radish Salad (page 101)
Four-Bean Salad (page 118)
Mediterranean Bean Salad with Artichokes and Lemon (page 118)
White Bean Salad with Tomatoes and Sage (page 120)

White Bean, Bell Pepper, and Caper Salad (page 120)
White Bean Salad with Roasted Zucchini and Radicchio (page 121)
Black Bean Salad with Roasted Corn and Poblanos (page 122)
Red Bean Salad with Queso Fresco (page 122)
Black Bean, Jicama, and Avocado Salad (page 122)
Black-eyed Pea Salad (page 124)

Lobster Rolls HIGH FIBER

makes 4 servings

Instead of cooking lobsters for these sandwiches, you can purchase 8 ounces of cooked lobster meat. If you're feeling less flush, you can substitute cooked, peeled, and deveined shrimp for the lobster. Coarsely chop the shrimp before making the sandwiches.

2 (1¼-pound) live lobsters
1 tablespoon mayonnaise
1 tablespoon plain low-fat yogurt
½ teaspoon grated lemon zest
2 teaspoons lemon juice
¼ teaspoon kosher salt
Pinch of freshly ground pepper
2 tablespoons minced celery
1 tablespoon minced scallion, green tops only
8 leaves Bibb lettuce
4 whole wheat hot dog buns, toasted
2 plum tomatoes, thinly sliced

1 Bring a large pot of water to a boil over high heat. Using tongs, carefully plunge the lobsters into the boiling water. Cover and boil 8 minutes. Using tongs, plunge the cooked lobsters into ice water and let stand 10 minutes. Drain and let cool completely.

2 Separate the tail and claws from the body and discard the body. Crack the shells and remove the meat. Coarsely chop the meat.

3 Stir together the mayonnaise, yogurt, lemon zest, lemon juice, salt, and pepper in a medium bowl. Add the lobster meat, celery, and scallion and toss gently to combine. Refrigerate, covered, at least 2 hours and up to 8 hours.

4 To serve, divide the lettuce leaves among the buns and top with the tomato slices. Spoon about ⅓ cup of the lobster mixture into each bun and serve at once.

Each serving: 25 g carb, 207 cal, 5 g fat, 1 g sat fat, 42 mg chol, 4 g fib, 16 g pro, 502 mg sod • Carb Choices: 1½; Exchanges: 1½ starch, 2 lean protein, ½ fat

Catfish Po Boys

QUICK | HIGH FIBER

makes 4 servings

Po boy sandwiches are a Louisiana tradition—and a not-so-healthy one. The sandwiches are usually made with fried seafood and loaded with tartar sauce. In this better-for-you version, the fish is sautéed in a minimum of oil and instead of tartar sauce, there's a light and crunchy slaw.

SLAW
1 tablespoon mayonnaise
1 tablespoon plain low-fat yogurt
1 teaspoon apple cider vinegar
¼ teaspoon kosher salt
Pinch of freshly ground pepper
2 cups thinly sliced cabbage
¼ cup coarsely shredded carrot
2 tablespoons minced red onion

FISH
¼ cup fine-grind yellow cornmeal
¼ cup unbleached all-purpose flour
1 teaspoon paprika
⅛ teaspoon ground cayenne
¼ cup low-fat buttermilk
4 (5-ounce) catfish or other mild fish fillets
½ teaspoon kosher salt
⅛ teaspoon freshly ground pepper
2 teaspoons canola oil
4 whole wheat hoagie rolls, split and toasted

1 To make the slaw, stir together the mayonnaise, yogurt, vinegar, salt, and pepper in a medium bowl. Add the cabbage, carrot, and onion and toss to coat. Refrigerate, covered, while you prepare the fish.

2 To make the fish, combine the cornmeal, flour, paprika, and cayenne in a shallow dish. Pour the buttermilk into a medium bowl. Sprinkle the fish fillets with the salt and pepper. Dip the fillets, one at a time into the buttermilk, then into the cornmeal mixture.

3 Heat a large nonstick skillet over medium heat. Add the oil and tilt the pan to coat the bottom evenly. Add the fish and cook, until the fish flakes when tested with a fork, 3 minutes on each side.

4 To serve, place a fish fillet on the bottom half of each roll and top with about ½ cup of the slaw. Cover with the top of each roll and serve at once.

Each serving: 37 g carb, 418 cal, 16 g fat, 4 g sat fat, 70 mg chol, 5 g fib, 30 g pro, 519 mg sod • Carb Choices: 2½; Exchanges: 2½ starch, 3 lean protein, 1 fat

Tuna Tartines QUICK

makes 4 servings

A tartine is a French open-face sandwich that can be topped with almost anything. This version uses a yogurt-lightened mayonnaise, peppery arugula, and an olive-spiked tuna salad to make a sandwich that is fresh and full-flavored.

2 (5-ounce) cans low-sodium chunk white albacore tuna in water, drained and flaked
6 Kalamata or niçoise olives, pitted and chopped
2 tablespoons chopped fresh Italian parsley
1 thin scallion, thinly sliced
2 teaspoons grated lemon zest
2 tablespoons lemon juice
¼ teaspoon freshly ground pepper
1 tablespoon mayonnaise
1 tablespoon plain low-fat yogurt
2 (6-inch) whole wheat French rolls, cut in half lengthwise and toasted
1½ cups loosely packed baby arugula
2 plum tomatoes, thinly sliced

1 Combine the tuna, olives, parsley, scallion, lemon zest, lemon juice, and pepper in a medium bowl and toss gently to coat.

2 Stir together the mayonnaise and yogurt in a small bowl. Spread the mixture evenly on the cut sides of the rolls. Top evenly with the arugula, the tomatoes, and the tuna mixture. Serve at once.

Each serving: 15 g carb, 200 cal, 7 g fat, 1 g sat fat, 23 mg chol, 2 g fib, 21 g pro, 280 mg sod • Carb Choices: 1; Exchanges: 1 starch, 3 lean protein, 1 fat

Grilled Vegetable and Goat Cheese Sandwiches

QUICK | HIGH FIBER

makes 6 servings

3 tablespoons plus ½ teaspoon extra virgin olive oil, divided
1 tablespoon balsamic vinegar
¼ teaspoon kosher salt
¼ teaspoon freshly ground pepper
1 large eggplant (about 1½ pounds), cut into ¼-inch slices
1 red bell pepper, thinly sliced
1 yellow bell pepper, thinly sliced
1 large sweet onion, halved lengthwise and thinly sliced
6 (6-inch) whole wheat baguettes
6 ounces goat cheese, softened
¾ cup loosely packed fresh basil leaves

1 Prepare the grill or heat a large grill pan over medium-high heat.

2 Whisk together 2 tablespoons of the oil, the vinegar, salt, and ground pepper in a large bowl. Set aside.

3 Combine the eggplant, bell peppers, and onion in another large bowl. Drizzle with 1 tablespoon of the remaining oil and toss to coat. Brush the grill rack or grill pan with the ½ teaspoon remaining oil. Place the vegetables on the grill rack or in the grill pan and grill, turning often, until the vegetables are browned, 8 to 10 minutes. Place the vegetables in the oil mixture and toss to coat.

4 Cut the baguettes in half lengthwise. Remove and discard the soft inner crumbs from each piece of bread. Spread the bottom halves of the bread with the goat cheese. Top with the basil, then with the vegetables. Cover with the top of each piece of bread and serve at once.

Each serving: 41 g carb, 368 cal, 19 g fat, 7 g sat fat, 22 mg chol, 9 g fib, 13 g pro, 460 mg sod • Carb Choices: 2½; Exchanges: 2 starch, 1 veg, 1 high-fat protein, 1½ fat

Portobello Mushroom, Feta, and Arugula Sandwiches QUICK | HIGH FIBER

makes 4 servings

When a mushroom sandwich is as delicious as this one, you won't miss the meat. A sharp feta cheese and yogurt sauce and peppery arugula give the earthy mushrooms amazing flavor.

4 large portobello mushrooms
1 tablespoon extra virgin olive oil
¼ teaspoon kosher salt, divided
¼ teaspoon freshly ground pepper, divided
2 ounces finely crumbled feta cheese (about ½ cup), at room temperature
2 tablespoons plain low-fat yogurt
2 tablespoons chopped fresh Italian parsley
½ teaspoon grated lemon zest
4 whole wheat kaiser rolls
2 cups loosely packed baby arugula or baby spinach

1 Preheat the oven to 400°F.

2 Cut away and discard the tough stems of the mushrooms. Using a spoon, gently scrape away and discard the dark gills on the underside of each mushroom.

3 Place the mushrooms on a large rimmed baking sheet. Brush both sides of each mushroom with the oil. Bake, turning once, until the mushrooms are tender, 25 to 30 minutes. Sprinkle the mushrooms with ⅛ teaspoon of the salt and ⅛ teaspoon of the pepper.

4 Meanwhile, stir together the feta, yogurt, parsley, lemon zest, the remaining ⅛ teaspoon salt, and the remaining ⅛ teaspoon pepper in a small bowl.

5 Cut the rolls in half lengthwise. Remove and discard the soft inner crumbs from each piece of bread. Toast the rolls. Spread the bottom halves of the bread evenly with the feta cheese mixture.

Top evenly with the arugula. Top with the mushrooms. Cover with the top half of each piece of bread and serve at once.

Each serving: 28 g carb, 219 cal, 9 g fat, 3 g sat fat, 13 mg chol, 5 g fib, 9 g pro, 448 mg sod • Carb Choices: 2; Exchanges: 1½ starch, 1 veg, 1½ fat

Open-Face Cheddar and Red Pepper Salad Sandwiches QUICK

makes 4 servings

In the South, versions of this salad are made with chopped pimentos instead of the roasted bell peppers—and with a lot more mayonnaise. This lightened version is just as satisfying.

¼ cup red Roasted Bell Peppers (page 21) or roasted red peppers from a jar
6 ounces coarsely shredded reduced-fat extra-sharp Cheddar cheese (about 1½ cups)
2 tablespoons chopped fresh basil
1 tablespoon minced scallion, green tops only
1 tablespoon mayonnaise
1 tablespoon plain low-fat yogurt
1 teaspoon white wine vinegar
½ teaspoon hot pepper sauce
4 thin slices whole wheat bread, toasted
1 large tomato, thinly sliced
½ hothouse (English) cucumber, thinly sliced
2 large radishes, cut into short, thin strips

1 Place the roasted peppers on layers of paper towels and blot dry. Chop the peppers and place in a medium bowl. Add the Cheddar, basil, scallion, mayonnaise, yogurt, vinegar, and pepper sauce and stir gently to mix well.

2 Place the bread on four plates. Top the bread evenly with the tomato slices and cucumber slices. Top evenly with the cheese mixture. Sprinkle with the radishes and serve at once.

Each serving: 15 g carb, 231 cal, 13 g fat, 7 g sat fat, 31 mg chol, 2 g fib, 13 g pro, 510 mg sod • Carb Choices: 1; Exchanges: ½ starch, 1 veg, 1 high-fat protein, ½ fat

Grilled Broccoli Rabe, Provolone, and Prosciutto Sandwiches QUICK

makes 4 servings

Eating cooked greens on a sandwich may seem odd, but give it a try, especially if you're a fan of broccoli rabe. The creamy provolone and salty prosciutto make the slight bitterness of the broccoli rabe disappear.

2 pounds broccoli rabe, tough stems removed, leaves and florets chopped

1 tablespoon extra virgin olive oil

1 tablespoon red wine vinegar

4 (4 x 4-inch) squares whole wheat focaccia, cut in half horizontally

2 ounces prosciutto

⅛ teaspoon crushed red pepper

4 thin slices provolone (about 2 ounces)

1 Bring a large pot of water to a boil. Add the broccoli rabe and cook until very tender, 8 minutes. Drain in a colander and press with a spatula to squeeze out as much water as possible.

2 Whisk together the oil and vinegar in a small bowl. Remove and discard the soft inner crumbs from each piece of bread. Brush the cut sides of the bread with the oil mixture.

3 Arrange the prosciutto evenly on the bottom halves of the bread. Top evenly with the broccoli rabe. Sprinkle the broccoli rabe with the crushed red pepper. Top with the provolone. Cover with the top half of each piece of bread.

4 Heat a large nonstick skillet over medium heat. Place the sandwiches in the pan and top with a heavy skillet. Cook, turning once, until well browned on each side, 4 to 5 minutes. Serve at once.

Each serving: 31 g carb, 292 cal, 11 g fat, 3 g sat fat, 23 mg chol, 3 g fib, 20 g pro, 609 mg sod • Carb Choices: 2; Exchanges: 1 starch, 2 veg, 1 medium-fat protein, ½ fat

Serrano Ham and Manchego Picnic Sandwich QUICK

makes 6 servings

This is a perfect portable sandwich for a picnic. Pack it up along with Roasted Mushroom Salad (page 96) and some fresh whole fruit for an easy alfresco meal.

1 tablespoon extra virgin olive oil

1 tablespoon red wine vinegar

½ teaspoon Dijon mustard

⅛ teaspoon freshly ground pepper

1 (8-inch) round whole wheat boule

4 ounces thinly sliced Serrano ham, trimmed of all visible fat

½ cup red Roasted Bell Peppers (page 21) or roasted red peppers from a jar

1 cup (4 ounces) shredded manchego

1 cup loosely packed baby spinach or thinly sliced romaine lettuce

1 Whisk together the oil, vinegar, mustard, and ground pepper in a small bowl.

2 Cut the boule in half crosswise. Remove and discard the soft inner crumbs from each piece of bread, leaving 1-inch bread shells. Brush the cut sides of bread with the oil mixture. Arrange half of the ham in the bottom of the bread. Top with half of the roasted peppers, manchego, and spinach. Repeat the layering using the remaining ingredients. Cover with the top half of the bread.

3 Serve immediately or wrap the sandwich in plastic wrap and refrigerate up to 4 hours. To serve, cut into 6 wedges.

Each serving: 15 g carb, 204 cal, 10 g fat, 4 g sat fat, 30 mg chol, 2 g fib, 12 g pro, 751 mg sod • Carb Choices: 1; Exchanges: 1 starch, 1 high-fat protein, ½ fat

Salads

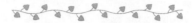

Leafy Salads

Caesar Salad

Greek Salad

Fattoush

Tri-Color Salad

Wilted Spinach–Mushroom Salad

Orchard Spinach Salad with Toasted Almonds

Spinach Salad with Nut-Crusted Goat Cheese

Mixed Green Salad with Marinated Tomatoes

Bibb Salad with Toasted Walnuts and Blue Cheese

Bibb and Whole Herb Salad

Arugula and Pear Salad with Walnuts and Blue Cheese

Arugula and Melon Salad with Crispy Prosciutto

Vegetable Salads

Creamy Coleslaw

Lemon–Poppy Seed Slaw

Waldorf Slaw

Cilantro-Sesame Slaw

Old-Fashioned Potato Salad

Cucumber-Dill Potato Salad

No-Mayo Potato Salad

Fingerling Potato and Green Bean Salad with Mustard Dressing

Sweet Potato Salad with Molasses

Marinated Cucumber and Sweet Onion Salad

Asian Cucumber Salad

Cucumber-Mango Salad

Asparagus Salad with Orange-Ginger Dressing

Roasted Beet and Green Bean Salad

Fennel, Apple, and Celery Salad

Fennel and Parmesan Salad

Roasted Mushroom Salad

Roasted Eggplant and Spinach Salad with Peanut Dressing

Celery Root Salad with Mustard Dressing

Mixed Tomato and Mozzarella Salad with Basil Dressing

Green Bean, Cherry Tomato, and Bacon Salad

Grilled Vegetable and Goat Cheese Salad

Layered Vegetable Salad

Chopped Salad

Greek Chopped Salad

Bread Salad

Lima Bean, Corn, and Tomato Salad

Edamame and Grape Tomato Salad

Asian Edamame and Radish Salad

Pasta Salads

Antipasto Pasta Salad

Roasted Vegetable and
Pasta Salad

Pasta and Pea Salad

Confetti Pasta Salad

Peanut Noodle Salad

Thai Rice Noodle Salad

Asian Pasta, Snow Pea, and
Radish Salad

Soba Salad with
Soy-Wasabi Vinaigrette

Grain Salads

Tabbouleh

Garbanzo Bean, Spinach,
and Feta Tabbouleh

Wheat Berry–Mango Salad

Wheat Berry, Fennel, and
Parsley Salad

Apricot-Orange
Wheat Berry Salad

Wheat Berry and
Almond Salad with Feta

Barley and Basil Salad

Tandoori-Spiced Barley and
Bean Salad

Southwestern Barley and
Avocado Salad

Quinoa and
Asparagus Salad

Quinoa, Zucchini, and
Mint Salad

Quinoa Salad with Mango,
Orange, and Basil

Cranberry-Maple Rice Salad

Rice Salad with Leeks and
Tomatoes

Rice and Red Bean Salad

Wild Rice, Fig, and
Gorgonzola Salad

Wild Rice, Raisin, and
Walnut Salad

Wild Rice Salad with
Apricots and Pecans

Bean Salads

Four-Bean Salad

Mediterranean Bean Salad
with Artichokes and Lemon

White Bean Salad with
Tomatoes and Sage

White Bean, Bell Pepper,
and Caper Salad

White Bean Salad with
Roasted Zucchini and
Radicchio

Black Bean Salad with
Roasted Corn and Poblanos

Black Bean, Jicama, and
Avocado Salad

Bean and Cornbread Salad

Black-eyed Pea Salad

Edamame and Bulgur Salad
with Basil

Lentil Salad with Walnut
Vinaigrette

Main Dish Salads

Classic Chicken Salad

Artichoke-Lemon
Chicken Salad

Oven-Fried Chicken Salad

Grilled Chicken Salad with
Miso-Basil Dressing

Warm Chicken and
Roasted Tomato Salad

Mediterranean Chicken,
Bean, and Pasta Salad

Thai Chicken Salad

Cobb Salad

Chef's Salad

Egg Salad

Taco Salad

Steak and Arugula Salad
with Lemon and Dill

Grilled Asian Flank
Steak Salad

Tuna Salad

Pesto–Red Pepper
Tuna Salad

No-Mayo Tuna Salad

Niçoise Salad

Niçoise Pasta Salad

Tuna and White Bean
Salad with Spinach

Warm Salmon and
Potato Salad

Creamy Salmon and
Pasta Salad

Shrimp, Mango, and
Avocado Salad

Ceviche-Style Shrimp Salad

Dressings and Croutons

Basic Vinaigrette

Herbed Vinaigrette

Sherry-Walnut Vinaigrette

Lemon Vinaigrette

Cilantro-Lime Vinaigrette

Honey–Poppy Seed
Vinaigrette

Feta-Oregano Vinaigrette

Balsamic Vinaigrette

Creamy Herb Dressing

Creamy Goat Cheese–
Chive Dressing

Creamy Blue Cheese–
Peppercorn Dressing

Creamy Parmesan Dressing

Roasted Red Pepper
Dressing

Sun-Dried Tomato–Basil
Dressing

Avocado Dressing

Soy-Sesame Dressing

Orange-Ginger Dressing

Peanut Dressing

Homemade Croutons

A salad can be as simple as lettuce tossed with a splash of vinaigrette or a complicated concoction of greens, numerous vegetables, and cheese. Salads don't even have to contain lettuce or greens—fiber-rich whole wheat pasta, grains, and beans all make delicious and healthful salads when tossed with fresh vegetables and a touch of dressing.

You'll find recipes here for all those and plenty in between. Of course, there are the classics (which I've lightened up) like Caesar Salad (page 84), Creamy Coleslaw (page 90), Old-Fashioned Potato Salad (page 91), and Egg Salad (page 130). I've included an abundance of leafy green salads and vegetable salads. Hardly anyone eats as many vegetables as they should, and colorful, flavorful, easy-to-prepare salads are a good way to incorporate more of these health-giving foods into every-day meals.

Salads are not just starters or accompaniments to an entrée either—many are meals in themselves. Try kid-friendly Taco Salad (page 131) or a gorgeous Shrimp, Mango, and Avocado Salad (page 137) that's perfect for easy entertaining.

At the end of the chapter, you'll find variety of salad dressing recipes for mixing up with the salads here or for dressing salad creations of your own. Be sure to read A Drizzle Will Do (page 139) for tips on making the most of a little dressing. And Keeping Greens Fresh (page 85) tells you how to keep washed greens fresh for a week.

If you're watching your weight—or even if you're not—consider making salads a part of every lunch and dinner. They are simple to make (most require no cooking); add crunch, color, and freshness to a meal; are good sources of fiber, vitamins, and minerals; and they fill you up with hardly any calories.

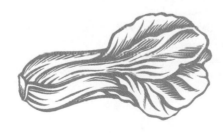

Leafy Salads

Caesar Salad QUICK

makes 8 servings

Blending grated Parmesan into this Caesar dressing gives it a creamy texture without using a raw egg. You can make the dressing ahead and refrigerate, covered, for up to a week. Let the dressing come to room temperature before using. Use it not just on this Caesar salad, but on any kind of simple salad of lettuce and vegetables.

¼ cup olive oil
1 ounce freshly grated Parmesan (about ¼ cup)
2 tablespoons white wine vinegar
2 canned anchovy fillets, drained
1 small garlic clove, chopped
½ teaspoon Dijon mustard
½ teaspoon Worcestershire sauce
¼ teaspoon kosher salt
⅛ teaspoon freshly ground pepper
16 cups loosely packed torn romaine lettuce
1 cup Homemade Croutons (page 144)
½ cup finely shredded Parmesan

1 To make the dressing, combine the oil, grated Parmesan, vinegar, anchovies, garlic, mustard, Worcestershire, salt, and pepper in a blender and process until smooth.

2 Place the lettuce in a large bowl. Add the dressing and croutons and toss to coat. Divide the salad evenly among 8 plates. Sprinkle evenly with the shredded Parmesan and serve at once.

Each serving: 10 g carb, 165 cal, 12 g fat, 3 g sat fat, 7 mg chol, 3 g fib, 6 g pro, 315 mg sod • Carb Choices: ½; Exchanges: ½ starch, 1 veg, 2 fat

Greek Salad QUICK

makes 4 servings

I prefer to use hothouse cucumbers because they have more flavor than regular cucumbers. Another flavorful type of cucumber are the small Kirby cukes. Kids love slices or spears of these tiny cucumbers to have with dip for a snack. If you substitute Kirbys for hothouse cucumbers, count on replacing 1 hothouse cucumber with 4 Kirbys.

1½ tablespoons extra virgin olive oil
1 tablespoon red wine vinegar
1 small garlic clove, crushed through a press
¼ teaspoon dried oregano
¼ teaspoon kosher salt
⅛ teaspoon freshly ground pepper
6 cups loosely packed torn romaine lettuce
2 plum tomatoes, each cut into 8 wedges
½ hothouse (English) cucumber, halved lengthwise and sliced
½ red bell pepper, cut into short, thin strips
¼ cup thinly sliced red onion
2 pepperoncini peppers, drained and chopped (optional)
1 ounce finely crumbled feta cheese (about ¼ cup)

1 Whisk together the oil, vinegar, garlic, oregano, salt, and ground pepper in a large bowl.

2 Add the remaining ingredients and toss to combine. Serve at once.

Each serving: 8 g carb, 107 cal, 8 g fat, 2 g sat fat, 8 mg chol, 3 g fib, 3 g pro, 185 mg sod • Carb Choices: ½; Exchanges: 1 veg, 1½ fat

Keeping Greens Fresh

Here's an easy way to wash and safely store a week's worth of salad in just a few minutes. It takes longer to describe how to do this than to actually do it, so don't be intimidated.

First, wash the greens by submerging them in a bowl of cold water. Lift them out and drain in a colander. Repeat, using fresh water, until no grit remains in the bottom of the bowl. Keep soft-leafed greens like leaf lettuce or Bibb whole and tear sturdier greens like romaine or radicchio into large pieces. Dry the greens well using a salad spinner. If you don't have a salad spinner, put the greens in a clean lingerie washing bag and, holding one end of the bag, whirl it around as fast as you can in the shower. Moisture is the main reason greens spoil, so get them as dry as possible.

Next, tear off two sheets of paper towels (still attached to each other) and put them inside a gallon-size resealable plastic bag with the perforated seam of the towels in the bottom of the bag. Open the bag with a sheet of the paper towel on each side of the plastic bag and place the greens inside. The paper towel absorbs any moisture that might remain on the greens. Seal the bag, squeezing out as much of the air as possible, so that you end up with what looks like a flat square. Air is another reason greens spoil, so squeeze out as much of it as possible. It's okay to crush the greens—they'll spring back when you take them out of the bag. Stored in this way, salad greens will keep for 5 to 7 days without losing freshness.

Fattoush QUICK

makes 4 servings

Fattoush is a Middle Eastern version of Italian bread salad. Fresh whole leaves of cilantro and mint make this version especially flavorful. In this recipe the pita is toasted, so it is crunchy like croutons. If you prefer softer bread, you can skip the toasting step.

1 (6-inch) whole wheat pita bread
1½ tablespoons extra virgin olive oil
1 teaspoon grated lemon zest
1 tablespoon lemon juice
1 small garlic clove, crushed through a press
¼ teaspoon kosher salt
⅛ teaspoon freshly ground pepper
2 cups cherry tomatoes, halved
1 hothouse (English) cucumber, halved lengthwise and cut into ½-inch slices
1 red or yellow bell pepper, coarsely chopped
¼ cup thinly sliced red onion
¼ cup fresh mint leaves
¼ cup fresh cilantro leaves
1 ounce finely crumbled feta cheese (about ¼ cup)

1 Preheat the oven to 350°F.

2 Split the pita in half to make 2 rounds and cut the rounds into ½-inch pieces. Place the pita on a medium baking sheet in a single layer and bake until lightly toasted, 10 to 12 minutes. Let cool.

3 Whisk together the oil, lemon zest, lemon juice, garlic, salt, and ground pepper in a large bowl.

4 Add the toasted pita and the remaining ingredients and toss to combine. Serve at once.

Each serving: 14 g carb, 131 cal, 7 g fat, 2 g sat fat, 6 mg chol, 3 g fib, 4 g pro, 215 mg sod • Carb Choices: 1; Exchanges: ½ starch, 1 veg, 1 fat

Tri-Color Salad QUICK

makes 4 servings

You can serve this versatile salad with almost any meal. The slight bitterness of the radic-chio and endive is offset by the nutty Parmesan shavings.

1 canned anchovy fillet, drained
1½ tablespoons extra virgin olive oil
1 tablespoon balsamic vinegar
1 garlic clove, crushed through a press
¼ teaspoon kosher salt
¼ teaspoon freshly ground pepper
4 cups loosely packed torn romaine lettuce
4 cups loosely packed torn radicchio
1 head Belgian endive, torn
¼ cup shaved Parmesan

1 Place the anchovy in a large bowl and use two forks to mash it into a paste. Add the oil, vinegar, garlic, salt, and pepper and whisk until smooth.

2 Add the romaine, radicchio, and endive and toss to coat. Divide the salad among 4 plates and sprinkle evenly with the Parmesan. Serve at once.

Each serving: 5 g carb, 96 cal, 7 g fat, 2 g sat fat, 4 mg chol, 2 g fib, 4 g pro, 206 mg sod • Carb Choices: 0; Exchanges: 1 veg, 1 fat

Wilted Spinach–Mushroom Salad QUICK

makes 4 servings

The warm smoky bacon dressing makes this a perfect cool weather salad.

8 cups loosely packed torn spinach
1 cup sliced white mushrooms
¼ cup thinly sliced red onion
2 strips smoked center-cut bacon
1 tablespoon water
1 tablespoon apple cider vinegar
½ teaspoon kosher salt
⅛ teaspoon freshly ground pepper
1 hard-boiled egg, chopped

1 Combine the spinach, mushrooms, and onion in a large bowl. Set aside.

2 Cook the bacon in a large skillet over medium-high heat until crisp. Drain on paper towels.

3 Add the water, vinegar, salt, and pepper to the bacon drippings, stirring to scrape up the browned bits. Pour the drippings mixture over the spinach mixture and toss to coat. Divide the salad among 4 plates and sprinkle evenly with the egg. Serve at once.

Each serving: 4 g carb, 57 cal, 3 g fat, 1 g sat fat, 56 mg chol, 2 g fib, 5 g pro, 271 mg sod • Carb Choices: 0; Exchanges: 1 veg, ½ fat

Orchard Spinach Salad with Toasted Almonds

QUICK

makes 4 servings

One of my favorite tricks to making a thick salad dressing with very little oil is to soften dried fruits and then puree them into the dressing. I use dried apricots here, which add a tart coun-terpoint to the sweet apple.

¼ cup orange juice
2 dried apricots, chopped
1 tablespoon white wine vinegar
1 tablespoon extra virgin olive oil
½ teaspoon kosher salt
¼ teaspoon freshly ground pepper
1 tablespoon minced red onion
8 cups loosely packed torn fresh spinach
1 apple, cored and thinly sliced
2 tablespoons golden raisins
2 tablespoons sliced almonds, toasted (page 4)

1 Pour the orange juice into a glass measuring cup. Add the apricots, cover with plastic wrap and microwave on high for 1 minute. Let cool slightly and place in a blender. Add the vinegar, oil, salt, and pepper and process until smooth. Transfer to a large bowl and stir in the onion.

2 Add the spinach, apple, raisins, and almonds and toss to coat. Serve at once.

Each serving: 15 g carb, 111 cal, 5 g fat, 1 g sat fat, 0 mg chol, 3 g fib, 3 g pro, 189 mg sod • Carb Choices: 1; Exchanges: 1 fruit, 1 fat

Spinach Salad with Nut-Crusted Goat Cheese QUICK

makes 8 servings

With fresh strawberries, baby spinach, and goat cheese, this salad says "Welcome Spring." It's a perfect beginning for any springtime lunch or dinner. I like to serve it at Easter with Rosemary-Garlic Roasted Rack of Lamb (page 320). To serve the nut-crusted goat cheese warm, place it in a small baking dish and bake at 350°F until it is just heated through, about 8 minutes.

¼ cup hazelnuts, toasted and finely chopped (page 4)
1 (8-ounce) log goat cheese
2 tablespoons seedless strawberry jam
2 tablespoons orange juice
1 tablespoon hazelnut oil or olive oil
1 tablespoon sherry vinegar or white wine vinegar
¼ teaspoon kosher salt
⅛ teaspoon freshly ground pepper
16 cups torn fresh spinach or baby spinach
2 cups fresh strawberries, hulled and halved

1 Place the hazelnuts in a shallow dish and roll the goat cheese in the nuts to coat, pressing to adhere.

2 Whisk together the jam, orange juice, oil, vinegar, salt, and pepper in a large bowl.

3 Add the spinach and strawberries and toss to coat. Divide the spinach among 8 plates. Cut the goat cheese into 8 slices and top each salad with a slice of cheese. Serve at once.

Each serving: 10 g carb, 186 cal, 13 g fat, 6 g sat fat, 22 mg chol, 3 g fib, 9 g pro, 229 mg sod • Carb Choices: ½; Exchanges: ½ carb, 1 high-fat protein, 1 fat

Mixed Green Salad with Marinated Tomatoes

makes 4 servings

Because the tomatoes marinate in a flavorful dressing, this is a good salad to make during the cold months when tomatoes lack flavor. You can use plum tomatoes, cut into wedges, instead of the cherry tomatoes if you prefer.

2 cups cherry tomatoes, halved
2 tablespoons Basic Vinaigrette (page 138)
4 cups loosely packed torn Bibb lettuce
4 cups loosely packed torn red leaf lettuce
2 tablespoons finely shredded Parmesan

1 Place the tomatoes in a large bowl. Drizzle with the vinaigrette and stir to coat. Let stand, stirring occasionally, at least 1 hour and up to 3 hours. Transfer the tomatoes to a small bowl using a slotted spoon.

2 Add the lettuces to the dressing remaining in the bowl and toss to coat. Divide the salad among 4 plates. Top evenly with the tomatoes and sprinkle with the Parmesan. Serve at once.

Each serving: 6 g carb, 76 cal, 5 g fat, 1 g sat fat, 2 mg chol, 2 g fib, 3 g pro, 97 mg sod • Carb Choices: ½; Exchanges: 1 veg, 1 fat

MIX AND MATCH GREEN SALADS

Combine ingredients from each column in a large bowl and toss to coat. The salad will serve 4 generously. Each serving has about 6 grams of carbs and about 100 calories.

Greens Choose 1 or 2 (4 cups total)	Vegetable Choose 1 or 2 (2 cups total)	Flavor Booster Choose 1	Dressing Choose 1	Finishing Touch Choose 1
Torn romaine lettuce	Plum tomatoes, quartered; or cherry tomatoes, halved	½ cup thinly sliced radishes	3 tablespoons Basic Vinaigrette (page 138)	1 chopped hard-boiled egg
Torn Bibb lettuce or red or green leaf lettuce	Thinly sliced red bell pepper	¼ cup thinly sliced scallions	3 tablespoons Mustard Vinaigrette (page 138)	¼ cup finely shredded reduced-fat extra-sharp Cheddar cheese
Mixed baby greens	Sliced cucumber	¼ cup thinly sliced red onion	3 tablespoons Lemon Vinaigrette (page 139)	¼ cup finely shredded Parmesan
Trimmed arugula or watercress	Cooked and chilled green beans or asparagus	¼ cup chopped fresh basil, dill, or Italian parsley	¼ cup Creamy Herb Dressing (page 141)	3 tablespoons crumbled feta or goat cheese
Torn spinach or baby spinach	Sliced white mushrooms	¼ cup thinly sliced dry-packed sun-dried tomatoes	¼ cup Creamy Parmesan Dressing (page 142)	¼ cup chopped pitted Kalamata olives
Torn frisée	Canned artichoke hearts, drained and quartered	½ cup thinly sliced roasted red bell peppers	¼ cup Sun-Dried Tomato–Basil Dressing (page 142)	3 strips crisp-cooked center-cut bacon, crumbled

Bibb Salad with Toasted Walnuts and Blue Cheese QUICK

makes 8 servings

Simplicity is the key to this sophisticated salad. Mild Bibb lettuce adds plenty of crunch, while the walnuts and cheese deliver great flavor. Serve it before a cool weather meal of roast pork or beef.

16 cups loosely packed torn Bibb lettuce
1 recipe Sherry-Walnut Vinaigrette (page 138)
2 ounces crumbled blue cheese (about ½ cup)
¼ cup walnuts, toasted and chopped (page 4)

Combine the lettuce and dressing in a large bowl and toss to coat. Divide the salad among 8 plates. Sprinkle evenly with the blue cheese and walnuts. Serve at once.

Each serving: 4 g carb, 112 cal, 10 g fat, 2 g sat fat, 6 mg chol, 1 g fib, 4 g pro, 166 mg sod • Carb Choices: 0; Exchanges: 1 veg, 2 fat

Bibb and Whole Herb Salad QUICK

makes 4 servings

Whole fresh herb leaves give this salad as서-tive flavor. Serve it alongside simply prepared salmon or chicken to make a mundane meal seem special. You can mix up the herbs, depending on what flavors you like best and what you have on hand.

2 tablespoons lemon juice
1½ tablespoons extra virgin olive oil
¼ teaspoon kosher salt
⅛ teaspoon freshly ground pepper
8 cups loosely packed torn Bibb lettuce
½ cup loosely packed fresh Italian parsley leaves
½ cup loosely packed fresh basil leaves, thinly sliced if large
¼ cup loosely packed small fresh dill sprigs

1 Whisk together the lemon juice, oil, salt, and pepper in a large bowl.

2 Add the lettuce, parsley, basil, and dill and toss to coat. Divide the salad among 4 plates. Serve at once.

Each serving: 4 g carb, 68 cal, 6 g fat, 1 g sat fat, 0 mg chol, 2 g fib, 2 g pro, 80 mg sod • Carb Choices: 0; Exchanges: 1 veg, 1 fat

Arugula and Pear Salad with Walnuts and Blue Cheese QUICK

makes 8 servings

Start any fall or winter dinner party—be it a casual get-together or a fancy meal—with this versatile salad. Using two varieties of pears makes it especially colorful and flavorful.

16 cups loosely packed arugula
1 red pear (such as Red Bartlett or Comice), cored and thinly sliced
1 green pear (such as Green Anjou or Bartlett), cored and thinly sliced
1 recipe Basic Vinaigrette (page 138)
2 ounces crumbled blue cheese (about ½ cup)
¼ cup walnuts, toasted and chopped (page 4)

Combine the arugula, pears, and dressing in a large bowl and toss to coat. Divide the salad among 8 plates. Sprinkle evenly with the blue cheese and walnuts. Serve at once.

Each serving: 9 g carb, 132 cal, 10 g fat, 2 g sat fat, 6 mg chol, 2 g fib, 3 g pro, 172 mg sod • Carb Choices: ½; Exchanges: ½ fruit, 2 fat

Arugula and Melon Salad with Crispy Prosciutto QUICK

makes 4 servings

Sweet melon, peppery arugula, and salty prosciutto make this salad a riot of flavor. The honey-sweetened dressing ties all the ingredients together.

4 ounces prosciutto, trimmed of all visible fat, cut into thin strips
2 tablespoons rice vinegar
1 tablespoon extra virgin olive oil
½ teaspoon honey
¼ teaspoon kosher salt
Pinch of freshly ground pepper
6 cups loosely packed arugula
¼ medium honeydew melon, seeded, peeled, and thinly sliced
¼ medium cantaloupe, seeded, peeled, and thinly sliced

1 Preheat the oven to 400°F.

2 Line a medium rimmed baking sheet with parchment paper. Place the prosciutto in the pan and bake until lightly browned, 8 to 10 minutes. Transfer the prosciutto to a paper towel–lined plate to cool.

3 Meanwhile, whisk together the vinegar, oil, honey, salt, and pepper in a large bowl. Add the arugula and toss to coat. Divide the salad evenly among 4 plates. Top evenly with the honeydew and cantaloupe and sprinkle evenly with the prosciutto. Serve at once.

Each serving: 13 g carb, 148 cal, 7 g fat, 2 g sat fat, 25 mg chol, 2 g fib, 9 g pro, 646 mg sod • Carb Choices: 1; Exchanges: 1 fruit, 1 medium-fat protein, 1 fat

Vegetable Salads

Creamy Coleslaw QUICK

makes 4 servings

This salad is a must-have at summer picnics to accompany everything from cold cut sandwiches to grilled chicken. If you're in a rush, you can make this with bagged coleslaw mix, though the flavor will not be as fresh.

2 tablespoons plain low-fat yogurt
2 tablespoons mayonnaise
1 teaspoon apple cider vinegar
1 teaspoon sugar
½ teaspoon kosher salt
⅛ teaspoon freshly ground pepper
3 cups thinly sliced green cabbage
1 small carrot, peeled and coarsely shredded
2 tablespoons coarsely shredded sweet onion (optional)

1 Whisk together the yogurt, mayonnaise, vinegar, sugar, salt, and pepper in a large bowl.

2 Add the cabbage, carrot, and onion, if using, and toss to coat. Serve the salad at room temperature or chilled. The salad tastes best on the day it is made, but it can be refrigerated, covered, for up to 2 days.

Each serving: 6 g carb, 79 cal, 6 g fat, 1 g sat fat, 3 mg chol, 2 g fib, 1 g pro, 61 mg sod • Carb Choices: ½; Exchanges: 1 veg, 1 fat

Lemon–Poppy Seed Slaw QUICK

makes 6 servings

The citrusy flavor of this slaw makes it perfect for serving with a fish sandwich or grilled shrimp.

2 tablespoons plain low-fat Greek yogurt or strained yogurt (page 11)
1 tablespoon honey
1 tablespoon lemon juice
½ teaspoon kosher salt
½ teaspoon poppy seeds
Pinch of freshly ground pepper
6 cups thinly sliced savoy or napa cabbage
1 small carrot, peeled and coarsely shredded
¼ cup thinly sliced red onion

Whisk together the yogurt, honey, lemon juice, salt, poppy seeds, and pepper in a large bowl. Add the cabbage, carrot, and onion and toss to coat. Serve the slaw at once or cover and chill up to 4 hours.

Each serving: 9 g carb, 40 cal, 0 g fat, 0 g sat fat, 0 mg chol, 3 g fib, 2 g pro, 121 mg sod • Carb Choices: ½; Exchanges: ½ carb

Waldorf Slaw QUICK

makes 6 servings

Apples and raisins add a touch of sweetness to this slaw. It goes great with roast pork tenderloin or barbecued chicken.

¼ cup plain low-fat Greek yogurt or strained yogurt (page 11)
1 tablespoon apple cider vinegar
1 tablespoon real maple syrup
½ teaspoon kosher salt
⅛ teaspoon freshly ground pepper
3 cups thinly sliced green cabbage
1 large red apple, cored and cut into thin strips
1 stalk celery, thinly sliced
¼ cup golden raisins

Whisk together the yogurt, vinegar, maple syrup, salt, and pepper in a large bowl. Add the cabbage, apple, celery, and raisins and toss to coat. Serve the slaw at once or cover and chill up to 4 hours.

Each serving: 15 g carb, 62 cal, 0 g fat, 0 g sat fat, 1 mg chol, 2 g fib, 2 g pro, 110 mg sod • Carb Choices: 1; Exchanges: 1 carb

Cilantro-Sesame Slaw QUICK

makes 4 servings

Try this spicy sesame slaw as a light and refreshing accompaniment to grilled salmon or chicken. Savoy or napa cabbage gives this slaw a more delicate texture than one made with green cabbage, but you can use it with delicious results.

2 tablespoons lime juice
2 tablespoons reduced-sodium soy sauce
2 teaspoons Asian sesame oil
1 teaspoon grated fresh ginger
½ teaspoon sugar
¼ to ½ teaspoon chili-garlic paste
4 cups thinly sliced savoy or napa cabbage
1 carrot, peeled and coarsely grated
¼ cup thinly sliced red onion
¼ cup chopped fresh cilantro

1 Whisk together the lime juice, soy sauce, oil, ginger, sugar, and chili-garlic paste in a large bowl.

2 Add the cabbage, carrot, onion, and cilantro and toss to combine. Serve the slaw at once or refrigerate, covered, for up to 4 hours.

Each serving: 8 g carb, 56 cal, 2 g fat, 0 g sat fat, 0 mg chol, 3 g fib, 2 g pro, 344 mg sod • Carb Choices: ½; Exchanges: 1 veg, ½ fat

Old-Fashioned Potato Salad

makes 4 servings

Plain yogurt lightens up this classic recipe and adds tangy flavor to an old favorite. Double or triple the recipe depending on the size of your picnic or cookout.

1 pound red-skinned or other waxy potatoes, well scrubbed
2 tablespoons mayonnaise
2 tablespoons plain low-fat yogurt
1 tablespoon white wine vinegar or apple cider vinegar
1 teaspoon kosher salt
⅛ teaspoon freshly ground pepper
2 stalks celery, chopped
2 tablespoons minced red onion
2 tablespoons chopped fresh Italian parsley

1 Place the potatoes in a large saucepan. Add water to cover and bring to a boil over high heat. Reduce the heat to low and simmer, uncovered, until the potatoes are tender, 15 to 20 minutes. Drain and let stand until cool enough to handle. Cut the potatoes into 1-inch pieces.

2 Meanwhile, whisk together the mayonnaise, yogurt, vinegar, salt, and pepper in a large bowl. Add the potatoes, celery, onion, and parsley and toss to combine. Serve the salad at room temperature or chilled. The salad tastes best on the day it is made, but it can be refrigerated, covered, for up to 1 day.

Each serving: 20 g carb, 140 cal, 6 g fat, 1 g sat fat, 3 mg chol, 2 g fib, 3 g pro, 347 mg sod • Carb Choices: 1; Exchanges: 1 starch, 1 fat

BACON-POTATO SALAD: Follow the Old-Fashioned Potato Salad recipe, above, adding 2 strips center-cut bacon, cooked until crisp and coarsely chopped, just before serving the salad.

Each serving: 20 g carb, 154 cal, 7 g fat, 1 g sat fat, 6 mg chol, 2 g fib, 4 g pro, 411 mg sod • Carb Choices: 1; Exchanges: 1½ starch, 1½ fat

Cucumber-Dill Potato Salad

makes 4 servings

When you want a potato salad that's a little out of the ordinary, serve this lemony version. The combination of cucumber and potato is delicious and the fresh dill adds a fresh summery accent.

1 pound red-skinned or other waxy potatoes, well scrubbed
2 tablespoons mayonnaise
2 tablespoons plain low-fat yogurt
1 tablespoon lemon juice
1 teaspoon kosher salt
⅛ teaspoon freshly ground pepper
½ hothouse (English) cucumber, halved lengthwise and thinly sliced
1 thin scallion, thinly sliced
2 tablespoons chopped fresh dill

1 Place the potatoes in a large saucepan. Add water to cover and bring to a boil over high heat. Reduce the heat to low and simmer, uncovered, until the potatoes are tender, 15 to 20 minutes. Drain and let stand until cool enough to handle. Cut the potatoes into 1-inch pieces.

2 Meanwhile, whisk together the mayonnaise, yogurt, lemon juice, salt, and pepper in a large bowl. Add the potatoes, cucumber, scallion, and dill and toss to combine. Serve the salad at room temperature or chilled. The salad tastes best on the day it is made, but it can be refrigerated, covered, for up to 1 day.

Each serving: 20 g carb, 142 cal, 6 g fat, 1 g sat fat, 3 mg chol, 2 g fib, 3 g pro, 331 mg sod • Carb Choices: 1; Exchanges: 1½ starch, 1 fat

No-Mayo Potato Salad

makes 4 servings

Who says potato salad has to have mayonnaise? This version is light and tart with just a touch of crunch from the scallions. To give the salad a fresh citrus flavor, replace the vinegar with lemon juice and add 1 teaspoon grated lemon zest.

1 pound small red-skinned or other waxy potatoes, well scrubbed
2 tablespoons white wine vinegar
1½ tablespoon extra virgin olive oil
1 teaspoon kosher salt
⅛ teaspoon freshly ground pepper
¼ cup thinly sliced scallions
2 tablespoons chopped fresh Italian parsley

1 Place the potatoes in a large saucepan. Add water to cover and bring to a boil over high heat. Reduce the heat to low and simmer, uncovered, until the potatoes are tender, 15 to 20 minutes. Drain and let stand until cool enough to handle. Thinly slice the potatoes.

2 Meanwhile, whisk together the vinegar, oil, salt, and pepper in a large bowl. Add the potatoes, scallions, and parsley and toss to combine. Serve the salad at room temperature or chilled. The salad tastes best on the day it is made, but it can be refrigerated, covered, for up to 1 day.

Each serving: 19 g carb, 129 cal, 5 g fat, 1 g sat fat, 0 mg chol, 2 g fib, 2 g pro, 289 mg sod • Carb Choices: 1; Exchanges: 1 starch, 1 fat

BLUE CHEESE POTATO SALAD: Follow the No-Mayo Potato Salad recipe, above, adding ¼ cup crumbled blue cheese with the potatoes in step 2.

Each serving: 19 g carb, 159 cal, 8 g fat, 2 g sat fat, 6 mg chol, 2 g fib, 4 g pro, 407 mg sod • Carb Choices: 1; Exchanges: 1 starch, 1½ fat

GREEK POTATO SALAD: Follow the No-Mayo Potato Salad recipe, above, adding ¼ cup finely crumbled feta and 2 tablespoons chopped pitted Kalamata olives with the potatoes in step 2.

Each serving: 19 g carb, 165 cal, 8 g fat, 2 g sat fat, 8 mg chol, 2 g fib, 4 g pro, 455 mg sod • Carb Choices: 1; Exchanges: 1 starch, 1½ fat

Fingerling Potato and Green Bean Salad with Mustard Dressing HIGH FIBER

makes 4 servings

If you find several varieties of fingerling potatoes at the farmers' market, buy a few different kinds and mix them up in this salad. For another fresh addition, you can toss 2 cups of baby arugula or baby spinach into the salad just before serving.

8 ounces green beans, trimmed and cut into 2-inch pieces
1 pound fingerling potatoes, well scrubbed
2 tablespoons whole grain mustard
1 tablespoon white wine vinegar
1 tablespoon extra virgin olive oil
½ teaspoon kosher salt
⅛ teaspoon freshly ground pepper
2 tablespoons diced red onion

1 Bring a large saucepan of water to a boil over high heat. Add the green beans, return to a boil, and cook just until crisp-tender, about 3 minutes. Using a slotted spoon, transfer the beans to a colander and rinse under cold running water until cool. Drain well.

2 Carefully add the potatoes to the saucepan and return to a boil. Reduce the heat to low and simmer, uncovered, until the potatoes are tender, 15 to 20 minutes. Drain and let stand until cool enough to handle. Cut each potato in half lengthwise.

3 Meanwhile, whisk together the mustard, vinegar, oil, salt, and pepper in a large bowl. Add the green beans, potatoes, and onion and toss gently to combine. Serve the salad at room temperature or chilled. The salad tastes best on the day it is made, but it can be refrigerated, covered, for up to 1 day.

Each serving: 23 g carb, 138 cal, 4 g fat, 1 g sat fat, 0 mg chol, 4 g fib, 4 g pro, 304 mg sod • Carb Choices: 1½; Exchanges: 1 starch, 1 veg, ½ fat

Sweet Potato Salad with Molasses

makes 8 servings

If you have pecan oil on hand, use it instead of olive oil. My favorite molasses is from Sand Mountain Sorghum, made in Scottsboro, Alabama. It has a gleaming dark amber color and just a hint of bitterness.

2 pounds sweet potatoes, peeled and cut into large cubes
2 teaspoons plus 1 tablespoon extra virgin olive oil, divided
2 teaspoons apple cider vinegar
2 teaspoons molasses
½ teaspoon Dijon mustard
½ teaspoon kosher salt
⅛ teaspoon freshly ground pepper
2 teaspoons chopped fresh sage or ½ teaspoon crumbled dried sage
¼ cup thinly sliced red onion
2 tablespoons pecans, toasted and chopped (page 4)

1 Preheat the oven to 425°F.

2 Place the potatoes in a large rimmed baking sheet. Drizzle with 2 teaspoons of the oil and toss to coat. Arrange in a single layer.

3 Bake, turning the potatoes once, until tender and browned, 30 to 35 minutes.

4 Meanwhile, whisk together the vinegar, remaining 1 tablespoon oil, molasses, mustard, salt, and pepper. Stir in the sage. Add the roasted potatoes and toss to coat. Cool to room temperature and stir in the onion. Stir in the pecans just before serving. Serve the salad at room temperature. The salad tastes best on the day it is made, but it can be refrigerated, covered, for up to 1 day. Let stand at room temperature 30 minutes before serving.

Each serving: 16 g carb, 108 cal, 4 g fat, 1 g sat fat, 0 mg chol, 3 g fib, 2 g pro, 103 mg sod • Carb Choices: 1; Exchanges: 1 starch, 1 fat

Marinated Cucumber and Sweet Onion Salad

makes 4 servings

Marinating the vegetables in mild vinegar makes them crisp and flavorful. This basic salad is refreshing and flavorful on its own, but if you have any fresh herbs on hand, by all means, add a couple tablespoons.

1 large hothouse (English) cucumber, thinly sliced
½ large sweet onion, thinly sliced
2 tablespoons rice vinegar or white wine vinegar
½ teaspoon kosher salt
⅛ teaspoon freshly ground pepper
Chopped fresh Italian parsley, basil, dill, or tarragon (optional)

Combine the cucumber, onion, and vinegar in a medium shallow dish. Refrigerate the salad, covered, stirring occasionally, until chilled, at least 2 hours and up to 12 hours. Just before serving, stir in the salt, pepper, and parsley, if using.

Each serving: 4 g carb, 17 cal, 0 g fat, 0 g sat fat, 0 mg chol, 1 g fib, 1 g pro, 142 mg sod • Carb Choices: 0; Exchanges: 1 veg

Asian Cucumber Salad

makes 4 servings

Serve this salad alongside Cilantro Chicken Salad Wraps (page 65) for an Asian-inspired picnic or at-work lunch. It makes a refreshing—and very low-calorie—afternoon snack, too.

1 large hothouse (English) cucumber, thinly sliced
2 tablespoons rice vinegar
2 scallions, thinly sliced
2 tablespoons chopped fresh cilantro
½ teaspoon kosher salt
¼ teaspoon Asian sesame oil
1 teaspoon toasted sesame seeds (page 4)

1 Combine the cucumber and vinegar in a medium shallow dish. Refrigerate, covered, stirring occasionally, until chilled, at least 2 hours and up to 12 hours.

2 To serve, add the scallions, cilantro, salt, and oil and toss to combine. Sprinkle with the sesame seeds and serve at once.

Each serving: 4 g carb, 25 cal, 1 g fat, 0 g sat fat, 0 mg chol, 1 g fib, 1 g pro, 143 mg sod • Carb Choices: 0; Exchanges: 1 veg

Cucumber-Mango Salad

QUICK

makes 4 servings

This salad is a riot of colors and textures—crunchy and colorful cucumber and bell pepper and soft yellow mango—all dressed in a spicy-sweet dressing. It's a great salad to serve with grilled salmon or shrimp, with any ordinary sandwich for lunch, or as part of a summer salad buffet when you entertain.

1 teaspoon grated lime zest
2 tablespoons lime juice
1 tablespoon canola oil
1 teaspoon honey
½ teaspoon kosher salt
¼ teaspoon ground cumin
¼ teaspoon ground coriander
Pinch of ground cayenne
1 large mango, peeled, pitted, and thinly sliced
1 hothouse (English) cucumber, halved lengthwise, seeded, and cut into thin strips
1 medium red bell pepper, thinly sliced
¼ cup chopped fresh cilantro

1 Whisk together the lime zest, lime juice, oil, honey, salt, cumin, coriander, and cayenne in a large bowl.

2 Add the mango, cucumber, bell pepper, and cilantro and toss to coat. Serve at once, or cover, and refrigerate up to 1 day. Let stand at room temperature 30 minutes before serving.

Each serving: 14 g carb, 88 cal, 4 g fat, 0 g sat fat, 0 mg chol, 2 g fib, 1 g pro, 143 mg sod • Carb Choices: 1; Exchanges: ½ fruit, 1 veg, ½ fat

Asparagus Salad with Orange-Ginger Dressing QUICK

makes 6 servings

To remove the tough ends of asparagus, bend each spear, and it will naturally snap off where the asparagus becomes tough.

1½ pounds asparagus, tough ends removed
2 tablespoons Orange-Ginger Dressing
    (page 144)
2 tablespoons thinly sliced scallions
½ teaspoon toasted sesame seeds (page 4)

1 Fill a large saucepan three-fourths full with water; bring to a boil over high heat. Add the asparagus and cook until crisp-tender, 3 to 4 minutes. Drain the asparagus and rinse under cold water until cool. Dry the asparagus with paper towels.

2 Arrange the asparagus on a serving platter. Drizzle with the dressing. Sprinkle with the scallions and sesame seeds and serve at room temperature within 2 hours.

Each serving: 3 g carb, 20 cal, 0 g fat, 0 g sat fat, 0 mg chol, 1 g fib, 1 g pro, 3 mg sod • Carb Choices: 0; Exchanges: 1 veg

Roasted Beet and Green Bean Salad HIGH FIBER

makes 8 servings

You can cook the beets and green beans for this salad a day ahead and simply assemble it before serving.

1 pound green beans, trimmed
1 head Bibb lettuce, separated into leaves
2 recipes Foil-Roasted Beets (page 447)
1 small red onion, thinly sliced
1 recipe Herbed Vinaigrette (page 138), made
    with dill or parsley
1 ounce finely crumbled feta cheese
    (about ¼ cup)

1 Bring a large saucepan of water to a boil over high heat. Add the green beans and cook until crisp-tender, 4 to 5 minutes. Drain in a colander and rinse with cold running water until cool. Pat the beans dry with paper towels and set aside.

2 Arrange the lettuce on a large platter. Cut the beets into ½-inch wedges and arrange on top of the lettuce. Top with the cooked green beans and onion. Drizzle with the vinaigrette and sprinkle with the feta. Serve at once.

Each serving: 12 g carb, 116 cal, 7 g fat, 1 g sat fat, 4 mg chol, 4 g fib, 3 g pro, 159 mg sod • Carb Choices: 1; Exchanges: 2 veg, 1 fat

Fennel, Apple, and Celery Salad QUICK HIGH FIBER

makes 4 servings

Fennel is one of my favorite vegetables and I am always looking for new ways to serve it. This is a much-loved fall salad that partners fennel with two kinds of apple—one tart and one sweet—and crunchy celery. A molasses-kissed dressing brings all the flavors together.

1½ tablespoons extra virgin olive oil
1 tablespoon apple cider vinegar
2 teaspoons molasses
½ teaspoon Dijon mustard
½ teaspoon kosher salt
¼ teaspoon freshly ground pepper
1 small bulb fennel, tough outer leaves
    removed, cored and thinly sliced
1 Granny Smith apple, cored and cut into thin
    strips
1 Gala apple, cored and cut into thin strips
1 stalk celery, thinly sliced

Whisk together the oil, vinegar, molasses, mustard, salt, and pepper in a large bowl. Add the fennel, apples, and celery and toss to coat. Serve the salad at once or cover and chill up to 4 hours.

Each serving: 16 g carb, 108 cal, 5 g fat, 1 g sat fat, 0 mg chol, 4 g fib, 1 g pro, 184 mg sod • Carb Choices: 1; Exchanges: 1 fruit, 1 fat

Fennel and Parmesan Salad QUICK

makes 8 servings

The fresh bright flavors of this salad make it a refreshing starter for a rich Italian meal of lasagna or pasta and meatballs.

2 medium bulbs fennel, tough outer leaves removed, cored and thinly sliced
1 large head Bibb lettuce, leaves torn
2 ounces finely shredded Parmesan (about ½ cup)
¼ cup chopped fresh fennel fronds (optional)
1 recipe Lemon Vinaigrette (page 139)

Combine the fennel, lettuce, Parmesan, and fennel fronds, if using, in a large bowl. Drizzle with the vinaigrette and toss to coat. Serve at once.

Each serving: 5 g carb, 99 cal, 7 g fat, 2 g sat fat, 5 mg chol, 2 g fib, 4 g pro, 195 mg sod • Carb Choices: 0; Exchanges: 1 veg, 1½ fat

Roasted Mushroom Salad

makes 8 servings

Adding the dressing to the mushrooms while they are hot gives them time to soak up the flavors of the vinaigrette as they cool. Serve them with grilled steak, or spoon them on top of mixed salad greens and sprinkle with grated Parmesan or crumbled blue cheese.

1 pound white mushrooms, quartered
1 pound cremini mushrooms, quartered
12 ounces shiitake mushrooms, stemmed and quartered
1 tablespoon extra virgin olive oil
½ teaspoon kosher salt
1 recipe Basic Vinaigrette (page 138)
¼ cup chopped fresh Italian parsley

1 Preheat the oven to 425°F.

2 Place the mushrooms in a large rimmed baking sheet. Drizzle with the oil, sprinkle with the salt, and toss to coat. Arrange the mushrooms in a single layer. Bake, stirring twice, until the mushrooms are tender and the liquid has evaporated, 45 minutes.

3 Place the vinaigrette in a medium bowl. Add the hot mushrooms and let stand until cooled to room temperature, stirring occasionally. Serve at once, or cover and refrigerate up to 1 day. Let stand at room temperature 30 minutes before serving. Stir in the parsley just before serving.

Each serving: 7 g carb, 108 cal, 7 g fat, 1 g sat fat, 0 mg chol, 2 g fib, 3 g pro, 122 mg sod • Carb Choices: ½; Exchanges: 1 veg, 1½ fat

Roasted Eggplant and Spinach Salad with Peanut Dressing HIGH FIBER

makes 4 servings

Peanut dressing makes an unexpected, yet delicious accompaniment to eggplant in this salad. Add grilled shrimp to make it an entrée.

1 tablespoon plus 1 teaspoon canola oil, divided
1 medium eggplant (about 1¼ pounds), cut into ½-inch rounds
¼ teaspoon kosher salt
6 cups loosely packed torn fresh spinach
1 recipe Peanut Dressing (page 144)
2 tablespoons chopped fresh cilantro

1 Preheat the oven to 425°F. Brush a large rimmed baking sheet with 1 teaspoon of the oil.

2 Brush the eggplant slices with the remaining 1 tablespoon oil. Sprinkle with the salt. Arrange in a single layer on the baking sheet. Bake, turning once, until tender and well browned, 35 to 40 minutes. Transfer to a platter and let cool to room temperature.

3 Place the spinach in a large bowl, drizzle with 2 tablespoons of the dressing, and toss to coat. Divide the spinach among 4 plates and top evenly with the eggplant. Drizzle the eggplant evenly with the remaining dressing, sprinkle with the cilantro, and serve at once.

Each serving: 13 g carb, 158 cal, 10 g fat, 1 g sat fat, 0 mg chol, 6 g fib, 5 g pro, 351 mg sod • Carb Choices: ½; Exchanges: ½ carb, 2 fat

Celery Root Salad with Mustard Dressing

makes 4 servings

If you've never known what to do with gnarly celery roots that appear every fall in grocery stores and farmers' markets, give this salad a try. Celery root tastes like rarefied celery—it's crunchy but not watery and not a string in sight. In this salad, it's dressed in classic French style, with whole grain mustard and fresh parsley—except I've used yogurt instead of mayonnaise. Serve it with any roast poultry or meat or with grilled fish or shellfish.

¼ cup plain low-fat Greek yogurt or strained yogurt (page 11)
1½ tablespoons lemon juice
2 teaspoons whole grain mustard
2 teaspoons extra virgin olive oil
¼ teaspoon kosher salt
Pinch of freshly ground pepper
1 large celery root, cut into long, thin strips (about 4 cups)
¼ cup chopped fresh Italian parsley

1 Whisk together the yogurt, lemon juice, mustard, oil, salt, and pepper in a large bowl.

2 Add the celery root and parsley and toss to coat. Refrigerate the salad, covered, until chilled, 2 hours or up to 1 day.

Each serving: 13 g carb, 88 cal, 3 g fat, 1 g sat fat, 1 mg chol, 2 g fib, 3 g pro, 250 mg sod • Carb Choices: 1; Exchanges: 2 veg, ½ fat

Mixed Tomato and Mozzarella Salad with Basil Dressing QUICK

makes 8 servings

To thinly slice the mozzarella, slice it while it is cold using a serrated knife. The flavor of the cheese is better if it is at room temperature, so let the cheese stand at room temperature once it's sliced for about 15 minutes before serving the salad. You can use any variety of fresh tomatoes in this salad—try heirloom varieties that are available at farmers' markets in the summer. Capers, sliced roasted red peppers, halved black olives, and sliced cucumbers all make delicious additions to this versatile salad.

8 ounces fresh mozzarella, thinly sliced
4 large tomatoes, sliced
1 cup red cherry tomatoes, halved
1 cup yellow cherry tomatoes, halved
1 recipe Herbed Vinaigrette (page 138), made with fresh basil
Thinly sliced fresh basil leaves

Arrange the mozzarella and sliced tomatoes in alternating layers on a large platter. Top with the cherry tomatoes. Drizzle with the vinaigrette and sprinkle with the basil. Serve at once.

Each serving: 4 g carb, 139 cal, 12 g fat, 3 g sat fat, 10 mg chol, 1 g fib, 6 g pro, 69 mg sod • Carb Choices: 0; Exchanges: 1 veg, 1 medium-fat protein, 1 fat

Green Bean, Cherry Tomato, and Bacon Salad

QUICK | HIGH FIBER

makes 4 servings

I would rather have half a slice of real bacon than a pound of turkey bacon. As you'll see from the small amount in this salad, that's all you need to add authentic flavor and irresistible crunch. You can also sprinkle the salad with the kernels from an ear of corn just before serving.

1 pound green beans, trimmed
2 strips smoked center-cut bacon
2 cups cherry tomatoes, halved
3 tablespoons Basic Vinaigrette (page 138)

1 Bring a large saucepan of water to a boil over high heat. Add the green beans and cook until crisp-tender, 4 to 5 minutes. Drain in a colander and rinse with cold running water until cool. (The beans may be cooked up to 1 day ahead and refrigerated.)

2 Meanwhile, cook the bacon in a large skillet over medium-high heat until crisp. Drain on paper towels and chop.

3 Arrange the green beans and tomatoes on a large serving platter. Drizzle with the vinaigrette and toss to coat. Sprinkle with the bacon and serve at once.

Each serving: 10 g carb, 114 cal, 7 g fat, 1 g sat fat, 3 mg chol, 4 g fib, 3 g pro, 122 mg sod • Carb Choices: ½; Exchanges: 2 veg, 1½ fat

Grilled Vegetable and Goat Cheese Salad

makes 6 servings

When summer vegetables are at their peak and I've run out of ideas for preparing them, I like to grill a big batch of vegetables and keep them in the refrigerator to use in pasta salads, sandwiches, or salads such as this one.

3 tablespoons plus ½ teaspoon extra virgin olive oil, divided
2 tablespoons white balsamic or white wine vinegar
1 garlic clove, crushed through a press
¾ teaspoon kosher salt
¼ teaspoon freshly ground pepper
4 plum tomatoes, quartered
2 medium zucchini, cut on the diagonal into ½-inch slices
2 medium yellow squash, cut on the diagonal into ½-inch slices
1 large red bell pepper, cut into 1-inch strips
1 large red onion, cut into thin wedges
2 tablespoons chopped fresh basil
2 ounces finely crumbled goat cheese (about ½ cup)
2 tablespoons pine nuts, toasted (page 4)

1 Prepare the grill or heat a large grill pan over medium-high heat.

2 To make the dressing, whisk together 2 tablespoons of the oil, the vinegar, garlic, salt, and ground pepper in a large bowl. Set aside.

3 Combine the tomatoes, zucchini, yellow squash, bell pepper, and onion in a separate large bowl. Drizzle with 1 tablespoon of the remaining oil and toss to coat. Brush the grill rack or grill pan with the remaining ½ teaspoon oil. Place the vegetables on the grill rack or in the grill pan, in batches, if necessary, and grill, turning often, until the vegetables are browned, 10 to 12 minutes for the zucchini, yellow squash, bell pepper, and onion, and 4 to 6 minutes for the tomatoes. Place the vegetables in the prepared dressing, add the basil, and toss to coat.

4 Arrange the vegetables on a serving platter. Sprinkle with the goat cheese and pine nuts. Serve warm or at room temperature.

Each serving: 12 g carb, 171 cal, 13 g fat, 3 g sat fat, 7 mg chol, 3 g fib, 5 g pro, 207 mg sod • Carb Choices: 1; Exchanges: 2 veg, 2 fat

Layered Vegetable Salad

makes 8 servings

I call this a "casserole salad" since it's layered in a dish and instead of a creamy sauce, it has a creamy dressing.

2 strips center-cut bacon
6 cups loosely packed torn romaine lettuce
1 large tomato, chopped
1 cup frozen petite green peas, thawed
2 ounces shredded reduced-fat extra-sharp Cheddar (about ½ cup)
½ cup thinly sliced red onion
1 large yellow or green bell pepper, chopped
1 cup thinly sliced red cabbage
1 recipe Creamy Herb Dressing (page 141)

1 Cook the bacon in a skillet over medium-high heat until crisp. Drain on paper towels and chop.

2 Place the lettuce in a large deep-sided glass bowl. Top with the tomato, peas, Cheddar, onion, bell pepper, cabbage, and bacon. Refrigerate the salad, covered, 2 hours or up to 4 hours.

3 Just before serving, drizzle the salad with the dressing and toss to coat.

Each serving: 7 g carb, 89 cal, 5 g fat, 2 g sat fat, 8 mg chol, 2 g fib, 5 g pro, 162 mg sod • Carb Choices: ½; Exchanges: 1 veg, ½ fat

Chopped Salad QUICK

makes 4 servings

A chopped salad is great to serve at a party where there might not be enough room for everyone to sit—you don't need a knife to eat it.

1 tablespoon red wine vinegar
1½ teaspoons extra virgin olive oil
¼ teaspoon kosher salt
⅛ teaspoon freshly ground pepper
4 plum tomatoes, chopped
1 hothouse (English) cucumber, chopped
½ cup diced red or yellow bell pepper
2 tablespoons diced red onion
2 tablespoons chopped fresh Italian parsley

1 Whisk together the vinegar, oil, salt, and ground pepper in a large bowl.

2 Add the tomatoes, cucumber, bell pepper, onion, and parsley and stir to coat. Serve the salad at room temperature or chilled. The salad tastes better on the day it is made, but it can be refrigerated, covered, for up to 2 days.

Each serving: 7 g carb, 45 cal, 2 g fat, 0 g sat fat, 0 mg chol, 2 g fib, 1 g pro, 77 mg sod • Carb Choices: ½; Exchanges: 1 veg, ½ fat

Greek Chopped Salad QUICK

makes 4 servings

In this salad, a small amount of high-calorie olives go a long way, since they are chopped before being added to the salad. I make this often for lunch and sometimes include canned garbanzo beans or canned tuna to add some protein.

2 teaspoons grated lemon zest
1 tablespoon lemon juice
1 tablespoon extra virgin olive oil
¼ teaspoon kosher salt
⅛ teaspoon freshly ground pepper
4 cups chopped romaine lettuce
2 cups cherry tomatoes, halved
2 pepperoncini peppers, drained and chopped
6 Kalamata olives, pitted and chopped
½ hothouse (English) cucumber, chopped
½ red or yellow bell pepper, chopped
1 ounce finely crumbled feta cheese (about ¼ cup)
2 tablespoons chopped fresh dill
2 tablespoons diced red onion

1 Whisk together the lemon zest, lemon juice, oil, salt, and ground pepper in a large bowl.

2 Add the remaining ingredients and toss to coat. Serve at once.

Each serving: 9 g carb, 107 cal, 7 g fat, 2 g sat fat, 6 mg chol, 3 g fib, 3 g pro, 296 mg sod • Carb Choices: ½; Exchanges: 1 veg, 1 fat

Bread Salad QUICK

makes 8 servings

This is a lightened version of a classic Italian salad called panzanella. The bread in this version is toasted like croutons, but you can skip the toasting step if you prefer. If you have an abundance of fresh basil or Italian parsley, add some whole leaves to the salad to give big bursts of vibrant flavor.

4 ounces whole grain bread, cut into ½-inch cubes (about 2½ cups)

4 cups loosely packed torn romaine lettuce

1 large tomato, chopped

1 large hothouse (English) cucumber, halved lengthwise and sliced

½ cup red Roasted Bell Peppers (page 21) or roasted red peppers from a jar, thinly sliced

¼ cup thinly sliced red onion

1 recipe Basic Vinaigrette (page 138)

1 ounce finely shredded Parmesan (about ¼ cup)

1 Preheat the oven to 350°F. Place the bread cubes in a single layer on a large rimmed baking sheet. Bake, stirring once, until lightly toasted, 8 minutes. Let cool to room temperature.

2 Combine the toasted bread cubes, lettuce, tomato, cucumber, roasted peppers, and onion in a large bowl. Drizzle with the vinaigrette and toss to coat. Divide the salad among 8 plates and sprinkle evenly with the Parmesan. Serve at once.

Each serving: 10 g carb, 107 cal, 7 g fat, 1 g sat fat, 3 mg chol, 3 g fib, 3 g pro, 141 mg sod • Carb Choices: ½; Exchanges: ½ carb, 1 fat

Lima Bean, Corn, and Tomato Salad QUICK | HIGH FIBER

makes 8 servings

I could have called this succotash salad, since it has all the ingredients of the vegetable side dish. If you're making this salad in summer, use fresh corn. Cut the kernels from two large ears of corn and cook as directed for the frozen corn.

1 (10-ounce) package frozen baby lima beans

1 (10-ounce) package frozen corn kernels

½ cup diced yellow or green bell pepper

1 large tomato, chopped

4 small scallions, thinly sliced

½ cup chopped fresh basil or Italian parsley

1 recipe Basic Vinaigrette or Herbed Vinaigrette (page 138)

1 Bring a large pot of water to a boil over high heat. Add the lima beans, return to a boil, and cook 2 minutes. Add the corn and cook 1 minute. Drain in a colander and rinse with cold running water until cool.

2 Combine the lima bean mixture and the remaining ingredients in a large bowl and toss to coat. Serve the salad at room temperature or chilled. The salad tastes best on the day it is made.

Each serving: 18 g carb, 136 cal, 6 g fat, 1 g sat fat, 0 mg chol, 4 g fib, 4 g pro, 65 mg sod • Carb Choices: 1; Exchanges: 1 starch, 1 fat

Edamame

If you'd like to get more of the lean protein goodness of soy, but you don't like tofu, try edamame. Edamame are young green soybeans that have a nutty mild flavor, much like a cross between a lima bean and a green pea. You can buy them frozen in most large supermarkets and they come in the pod or shelled.

The ones in the pod make a healthy snack (and slow down your eating, because you have to peel them first). The shelled ones can be eaten on their own seasoned only with a little sesame or olive oil and a sprinkle of salt. Add them to salads, soups, or stews—they're a delicious way to eat more healthful soy. A ½ cup of shelled edamame has ½ a Carb Choice (9 grams of carbs), 100 calories, 8 grams of protein, and 4 grams of fiber.

Edamame and Grape Tomato Salad QUICK | HIGH FIBER

makes 8 servings

If you haven't tried edamame, this salad is a delicious introduction. You can use frozen baby lima beans instead of the edamame if you prefer. Using baby limas will increase the carbohydrates to 16 grams and the Carb Choices will be 1.

1 pound frozen shelled edamame
2 tablespoons white wine vinegar
2 tablespoons extra virgin olive oil
1 garlic clove, crushed through a press
½ teaspoon kosher salt
⅛ teaspoon freshly ground pepper
1 cup grape tomatoes, halved
1 small red or green bell pepper, diced
½ hothouse (English) cucumber, diced
¼ cup chopped fresh Italian parsley
2 tablespoons minced red onion

1 Bring a large saucepan of water to a boil over high heat. Add the edamame and cook until tender, about 5 minutes. Drain in a colander and rinse with cold running water until cool.

2 Meanwhile, whisk together the vinegar, oil, garlic, salt, and ground pepper in a large bowl. Add the edamame, tomatoes, bell pepper, cucumber, parsley, and onion and stir to combine. Serve the salad at room temperature or chilled. The salad tastes best on the day it is made, but it can be refrigerated, covered, for up to 2 days.

Each serving: 7 g carb, 108 cal, 6 g fat, 1 g sat fat, 0 mg chol, 4 g fib, 7 g pro, 76 mg sod • Carb Choices: ½; Exchanges: ½ carb, 1 plant-based protein, 1 fat

Asian Edamame and Radish Salad QUICK

makes 4 servings

This is one of my favorite ways to use edamame. I love the ginger and lime dressing and I can keep the salad in the refrigerator for a couple of days to have for a healthful lunch or an afternoon snack. Rice vinegar is milder than other vinegars and is a good pantry staple to have on hand for making salad dressings and brightening the flavor of soups and dips.

2 cups frozen shelled edamame
1½ tablespoons canola oil
1 tablespoon rice vinegar
1 tablespoon lime juice
1 tablespoon reduced-sodium soy sauce
½ teaspoon kosher salt
¼ teaspoon Asian sesame oil
2 teaspoons minced fresh ginger
6 radishes, thinly sliced
½ cup diced yellow or green bell pepper
½ cup diced hothouse (English) cucumber
¼ cup chopped fresh cilantro or 2 tablespoons chopped fresh mint

1 Bring a medium saucepan of water to a boil over high heat. Add the edamame and cook until tender, about 5 minutes. Drain in a colander and rinse with cold running water until cool.

2 Meanwhile, whisk together the canola oil, vinegar, lime juice, soy sauce, salt, sesame oil, and ginger in a large bowl. Add the edamame, radishes, bell pepper, cucumber, and cilantro and stir to combine. Serve the salad at room temperature or chilled. The salad tastes best on the day it is made, but it can be refrigerated, covered, for up to 2 days.

Each serving: 7 g carb, 125 cal, 8 g fat, 0 g sat fat, 0 mg chol, 3 g fib, 7 g pro, 299 mg sod • Carb Choices: ½; Exchanges: ½ carb, 1 plant-based protein, 1 fat

Pasta Salads

Antipasto Pasta Salad

QUICK | HIGH FIBER

makes 8 servings

This salad is a great example of how a very small amount of a high-fat ingredient such as salami can flavor an entire dish. When it is cut into thin slices and tossed with whole wheat pasta and loads of vegetables, there's enough to flavor the dish, yet not enough to send you to your cardiologist. Be sure to blot the artichokes with paper towels to remove the excess moisture and to prevent diluting the flavors of the salad.

8 ounces whole wheat penne or other short pasta (about 2⅔ cups)
1 (14-ounce) can artichoke hearts
1½ tablespoons extra virgin olive oil
1 tablespoon red wine vinegar
¼ teaspoon kosher salt
⅛ teaspoon freshly ground pepper
2 ounces hard salami, cut into thin strips
2 ounces fresh mozzarella, diced
1 cup cherry or grape tomatoes, halved
½ hothouse (English) cucumber, halved lengthwise and sliced
½ cup red Roasted Bell Peppers (page 21) or roasted red peppers from a jar, sliced
¼ cup Kalamata olives, pitted and quartered
¼ cup chopped fresh basil or Italian parsley

1 Cook the pasta according to the package directions. Drain in a colander and rinse under cold running water until cool. Drain well.

2 Meanwhile, drain the artichoke hearts and cut into quarters. Place the artichokes on several thicknesses of paper towels and gently blot dry. Set aside.

3 Whisk together the oil, vinegar, salt, and ground pepper in a large bowl. Add the cooked pasta, artichoke hearts, salami, mozzarella, tomatoes, cucumber, roasted peppers, olives, and basil and toss to combine. Serve the salad at room temperature. The salad tastes best on the day it is made, but it can be refrigerated, covered, for up to 2 days. Let stand at room temperature 30 minutes before serving.

Each serving: 22 g carb, 195 cal, 8 g fat, 2 g sat fat, 9 mg chol, 4 g fib, 9 g pro, 342 mg sod • Carb Choices: 1; Exchanges: 1 starch, 1 veg, 1½ fat

Roasted Vegetable and Pasta Salad HIGH FIBER

makes 6 servings

The fantastic flavor of this salad belies its simple ingredients. Roasting the vegetables sweetens and concentrates their flavor and the fresh mint is an unexpected surprise. Roast double the amount of zucchini and bell pepper when you make this salad and serve the leftover vegetables as a side dish later in the week.

1 pound zucchini, halved lengthwise and cut into ½-inch slices
1 large red bell pepper, thinly sliced
2 teaspoons plus 1½ tablespoon extra virgin olive oil, divided
½ teaspoon kosher salt, divided
¼ teaspoon freshly ground pepper, divided
6 ounces whole wheat penne or other short pasta (about 2 cups)
2 tablespoons white wine vinegar
1 ounce finely crumbled feta cheese (about ¼ cup)
2 tablespoons chopped fresh mint or Italian parsley

1 Preheat the oven to 425°F.

2 Place the zucchini and bell pepper in a large roasting pan. Drizzle with 2 teaspoons of the oil and sprinkle with ¼ teaspoon of the salt and

⅛ teaspoon of the ground pepper. Toss to coat. Arrange the vegetables in a single layer. Bake, stirring once, until tender and lightly browned, 25 to 30 minutes. Transfer to a plate to cool.

3 Meanwhile, cook the pasta according to the package directions. Drain in a colander and rinse under cold running water until cool. Drain well.

4 Whisk together the vinegar, remaining 1½ tablespoons oil, remaining ¼ teaspoon salt, and remaining ⅛ teaspoon ground pepper in a large bowl. Add the pasta, zucchini and bell peppers, feta, and mint and toss to coat. Serve at once, or refrigerate, covered, for up to 4 hours.

Each serving: 24 g carb, 171 cal, 7 g fat, 2 g sat fat, 4 mg chol, 5 g fib, 6 g pro, 157 mg sod • Carb Choices: 1½; Exchanges: 1½ starch, 1 veg, 1½ fat

Pasta and Pea Salad

QUICK | HIGH FIBER

makes 6 servings

Simple, but oh, so good. Especially if you make this in the springtime with fresh peas from the farmers' market. If you use fresh peas, you'll need about 1 pound of English peas to get 1 cup shelled peas. Adding a pound of cooked shrimp will turn this side dish into an entrée.

6 ounces whole wheat rotini or other short pasta (about 2 cups)
6 ounces fresh sugar snap peas, trimmed (about 2 cups)
1 cup shelled fresh English peas or unthawed frozen green peas
3 tablespoons white wine vinegar
1 tablespoon extra virgin olive oil
¾ teaspoon kosher salt
⅛ teaspoon freshly ground pepper
2 tablespoons finely crumbled feta cheese
2 tablespoons chopped fresh dill

1 Bring a large pot of water to a boil over high heat; add the pasta, return to a boil and cook 8 minutes. Add the snap peas and English peas

Pasta Salads Are Carb Smart

Pasta salads are not off-limits for carb counters. If you prepare them with fiber- and nutrient-rich whole grain pasta, load them up with fresh vegetables, and toss lightly with a dressing made with a healthy oil like olive oil or canola oil, pasta salads make a flavorful, nutritious, and easily manageable addition to any meal plan.

For those in your family who don't love veggies, adding them to pasta salads is a wonderful way to make almost any vegetable more appealing. Everyone loves pasta (even the pickiest child) and when it's tossed with fresh vegetables and a drizzle of flavorful dressing, you've got a universally appealing dish that's healthy and wholesome.

A good rule of thumb for keeping the carbs in check in a pasta salad is to use the same volume of vegetables as you do cooked pasta. If you use 4 cups of cooked pasta, add 4 cups of vegetables. This ratio is used in the Mix and Match Pasta Salads (page 104) to make all kinds of pasta salads for just 1½ Carb Choices each.

and cook 1 minute. Drain in a colander and rinse under cold running water until cool. Drain well.

2 Meanwhile, whisk together the vinegar, oil, salt, and pepper in a large bowl. Add the pasta mixture, feta, and dill and toss to coat. Serve the salad at room temperature. The salad tastes best on the day it is made, but it can be refrigerated, covered, for up to 2 days. Let stand at room temperature 30 minutes before serving.

Each serving: 23 g carb, 158 cal, 4 g fat, 1 g sat fat, 3 mg chol, 5 g fib, 7 g pro, 181 mg sod • Carb Choices: 1½; Exchanges: 1½ starch, ½ fat

MIX AND MATCH PASTA SALADS

Cook 8 ounces (about 2⅔ cups) short whole wheat pasta (such as penne, cavatappi, macaroni, or fusilli) according to the package directions. Combine the cooked pasta (you'll have about 4 cups) with one ingredient from each column in the chart below. The salads make enough to serve 8 as a side dish. Each serving has 1½ Carb Choices (about 23 grams of carbs) and around 160 calories.

Vegetable 1	Vegetable 2	Flavor Booster	Dressing	Finishing Touch
2 cups peeled, seeded, sliced cucumber	2 cups chopped zucchini	¼ cup finely crumbled goat cheese	1 recipe Basic Vinaigrette (page 138)	¼ cup chopped fresh Italian parsley
¾ cup cherry or grape tomatoes, halved	2 cups chopped yellow squash	¼ cup finely crumbled feta cheese	1 recipe Mustard Vinaigrette (page 138)	¼ cup chopped fresh basil
2 cups chopped bell pepper	1 cup cooked green beans, cut into 1-inch pieces	¼ cup finely shredded Parmesan	1 recipe Lemon Vinaigrette (page 139)	1 tablespoon chopped fresh rosemary
2 cups small broccoli florets	2 cups 1-inch pieces cooked asparagus	3 tablespoons finely crumbled blue cheese	1 recipe Creamy Herb Dressing (page 141)	2 tablespoons capers, rinsed and drained
2 cups small cauliflower florets	1½ cups chopped fresh fennel	¼ cup brine-cured black or green olives, pitted and chopped	1 recipe Creamy Parmesan Dressing (page 142)	2 pepperoncini peppers, drained and chopped
¾ cup canned artichoke hearts, drained and quartered	2 cups sliced white mushrooms	3 strips crisp-cooked center-cut bacon, crumbled	1 recipe Roasted Red Pepper Dressing (page 142)	2 tablespoons minced scallions

Confetti Pasta Salad QUICK

makes 6 servings

Adding vegetables to pasta during the last few minutes of cooking is a timesaving idea. Instead of green beans, try chopped zucchini, adding it during the last 1 to 2 minutes of cooking.

6 ounces whole wheat orzo (about 1 cup)

4 ounces green beans, trimmed and cut into ¼-inch pieces

2 tablespoons white wine vinegar

1½ tablespoons extra virgin olive oil

¾ teaspoon kosher salt

⅛ teaspoon freshly ground pepper

½ hothouse (English) cucumber, diced

1 small yellow bell pepper, diced

2 tablespoons diced red onion

¼ cup chopped fresh basil

1 Cook the orzo according to the package directions, adding the green beans during the last 3 minutes of cooking. Drain in a colander and rinse under cold running water until cool. Drain well.

2 Meanwhile, whisk together the vinegar, oil, salt, and ground pepper in a large bowl. Add the cucumber, bell pepper, onion, basil, and orzo mixture. Toss to coat. Serve the salad at room temperature. The salad tastes best on the day it is made, but it can be refrigerated, covered, for up to 2 days. Let stand at room temperature 30 minutes before serving.

Each serving: 24 g carb, 141 cal, 4 g fat, 1 g sat fat, 0 mg chol, 3 g fib, 5 g pro, 144 mg sod • Carb Choices: 1½; Exchanges: 1 starch, 1 veg, ½ fat

Peanut Noodle Salad

QUICK | HIGH FIBER

makes 8 servings

I don't make this salad too often because I eat it all. I am a peanut lover and if you've got little ones at your house who are, too, this might be a good dish for getting them to eat their vegetables. Cutting the cucumber and bell pepper into long thin strips makes them easier to eat with the spaghetti.

8 ounces whole wheat spaghetti or capellini
1 hothouse (English) cucumber, cut into long, thin strips
1 red bell pepper, thinly sliced
1 carrot, peeled and coarsely shredded
¼ cup thinly sliced scallions
¼ cup chopped fresh cilantro
2 recipes Peanut Dressing (page 144)

1 Cook the pasta according to the package directions. Drain in a colander and rinse under cold running water until cool. Drain well.

2 Combine the cooked pasta, cucumber, bell pepper, carrot, scallions, and cilantro in a large bowl. Drizzle with the dressing and toss to coat. Serve the salad at room temperature. The salad tastes best on the day it is made, but it can be refrigerated, covered, for up to 2 days. Let stand at room temperature 30 minutes before serving.

Each serving: 27 g carb, 170 cal, 5 g fat, 1 g sat fat, 0 mg chol, 5 g fib, 7 g pro, 193 mg sod • Carb Choices: 2; Exchanges: 1½ starch, ½ carb, 1 fat

Thai Rice Noodle Salad

QUICK

makes 6 servings

Every time I make this salad—or anything with fish sauce—my husband runs from the kitchen. He can't stand the smell of the fish sauce. But, once I've prepared whatever I'm making, he usually loves it. Don't judge Asian fish sauce by its aroma. Once it's incorporated into a dish, it mellows and adds a nuanced flavor that's not at all fishy.

6 ounces thin rice noodles
3 tablespoons lime juice
2 tablespoons Asian fish sauce
1 tablespoon canola oil
½ teaspoon sugar
¼ teaspoon chili-garlic paste
1 carrot, peeled and coarsely shredded
1 shallot, thinly sliced or ¼ cup thinly sliced red onion
½ medium hothouse (English) cucumber, diced
2 tablespoons chopped fresh mint
2 tablespoons chopped fresh cilantro
3 tablespoons dry-roasted peanuts, chopped

1 Cook the noodles according to the package directions. Drain in a colander and rinse under cold running water until cool. Drain well.

2 Meanwhile, whisk together the lime juice, fish sauce, oil, sugar, and chili-garlic paste in a large bowl. Add the cooked noodles, carrot, shallot, cucumber, mint, and cilantro and toss to coat. Refrigerate the salad, covered, until chilled, 2 hours or up to 1 day. Sprinkle with the peanuts just before serving.

Each serving: 31 g carb, 177 cal, 5 g fat, 1 g sat fat, 0 mg chol, 1 g fib, 4 g pro, 482 mg sod • Carb Choices: 2; Exchanges: 1½ starch, 1 veg, 1 fat

Asian Pasta, Snow Pea, and Radish Salad [QUICK]

makes 6 servings

Soba noodles are made from buckwheat and they are a nice change from whole wheat noodles. If you don't have them on hand, you can make this salad with whole wheat spaghetti or capellini.

6 ounces soba noodles
8 ounces snow peas, trimmed and cut in half on the diagonal
2 tablespoons lime juice
2 tablespoons reduced-sodium soy sauce
1 tablespoon canola oil
2 teaspoons grated fresh ginger
1 teaspoon chili-garlic paste
4 large radishes, thinly sliced
1 scallion, thinly sliced

1 Cook the soba according to the package directions, adding the snow peas during the last 1 minute of cooking. Drain in a colander and rinse under cold running water until cool. Drain well.

2 Meanwhile, whisk together the lime juice, soy sauce, oil, ginger, and chili-garlic paste in a large bowl. Add the soba mixture, radishes, and scallion to the lime juice mixture and toss to combine. Serve the salad at room temperature. The salad tastes best on the day it is made, but it can be refrigerated, covered, for up to 1 day. Let stand at room temperature 30 minutes before serving.

Each serving: 27 g carb, 154 cal, 2 g fat, 0 g sat fat, 0 mg chol, 2 g fib, 7 g pro, 271 mg sod • Carb Choices: 2; Exchanges: 2 starch

Soba Salad with Soy-Wasabi Vinaigrette [QUICK]

makes 4 servings

Hearty enough for a light lunch, this soba salad has a kick of wasabi. Look for the wasabi paste in tubes or small jars in the Asian section of the supermarket. A sprinkle of chopped fresh mint, cilantro, or basil makes a nice addition to the salad.

6 ounces soba noodles
1 cup frozen shelled edamame
3 tablespoons reduced-sodium soy sauce
2 tablespoons rice vinegar
1 tablespoon canola oil
1 teaspoon grated fresh ginger
2 teaspoons prepared wasabi paste
1 large carrot, peeled and cut into long, thin strips
1 hothouse (English) cucumber, halved lengthwise, seeded, and cut into long, thin strips
2 scallions, thinly sliced

1 Cook the soba according to the package directions, adding the edamame along with the noodles while cooking. Drain in a colander and rinse under cold running water until cool. Drain well.

2 Meanwhile, whisk together the soy sauce, vinegar, oil, ginger, and wasabi paste in a large bowl. Add the soba mixture, carrot, cucumber, and scallions to the soy sauce mixture and toss to combine. Serve the salad at room temperature. The salad tastes best on the day it is made, but it can be refrigerated, covered, for up to 1 day. Let stand at room temperature 30 minutes before serving.

Each serving: 26 g carb, 156 cal, 3 g fat, 0 g sat fat, 0 mg chol, 2 g fib, 7 g pro, 537 mg sod • Carb Choices: 2; Exchanges: 2 starch

Grain Salads

Tabbouleh HIGH FIBER

makes 4 servings

I often make this Middle Eastern bulgur salad for lunch or a light dinner with fish or chicken. If you like, replace ¼ cup parsley with chopped fresh mint.

1 cup water
¾ cup uncooked fine-grind bulgur
1 teaspoon grated lemon zest
3 tablespoons lemon juice
1 tablespoon extra virgin olive oil
1 small garlic clove, crushed through a press
½ teaspoon kosher salt
⅛ teaspoon freshly ground pepper
1 medium tomato, chopped
½ hothouse (English) cucumber, chopped
¾ cup chopped fresh Italian parsley

1 Pour the water in a small saucepan and bring to a boil over high heat. Remove from the heat and add the bulgur. Cover and let stand until the water is absorbed, 25 minutes.

2 Meanwhile, whisk together the lemon zest, lemon juice, oil, garlic, salt, and pepper in a large bowl. Add the cooked bulgur and stir to combine. Let stand to cool to room temperature, stirring occasionally. Stir in the tomato, cucumber, and parsley. Serve at room temperature or chilled. The salad tastes best on the day it is made, but it can be refrigerated, covered, for up to 2 days.

Each serving: 25 g carb, 142 cal, 4 g fat, 1 g sat fat, 0 mg chol, 6 g fib, 4 g pro, 154 mg sod • Carb Choices: 1½; Exchanges: 1 starch, 1 veg, ½ fat

TUNA TABBOULEH: Follow the Tabbouleh recipe, above, adding a 5-ounce can chunk light tuna packed in water in water, drained and broken into bite-size pieces, to the salad.

Each serving: 25 g carb, 177 cal, 5 g fat, 1 g sat fat, 15 mg chol, 6 g fib, 12 g pro, 269 mg sod • Carb Choices: 1½; Exchanges: 1 starch, 1 veg, 1 lean protein, ½ fat

Garbanzo Bean, Spinach, and Feta Tabbouleh HIGH FIBER

makes 4 servings

This hearty version of tabbouleh is filling enough for a light lunch. Tossing in baby spinach just before serving lightens the salad and adds more texture—and nutrients.

1 cup water
¾ cup uncooked fine-grind bulgur
1 teaspoon grated lemon zest
3 tablespoons lemon juice
1 tablespoon extra virgin olive oil
1 small garlic clove, crushed through a press
½ teaspoon kosher salt
⅛ teaspoon freshly ground pepper
1 cup grape tomatoes, halved
½ hothouse (English) cucumber, chopped
1 (15-ounce) can no-salt-added garbanzo beans, rinsed and drained
½ cup chopped fresh Italian parsley
¼ cup chopped fresh mint
2 cups loosely packed fresh baby spinach
1 ounce finely crumbled feta cheese (about ¼ cup)

1 Pour the water in a small saucepan and bring to a boil over high heat. Remove from the heat and add the bulgur. Cover and let stand until the water is absorbed, 25 minutes.

2 Meanwhile, whisk together the lemon zest, lemon juice, oil, garlic, salt, and pepper in a large bowl. Add the bulgur and stir to combine. Let stand to cool to room temperature, stirring occasionally. Stir in the tomatoes, cucumber, beans, parsley, and mint. Toss in the spinach and feta just before serving. Serve at room temperature or chilled. The salad tastes best on the day it is made, but it can be refrigerated, covered, for up to 2 days.

Each serving: 45 g carb, 272 cal, 6 g fat, 2 g sat fat, 6 mg chol, 10 g fib, 11 g pro, 257 mg sod • Carb Choices: 2½; Exchanges: 2 starch, 1 veg, 1 plant-based protein, 1 fat

COOKING WHOLE GRAINS

Combine 1 cup of the grain, the amount of water specified, and ½ teaspoon kosher salt in a medium saucepan. Bring to a boil over high heat, reduce the heat, and simmer, covered for the amount of time specified (see the exception with bulgur). Cooked grains can be stored in the refrigerator and covered, for up to 5 days. Freezing cooked grains is not recommended.

Grain (1 cup)	Water	Cooking Time	Makes	Carbs (grams) (½ cup)	Calories (½ cup)	Fiber (grams) (½ cup)
Bulgur	2 cups	Bring the water and salt to a boil and add the bulgur. Remove from the heat, cover, and let stand 25 minutes.	2½ cups	17 1 Carb Choice	76	4
Pearl barley	4 cups	25 to 30 minutes (drain, if necessary)	3½ cups	22 1½ Carb Choices	97	3
Wheat berries, farro, kamut, and spelt	4 cups	45 to 60 minutes (drain, if necessary)	2½ to 3 cups	27 2 Carb Choices	129	4
Quinoa	1½ cups	12 to 15 minutes (drain, if necessary)	2½ cups	23 1½ Carb Choices	127	2
Long-grain brown rice	2 cups	35 to 40 minutes	2½ cups	22 1½ Carb Choices	108	2
Short-grain brown rice	2 cups	40 to 45 minutes	2½ cups	23 1½ Carb Choices	109	2
Brown basmati rice	2 cups	30 minutes	2½ cups	29 2 Carb Choices	133	2
Wild rice	2 cups	45 minutes (drain, if necessary)	2 cups	18 1 Carb Choice	83	2

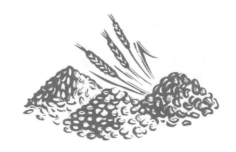

Wheat Berry–Mango Salad HIGH FIBER

makes 6 servings

Cumin and coriander give this salad a Moroccan twist. Wheat berries are nothing new—they are what is ground up to make flour. Farro, kamut, and spelt are all varieties of wheat.

1 cup wheat berries, farro, kamut, or spelt
4 cups water
¾ teaspoon kosher salt, divided
1 teaspoon grated lemon zest
¼ cup lemon juice
1 tablespoon extra virgin olive oil
1 tablespoon honey
½ teaspoon ground cumin
½ teaspoon ground coriander
⅛ teaspoon freshly ground pepper
1 mango, peeled, pitted, and chopped
¼ cup diced carrot
2 tablespoons minced red onion
2 tablespoons chopped fresh Italian parsley
3 tablespoons slivered almonds, toasted (page 4)

1 Combine the wheat berries, water, and ½ teaspoon of the salt in a medium saucepan and bring to a boil over high heat. Reduce the heat to low, cover, and simmer until tender yet firm to the bite, 45 minutes to 1 hour. Drain.

2 Meanwhile, whisk together the lemon zest, lemon juice, oil, honey, cumin, coriander, remaining ¼ teaspoon salt, and the pepper in a large bowl. Stir in the hot cooked wheat berries and let stand to cool to room temperature, stirring occasionally. Stir in the mango, carrot, onion, and parsley. Stir in the almonds just before serving. Serve the salad at room temperature or chilled. The salad tastes best on the day it is made, but it can be refrigerated for up to 2 days.

Each serving: 32 g carb, 188 cal, 5 g fat, 0 g sat fat, 0 mg chol, 4 g fib, 6 g pro, 146 mg sod • Carb Choices: 2; Exchanges: 1½ starch, ½ carb, 1 fat

Wheat Berry, Fennel, and Parsley Salad HIGH FIBER

makes 6 servings

Whole parsley leaves give this salad a wonderful herbal flavor. Serve any kind of grilled or baked fish fillet or chicken breast atop this salad for an easy and pretty meal. Or add cannellini beans and a sprinkle of finely crumbled feta cheese to make it a vegetarian main dish.

1 cup wheat berries, farro, kamut, or spelt
4 cups water
¾ teaspoon kosher salt, divided
2 teaspoons grated lemon zest
¼ cup lemon juice
1 tablespoon extra virgin olive oil
¼ teaspoon freshly ground pepper
1 large bulb fennel
1 cup loosely packed fresh Italian parsley leaves

1 Combine the wheat berries, water, and ½ teaspoon of the salt in a medium saucepan and bring to a boil over high heat. Reduce the heat to low, cover, and simmer until tender yet firm to the bite, 45 minutes to 1 hour. Drain.

2 Meanwhile, whisk together the lemon zest, lemon juice, oil, remaining ¼ teaspoon salt, and the pepper in a large bowl. Stir in the hot cooked wheat berries and let stand to cool to room temperature, stirring occasionally.

3 Trim the tough outer stalks from the fennel. Cut the fennel bulb in half vertically and cut away and discard the core. Cut each half lengthwise into ⅛-inch slices. Add the fennel and parsley to the wheat berry mixture and stir to combine. Serve at room temperature or refrigerate, covered, for up to 4 hours.

Each serving: 26 g carb, 153 cal, 3 g fat, 0 g sat fat, 0 mg chol, 5 g fib, 6 g pro, 167 mg sod • Carb Choices: 2; Exchanges: 1½ starch, ½ fat

Apricot-Orange Wheat Berry Salad HIGH FIBER

makes 6 servings

This sturdy fruit-and-nut-packed salad is great for serving at a Thanksgiving buffet or a holiday open house, where guests may be grazing for several hours.

1 cup wheat berries, farro, kamut, or spelt
4 cups water
1 teaspoon kosher salt, divided
2 large navel oranges
¼ cup diced dried apricots
¼ cup dried cranberries
2 tablespoons extra virgin olive oil
2 tablespoons white wine vinegar
¼ teaspoon freshly ground pepper
1 stalk celery, diced
¼ cup minced red onion
¼ cup pecans, toasted and chopped (page 4)

1 Combine the wheat berries, water, and ½ teaspoon of the salt in a large saucepan and bring to a boil over high heat. Reduce the heat to low, cover, and simmer until tender yet firm to the bite, 45 minutes to 1 hour. Drain.

2 Meanwhile grate 2 teaspoons of zest from the oranges and set aside. Squeeze the juice from oranges and place in a medium saucepan. Bring the juice to a boil over medium-high heat, remove from the heat, and stir in the apricots and cranberries. Cover and let stand 15 minutes.

3 Whisk together the oil, vinegar, remaining ½ teaspoon salt, and the pepper in a large bowl. Stir in the orange zest, celery, onion, the apricot mixture (with the juice), and the cooked wheat berries; stir to combine. Stir in pecans just before serving. Serve at room temperature. The salad tastes best on the day it is made, but it can be refrigerated for up to 1 day. Let stand at room temperature 30 minutes before serving.

Each serving: 34 g carb, 243 cal, 9 g fat, 1 g sat fat, 0 mg chol, 6 g fib, 6 g pro, 197 mg sod • Carb Choices: 2; Exchanges: 1½ starch, ½ fruit, 1 fat

Wheat Berry and Almond Salad with Feta HIGH FIBER

makes 6 servings

This salad takes wheat berries in a Middle Eastern direction with ginger, cumin, and honey flavoring the chewy fiber-rich grains.

1 cup wheat berries, farro, kamut, or spelt
4 cups water
1 teaspoon kosher salt, divided
2 tablespoons extra virgin olive oil
1 teaspoon grated fresh lemon zest
2 tablespoons lemon juice
2 teaspoons honey
½ teaspoon grated fresh ginger
½ teaspoon ground cumin
¼ cup currants
¼ cup thinly sliced scallions
2 tablespoons chopped fresh cilantro
3 tablespoons slivered almonds, toasted (page 4)
1 ounce finely crumbled feta cheese (about ¼ cup)

1 Combine the wheat berries, water, and ½ teaspoon of the salt in a large pot and bring to a boil over high heat. Reduce the heat to low, cover, and simmer until tender yet firm to the bite, 45 minutes to 1 hour. Drain.

2 Meanwhile, whisk together the oil, lemon zest, lemon juice, honey, ginger, cumin, and the remaining ½ teaspoon salt in a large bowl. Add the hot cooked wheat berries and the currants and stir to combine. Let stand to cool to room temperature, stirring occasionally.

3 Stir in the scallions and cilantro. Stir in the almonds and sprinkle with the feta just before serving. Serve at room temperature. The salad tastes best on the day it is made, but it can be refrigerated, covered, for up to 1 day. Let stand at room temperature 30 minutes before serving.

Each serving: 30 g carb, 214 cal, 8 g fat, 1 g sat fat, 4 mg chol, 4 g fib, 6 g pro, 242 mg sod • Carb Choices: 2; Exchanges: 2 starch, 1½ fat

Barley and Basil Salad

HIGH FIBER

makes 6 servings

If your only exposure to barley is a beefy barley soup, this salad will introduce you to the lighter side of this healthful grain. Be sure to rinse the barley after cooking to remove the excess starch from the grains.

3 cups water
1 cup pearled barley
1 teaspoon kosher salt, divided
2 tablespoons white balsamic or white wine vinegar
1½ tablespoons extra virgin olive oil
⅛ teaspoon freshly ground pepper
4 scallions, thinly sliced
1 cup grape tomatoes, halved
½ yellow or red bell pepper, diced
¼ cup chopped fresh basil

1 Combine the water, barley, and ½ teaspoon of the salt in a medium saucepan and bring to a boil over high heat. Reduce the heat to low, cover, and simmer until the barley is tender, yet firm to the bite, 25 to 30 minutes. Drain and rinse under cold running water until cool.

2 Meanwhile, whisk together the vinegar, oil, remaining ½ teaspoon salt, and the ground pepper in a large bowl. Stir in the cooked barley, scallions, tomatoes, bell pepper, and basil. Serve at room temperature. The salad tastes best on the day it is made, but it can be refrigerated, covered, for up to 1 day. Let stand at room temperature 30 minutes before serving.

Each serving: 29 g carb, 163 cal, 4 g fat, 1 g sat fat, 0 mg chol, 6 g fib, 4 g pro, 194 mg sod • Carb Choices: 2; Exchanges: 2 starch, 1 fat

Tandoori-Spiced Barley and Bean Salad

HIGH FIBER

makes 8 servings

If you love the flavor of Indian spices, here's an unusual way to use them—in a fresh, fiber-rich barley salad. It's delicious as an accompaniment to grilled chicken or salmon.

3 cups water
1 cup pearl barley
1¼ teaspoons kosher salt, divided
¼ cup lemon juice
1 tablespoon canola oil
1 teaspoon grated fresh ginger
¾ teaspoon curry powder
½ teaspoon ground cumin
¼ teaspoon ground coriander
¼ teaspoon paprika
1 (15-ounce) can no-salt-added garbanzo beans, rinsed and drained
1 cup chopped hothouse (English) cucumber
1 red bell pepper, chopped
2 scallions, thinly sliced
¼ cup chopped fresh cilantro

1 Combine the water, barley, and ½ teaspoon of the salt in a medium saucepan and bring to a boil over high heat. Reduce the heat to low, cover, and simmer until the barley is tender, yet firm to the bite, 25 to 30 minutes. Drain and rinse under cold running water until cool.

2 Meanwhile, whisk together the lemon juice, oil, ginger, curry powder, cumin, coriander, paprika, and the remaining ¾ teaspoon salt in a large bowl. Stir in the cooked barley, beans, cucumber, bell pepper, scallions, and cilantro. Serve at room temperature. The salad tastes best on the day it is made, but it can be refrigerated, covered, for up to 1 day. Let stand at room temperature 30 minutes before serving.

Each serving: 32 g carb, 172 cal, 3 g fat, 0 g sat fat, 0 mg chol, 7 g fib, 6 g pro, 182 mg sod • Carb Choices: 2; Exchanges: 2 starch

Southwestern Barley and Avocado Salad [HIGH FIBER]

makes 6 servings

In this salad, flecked with avocado and tomatoes, barley soaks up a chipotle-spiked orange dressing.

3 cups water
1 cup pearl barley
1¼ teaspoons kosher salt, divided
1 teaspoon grated orange zest
¼ cup orange juice
1½ tablespoons white wine vinegar
1 tablespoon canola oil
½ teaspoon minced chipotle in adobo
    sauce
½ teaspoon ground cumin
1 cup grape tomatoes, halved
1 avocado, pitted, peeled, and chopped
½ hothouse (English) cucumber, peeled
    and chopped
¼ cup minced red onion
¼ cup chopped fresh cilantro

1 Combine the water, barley, and ½ teaspoon of the salt in a medium saucepan and bring to a boil over high heat. Reduce the heat to low, cover, and simmer until the barley is tender, yet firm to the bite, 25 to 30 minutes. Drain and rinse under cold running water until cool.

2 Meanwhile, whisk together the orange zest, orange juice, vinegar, oil, chipotle, cumin, and the remaining ¾ teaspoon salt in a large bowl. Stir in the cooked barley, tomatoes, avocado, cucumber, onion, and cilantro. Serve at room temperature. The salad tastes best on the day it is made, but it can be refrigerated, covered, for up to 1 day. Let stand at room temperature 30 minutes before serving.

Each serving: 32 g carb, 207 cal, 8 g fat, 1 g sat fat, 0 mg chol,
8 g fib, 5 g pro, 241 mg sod • Carb Choices: 2; Exchanges: 2 starch,
1½ fat

Quinoa and Asparagus Salad

makes 6 servings

Crisp green asparagus paired with quinoa and dressed with a tangy lemon dressing makes a simple springtime salad. Always rinse quinoa before cooking to wash away a naturally occurring substance called saponin, which can make the quinoa taste bitter.

1½ cups water
1 cup quinoa, rinsed
¾ teaspoon kosher salt, divided
2 teaspoons grated lemon zest
2 tablespoons lemon juice
1½ tablespoons extra virgin olive oil
¼ teaspoon freshly ground pepper
8 ounces asparagus, tough ends removed, cut
    into ½-inch pieces
1 scallion, thinly sliced
2 tablespoons chopped fresh Italian parsley,
    dill, or basil

1 Combine the water, quinoa, and ½ teaspoon of the salt in a medium saucepan and bring to a boil over high heat. Reduce the heat to low, cover, and simmer until the quinoa is tender, 12 to 15 minutes. Drain and keep warm.

2 Meanwhile, whisk together the lemon zest, lemon juice, oil, remaining ¼ teaspoon salt, and the pepper in a large bowl. Stir in the hot cooked quinoa and let stand to cool to room temperature, stirring occasionally.

3 Bring a large saucepan of water to a boil over high heat. Add the asparagus and cook until crisp-tender, 3 to 4 minutes. Drain the asparagus and rinse under cold running water until cool.

4 Add the cooked asparagus, scallion, and parsley to the quinoa mixture and stir to combine. Serve at room temperature or chilled. The salad tastes best on the day it is made.

Each serving: 21 g carb, 145 cal, 5 g fat, 1 g sat fat, 0 mg chol, 2 g fib,
4 g pro, 148 mg sod • Carb Choices: 1½; Exchanges: 1½ starch, 1 fat

Quinoa, Zucchini, and Mint Salad

makes 6 servings

When the first small tender zucchini of the summer arrive, I love to eat them raw in salads such as this one. Fresh lime juice and mint give this most ordinary of vegetables a flavorful showcase in this healthful salad.

1½ cups water

1 cup quinoa, rinsed

¾ teaspoon kosher salt, divided

1 teaspoon grated lime zest

2 tablespoons lime juice

1½ tablespoons extra virgin olive oil

¼ teaspoon freshly ground pepper

2 small zucchini, quartered lengthwise and thinly sliced

2 tablespoons chopped fresh mint

2 tablespoons pine nuts, toasted (page 4)

1 Combine the water, quinoa, and ½ teaspoon of the salt in a medium saucepan and bring to a boil over high heat. Reduce the heat to low, cover, and simmer until the quinoa is tender, 12 to 15 minutes. Drain and keep warm.

2 Meanwhile, whisk together the lime zest, lime juice, oil, remaining ¼ teaspoon salt, and the pepper in a large bowl. Stir in the hot cooked quinoa and let stand to cool to room temperature, stirring occasionally.

3 Add the zucchini and mint and stir to combine. Stir in the pine nuts just before serving. Serve at room temperature or chilled. The salad tastes best on the day it is made.

Each serving: 22 g carb, 165 cal, 7 g fat, 1 g sat fat, 0 mg chol, 2 g fib, 5 g pro, 151 mg sod • Carb Choices: 1½; Exchanges: 1 starch, 1 veg, 1 fat

Quinoa Salad with Mango, Orange, and Basil

makes 6 servings

Mango and basil is one of my favorite flavor combinations. In this salad, I've added a bit of spicy jalapeño and a mixture of citrus juices to liven up mild-flavored quinoa. To give the salad a kick of heat, leave some of the seeds in the jalapeño. Serve this salad as a bed for grilled chicken, shrimp, or salmon.

1½ cups water

1 cup quinoa, rinsed

¾ teaspoon kosher salt, divided

2 teaspoons grated orange zest

3 tablespoons orange juice

2 tablespoons lime juice

1½ tablespoons extra virgin olive oil

1 jalapeño, seeded and chopped

1 garlic clove, minced

1 mango, peeled, pitted, and chopped

¼ cup chopped fresh basil

1 Combine the water, quinoa, and ½ teaspoon of the salt in a medium saucepan and bring to a boil over high heat. Reduce the heat to low, cover, and simmer until the quinoa is tender, 12 to 15 minutes. Drain and keep warm.

2 Meanwhile, combine the orange zest, orange juice, lime juice, oil, jalapeño, garlic, and remaining ¼ teaspoon salt in a blender and process until pureed. Transfer to a large bowl. Stir in the hot cooked quinoa and let stand to cool to room temperature, stirring occasionally.

3 Add the mango and basil to the quinoa mixture and stir to combine. Serve at room temperature or chilled. The salad tastes best on the day it is made.

Each serving: 26 g carb, 162 cal, 5 g fat, 1 g sat fat, 0 mg chol, 2 g fib, 4 g pro, 147 mg sod • Carb Choices: 2; Exchanges: 1½ starch, ½ fruit, 1 fat

Cranberry-Maple Rice Salad

makes 8 servings

Fresh cranberries, sweetened with orange juice and a touch of maple syrup, make a fresh and festive dressing for this salad. Of course, it's perfect for serving during the winter holidays. You can make it with any variety of brown rice, wheat berries, farro, or spelt.

3 cups water

1½ cups long-grain brown rice

1 teaspoon kosher salt, divided

1 cup fresh cranberries or unthawed frozen cranberries

2 tablespoons real maple syrup

⅓ cup orange juice

2 tablespoon extra virgin olive oil

1 tablespoon white wine vinegar

2 teaspoons Dijon mustard

2 teaspoons grated orange zest

¼ teaspoon freshly ground pepper

½ cup diced celery

2 scallions, thinly sliced

¼ cup chopped fresh Italian parsley

¼ cup walnuts, toasted and chopped (page 4)

1 Combine the water, rice, and ½ teaspoon of the salt in a medium saucepan and bring to a boil over high heat. Reduce the heat to low, cover, and simmer until the rice is tender, 35 to 40 minutes. Drain and cool.

2 Meanwhile, combine the cranberries and maple syrup in a small saucepan; bring to a boil over medium heat. Cook, stirring often, until most of the berries pop, about 5 minutes. Transfer to a large bowl to cool.

3 Stir the orange juice, oil, vinegar, mustard, orange zest, pepper, and remaining ½ teaspoon salt into the cranberry mixture.

4 Add the cooked rice, celery, scallions, and parsley and stir to coat. Stir in the walnuts just before serving. Serve the salad at room temperature. The salad tastes best on the day it is made, but it can be refrigerated, covered, for up to 1 day. Let stand at room temperature 30 minutes before serving.

Each serving: 34 g carb, 212 cal, 7 g fat, 1 g sat fat, 0 mg chol, 3 g fib, 4 g pro, 184 mg sod • Carb Choices: 2; Exchanges: 2 starch, 1½ fat

Rice Salad with Leeks and Tomatoes

makes 6 servings

Steamed leeks are an unexpected salad ingredient, but once you discover their sweet flavor you'll be a convert. Grilled or broiled fish or shrimp are delicious with this salad.

2 cups water

1 cup long-grain brown rice

¾ teaspoon kosher salt, divided

2 medium leeks, cut in half lengthwise, sliced into ¼-inch slices

2 tablespoons sherry vinegar or white wine vinegar

1½ tablespoon extra virgin olive oil

⅛ teaspoon freshly ground pepper

2 cups cherry tomatoes, halved, or 1 large tomato, chopped

1 tablespoon chopped fresh thyme or 1 teaspoon dried thyme

1 Combine the water, rice, and ½ teaspoon of the salt in a medium saucepan and bring to a boil over high heat. Reduce the heat to low,

cover, and simmer until the rice is tender, 35 to 40 minutes. Drain and cool.

2 Meanwhile, submerge the sliced leeks in a large bowl of water, lift them out, and drain in a colander. Repeat, using fresh water, until no grit remains in the bottom of the bowl. In a saucepan fitted with a steamer basket, bring 1 inch of water to a boil over high heat. Add the leeks, cover, and steam until tender, about 8 minutes. Transfer to a plate to cool.

3 Whisk together the vinegar, oil, remaining ¼ teaspoon salt, and the pepper in a large bowl. Add the rice, leeks, tomatoes, and thyme. Serve the salad at room temperature. The salad tastes best on the day it is made, but it can be refrigerated, covered, for up to 1 day. Let stand at room temperature 30 minutes before serving.

Each serving: 30 g carb, 174 cal, 5 g fat, 1 g sat fat, 0 mg chol, 3 g fib, 4 g pro, 107 mg sod • Carb Choices: 2; Exchanges: 1½ starch, 1 veg, 1 fat

Making Salads Ahead of Time

All salads certainly look and taste best as soon as they are made or after a brief chill in the refrigerator. Green leafy salads, of course, must be served as soon as they are made. So, how can you make vegetable, bean, pasta, and grain salads ahead and still have them taste and look great? Here are a few tricks.

Cook or prepare all the salad ingredients separately, refrigerate them, and toss together 30 minutes to an hour before serving. The acidic ingredients in salad dressing (vinegar or lemon juice) cause crisp vegetables to soften upon standing, and they turn bright green vegetables like broccoli or asparagus an unappetizing olive-drab color in a matter of hours. Keeping the acidic ingredients away from the salad until just before serving will maintain the vibrant green color and crisp texture.

If the salad has fresh herbs, add those at the last minute, as they tend to turn color even quicker than green vegetables do. Also, add any ingredient that gets soggy quickly, like chopped bacon or nuts, to the salad just before serving.

Always serve starchy salads, such as pasta, rice, or whole grain salads, at room temperature. When starchy grains and pasta are chilled, they become hard and unpleasantly chewy. The starch molecules, which loosened during cooking, firm up again when they are chilled. For this reason, even if you have made the salad ahead, let starchy salads stand at room temperature for 20 to 30 minutes before serving.

If you do assemble a salad a few hours ahead, stir it and taste before serving. You'll probably find that it needs a few additional drops of whatever the acid is in the dressing (citrus juice or vinegar) and a pinch of additional salt to brighten the flavors, which can dull upon standing.

Rice and Red Bean Salad

HIGH FIBER

makes 6 servings

The classic Louisiana rice and beans dish is turned into a crunchy and colorful salad in this recipe. This salad holds up well, so it's great for a picnic or a potluck. Different brands of Cajun seasoning vary widely. Check the label and if yours contains salt, then omit the salt in this recipe.

1 cup water
½ cup long-grain brown rice
¾ teaspoon kosher salt, divided
2 tablespoons red wine vinegar
1½ tablespoons extra virgin olive oil
2 teaspoons no-salt Cajun seasoning
1 (15-ounce) can no-salt-added red beans, drained and rinsed
1 large tomato, chopped
1 small green bell pepper, diced
1 stalk celery, diced
¼ cup diced sweet onion
¼ cup chopped fresh Italian parsley

1 Combine the water, rice, and ¼ teaspoon of the salt in a medium saucepan and bring to a boil over high heat. Reduce the heat to low, cover, and simmer until the rice is tender, 35 to 40 minutes. Drain and cool.

2 Meanwhile, whisk together the vinegar, oil, Cajun seasoning, and remaining ½ teaspoon salt in a large bowl. Add the cooked rice, beans, tomato, bell pepper, celery, onion, and parsley. Serve the salad at room temperature. The salad tastes best on the day it is made, but it can be refrigerated, covered, for up to 2 days. Let stand at room temperature 30 minutes before serving.

Each serving: 24 g carb, 157 cal, 4 g fat, 1 g sat fat, 0 mg chol, 5 g fib, 5 g pro, 166 mg sod • Carb Choices: 1½; Exchanges: 1½ starch, 1 fat

Wild Rice, Fig, and Gorgonzola Salad

makes 8 servings

Salty blue cheese and sweet fruit is a classic pairing for good reason—it tastes great. If you don't like the texture of dried figs, you can use dried apricots or golden raisins in this salad.

3 cups water
1½ cups wild rice
¾ teaspoon kosher salt, divided
½ cup unsweetened apple juice
4 dried figs, each cut into eighths
1½ tablespoons extra virgin olive oil
1 teaspoon Dijon mustard
¼ teaspoon freshly ground pepper
¼ cup chopped fresh Italian parsley
1 ounce crumbled Gorgonzola or other blue cheese (about ¼ cup)

1 Combine the water, rice, and ½ teaspoon of the salt in a medium saucepan and bring to a boil over high heat. Reduce the heat to low, cover, and simmer until the rice is tender, about 45 minutes. Drain and cool.

2 Meanwhile, place the apple juice and figs in a medium saucepan and bring to a boil over high heat. Remove from the heat, cover, and let stand 15 minutes. Transfer to a large bowl to cool completely.

3 Add the oil, mustard, remaining ¼ teaspoon salt, and the pepper to the fig mixture and stir to combine. Add the cooked rice and parsley and toss to coat. Stir in the Gorgonzola just before serving. Serve the salad at room temperature. The salad tastes best on the day it is made, but it can be refrigerated, covered, for up to 1 day. Let stand at room temperature 30 minutes before serving.

Each serving: 33 g carb, 186 cal, 4 g fat, 1 g sat fat, 3 mg chol, 3 g fib, 6 g pro, 126 mg sod • Carb Choices: 2; Exchanges: 2 starch, 1 fat

Wild Rice, Raisin, and Walnut Salad

makes 8 servings

Flavored with orange and fresh thyme, this makes a lovely salad for fall and winter entertaining. It's sturdy enough to look attractive on a buffet table for hours and tastes great with anything from grilled salmon to roast turkey.

3 cups water
1½ cups wild rice
¾ teaspoon kosher salt, divided
½ cup orange juice
⅓ cup golden raisins
1½ tablespoons extra virgin olive oil
1 tablespoon chopped fresh thyme
2 teaspoons grated orange zest
¼ teaspoon freshly ground pepper
¼ cup walnuts, toasted and chopped
    (page 4)

1 Combine the water, rice, and ½ teaspoon of the salt in a medium saucepan and bring to a boil over high heat. Reduce the heat to low, cover, and simmer until the rice is tender, about 45 minutes. Drain and cool.

2 Meanwhile, place the orange juice and raisins in a medium saucepan and bring to a boil over high heat. Remove from the heat, cover, and let stand 15 minutes. Transfer to a large bowl to cool completely.

3 Add the cooked rice, oil, thyme, orange zest, remaining ¼ teaspoon salt, and the pepper to the raisin mixture and stir to combine. Stir in the walnuts just before serving. Serve the salad at room temperature. The salad tastes best on the day it is made, but it can be refrigerated, covered, for up to 1 day. Let stand at room temperature 30 minutes before serving.

Each serving: 33 g carb, 193 cal, 5 g fat, 1 g sat fat, 0 mg chol, 3 g fib, 6 g pro, 110 mg sod • Carb Choices: 2; Exchanges: 2 starch, 1 fat

Wild Rice Salad with Apricots and Pecans

makes 8 servings

This pecan-crazy salad reflects on my Southern heritage. If you can find toasted pecan oil, it's worth the investment.

3 cups water
1½ cups wild rice
¾ teaspoon kosher salt, divided
½ cup orange juice
½ cup diced dried apricots
2 tablespoons sherry vinegar
2 tablespoons toasted pecan oil or extra virgin
    olive oil
1 stalk celery, minced
1 large shallot, minced
¼ cup chopped fresh Italian parsley
½ teaspoon freshly ground pepper
¼ cup pecans, toasted and chopped (page 4)

1 Combine the water, rice, and ½ teaspoon of the salt in a medium saucepan and bring to a boil over high heat. Reduce the heat to low, cover, and simmer until the rice is tender, about 45 minutes. Drain and cool.

2 Meanwhile, place the orange juice and apricots in a medium saucepan and bring to a boil over medium-high heat. Remove from the heat, cover, and let stand 15 minutes. Transfer to a large bowl to cool completely.

3 Add the cooked rice, vinegar, oil, celery, shallot, parsley, remaining ¼ teaspoon salt, and the pepper to the apricot mixture and stir to combine. Stir in the pecans just before serving. Serve the salad at room temperature. The salad tastes best on the day it is made, but it can be refrigerated, covered, for up to 1 day. Let stand at room temperature 30 minutes before serving.

Each serving: 33 g carb, 205 cal, 6 g fat, 1 g sat fat, 0 mg chol, 3 g fib, 6 g pro, 115 mg sod • Carb Choices: 2; Exchanges: 2 starch, 1 fat

Bean Salads

Four-Bean Salad

QUICK | HIGH FIBER

makes 8 servings

Sturdy and transportable, this salad is perfect for potlucks. You can switch up the canned beans and use black beans, navy beans, garbanzo beans, or pinto beans.

1 (10-ounce) package frozen baby lima beans
8 ounces green beans, trimmed and cut
    into 1-inch pieces
2 tablespoons white wine vinegar
1½ tablespoons extra virgin olive oil
½ teaspoon kosher salt
¼ teaspoon freshly ground pepper
1 (15-ounce) can no-salt-added black beans,
    rinsed and drained
1 (15-ounce) can no-salt-added kidney beans,
    rinsed and drained
1 small red bell pepper, diced
¼ cup diced red onion
¼ cup chopped fresh Italian parsley

1 Fill a large saucepan half full with water and bring to a boil over high heat. Add the lima beans and green beans, return to a boil, and cook just until crisp-tender, about 3 minutes. Drain and rinse under cold running water until cool.

2 Meanwhile, whisk together the vinegar, oil, salt, and ground pepper in a large bowl. Add the lima bean mixture, black beans, kidney beans, bell pepper, onion, and parsley. Serve the salad at room temperature. The salad tastes best on the day it is made, but it can be refrigerated, covered, for up to 2 days. Let stand at room temperature 30 minutes before serving.

Each serving: 26 g carb, 164 cal, 3 g fat, 0 g sat fat, 0 mg chol, 10 g fib, 9 g pro, 104 mg sod • Carb Choices: 1½; Exchanges: 1½ starch, 1 plant-based protein, ½ fat

Mediterranean Bean Salad with Artichokes and Lemon QUICK | HIGH FIBER

makes 4 servings

Use this salad as a bed for serving salmon fillets, or serve the salad on a bed of greens. You can sprinkle the salad with a couple tablespoons crumbled feta or goat cheese just before serving if you wish.

1 (14-ounce) can artichoke hearts
1 teaspoon grated lemon zest
2 tablespoons lemon juice
1½ tablespoon extra virgin olive oil
1 garlic clove, minced
1 teaspoon Dijon mustard
¼ teaspoon kosher salt
⅛ teaspoon freshly ground pepper
1 (15-ounce) can no-salt-added cannellini
    beans, rinsed and drained
½ cup red Roasted Bell Peppers (page 21) or
    roasted red peppers from a jar, chopped
¼ cup thinly sliced red onion
2 teaspoons chopped fresh rosemary or 1
    tablespoon chopped fresh Italian parsley

1 Drain the artichokes and cut into quarters. Place the artichokes on several thicknesses of paper towels and gently blot dry. Set aside.

2 Whisk together the lemon zest, lemon juice, oil, garlic, mustard, salt, and ground pepper in a large bowl. Add the artichokes, beans, roasted peppers, onion, and rosemary and toss gently to coat. Serve the salad at room temperature. The salad tastes best on the day it is made, but it can be refrigerated, covered, for up to 1 day. Let stand at room temperature 30 minutes before serving.

Each serving: 23 g carb, 180 cal, 6 g fat, 1 g sat fat, 0 mg chol, 5 g fib, 8 g pro, 355 mg sod • Carb Choices: 1½; Exchanges: 1 starch, 1 veg, 1 plant-based protein, 1 fat

COOKING DRIED BEANS

Dried beans do not have to be soaked. Soaking reduces the cooking time by less than 30 minutes, and the texture and flavor are the same whether the beans are soaked or not. To cook dried beans, combine the beans, the amount of water specified, 1 teaspoon kosher salt, and the following aromatics in a large pot: 1 large onion, halved; 2 stalks celery, cut into 3-inch pieces; and 1 bay leaf. Bring to a boil over high heat, reduce the heat to low and simmer, covered, for the amount of time specified, stirring occasionally and adding additional water, if necessary. When the beans are done, remove and discard the aromatics. Cooked dried beans can be stored in the refrigerator, covered, for up to 3 days. They can be frozen up to 6 months. To prevent the beans from bursting, make sure they are covered with cooking liquid or with water before freezing. If you want to substitute home-cooked beans for canned, a 15-ounce can of beans is about 1¾ cups.

Bean (1 pound)	Water	Cooking Time	Makes	Carbs (grams) (½ cup)	Calories (½ cup)	Fiber (grams) (½ cup)
Black beans	8 cups	1½ hours	6 cups	20 1 Carb Choice	114	7
Cannellini beans	8 cups	1 hour	6½ cups	19 1 Carb Choice	104	6
Black-eyed peas	6 cups	45 minutes to 1 hour	7 cups	18 1 Carb Choice	100	6
Garbanzo beans	8 cups	2 hours	6 cups	22 1½ Carb Choices	134	6
Kidney beans	8 cups	1½ to 2 hours	6½ cups	20 1 Carb Choice	112	7
Lima beans	8 cups	1 hour	6 cups	20 1 Carb Choice	108	7
Brown lentils	5 cups	30 minutes	7 cups	20 1 Carb Choice	115	8
Green lentils	5 cups	20 to 25 minutes	4 cups	27 2 Carb Choices	150	7
Navy beans	8 cups	1 hour	6 cups	24 1½ Carb Choices	127	10
Green split peas	6 cups	30 to 45 minutes	5½ cups	21 1½ Carb Choices	116	8
Pinto beans	8 cups	1 hour 15 minutes	6 cups	22 1½ Carb Choices	122	8

White Bean Salad with Tomatoes and Sage

QUICK | HIGH FIBER

makes 4 servings

Fresh sage can taste harsh and sometimes bitter. For this salad, I've warmed the sage along with garlic in extra virgin olive oil to mellow the flavors. The sage makes and excellent complement to the creamy beans and tangy tomatoes.

2 tablespoon extra virgin olive oil
1 garlic clove, minced
1 tablespoon minced fresh sage or 1 teaspoon crumbled dried sage
2 tablespoons red wine vinegar
1 teaspoon Dijon mustard
½ teaspoon kosher salt
⅛ teaspoon freshly ground pepper
1 (15-ounce) can no-salt-added cannellini beans, rinsed and drained
2 plum tomatoes, each cut into 8 wedges

1 Combine the oil, garlic, and sage in a small saucepan. Set over medium-low heat and cook, stirring often, until the oil is warmed and the garlic and sage are fragrant, about 3 minutes. Transfer to a large bowl to cool.

2 Whisk the vinegar, mustard, salt, and pepper into the oil mixture. Add the beans and tomatoes and toss gently to combine. Serve the salad at room temperature. The salad tastes best on the day it is made, but it can be refrigerated, covered, for up to 1 day. Let stand at room temperature 30 minutes before serving.

Each serving: 17 g carb, 160 cal, 8 g fat, 1 g sat fat, 0 mg chol, 5 g fib, 6 g pro, 207 mg sod • Carb Choices: 1; Exchanges: 1 starch, 1 plant-based protein, 1½ fat

White Bean, Bell Pepper, and Caper Salad

QUICK | HIGH FIBER

makes 4 servings

You can make this flavorful salad even when you think the cupboard is bare—all the ingredients are pantry staples. Other additions you might add include chopped cucumbers or halved cherry tomatoes.

1 teaspoon grated lemon zest
2 tablespoons lemon juice
1 tablespoon extra virgin olive oil
1 garlic clove, crushed through a press
½ teaspoon kosher salt
⅛ teaspoon freshly ground pepper
1 (15-ounce) can no-salt-added cannellini beans
½ cup red or yellow Roasted Bell Peppers (page 21) or roasted red peppers from a jar, cut into short, thin strips
2 tablespoons chopped fresh Italian parsley
1 tablespoon capers, rinsed and drained

1 Whisk together the lemon zest, lemon juice, oil, garlic, salt, and ground pepper in a large bowl.

2 Add the beans, roasted peppers, parsley, and capers and toss to combine. Serve the salad at room temperature. The salad tastes best on the day it is made, but it can be refrigerated, covered, for up to 1 day. Let stand at room temperature 30 minutes before serving.

Each serving: 17 g carb, 128 cal, 4 g fat, 1 g sat fat, 0 mg chol, 5 g fib, 6 g pro, 240 mg sod • Carb Choices: 1; Exchanges: 1 starch, 1 plant-based protein, 1 fat

White Bean Salad with Roasted Zucchini and Radicchio HIGH FIBER

makes 4 servings

This salad is an unusual use for summer zucchini. Roasting it gives it a sweet and slightly smoky flavor that pairs well with the creamy beans and bitter greens. If you are not fond of radicchio, you can use baby spinach or arugula in this salad instead.

2 medium zucchini, halved lengthwise and cut into ½-inch slices

2 teaspoons plus 1 tablespoon extra virgin olive oil, divided

⅛ teaspoon plus ½ teaspoon kosher salt, divided

4 teaspoons red wine vinegar

½ teaspoon Dijon mustard

1 garlic clove, crushed through a press

⅛ teaspoon freshly ground pepper

1 (15-ounce) can no-salt-added cannellini beans, rinsed and drained

2 cups thinly sliced radicchio

1 Preheat the oven to 425°F.

2 Place the zucchini on a large rimmed baking sheet. Drizzle with 2 teaspoons of the oil and sprinkle with ⅛ teaspoon of the salt. Toss to coat. Arrange in a single layer.

3 Bake, stirring the zucchini once, until tender and browned, 25 to 30 minutes.

4 Meanwhile, whisk together the remaining 1 tablespoon oil, the vinegar, mustard, garlic, pepper, and the remaining ½ teaspoon salt in a large bowl. Add the beans, roasted zucchini, and radicchio and toss to combine. Serve at once.

Each serving: 19 g carb, 163 cal, 7 g fat, 1 g sat fat, 0 mg chol, 6 g fib, 7 g pro, 65 mg sod • Carb Choices: 1; Exchanges: 1 starch, 1 plant-based protein, 1 fat

Canned Beans and Sodium

Canned beans vary greatly in sodium from brand to brand. It definitely pays to read the label. The lowest-sodium beans are those labeled "no-salt-added." Brands to look for are Eden, 365 (Whole Foods), and Health Valley.

Low-sodium beans are also available. They have about two-thirds less sodium than regular canned beans. Look for Eden, Goya, and S&W brands.

Rinsing regular canned beans before eating reduces the sodium by about 40 percent, so if you don't buy low-sodium canned beans or cook your own, always rinse canned beans in a colander under cold running water before eating.

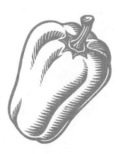

Black Bean Salad with Roasted Corn and Poblanos HIGH FIBER

makes 6 servings

You can serve this salad like you would a salsa— as an accompaniment for grilled chicken or pork chops or as a dip for baked corn chips. A larger serving makes an ideal hot weather dinner.

2 large ears corn, kernels cut from the cob, or 1½ cups frozen corn kernels

4 poblano chiles, chopped

1 jalapeño, halved lengthwise and seeded

2 teaspoons plus 1 tablespoon extra virgin olive oil, divided

¾ teaspoon kosher salt, divided

¼ cup lime juice

1 teaspoon ground cumin

1 (15-ounce) can no-salt-added black beans, rinsed and drained

⅓ cup minced red onion

¼ cup chopped fresh cilantro

1 Preheat the oven to 425°F.

2 Place the corn, poblanos, and jalapeño on a large rimmed baking sheet. Drizzle with 2 teaspoons of the oil and sprinkle with ¼ teaspoon of the salt. Toss to coat. Scatter the vegetables in a single layer. Bake, stirring the corn and peppers, and turning the jalapeño once, until tender and lightly browned, 15 to 20 minutes. Transfer the corn and poblano to a large bowl and let cool.

3 To make the dressing, place the jalapeño in a small bowl and let stand until cool enough to handle. Peel the jalapeño and mash it into a paste using a fork. Add the lime juice, cumin, remaining 1 tablespoon oil, and remaining ½ teaspoon salt and whisk to mix well.

4 Add the beans, onion, and cilantro to the corn and poblanos. Add the dressing and toss to coat. Serve the salad at room temperature. The salad tastes best on the day it is made, but it can be refrigerated, covered, for up to 1 day. Let stand at room temperature 30 minutes before serving.

Each serving: 19 g carb, 149 cal, 5 g fat, 1 g sat fat, 0 mg chol, 5 g fib, 6 g pro, 212 mg sod • Carb Choices: 1½; Exchanges: 1½ starch, 1 plant-based protein, 1 fat

RED BEAN SALAD WITH QUESO FRESCO HIGH FIBER : Follow the Black Bean Salad with Roasted Corn and Poblanos recipe, at left, substituting red beans for the black beans and stirring 1 ounce (about ¼ cup) finely crumbled queso fresco or feta cheese into the salad just before serving.

Each serving: 21 g carb, 150 cal, 5 g fat, 1 g sat fat, 2 mg chol, 4 g fib, 6 g pro, 169 mg sod • Carb Choices: 1½; Exchanges: 1½ starch, 1 plant-based protein, 1 fat

Black Bean, Jicama, and Avocado Salad QUICK HIGH FIBER

makes 6 servings

This is such a versatile salad. Serve it as a salsa, on salad greens topped with crumbled queso fresco for a light lunch, or as a side dish with grilled steak, salmon, or shrimp. The jicama adds a lovely crunch to the salad, but if you can't find it, add a stalk of chopped celery to the salad.

1 teaspoon grated lime zest

2 tablespoons lime juice

1½ tablespoons extra virgin olive oil

1 garlic clove, crushed through a press

½ teaspoon ground cumin

½ teaspoon kosher salt

⅛ teaspoon freshly ground pepper

1 (15-ounce) can no-salt-added black beans

1 small jicama, peeled and chopped

1 small avocado, pitted, peeled, and diced

3 tablespoons diced red onion

¼ cup chopped fresh cilantro

1 Whisk together the lime zest, lime juice, oil, garlic, cumin, salt, and pepper in a large bowl.

2 Add the beans, jicama, avocado, onion, and cilantro and toss to coat. Serve the salad at room temperature. The salad tastes best on the day it is made, but it can be refrigerated, covered, for up to 1 day. Let stand at room temperature 30 minutes before serving.

Each serving: 17 g carb, 161 cal, 9 g fat, 1 g sat fat, 0 mg chol, 7 g fib, 5 g pro, 162 mg sod • Carb Choices: 1; Exchanges: 1 starch, ½ plant-based protein, 1½ fat

Bean and Cornbread Salad HIGH FIBER

makes 8 servings

This is my Southern version of the Italian bread salad, panzanella. Any kind of bread tossed with a tart vinaigrette and colorful mixture of vegetables is delicious, no matter what part of the world you are from. If you are using purchased cornbread, look for one without a lot of added sugar, or your salad will be sweet.

4 cups ½-inch cubes Southern Cornbread (page 508) or purchased cornbread

2 large ears corn, kernels cut from the cob, or ¾ cup frozen corn kernels

2 tablespoons extra virgin olive oil

1 tablespoon apple cider vinegar

1 teaspoon Dijon mustard

½ teaspoon kosher salt

¼ teaspoon freshly ground pepper

4 scallions, thinly sliced

2 cups cherry tomatoes, quartered

1 (15-ounce) can no-salt-added pinto beans, rinsed and drained

4 ounces shredded reduced-fat sharp Cheddar cheese (about 1 cup)

1 large green or red bell pepper, cut into 1-inch strips

½ cup chopped fresh Italian parsley

1 Preheat the oven to 350°F. Place the bread cubes in a single layer on a large rimmed baking sheet. Bake, stirring once, until the cubes are lightly toasted, 20 to 25 minutes. Set aside to cool.

2 Meanwhile, fill a medium saucepan half full with water and bring to a boil over high heat. Add the corn and cook 2 minutes. Drain and transfer to a plate to cool.

3 Whisk together the oil, vinegar, mustard, salt, and ground pepper in a large bowl. Add the toasted bread cubes, cooked corn, scallions, tomatoes, beans, Cheddar, bell pepper, and parsley and toss to coat. Serve at once.

Each serving: 24 g carb, 235 cal, 10 g fat, 3 g sat fat, 29 mg chol, 5 g fib, 10 g pro, 353 mg sod • Carb Choices: 1½; Exchanges: 1½ starch, 1 plant-based protein, 2 fat

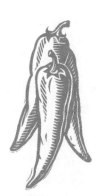

Black-eyed Pea Salad

QUICK | HIGH FIBER

makes 6 servings

In the South, black-eyed peas and greens are thought to bring you luck for the whole year if you eat them on New Year's Day. They are always cooked with lots of salt pork. This healthful recipe turns tradition on its head by using the traditional ingredients in a fresh-tasting salad—with just a sprinkle of bacon. Be sure to slice the sturdy kale leaves into very thin strips. You can use any kind of greens instead of kale—mustard greens, collards, or spinach all work well.

2 strips center-cut bacon
2 tablespoons apple cider vinegar
1½ tablespoons extra virgin olive oil
1 teaspoon Dijon mustard
½ teaspoon kosher salt
⅛ teaspoon ground cayenne
2 (15-ounce) cans no-salt-added black-eyed peas, rinsed and drained
2 cups thinly sliced kale
1 large tomato, chopped
¼ cup thinly sliced red onion

1 Cook the bacon in a large skillet over medium-high heat until crisp. Drain on paper towels and coarsely chop.

2 Meanwhile, whisk together the vinegar, oil, mustard, salt, and cayenne in a large bowl.

3 Add the peas, kale, tomato, and onion and toss to coat. Stir in the bacon just before serving. Serve the salad at room temperature. The salad tastes best on the day it is made, but it can be refrigerated, covered, for up to 1 day. Let stand at room temperature 30 minutes before serving.

Each serving: 19 g carb, 158 cal, 6 g fat, 1 g sat fat, 2 mg chol, 5 g fib, 8 g pro, 201 mg sod • Carb Choices: 1; Exchanges: 1 starch, 1 veg, 1 plant-based protein, 1 fat

Edamame and Bulgur Salad with Basil   HIGH FIBER

makes 6 servings

When you need an easy and colorful salad for summer barbecues, picnics, or potlucks, this one will please any crowd. Who doesn't love loads of fresh tomatoes and basil? If you have them, use both red and yellow cherry tomatoes to add even more color.

1 cup water
¾ cup fine bulgur
1 pound frozen shelled edamame
2 tablespoons white wine vinegar
2 tablespoons extra virgin olive oil
1 garlic clove, minced
¾ teaspoon kosher salt
¼ teaspoon freshly ground pepper
2 cups cherry tomatoes, halved, or quartered if large
¼ cup minced red onion
½ cup chopped fresh basil

1 Pour the water in a small saucepan and bring to a boil over high heat. Remove from the heat and add the bulgur. Cover and let stand until the water is absorbed, 25 minutes. Transfer to a bowl and let stand to cool to room temperature.

2 Meanwhile, bring a medium saucepan of water to a boil over high heat. Add the edamame and cook until tender, about 5 minutes. Drain in a colander and rinse with cold running water until cool.

3 Whisk together the vinegar, oil, garlic, salt, and pepper in a large bowl. Add the cooked bulgur, cooked edamame, salt, and pepper and stir to combine. Add the tomatoes, onion, and basil and toss gently to combine. Serve the salad at room temperature or chilled. The salad tastes best on the day it is made, but it can be refrigerated, covered, for up to 1 day.

Each serving: 19 g carb, 198 cal, 9 g fat, 1 g sat fat, 0 mg chol, 8 g fib, 11 g pro, 150 mg sod • Carb Choices: 1; Exchanges: 1 starch, 1 plant-based protein, 1 fat

Lentil Salad with Walnut Vinaigrette HIGH FIBER

makes 6 servings

Green lentils have an affinity for walnut oil, but you can certainly make this with olive oil instead. Check the lentils often when they are almost done. They go from perfectly cooked to overcooked in just a few minutes. They should be tender, but firm to the bite, and they should not split.

2½ cups water

1 cup dried French green lentils

¾ teaspoon kosher salt, divided

2 tablespoons sherry vinegar or white wine vinegar

1½ tablespoons walnut oil or extra virgin olive oil

⅛ teaspoon freshly ground pepper

1 cup peeled, diced hothouse (English) cucumber

2 tablespoon minced red onion

3 tablespoons chopped fresh dill or Italian parsley

1 Combine the water, lentils, and ½ teaspoon of the salt in a medium saucepan. Bring to a boil over high heat, reduce the heat to low, and simmer, covered, until the lentils are tender, 20 to 25 minutes. Drain.

2 Meanwhile, whisk together the vinegar, oil, remaining ¼ teaspoon salt, and the pepper in a large bowl. Stir in the hot cooked lentils and let stand to cool to room temperature, stirring occasionally. Stir in the cucumber, onion, and dill. Serve the salad at room temperature. The salad tastes best on the day it is made, but it can be refrigerated, covered, for up to 1 day. Let stand at room temperature 30 minutes before serving.

Each serving: 19 g carb, 134 cal, 4 g fat, 0 g sat fat, 0 mg chol, 4 g fib, 7 g pro, 144 mg sod • Carb Choices: 1; Exchanges: 1 starch, 1 plant-based protein, ½ fat

LENTIL AND GOAT CHEESE SALAD HIGH FIBER : Follow the Lentil Salad with Walnut Vinaigrette recipe, at left, stirring in 3 tablespoons (1½ ounces) finely crumbled goat cheese just before serving.

Each serving: 19 g carb, 160 cal, 6 g fat, 2 g sat fat, 6 mg chol, 5 g fib, 8 g pro, 181 mg sod • Carb Choices: 1; Exchanges: 1 starch, 1 plant-based protein, ½ fat

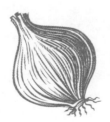

Main Dish Salads

Classic Chicken Salad QUICK

makes 4 servings

Creamy chicken salad is almost always a nutritional nightmare—or if it's not, it's dry and flavorless. This one strikes a balance as it has some mayonnaise, but it's lightened with yogurt and has flavorful lemon and scallions. It's quite delicious and no one will guess that it's as light and healthy as it is. Use it for making sandwiches or serve it over salad greens or alongside ripe summer tomatoes.

2 tablespoons mayonnaise
2 tablespoons low-fat yogurt
2 teaspoons lemon juice
¼ teaspoon kosher salt
Dash of hot sauce
12 ounces chopped cooked chicken breast
    (about 2 cups)
¾ cup chopped celery
2 tablespoons minced scallion
2 tablespoons chopped fresh Italian parsley
    (optional)

1 Stir together the mayonnaise, yogurt, lemon juice, salt, and hot sauce in a medium bowl.

2 Add the chicken, celery, scallion, and parsley, if using, and stir to coat. Cover and refrigerate until chilled, at least 2 hours and up to 2 days.

Each serving: 2 g carb, 200 cal, 9 g fat, 2 g sat fat, 75 mg chol, 0 g fib, 27 g pro, 196 mg sod • Carb Choices: 0; Exchanges: 4 lean protein, 1 fat

CURRIED CHICKEN SALAD QUICK: Follow the Classic Chicken Salad recipe, above, stirring 1 teaspoon curry powder in with the mayonnaise mixture in step 1. Stir in ¼ cup raisins and 2 tablespoons slivered almonds, toasted (page 4), with the chicken in step 2 and proceed as directed.

Each serving: 10 g carb, 249 cal, 11 g fat, 2 g sat fat, 75 mg chol, 1 g fib, 28 g pro, 198 mg sod • Carb Choices: ½; Exchanges: ½ fruit, 4 lean protein, 1½ fat

CRANBERRY-PECAN CHICKEN SALAD QUICK: Follow the Classic Chicken Salad recipe, at left, adding 3 tablespoons dried cranberries and 2 tablespoons pecans, toasted and chopped (page 4), with the chicken in step 2, and proceed as directed.

Each serving: 7 g carb, 245 cal, 11 g fat, 2 g sat fat, 75 mg chol, 1 g fib, 27 g pro, 196 mg sod • Carb Choices: ½; Exchanges: ½ carb, 4 lean protein, 1½ fat

Artichoke-Lemon Chicken Salad QUICK

makes 4 servings

When you need a dressed-up chicken salad, this is a great recipe to turn to. The artichokes and fresh basil give it a lift beyond the ordinary. Serve it as an open-face sandwich on hearty country bread with cups of Carrot-Ginger Soup (page 164) for a casual lunch get-together.

1 (14-ounce) can artichoke hearts
2 tablespoons mayonnaise
2 tablespoons low-fat yogurt
1 teaspoon grated lemon zest
2 teaspoons lemon juice
12 ounces chopped cooked chicken breast
    (about 2 cups)
¾ cup chopped celery
2 tablespoons minced red onion
2 tablespoons chopped fresh basil

1 Drain the artichokes and cut into quarters. Place the artichokes on several thicknesses of paper towels and gently blot dry. Set aside.

2 Stir together the mayonnaise, yogurt, lemon zest, and lemon juice in a medium bowl.

3 Add the artichokes, chicken, celery, onion, and basil and toss gently to coat. Cover and refrigerate until chilled, at least 2 hours and up to 2 days.

Each serving: 7 g carb, 233 cal, 9 g fat, 2 g sat fat, 75 mg chol, 0 g fib, 29 g pro, 345 mg sod • Carb Choices: ½; Exchanges: 1 veg, 4 lean protein, 1½ fat

Oven-Fried Chicken Salad

HIGH FIBER

makes 4 servings

Every suburban chain restaurant has a version of this salad—and I love them all. This much healthier version doesn't compromise on flavor, but cuts back on the fat and calories by baking the "fried" chicken and using a yogurt-based dressing. Serve it with chilled wedges of cantaloupe or honeydew melon for a light summer meal.

½ teaspoon canola oil
½ cup plain dry breadcrumbs
1 ounce freshly grated Parmesan (about ¼ cup)
1 tablespoon Dijon mustard
½ teaspoon hot sauce
4 (4-ounce) boneless skinless chicken breasts
6 cups loosely packed torn romaine lettuce
4 plum tomatoes, quartered
1 hothouse (English) cucumber, sliced
¼ cup thinly sliced red onion
6 tablespoons Creamy Herb Dressing (page 141), divided

1 Preheat the oven to 375°F. Brush a medium rimmed baking sheet with the oil.

2 Combine the breadcrumbs and Parmesan in a shallow dish and stir to mix well. Combine the mustard and hot sauce in a medium bowl.

3 Place the chicken in the mustard mixture and turn to coat. Working with one piece at a time, dredge the chicken in the breadcrumb mixture, pressing to adhere crumbs. Arrange the chicken on the prepared baking sheet. Bake until the juices run clear, about 15 minutes.

4 Meanwhile, combine the lettuce, tomatoes, cucumber, and onion in a large bowl. Add 4 tablespoons of the dressing and toss to coat. Divide the salad evenly among 4 plates. Top each salad with a chicken breast. Drizzle the chicken evenly with the remaining 2 tablespoons dressing. Serve at once.

Each serving: 21 g carb, 289 cal, 9 g fat, 2 g sat fat, 70 mg chol, 4 g fib, 30 g pro, 431 sod • Carb Choices: 1½; Exchanges: ½ starch, 2 veg, 3 lean protein, 1 fat

Grilled Chicken Salad with Miso-Basil Dressing HIGH FIBER

makes 4 servings

If you've had a miso-dressed salad in a Japanese restaurant and loved the earthy salty flavor, try making this easy version at home.

2 tablespoons white miso paste
2 tablespoons cold water
2 tablespoons rice vinegar
1 tablespoon plus ½ teaspoon canola oil
2 teaspoons grated fresh ginger
½ teaspoon chili-garlic paste
4 (4-ounce) boneless skinless chicken breasts
6 cups loosely packed torn romaine lettuce
1 cup cherry tomatoes, halved
½ large hothouse (English) cucumber, thinly sliced
¼ cup thinly sliced red onion
2 tablespoons chopped fresh basil

1 Prepare the grill or heat a large grill pan over medium-high heat.

2 Whisk together the miso, water, vinegar, 1 tablespoon of the oil, ginger, and chili-garlic paste in a small bowl. Spoon 2 tablespoons of the miso mixture into a shallow dish. Add the chicken and turn to coat. Let stand at room temperature for 15 minutes.

3 Brush the grill rack or grill pan with the remaining ½ teaspoon oil. Remove the chicken from the marinade and discard the marinade. Grill the chicken, turning often, until the juices of the chicken run clear, 8 to 10 minutes.

4 Meanwhile, combine the lettuce, tomatoes, cucumber, and onion in a large bowl. Stir the basil into the remaining miso mixture. Drizzle the salad with 2 tablespoons of the miso mixture and toss to coat. Divide the salad evenly among 4 plates. Top each salad with a chicken breast. Drizzle the chicken evenly with the remaining miso mixture. Serve at once.

Each serving: 9 g carb, 203 cal, 7 g fat, 1 g sat fat, 63 mg chol, 4 g fib, 26 g pro, 334 mg sod • Carb Choices: ½; Exchanges: 1 veg, 3 lean protein, 1 fat

Warm Chicken and Roasted Tomato Salad

makes 4 servings

Roasted plum tomatoes make an everyday chicken salad something special.

8 plum tomatoes, halved lengthwise
4 teaspoons extra virgin olive oil, divided
½ teaspoon kosher salt, divided
¼ teaspoon freshly ground pepper, divided
4 (4-ounce) boneless skinless chicken breasts
6 cups loosely packed mixed baby greens
4 tablespoons Herbed Vinaigrette (page 138), made with fresh basil, divided
2 tablespoons freshly grated Parmesan

1 Preheat the oven to 400°F.

2 Place the tomatoes on a large rimmed baking sheet. Drizzle with 2 teaspoons of the oil, and sprinkle with ¼ teaspoon of the salt and ⅛ teaspoon of the pepper. Arrange the tomatoes skin side down in a single layer. Bake until the tomatoes are soft and the bottoms are well browned, 40 to 45 minutes. Let the tomatoes cool slightly.

3 Meanwhile, sprinkle the chicken with the remaining ¼ teaspoon salt and remaining ⅛ teaspoon pepper. Heat a large nonstick skillet over medium-high heat. Add the remaining 2 teaspoons oil and tilt the pan to coat the bottom evenly. Cook the chicken until the juices run clear, about 4 minutes on each side. Transfer to a plate and let cool slightly.

4 Combine the greens and 2 tablespoons of the vinaigrette in a large bowl and toss to coat. Divide the salad evenly among 4 plates. Cut each chicken breast into thin slices and arrange on the salad. Arrange 4 tomato halves on each salad. Drizzle the chicken and tomatoes evenly with the remaining 2 tablespoons dressing. Sprinkle evenly with the Parmesan and serve at once.

Each serving: 10 g carb, 289 cal, 16 g fat, 3 g sat fat, 65 mg chol, 3 g fib, 26 g pro, 339 mg sod • Carb Choices: ½; Exchanges: 2 veg, 3 lean protein, 2½ fat

Mediterranean Chicken, Bean, and Pasta Salad

HIGH FIBER

makes 6 servings

When you cook chicken breasts, make extra so you can use the leftovers to make this salad later in the week. Full of flavorful ingredients, this salad is really healthy and perfect for those nights when you need dinner in a hurry. You can also make it using Basic Vinaigrette (page 138).

4½ ounces whole wheat penne or other short pasta (about 1½ cups)
12 ounces shredded cooked chicken breast (about 2 cups)
1 (15-ounce) can no-salt-added garbanzo beans, rinsed and drained
1 large tomato, chopped
¼ cup Kalamata olives, pitted and chopped
2 tablespoons minced red onion
1 recipe Sun-Dried Tomato–Basil Dressing (page 142)
4 cups loosely packed fresh baby spinach
2 tablespoons pine nuts, toasted (page 4)

1 Cook the pasta according to the package directions. Drain and rinse with cold running water.

2 Combine the pasta, chicken, beans, tomato, olives, and onion in a large bowl. Drizzle with the dressing and toss to coat. Stir in the spinach and pine nuts just before serving. Serve the salad at room temperature. The salad tastes best on the day it is made, but it can be refrigerated, covered, for up to 1 day. Let stand at room temperature 30 minutes before serving.

Each serving: 31 g carb, 336 cal, 11 g fat, 2 g sat fat, 48 mg chol, 6 g fib, 26 g pro, 254 mg sod • Carb Choices: 2; Exchanges: 2 starch, 3 lean protein, 1½ fat

Thai Chicken Salad QUICK

makes 4 servings

An alternative way to serve this salad is to scoop the chicken mixture (step 1 of the instructions) into Bibb lettuce leaves and sprinkle with sliced scallions, mint, and cilantro. Let diners roll up the leaves to eat the salad.

3 tablespoons lime juice
2 tablespoons Asian fish sauce
1 teaspoon grated lime zest
½ teaspoon chili-garlic paste
½ teaspoon sugar
12 ounces shredded cooked chicken breast (about 2 cups)
1 large head Bibb lettuce, separated into leaves and thinly sliced
1 hothouse (English) cucumber, halved lengthwise and sliced
4 radishes, halved and sliced
¼ cup thinly sliced scallions
¼ cup whole fresh mint leaves
¼ cup whole fresh cilantro leaves

1 Whisk together the lime juice, fish sauce, limezest, chili-garlic paste, and sugar in a large bowl. Place the chicken in a medium bowl, drizzle with 2 tablespoons of the fish sauce mixture, and toss to coat.

2 Add the lettuce, cucumber, radishes, scallions, mint, and cilantro to the fish sauce mixture remaining in the large bowl and toss to coat. Divide the salad among 4 plates. Top with the chicken and serve at once.

Each serving: 7 g carb, 174 cal, 3 g fat, 1 g sat fat, 72 mg chol, 2 g fib, 29 g pro, 787 mg sod • Carb Choices: ½; Exchanges: 1 veg, 3½ lean protein

Cobb Salad QUICK

makes 4 servings

Essentially a resourceful meal of leftovers, this salad was invented in the 1930s by Los Angeles restaurateur Robert Cobb, owner of the Brown Derby restaurant, to use ingredients he had on hand.

2 strips center-cut bacon
4 cups chopped romaine lettuce
2 cups chopped Bibb lettuce
6 ounces diced cooked chicken breast (about 1 cup)
1 medium tomato, chopped
1 hard-boiled egg, chopped
½ avocado, pitted, peeled, and chopped
3 tablespoons crumbled blue cheese
3 tablespoons Basic Vinaigrette (page 138)

1 Cook the bacon in a large skillet over medium-high heat until crisp. Drain on paper towels and coarsely chop.

2 Combine the romaine and Bibb lettuces in a large serving bowl. Arrange the bacon, chicken, tomato, egg, avocado, and blue cheese decoratively over the lettuce.

3 Drizzle with the vinaigrette and toss to coat. Serve at once.

Each serving: 6 g carb, 234 cal, 15 g fat, 4 g sat fat, 97 mg chol, 3 g fib, 19 g pro, 259 mg sod • Carb Choices: ½; Exchanges: 1 veg, 2½ lean protein, 2 fat

Chef's Salad QUICK HIGH FIBER

makes 4 servings

A no-cook summer supper standby, a chef's salad is great for using up leftovers and using your imagination. Change the meats, cheese, vegetables, and salad dressing depending on what's in season and on hand—the results will always be delicious.

6 cups chopped romaine lettuce
¼ cup thinly sliced red onion
1 hothouse (English) cucumber, halved lengthwise and sliced
1 red bell pepper, thinly sliced
4 ounces cooked chicken or turkey breast, cut into thin strips
4 ounces lean reduced-sodium ham, cut into thin strips
2 ounces Swiss cheese, cut into thin strips
4 plum tomatoes, cut into wedges
2 hard-boiled eggs, quartered
¼ cup Basic Vinaigrette (page 138) or ⅓ cup Creamy Herb Dressing (page 141)

1 Combine the lettuce, onion, cucumber, and bell pepper in a large serving bowl and toss to distribute the vegetables evenly. Arrange the chicken, ham, Swiss cheese, tomatoes, and eggs decoratively on the lettuce.

2 Drizzle with the vinaigrette and toss to coat. Serve at once.

Each serving: 12 g carb, 290 cal, 17 g fat, 6 g sat fat, 157 mg chol, 4 g fib, 23 g pro, 394 mg sod • Carb Choices: 1; Exchanges: 2 veg, ½ high-fat protein, ½ medium-fat protein, 2 lean protein, 1½ fat

Egg Salad

makes 6 servings

This is classic egg salad, lightened up by using fewer yolks and substituting yogurt for part of the mayonnaise. It makes a great egg salad sandwich on toasted Caraway Beer Bread (page 525).

10 large eggs
2 tablespoons mayonnaise
2 tablespoons plain low-fat yogurt
¼ cup minced celery
2 tablespoons minced scallions
2 tablespoons chopped fresh Italian parsley (optional)
1 teaspoon lemon juice
¾ teaspoon kosher salt
⅛ teaspoon freshly ground pepper

1 Place the eggs in a large saucepan and cover with cold water. Cover and bring to a boil over medium heat. Turn off the heat and let the eggs stand 12 minutes. Drain and peel under cold running water.

2 Remove and discard 4 of the egg yolks. Chop the remaining egg whites and eggs and place in a medium bowl. Add the mayonnaise, yogurt, celery, scallions, parsley, if using, lemon juice, salt, and pepper and stir to mix well. Cover and refrigerate until chilled at least 2 hours and up to 2 days.

Each serving: 1 g carb, 121 cal, 9 g fat, 2 g sat fat, 213 mg chol, 0 g fib, 9 g pro, 280 mg sod • Carb Choices: 0; Exchanges: 1 medium-fat protein, 1 fat

Taco Salad HIGH FIBER

makes 4 servings

There's a reason taco salads are so popular—
they're delicious! This version has a long list of
ingredients, but all of them are pantry staples
and the salad comes together quickly. If you
make it for the kids, I guarantee you'll love it as
much as they do.

3 (6-inch) corn tortillas, cut in half and into thin
strips
¾ teaspoon plus 1 tablespoon chili powder,
divided
8 ounces 95% lean ground beef
½ cup diced green or red bell pepper
½ cup diced onion
1 garlic clove, minced
1 teaspoon ground cumin
1 teaspoon kosher salt, divided
1 (14½-ounce) can no-salt-added diced tomatoes
1 (15-ounce) can no-salt-added black beans or
kidney beans, rinsed and drained
2 tablespoons lime juice
1 tablespoon extra virgin olive oil
6 cups thinly sliced iceberg lettuce
1 large tomato, chopped
2 scallions, thinly sliced
¼ cup chopped fresh cilantro
2 ounces shredded reduced-fat sharp Cheddar
or Colby cheese (about ¼ cup)

1 Preheat the oven to 350°F. Place the tortilla
strips on a large rimmed baking sheet, sprinkle
with ½ teaspoon of the chili powder and toss
to coat. Bake until lightly browned and crisp,
10 minutes.

2 Meanwhile, combine the beef, bell pepper,
and onion in a large nonstick skillet and set over
medium-high heat. Cook, stirring often, until
the beef is browned and the vegetables are
softened, about 8 minutes. Stir in 1 tablespoon
of the remaining chili powder, the garlic, cumin,
and ½ teaspoon of the salt and cook, stirring
constantly until fragrant, 30 seconds. Add the
diced tomatoes and beans, and bring to a boil.
Cook, stirring occasionally, until most of the liquid has evaporated, about 5 minutes.

3 Meanwhile, whisk together the lime juice, oil,
remaining ½ teaspoon salt, and the remaining
¼ teaspoon chili powder in a large bowl. Add the
lettuce, chopped tomato, scallions, cilantro, and
tortilla strips and toss to coat. Divide the salad
mixture evenly among four plates. Top evenly
with the beef mixture. Sprinkle evenly with the
Cheddar and serve at once.

Each serving: 31 g carb, 327 cal, 12 g fat, 5 g sat fat, 48 mg chol, 9 g fib,
23 g pro, 247 mg sod • Carb Choices: 2; Exchanges: 1 starch, 2 veg,
½ high-fat protein, 2 lean protein, ½ fat

Steak and Arugula Salad with Lemon and Dill QUICK

makes 4 servings

Arugula and dill give a fresh counterpoint to the rich beef in this dish. To make a heartier meal, toss halved roasted baby potatoes with the salad greens. For variety, serve salmon fillets, shrimp, or chicken breasts over this flavorful salad for a quick meal.

2 tablespoons lemon juice
1½ tablespoons plus 2 teaspoons extra virgin olive oil, divided
¾ teaspoon kosher salt, divided
¼ teaspoon freshly ground pepper
2 tablespoons chopped fresh dill
4 (4-ounce) filets mignons
8 cups loosely packed baby arugula or torn regular arugula

1 To make the dressing, whisk together the lemon juice, 1½ tablespoons of the oil, ½ teaspoon of the salt, and ⅛ teaspoon of the pepper in a large bowl. Stir in the dill.

2 Sprinkle the steaks with the remaining ¼ teaspoon salt and ⅛ teaspoon pepper. Heat a large heavy-bottomed skillet over medium-high heat. Add the remaining 2 teaspoons oil and tilt the pan to coat the bottom evenly. Add the steaks and cook, turning once, 2 minutes on each side for medium-rare, or to the desired degree of doneness.

3 Add the arugula to the dressing and toss to coat. Divide the salad among 4 plates and top each one with a steak. Serve at once.

Each serving: 2 g carb, 222 cal, 13 g fat, 3 g sat fat, 52 mg chol, 1 g fib, 23 g pro, 268 mg sod • Carb Choices: 0; Exchanges: 3 lean protein, 1½ fat

Grilled Asian Flank Steak Salad

makes 4 servings

Lime juice and sesame oil make a simple, yet intensely flavored marinade for this steak salad. Instead of serving it in a salad, try the steak on its own with a side of Roasted Sweet Potatoes with Ginger and Lime (page 488).

1 (1-pound) flank steak, trimmed of all visible fat
¼ cup lime juice
1 teaspoon Asian sesame oil
⅛ teaspoon ground cayenne
½ teaspoon kosher salt
½ teaspoon canola oil
6 cups loosely packed torn Bibb lettuce
1 large red bell pepper, cut into short, thin strips
1 hothouse (English) cucumber, cut into short, thin strips
½ cup loosely packed fresh basil leaves
¼ cup loosely packed fresh mint leaves
¼ cup thinly sliced red onion
1 recipe Soy-Sesame Dressing (page 143), divided

1 Place the steak in a shallow dish, add the lime juice, sesame oil, and cayenne, and turn to coat. Cover and refrigerate at least 6 hours or up to 12 hours.

2 Prepare the grill or heat a large grill pan over medium-high heat.

3 Remove the steak from the marinade and discard the marinade. Pat dry with paper towels. Sprinkle the steak with the salt.

4 Brush the grill rack or grill pan with the canola oil. Place the steak on the grill rack or in the grill pan and grill, turning once, 4 minutes on each side for medium-rare, or to the desired degree of doneness.

5 Transfer the steak to a cutting board, cover loosely with foil, and let stand 5 minutes. Cut across the grain into thin slices.

6 To assemble the salad, combine the lettuce, bell pepper, cucumber, basil, mint, and onion in a large bowl. Drizzle with 2 tablespoons of the dressing and toss to coat. Divide the salad among 4 plates and top evenly with the steak. Drizzle the steak with the remaining dressing. Serve at once.

Each serving: 10 g carb, 281 cal, 15 g fat, 3 g sat fat, 37 mg chol, 3 g fib, 27 g pro, 364 mg sod • Carb Choices: ½; Exchanges: 2 veg, 3 lean protein, 1½ fat

Tuna Salad QUICK

makes 4 servings

If you love creamy tuna salad, this is a healthful spin on the classic version using a combination of yogurt and mayonnaise for the dressing. My favorite way to serve tuna salad is to spoon a scoop of it inside a fresh tomato. It's very retro, but it tastes terrific for a late-summer lunch. This traditional recipe or the curried version are good for sandwiches, for stuffing a summer tomato, or for serving on top of salad greens.

2 tablespoons plain low-fat yogurt
1 tablespoon mayonnaise
1 teaspoon lemon juice
¼ teaspoon kosher salt
⅛ teaspoon freshly ground pepper
2 (5-ounce) cans low-sodium chunk white alba-
   core tuna in water, drained and flaked
¼ cup diced celery
2 tablespoons thinly sliced scallions
1 tablespoon chopped fresh Italian parsley
   (optional)

1 Stir together the yogurt, mayonnaise, lemon juice, salt, and pepper in a medium bowl.

2 Add the tuna, celery, scallions, and parsley, if using, and stir to combine. Serve at once, or refrigerate, covered, for up to 2 days.

Each serving: 1 g carb, 94 cal, 4 g fat, 0 g sat fat, 27 mg chol, 0 g fib, 16 g pro, 136 mg sod • Carb Choices: 0; Exchanges: 2 lean protein, ½ fat

CURRIED TUNA SALAD WITH APPLE QUICK: Follow the Tuna Salad recipe, at left, stirring in 1 medium Granny Smith apple, cored and chopped, and 1 teaspoon curry powder.

Each serving: 7 g carb, 114 cal, 4 g fat, 0 g sat fat, 27 mg chol, 1 g fib, 16 g pro, 136 mg sod • Carb Choices: ½; Exchanges: ½ fruit, 2 lean protein, ½ fat

Pesto–Red Pepper Tuna Salad QUICK

makes 4 servings

Canned tuna lends itself to almost any kind of flavoring—even assertive ones like the pesto and red pepper in this recipe. If you'd like to make this salad ahead of time, leave out the roasted peppers and stir them in just before serving to prevent them from discoloring the other ingredients.

2 tablespoons plain low-fat yogurt
1 tablespoon mayonnaise
1 tablespoon Basil Pesto (page 597) or
   purchased pesto
1 teaspoon lemon juice
¼ teaspoon kosher salt
⅛ teaspoon freshly ground pepper
2 (5-ounce) cans low-sodium chunk white alba-
   core tuna in water, drained and flaked
⅓ cup red Roasted Bell Peppers (page 21) or
   roasted red peppers from a jar, chopped
¼ cup diced hothouse (English) cucumber
2 tablespoons minced red onion

1 Stir together the yogurt, mayonnaise, pesto, lemon juice, salt, and ground pepper in a medium bowl.

2 Add the tuna, roasted peppers, cucumber, and onion and stir to combine. Serve at once.

Each serving: 3 g carb, 137 cal, 5 g fat, 1 g sat fat, 23 mg chol, 1 g fib, 19 g pro, 145 mg sod • Carb Choices: 0; Exchanges: 2 lean protein, 1 fat

No-Mayo Tuna Salad QUICK

makes 4 servings

In the summer, serve this salad over fresh sliced beefsteak tomatoes, or in winter alongside a handful of sweet grape tomatoes. Use it to make sandwiches, too. There's so much flavor here from the capers, red onion, and lemon that you won't miss the mayo.

2 (5-ounce) cans low-sodium chunk white alba-core tuna in water, drained and flaked

1 stalk celery, diced

2 tablespoons chopped fresh Italian parsley

2 tablespoons capers, rinsed and drained

2 tablespoons minced red onion

1 tablespoon extra virgin olive oil

1 tablespoon lemon juice

⅛ teaspoon freshly ground pepper

Combine all the ingredients in a medium bowl and toss to mix well. Serve at once, or refrigerate, covered for up to 2 days.

Each serving: 2 g carb, 99 cal, 5 g fat, 1 g sat fat, 25 mg chol, 1 g fib, 16 g pro, 176 mg sod • Carb Choices: 0; Exchanges: 2 lean protein, ½ fat

ARTICHOKE-OLIVE TUNA SALAD QUICK: Follow the No-Mayo Tuna Salad recipe, above, stirring in 1 cup canned artichoke hearts, drained and chopped, and 2 tablespoons chopped pitted Kalamata olives.

Each serving: 5 g carb, 129 cal, 6 g fat, 1 g sat fat, 25 mg chol, 1 g fib, 17 g pro, 362 mg sod • Carb Choices: 0; Exchanges: 1 veg, 2 lean protein, 1 fat

Niçoise Salad HIGH FIBER

makes 4 servings

To make the salad more special, though it's not traditional, you can use fresh tuna steaks that are grilled or pan-seared.

12 ounces small red-skinned potatoes, well scrubbed

12 ounces green beans, trimmed

3 tablespoons Basic Vinaigrette (page 138), divided

1 large head Bibb lettuce, separated into leaves

2 (5-ounce) cans low-sodium chunk white alba-core tuna in water, drained and flaked

2 plum tomatoes, quartered

2 hard-boiled eggs, quartered

¼ cup niçoise or other oil-cured black olives, pitted and halved

2 tablespoons capers, rinsed and drained

4 canned anchovy fillets, drained (optional)

1 Place the potatoes in a large saucepan. Add water to cover and bring to a boil over high heat. Reduce the heat to low and simmer, uncovered, until the potatoes are tender, about 10 minutes. Remove the potatoes using a slotted spoon. Let stand until cool enough to handle. Add the green beans to the saucepan and cook until crisp-tender, about 4 minutes. Drain in a colander and rinse with cold running water until cool.

2 Cut the potatoes into ½-inch slices. Drizzle with 1 tablespoon of the vinaigrette and let stand while you assemble the salad.

3 To serve, arrange the lettuce leaves on a large platter. Arrange the potatoes, green beans, tuna, tomatoes, eggs, and olives on the lettuce. Sprinkle with the capers. Drizzle with the remaining 2 tablespoons vinaigrette. Top with the anchovies, if using. Serve at once.

Each serving: 23 g carb, 247 cal, 12 g fat, 2 g sat fat, 118 mg chol, 5 g fib, 15 g pro, 397 mg sod • Carb Choices: 1½; Exchanges: 1 starch, 2 veg, ½ medium-fat protein, 1 lean protein, 1½ fat

Niçoise Pasta Salad

QUICK | HIGH FIBER

makes 6 servings

This salad is a quick and easy way to get all the flavors of a classic niçoise salad in a hurry. You cook the pasta and beans in the same pan, so clean up is easy. For a change of flavors, you can make this salad with canned boneless skinless salmon instead of the tuna.

6 ounces whole wheat penne or other short pasta (about 2 cups)

8 ounces green beans, trimmed and cut into 2-inch pieces

2 (5-ounce) cans low-sodium chunk white albacore tuna in water, drained and flaked

1½ cups cherry or grape tomatoes, halved

¼ cup niçoise or other oil-cured black olives, pitted and halved

¼ cup chopped fresh Italian parsley

3 tablespoons minced red onion

3 tablespoons capers, rinsed and drained

1 recipe Basic Vinaigrette (page 138)

1 Cook the pasta according to the package directions, adding the green beans during the last 4 minutes of cooking. Drain in a colander and rinse with cold running water until cool.

2 Combine the pasta and beans, tuna, tomatoes, olives, parsley, onion, and capers in a large bowl. Drizzle with the vinaigrette and toss to coat. Serve the salad at room temperature. The salad tastes best on the day it is made, but it can be refrigerated, covered, for up to 1 day. Let stand at room temperature 30 minutes before serving.

Each serving: 26 g carb, 208 cal, 7 g fat, 1 g sat fat, 17 mg chol, 4 g fib, 16 g pro, 273 mg sod • Carb Choices: 2; Exchanges: 1½ starch, 1 veg, 1 lean protein, 1½ fat

Tuna and White Bean Salad with Spinach

QUICK | HIGH FIBER

makes 4 servings

With canned beans in the pantry, you can make all sorts of wonderful meals. This is one of them. Dressed with a fresh lemon dressing and served on a bed of baby spinach, it's nice enough to serve to company for a weekend lunch. You can turn it into a sandwich, too—just put all the ingredients (minus the spinach) into halved whole wheat pita breads.

2 (5-ounce) cans low-sodium chunk white albacore tuna in water, drained and flaked

1 (15-ounce) can no-salt-added cannellini or navy beans, rinsed and drained

1 cup chopped hothouse (English) cucumber

¼ cup diced red onion

2 tablespoons chopped fresh Italian parsley

1 tablespoon capers, rinsed and drained

4 tablespoons Lemon Vinaigrette (page 139), divided

6 cups loosely packed fresh baby spinach

4 plum tomatoes, quartered

1 Combine the tuna, beans, cucumber, onion, parsley, and capers in a medium bowl. Drizzle with 2 tablespoons of the vinaigrette and toss to coat. The salad can be made up to this point and refrigerated, covered, for up to 2 days.

2 Place the spinach in a large bowl. Drizzle with the remaining vinaigrette and toss to coat. Divide the spinach evenly among 4 plates. Top evenly with the tuna mixture and top evenly with the tomatoes. Serve at once.

Each serving: 27 g carb, 268 cal, 10 g fat, 1 g sat fat, 25 mg chol, 10 g fib, 21 g pro, 267 mg sod • Carb Choices: 1½; Exchanges: 1 starch, 2 veg, 2 lean protein, 1½ fat

Warm Salmon and Potato Salad [HIGH FIBER]

makes 4 servings

Double or triple this salad and serve it on a platter for an impressive addition to a warm weather buffet. It's perfect for entertaining, since it's a meal in itself. Serve Chilled Cucumber-Mint Soup (page 194) as a starter and Chocolate-Raspberry Chiffon Pie (page 551) for dessert and you've got a stunning summer menu.

12 ounces small red-skinned potatoes, well scrubbed
3 tablespoons Lemon Vinaigrette (page 139), divided
4 (4-ounce) salmon fillets
¼ teaspoon kosher salt
⅛ teaspoon freshly ground pepper
2 teaspoons extra virgin olive oil
6 cups loosely packed mixed baby greens or baby spinach
2 tablespoons capers, rinsed and drained

1 Place the potatoes in a large saucepan. Add water to cover and bring to a boil over high heat. Reduce the heat to low and simmer, uncovered, until the potatoes are tender, 15 to 20 minutes. Drain and let stand until cool enough to handle. Cut the potatoes into 1-inch pieces. Drizzle with 1 tablespoon of the vinaigrette.

2 Sprinkle the salmon with the salt and pepper. Heat a large nonstick skillet over medium-high heat. Add the oil and tilt the pan to coat the bottom evenly. Place the salmon in the skillet skin side up and cook until opaque in the center, 3 to 4 minutes on each side. Transfer to a plate and let cool slightly.

3 To assemble the salads, place the greens in a large bowl, drizzle with the remaining 2 tablespoons vinaigrette, and toss to coat. Divide the greens mixture evenly among 4 plates. Remove the skin from the salmon and place on top of the greens. Arrange the potatoes evenly on the salads. Sprinkle evenly with the capers and serve at once.

Each serving: 18 g carb, 335 cal, 17 g fat, 2 g sat fat, 72 mg chol, 4 g fib, 28 g pro, 338 mg sod • Carb Choices: 1; Exchanges: 1 starch, 1 veg, 3 lean protein, 1½ fat

Creamy Salmon and Pasta Salad

makes 6 servings

Fresh salmon is delicious in this salad, but if you're crunched for time, you can make it with canned skinless boneless salmon. To add some healthful greens, toss in 2 cups of baby arugula or baby spinach just before serving.

2 (5-ounce) salmon fillets
¼ teaspoon kosher salt
Pinch of freshly ground pepper
2 teaspoons extra virgin olive oil
6 ounces whole wheat penne or other short pasta (about 2 cups)
1 hothouse (English) cucumber, chopped
1 cup cherry tomatoes, halved
¼ cup thinly sliced scallions
¼ cup Creamy Herb Dressing (page 141)

1 Sprinkle the salmon with the salt and pepper. Heat a large nonstick skillet over medium-high heat. Add the oil and tilt the pan to coat the bottom evenly. Place the salmon in the skillet skin side up and cook until opaque in the center, 3 to 4 minutes on each side. Transfer to a plate and let cool to room temperature. Remove the skin from the salmon and flake with a fork.

2 Meanwhile, cook the pasta according to the package directions. Drain and rinse with cold running water.

3 Combine the pasta, salmon, cucumber, tomatoes, and scallions in a large bowl. Add the dressing and toss to coat. Serve the salad at room temperature. The salad tastes best on the day it is made, but it can be refrigerated, covered, for up to 1 day. Let stand at room temperature 30 minutes before serving.

Each serving: 24 g carb, 196 cal, 6 g fat, 1 g sat fat, 22 mg chol, 3 g fib, 13 g pro, 103 mg sod • Carb Choices: 1½; Exchanges: 1½ starch, 1 veg, 1 lean protein, ½ fat

Shrimp, Mango, and Avocado Salad QUICK

makes 4 servings

When you need an impressive lunch or light dinner without much fuss, this salad, with its out-of-the-ordinary blend of flavors, colors, and textures is a gorgeous option.

12 ounces medium cooked peeled deveined shrimp

1 large mango, peeled, pitted, and thinly sliced

1 hothouse (English) cucumber, cut in half lengthwise and thinly sliced

½ avocado, pitted, peeled, and thinly sliced

2 scallions, thinly sliced

4 tablespoons Honey–Poppy Seed Vinaigrette (page 140), divided

6 cups loosely packed baby arugula or fresh baby spinach

1 Combine the shrimp, mango, cucumber, avocado, and scallions in a medium bowl. Drizzle with 2 tablespoons of the vinaigrette and toss to coat.

2 Place the arugula in a large bowl. Drizzle with the remaining vinaigrette and toss to coat. Divide the arugula evenly among 4 plates. Top evenly with the shrimp mixture and serve at once.

Each serving: 18 g carb, 262 cal, 13 g fat, 2 g sat fat, 166 mg chol, 3 g fib, 20 g pro, 270 mg sod • Carb Choices: 1; Exchanges: ½ fruit, 1 veg, 3 lean protein, 2 fat

Ceviche-Style Shrimp Salad

makes 4 servings

This salad gives you the flavors of ceviche—citrus, chile, and cilantro—but using cooked shrimp instead of raw. Make the salad with small shrimp instead of large and serve it in endive spears as an hors d'oeuvre.

¼ cup orange juice

2 tablespoons lime juice

1½ tablespoons extra virgin olive oil

½ teaspoon kosher salt

12 ounces large cooked peeled deveined shrimp

1 hothouse (English) cucumber, halved lengthwise and sliced

1 red bell pepper, cut into short, thin strips

¼ cup chopped fresh cilantro

2 tablespoons diced red onion

1 tablespoon minced jalapeño, including seeds (or to taste)

Whisk together the orange juice, lime juice, oil, and salt in a large bowl. Add the shrimp, cucumber, bell pepper, cilantro, onion, and jalapeño and toss to coat. Refrigerate the salad, covered, until chilled, at least 2 hours and up to 4 hours.

Each serving: 8 g carb, 162 cal, 6 g fat, 1 g sat fat, 166 mg chol, 1 g fib, 19 g pro, 334 mg sod • Carb Choices: ½; Exchanges: ½ carb, 3 lean protein, 1 fat

Dressings and Croutons

Basic Vinaigrette QUICK

makes ⅓ cup

This basic vinaigrette is just that—basic. It's simple to make with ordinary pantry ingredients and tastes better than any vinaigrette you buy. Use it to dress greens, pasta, or meat or seafood salads. It also makes a great marinade for beef, pork, or lamb. It's basic, but very versatile.

3 tablespoons extra virgin olive oil
2 tablespoons white wine vinegar
½ teaspoon Dijon mustard
¼ teaspoon kosher salt
⅛ teaspoon freshly ground pepper

Whisk together all the ingredients in a small bowl. The dressing can be refrigerated, covered, for up to 3 days.

Each serving (about 2 teaspoons): 0 g carb, 48 cal, 5 g fat, 1 g sat fat, 0 mg chol, 0 g fib, 0 g pro, 43 mg sod • Carb Choices: 0; Exchanges: 1 fat

MUSTARD VINAIGRETTE QUICK : Follow the Basic Vinaigrette recipe, above, substituting 1 teaspoon whole grain Dijon mustard for the Dijon.

Each serving (about 2 teaspoons): 0 g carb, 49 cal, 5 g fat, 1 g sat fat, 0 mg chol, 0 g fib, 0 g pro, 50 mg sod • Carb Choices: 0; Exchanges: 1 fat

FRESH TOMATO VINAIGRETTE QUICK : Follow the Basic Vinaigrette recipe, above, stirring in ¼ cup seeded diced tomato.

Each serving (about 2 teaspoons): 0 g carb, 49 cal, 5 g fat, 1 g sat fat, 0 mg chol, 0 g fib, 0 g pro, 45 mg sod • Carb Choices: 0; Exchanges: 1 fat

Herbed Vinaigrette QUICK

makes ⅓ cup

If you have an herb garden, play with this dressing, adding different herbs depending on what's growing and what's cooking. For a salmon fillet or shrimp, use fresh dill. For a steak, use Italian parsley. For chicken, try tarragon.

3 tablespoons extra virgin olive oil
2 tablespoons red or white wine vinegar
½ teaspoon Dijon mustard
¼ teaspoon kosher salt
⅛ teaspoon freshly ground pepper
2 tablespoons chopped fresh basil, dill, tarragon, or Italian parsley

Combine all the ingredients in a blender or mini food processor and process until smooth. The dressing can be refrigerated, covered, for up to 3 days.

Each serving (about 2 teaspoons): 0 g carb, 49 cal, 5 g fat, 1 g sat fat, 0 mg chol, 0 g fib, 0 g pro, 43 mg sod • Carb Choices: 0; Exchanges: 1 fat

Sherry-Walnut Vinaigrette QUICK

makes ⅓ cup

This is my absolute favorite salad dressing. I love this on any mix of salad greens, drizzled on roasted winter squash, or as a sauce drizzled over sliced roasted pork tenderloin.

3 tablespoons toasted walnut oil
2 tablespoons sherry vinegar
½ teaspoon Dijon mustard
¼ teaspoon kosher salt
⅛ teaspoon freshly ground pepper

Whisk together all the ingredients in a small bowl. The dressing can be refrigerated, covered, for up to 3 days.

Each serving (about 2 teaspoons): 0 g carb, 47 cal, 5 g fat, 0 g sat fat, 0 mg chol, 0 g fib, 0 g pro, 43 mg sod • Carb Choices: 0; Exchanges: 1 fat

Lemon Vinaigrette QUICK

makes ⅓ cup

Bright and puckery, you'll find endless uses for this dressing. Naturally, it pairs well with any kind of fish or shellfish, but it also wakes up the flavor of chicken breast and makes pasta and bean salads sing. You can use it as a marinade for fish, shrimp, or chicken, as well.

3 tablespoons extra virgin olive oil
½ teaspoon grated lemon zest
2 tablespoons lemon juice
½ teaspoon Dijon mustard
¼ teaspoon kosher salt
⅛ teaspoon freshly ground pepper

Whisk together all the ingredients in a small bowl. The dressing can be refrigerated, covered, for up to 3 days.

Each serving (about 2 teaspoons): 0 g carb, 49 cal, 5 g fat, 1 g sat fat, 0 mg chol, 0 g fib, 0 g pro, 43 mg sod • Carb Choices: 0; Exchanges: 1 fat

Cilantro-Lime Vinaigrette QUICK

makes ⅓ cup

Great for bean salads or pasta salads, this dressing has just a bit of honey to round out the tart citrus flavor. It's also refreshing to drizzle over salmon, sliced avocado, or sliced honeydew melon.

3 tablespoons canola oil
½ teaspoon grated lime zest
2 tablespoons lime juice
2 tablespoons chopped fresh cilantro
½ teaspoon honey
¼ teaspoon kosher salt
¼ teaspoon ground cumin
⅛ teaspoon freshly ground pepper

A Drizzle Will Do

The dressing on a salad—whether it be a green salad or pasta, bean, or grain salad—should be just enough that the flavors of the dressing and the ingredients complement each other. There should not be so much dressing that the dressing is all you taste—the flavor of the salad ingredients should shine through.

The salad dressing recipes you'll find here have highly concentrated flavors from flavorful ingredients such as extra virgin olive oil, Dijon mustard, garlic, and fresh herbs. If you taste them on their own, you may think they will overpower a salad. If used judiciously, you'll find that they balance a salad without dominating the flavor.

To use the least amount of dressing for a green salad, always combine the greens and other salad ingredients with the dressing in a large bowl and toss them to coat. You will use far less dressing than if you drizzle the dressing over the salad at the table. As a rule of thumb, use 2 teaspoons of a vinaigrette dressing or 1 tablespoon of a creamy dressing to coat 2 cups of salad greens.

Whisk together all the ingredients in a small bowl. The dressing can be refrigerated, covered, for up to 3 days.

Each serving (about 2 teaspoons): 1 g carb, 49 cal, 5 g fat, 0 g sat fat, 0 mg chol, 0 g fib, 0 g pro, 35 mg sod • Carb Choices: 0; Exchanges: 1 fat

Honey–Poppy Seed Vinaigrette QUICK

makes ⅓ cup

Poppy seeds tend to turn rancid rather quickly. Give your jar a sniff before you make this dressing—your nose will know if the seeds are past their prime. Drizzle this lightly sweet dressing over fruit salad, chicken breast, salmon, or roasted sweet potatoes.

3 tablespoons extra virgin olive oil
2 tablespoons champagne vinegar or white wine vinegar
1 tablespoon honey
½ teaspoon Dijon mustard
½ teaspoon poppy seeds
¼ teaspoon kosher salt
⅛ teaspoon freshly ground pepper

Whisk together all the ingredients in a small bowl. The dressing can be refrigerated, covered, for up to 3 days.

Each serving (about 2 teaspoons): 2 g carb, 57 cal, 5 g fat, 1 g sat fat, 0 mg chol, 0 g fib, 0 g pro, 43 mg sod • Carb Choices: 0; Exchanges: 1 fat

Feta-Oregano Vinaigrette QUICK

makes ⅓ cup

Serve grilled steak or chicken breast over a bed of greens drizzled with this vinaigrette for a flavor-packed meal with hardly any effort. The dressing is also good over steamed or roasted potatoes, sliced tomatoes, or grilled lamb.

3 tablespoons extra virgin olive oil
2 tablespoons red or white wine vinegar
½ teaspoon Dijon mustard
¼ teaspoon kosher salt
¼ teaspoon dried oregano
⅛ teaspoon freshly ground pepper
2 tablespoons finely crumbled feta cheese

Whisk together all the ingredients except the feta in a small bowl. Stir in the feta and serve at once.

Each serving (about 2 teaspoons): 0 g carb, 55 cal, 6 g fat, 1 g sat fat, 2 mg chol, 0 g fib, 0 g pro, 69 mg sod • Carb Choices: 0; Exchanges: 1 fat

Balsamic Vinaigrette QUICK

makes ⅓ cup

Balsamic vinegar—even the cheap kind that I always use—is a little bit sweet. I've added a touch of honey here to round out the flavor (it could be my cheap vinegar), so taste your dressing before you add the honey—it may not need it, especially if you are using a more expensive variety. Drizzle this over salad greens, toss it in bean salads, or use it as a marinade for steak or pork chops.

3 tablespoons extra virgin olive oil
2 tablespoons balsamic vinegar
1 tablespoon minced shallots
1 teaspoon honey
½ teaspoon Dijon mustard
¼ teaspoon kosher salt
⅛ teaspoon freshly ground pepper

Whisk together all the ingredients in a small bowl. The dressing can be refrigerated, covered, for up to 3 days.

Each serving: 2 g carb, 54 cal, 5 g fat, 1 g sat fat, 0 mg chol, 0 g fib, 0 g pro, 39 mg sod • Carb Choices: 0; Exchanges: 1 fat

Creamy Herb Dressing [QUICK]

makes generous ½ cup

This basic ranch-style dressing has infinite uses as a dressing for green salad, pasta salad, or chicken salad. But that's just the beginning. Try it in coleslaw or potato salad, as a sandwich spread, or as a dip for fresh raw vegetables.

½ cup plain low-fat yogurt
2 tablespoons mayonnaise
1 teaspoon white wine vinegar
1 small garlic clove, crushed through a press
¼ teaspoon kosher salt
⅛ teaspoon freshly ground pepper
2 tablespoons chopped fresh basil or dill

Whisk together all the ingredients except the basil in a small bowl. Stir in the basil. The dressing can be refrigerated, covered, for up to 3 days.

Each serving (about 1 tablespoon): 1 g carb, 35 cal, 3 g fat, 1 g sat fat, 2 mg chol, 0 g fib, 1 g pro, 65 mg sod • Carb Choices: 0; Exchanges: ½ fat

Creamy Goat Cheese–Chive Dressing [QUICK]

makes generous ½ cup

The distinctive tart flavor of goat cheese brings great flavor to spinach salad, potato salad, grilled chicken, or steamed vegetables. Instead of the chives, try it with chopped fresh basil or dill.

½ cup plain low-fat yogurt
2 tablespoons mayonnaise
2 tablespoons finely crumbled soft goat cheese
1 teaspoon white wine vinegar
1 small garlic clove, crushed through a press
¼ teaspoon kosher salt
⅛ teaspoon freshly ground pepper
2 tablespoons minced fresh chives

Whisk together all the ingredients except the chives in a small bowl until smooth. Stir in the chives. The dressing can be refrigerated, covered, for up to 3 days.

Each serving (about 1 tablespoon): 1 g carb, 42 cal, 4 g fat, 1 g sat fat, 4 mg chol, 0 g fib, 1 g pro, 74 mg sod • Carb Choices: 0; Exchanges: ½ fat

Creamy Blue Cheese–Peppercorn Dressing [QUICK]

makes generous ½ cup

Crumble the blue cheese straight from the refrigerator while it is very cold. When it's cold, you can crumble it more finely so a little bit does go a long way. Use this rich dressing on sturdy greens like romaine or iceberg, drizzle it over roasted or steamed potatoes, or serve it as a dip.

6 whole black peppercorns
½ cup plain low-fat yogurt
2 tablespoons mayonnaise
1 teaspoon white wine vinegar
1 small garlic clove, crushed through a press
¼ teaspoon kosher salt
2 tablespoons finely crumbled blue cheese

1 Place the peppercorns in a mortar and crush with a pestle. Alternatively, place them in a small resealable plastic bag. Seal the bag, place on a cutting board, and crush using a meat mallet or the back of a large spoon.

2 Place the peppercorns and the remaining ingredients except the blue cheese in a small bowl and whisk until smooth. Stir in the cheese. The dressing can be refrigerated, covered, for up to 3 days.

Each serving (about 1 tablespoon): 1 g carb, 42 cal, 4 g fat, 1g sat fat, 4 mg chol, 0 g fib, 1 g pro, 89 mg sod • Carb Choices: 0; Exchanges: ½ fat

Creamy Parmesan Dressing QUICK

makes generous ½ cup

The cheese makes the dressing in this recipe, so use good quality Parmesan cheese, or substitute Pecorino Romano. Use it with just about anything—greens, sliced tomatoes, steamed vegetables, or grilled chicken.

½ cup plain low-fat yogurt
2 tablespoons mayonnaise
1 teaspoon white wine vinegar
1 small garlic clove, crushed through a press
¼ teaspoon kosher salt
⅛ teaspoon freshly ground pepper
2 tablespoons freshly grated Parmesan cheese, preferably Parmigiano-Reggiano
2 tablespoons chopped fresh Italian parsley

Whisk together all the ingredients except the parsley in a small bowl. Stir in the parsley. The dressing can be refrigerated, covered, for up to 3 days.

Each serving (about 1 tablespoon): 1 g carb, 41 cal, 3 g fat, 1 g sat fat, 3 mg chol, 0 g fib, 1 g pro, 84 mg sod • Carb Choices: 0; Exchanges: ½ fat

Roasted Red Pepper Dressing QUICK

makes ⅓ cup

The gorgeous ruby color of this dressing makes it a good choice for dishes where you use it as a drizzle rather than tossing it with the ingredients. Try it over a platter of sliced yellow tomatoes, fresh mozzarella, and fresh basil leaves for a colorful peak-of-summer supper.

¼ cup red Roasted Bell Peppers (page 21) or roasted red peppers from a jar, chopped
2 tablespoons extra virgin olive oil
1½ tablespoons red wine vinegar
1 small garlic clove, crushed through a press
¼ teaspoon kosher salt
⅛ teaspoon freshly ground pepper

Combine all the ingredients in a blender and process until smooth. The dressing can be refrigerated, covered, for up to 5 days.

Each serving (about 2 teaspoons): 0 g carb, 34 cal, 4 g fat, 0 g sat fat, 0 mg chol, 0 g fib, 0 g pro, 35 mg sod • Carb Choices: 0; Exchanges: ½ fat

Sun-Dried Tomato–Basil Dressing QUICK

makes ¼ cup

Pureed sun-dried tomatoes give this dressing rich color, intense flavor, and a thick consistency. Use this to make bean or pasta salad, or drizzle it over grilled or broiled steaks or chicken.

2 dry-packed sun-dried tomatoes, thinly sliced
2 tablespoons water
2 tablespoons extra virgin olive oil
2 tablespoons balsamic vinegar
1 small garlic clove, crushed through a press
¼ teaspoon kosher salt
⅛ teaspoon freshly ground pepper
1 tablespoon chopped fresh basil

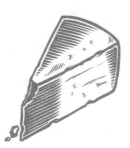

1 Combine the tomatoes and water in a small saucepan. Set over medium heat and bring to a boil. Remove from the heat, cover, and let stand until cooled, 15 minutes.

2 Transfer the tomatoes and any remaining water to a blender. Add the oil, vinegar, garlic, salt, and pepper and process until smooth. Transfer to a bowl and stir in the basil. The dressing can be refrigerated, covered, for up to 3 days.

Each serving (about 2 teaspoons): 1 g carb, 49 cal, 5 g fat, 1 g sat fat, 0 mg chol, 0 g fib, 0 g pro, 62 mg sod • Carb Choices: 0; Exchanges: 1 fat

Dry-Packed Sun-Dried Tomatoes

Dry-packed sun-dried tomatoes come in plastic bags like dried apricots or dried plums. You'll find them in the produce section or in the dried fruit section of the supermarket. Since they're not packed in oil, they are lower in calories and they retain more of the fresh tomato flavor than the oil-packed variety.

When purchasing dry-packed sun-dried tomatoes, make sure they are supple and pliable, not crisp. To use them in salads, soak them in a small amount of boiling water for about 15 minutes, then drain and slice or chop. To use them in soups or stews, soaking isn't necessary, as the broth from these dishes will soften the tomatoes as the dish cooks. Don't buy more than you'll use within a month or so, as their vibrant red color and their flavor fade quickly. They're a healthful way to add a lot of flavor to many dishes.

Avocado Dressing QUICK

makes ⅔ cup

This rich dressing turns even the simplest salad into a luxury. Drizzle it over sliced mangoes and red bell peppers or sliced tomatoes and sweet onions.

½ avocado, pitted, peeled, and chopped
½ cup loosely packed cilantro leaves
⅓ cup cold water
1 small jalapeño, seeded and chopped
1 small garlic clove, chopped
2 tablespoons lime juice
¼ teaspoon ground cumin
¼ teaspoon kosher salt

Combine all the ingredients in a blender and process until smooth. The dressing can be refrigerated, covered, for up to 3 days. The dressing thickens upon standing. Thin it with a little cold water, if necessary, before serving.

Each serving (about 1 tablespoon): 1 g carb, 16 cal, 1 g fat, 0 g sat fat, 0 mg chol, 1 g fib, 0 g pro, 29 mg sod • Carb Choices: 0; Exchanges: None

Soy-Sesame Dressing QUICK

makes ⅓ cup

If you'd like to give some spice to this dressing, add ½ teaspoon chili-garlic paste. Use it to dress salad greens or pasta salad, or as a dip for vegetables or summer rolls.

2 tablespoons canola oil
1 tablespoon rice vinegar
1 tablespoon lime juice
1 tablespoon reduced-sodium soy sauce
½ teaspoon grated fresh ginger
½ teaspoon honey
⅛ teaspoon Asian sesame oil

Whisk together all the ingredients in a small bowl. The dressing can be refrigerated, covered, for up to 5 days.

Each serving (about 2 teaspoons): 1 g carb, 35 cal, 4 g fat, 0 g sat fat, 0 mg chol, 0 g fib, 0 g pro, 76 mg sod • Carb Choices: 0; Exchanges: 1 fat

Orange-Ginger Dressing

QUICK

makes ¼ cup

Cooking the orange juice concentrates its flavor, giving this dressing a vivid punch of citrus. Serve this over any blend of greens, grilled salmon or shrimp, or chicken.

2 large navel oranges
2 tablespoons extra virgin olive oil
1 tablespoon champagne vinegar or white
    wine vinegar
½ teaspoon grated fresh ginger
⅛ teaspoon kosher salt
Pinch of freshly ground pepper

1 Grate ½ teaspoon zest from one of the oranges and set aside. Squeeze ¾ cup juice from the oranges. Put the juice in a small saucepan and bring to a boil over medium-high heat. Cook, stirring occasionally, until the juice is reduced to 2 tablespoons. Transfer the juice to a small bowl to cool.

2 Whisk the orange zest, oil, vinegar, ginger, salt, and pepper into the orange juice. Refrigerate, covered, for up to 3 days.

Each serving (about 2 teaspoons): 3 g carb, 57 cal, 5 g fat, 1 g sat fat, 0 mg chol, 0 g fib, 0 g pro, 24 mg sod • Carb Choices: 0; Exchanges: 1 fat

Peanut Dressing   QUICK

makes ⅓ cup

This delicious dressing will put an Asian spin on any mix of greens, grains, or pasta. It looks curdled when you first start whisking, but once mixed it will smooth out to a creamy dressing. It makes a great vegetable dip if your children like peanut butter. Omit the cayenne for the young ones.

2 tablespoons natural creamy
    peanut butter
1 tablespoon water
1 tablespoon apple cider vinegar
1 tablespoon reduced-sodium soy sauce
1 teaspoon minced fresh ginger
1 teaspoon light brown sugar
1 garlic clove, crushed through a press
Pinch of ground cayenne

Whisk together all the ingredients in a small bowl. Refrigerate, covered, for up to 3 days.

Each serving (about 1 tablespoon): 4 g carb, 59 cal, 4 g fat, 1 g sat fat, 0 mg chol, 1 g fib, 2 g pro, 182 mg sod • Carb Choices: 0; Exchanges: ½ fat

Homemade Croutons   QUICK

makes 8 servings

Croutons are a great way to use up day-old bread and these are effortless to make. Here's a basic recipe, but you can toss the croutons with ¼ teaspoon crumbled dried thyme or rosemary before baking, too. Keep them on hand to add crunch to green salads.

2 cups ½-inch cubes whole grain bread
    (about 3½ ounces)
1 tablespoon extra virgin olive oil
⅛ teaspoon salt

1 Preheat the oven to 350°F.

2 Place the bread cubes on a large rimmed baking sheet. Drizzle with the oil, sprinkle with the salt, and toss to coat. Bake, stirring once, until lightly browned and crisp, 15 to 20 minutes. Cool on a wire rack. Store in an airtight container at room temperature for up to 1 week.

Each serving: 6 g carb, 48 cal, 2 g fat, 0 g sat fat, 0 mg chol, 1 g fib, 1 g pro, 103 mg sod • Carb Choices: ½; Exchanges: ½ starch

Soups

Easy Homemade Stocks

Vegetable Stock

Chicken Stock

Leftover-Chicken Chicken Stock

Smoked Turkey Stock

Beef Stock

Ham Hock Stock

Shrimp Stock

Vegetable Soups

Homemade Tomato Soup

Tomato and Fennel Soup

Summer Squash and Tomato Soup

Root Vegetable Soup

Roasted Vegetable Soup

Roasted Yellow Bell Pepper Soup

Easy Vegetable Minestrone

Chile-Spiced Vegetable Soup

Creamy Vegetable Chowder

Pumpkin and Roasted Red Pepper Soup

Curried Cauliflower Apple Soup

Garden Pea Soup with Dill

Beet Soup with Fennel and Apple

Potato-Leek Soup

Sweet Potato–Apple Soup

Carrot-Ginger Soup

Orange-Carrot Soup

Butternut Squash Soup

Butternut Squash Soup with Red Curry and Coconut

Celery–Celery Root Soup

Parsnip-Pear Soup

Spinach Stracciatella

French Onion Soup with Gruyère Croutons

Hot-and-Sour Soup

Miso-Vegetable Soup

Egg Drop Soup

Bean Soups

Black Bean Soup

Quick Black Bean Soup

Pinto Bean Soup

Bean and Butternut Squash Mole Soup

Black-eyed Pea and Greens Soup

White Bean Soup

White Bean and Roasted Tomato Soup

Two-Bean Minestrone

Curried Lentil Soup

Split Pea Soup

Slow-Cooker Split Pea Soup

Italian Split Pea Soup

Chicken and Turkey Soups

Classic Chicken Noodle Soup

Quick and Easy Chicken Noodle Soup

Lemony Chicken Soup with Orzo and Spinach

Spring Chicken Soup with Potatoes and Asparagus

Chicken Tortilla Soup

Coconut Curry Chicken Soup

Italian Turkey Sausage and White Bean Soup

Turkey, Shiitake Mushroom, and Rice Soup

Spicy Turkey and Black Bean Soup

Meaty Soups

Vegetable Beef Soup

Beef Barley Soup with Mushrooms

Italian Meatball Soup

Lemon-Mint Meatball Soup

Vietnamese Beef Noodle Soup

Pork and Hominy Soup

Lentil and Chorizo Soup

Pork Dumplings in Ginger Broth

Moroccan Harira

Seafood Soups

New England Clam Chowder

Manhattan Clam Chowder

Cioppino

Shrimp Gumbo

Shrimp and Black Bean Soup with Chile and Lime

Coconut Shrimp Soup with Basmati Rice

Chilled Soups

Chunky Gazpacho

White Gazpacho

Cucumber-Buttermilk Vichyssoise

Chilled Cucumber-Mint Soup

Chilled Zucchini-Dill Soup

Chilled Avocado-Lime Soup

Chilled Tomatillo Soup

Icy Cold Melon-Mint Soup

Soups are a natural health food. They require very little added fat, usually just a drizzle for the initial cooking of the vege- tables and seasonings. Lean meats like sirloin, pork chops, chicken breast, or turkey breast that tend to be dry if only slightly overcooked are perfect for soups, since there's lots of flavor and moisture from the other ingredients.

A comforting bowl of soup can be a sneaky vehicle for all manner of healthy foods (vegetables, dried beans, whole wheat pastas) that many people wouldn't eat if they were served on their own. You'll find an abundance of vegetable soups in this chapter just for that reason. If picky eaters in your family won't eat parsnips or beets, you might have better luck with Parsnip-Pear Soup (page 167) or Beet Soup with Fennel and Apple (page 162).

Soups are easy on the cook, too. After the initial chopping of the vegetables, most soups come together pretty quickly and you don't have to hover over them while they cook. Many soups can be frozen, so if you make a double batch, you can freeze one for effortless lunches or dinners in the future (see Freezing Soups on page 157).

If you've never made your own stocks before, there are easy recipes here for making them— even super-simple slow-cooker versions. If you use purchased stocks or broths for soups, read the label carefully and choose those with the least amount of sodium. Read the ingredient list, too. There should be nothing on the list that you would not cook with at home.

Easy Homemade Stocks

Making your own stock is easier than you realize. All you do is throw vegetables, meaty poultry or beef bones, or shrimp shells in a pot with a few seasonings plus water and simmer them. Strain the flavorful stock and you are done (I like to chill meat or poultry stocks first to let the fat solidify and remove and discard it to cut down on fat and calories).

This simple kitchen technique results in stocks that are infinitely more flavorful than store-bought versions. Homemade stock has the wholesome flavor of the ingredients you use. Since some brands of broths contain dubious ingredients like cane juice, dextrose, MSG, hydrogenated oil, or wheat gluten, it's easy to understand why many of them taste so bad. Commercial stocks and broths are also typically high in sodium, and if you make your own, you control the amount of salt you add. Soups are, of course, the natural use for broths, but you can use them for braising meats, making risotto, or cooking rice and other grains.

Stocks can be frozen for up to 6 months, so it's easy to make a big batch in a single afternoon that will provide you with many months of meals. You can double or triple any of the stock recipes here, depending on how much stock you use and how much freezer space you have. There are slow-cooker versions of the slow-simmered stocks so that you can make them while you're busy with other things. The Leftover-Chicken Chicken Stock (page 150) is a must try—you make it with the carcass of a roasted chicken and basic vegetables you already have on hand.

When you make stock, keep it at a very low simmer with bubbles just breaking the surface at the center of the pot. Once it's done, strain the stock twice—once through a colander to remove big pieces of meat and vegetables, then through a fine wire mesh strainer to get rid of smaller particles. Strain the stock while it is hot so it will easily pour through the strainer. Once meat or poultry stocks cool, they become thicker (this is from the gelatin that is extracted from the bones as they simmer).

To safely strain hot stock, place a colander inside a large bowl and place the bowl in the sink. I find that it's easier to pour down into the sink than into a bowl at counter level. An added advantage is that if any splashes occur, they will land in the sink, not on your arms or the kitchen counter.

Vary the ingredients in your stocks depending on the kind of cooking you do. If you cook a lot of Asian dishes, add a couple slices of ginger; throw in some cilantro for Mexican dishes; or add corn cobs if you're going to use the stock for a summer vegetable soup. You can also include the leftover rind from a piece of Parmesan to add richer flavor—a great idea for stocks you'll use to make risotto or minestrone. The only vegetables I would advise not using would be cabbage-flavored ones: any cabbages, cauliflower, broccoli, turnips, and rutabagas. And don't add any vegetables that are aged or bruised to the point that you wouldn't eat them on their own.

What's the difference between a stock and a broth? Apparently very little. Some cooks say that if it's made with beef or poultry bones it's a stock and if it's made only with the beef or poultry flesh, it's a broth. Some say if you make it yourself it's a stock, if you buy it, it's a broth. Whatever you call them, stocks (or broths) are worth taking the time to make at home.

Vegetable Stock

makes 8 cups

This is a basic, easy vegetable stock that tastes better and has less sodium than any canned variety. For richer flavor and color, you can take an extra step and lightly brown the carrots, celery, and onion in a couple of teaspoons of olive oil before adding the other ingredients.

12 cups cold water
2 large carrots, peeled and cut into 1-inch chunks
2 stalks celery, cut into 1-inch chunks
1 large onion, chopped
4 sprigs Italian parsley
2 garlic cloves, smashed
8 black peppercorns
2 bay leaves
1 teaspoon kosher salt

1 Combine all the ingredients in a large pot. Bring just to a simmer over medium heat. Reduce the heat to low and simmer, partially covered, with bubbles gently coming to the surface in the center of the pot, 1 hour.

2 Place a colander in a large bowl and pour in the stock. Discard the vegetables and seasonings. Use the stock at once or let stand to cool to room temperature. The cooled stock can be refrigerated, covered, for up to 4 days or frozen for up to 6 months.

Each serving (½ cup): 2 g carb, 10 cal, 0 g fat, 0 g sat fat, 0 mg chol, 0 g fib, 0 g pro, 70 mg sod • Carb Choices: 0; Exchanges: None

Chicken Stock

makes 10 cups

If you make this once and realize how easy it is and how great it tastes, you'll be a convert. Everything you make with homemade chicken stock—from soups to stews to sauces—will taste fresher and more natural than when made with canned stock.

4 pounds any combination chicken wings, backs, necks, and legs
12 cups cold water
2 large carrots, peeled and cut into 1-inch chunks
2 stalks celery, cut into 1-inch chunks
1 large onion, chopped
4 sprigs Italian parsley
2 garlic cloves, smashed
8 black peppercorns
2 bay leaves
1 teaspoon kosher salt

1 Combine all the ingredients in a large pot. Bring just to a simmer over medium heat. Reduce the heat to low and simmer, partially covered, with bubbles gently coming to the surface in the center of the pot, 2 hours. Do not stir the stock while it cooks.

2 Place a colander in a large bowl and pour in the stock. Discard the chicken, vegetables, and seasonings. Strain the stock through a fine wire mesh strainer.

3 Let stand to cool to room temperature. Cover and refrigerate until the fat rises to the top of the stock. Remove and discard the fat. Use the stock at once or refrigerate, covered, for up to 4 days or freeze for up to 6 months.

Each serving (½ cup): 1 g carb, 13 cal, 0 g fat, 0 g sat fat, 3 mg chol, 0 g fib, 2 g pro, 70 mg sod • Carb Choices: 0; Exchanges: None

SLOW-COOKER VERSION: Follow the Chicken Stock recipe, above, using a 6-quart slow cooker. Reduce the water to 7 cups. Cook on high for 8 hours and proceed with steps 2 and 3. Makes 6 cups.

Leftover-Chicken Chicken Stock

makes 10 cups

Don't let the carcass of a leftover roasted chicken or a purchased rotisserie chicken go to waste. You can add a few vegetables and seasonings, simmer it for a few hours, and have great-tasting chicken stock. Try the slow-cooker version and you can make it while you're at work. You can make this with a leftover turkey carcass or a turkey breast carcass, too.

1 leftover chicken carcass
12 cups cold water
2 large carrots, peeled and cut into 1-inch
    chunks
2 stalks celery, cut into 1-inch chunks
1 large onion, chopped
4 sprigs Italian parsley
2 garlic cloves, smashed
8 black peppercorns
2 bay leaves
1 teaspoon kosher salt

1 Combine all the ingredients in a large pot. Bring just to a simmer over medium heat. Reduce the heat to low and simmer, partially covered, with bubbles gently coming to the surface in the center of the pot, 2 hours. Do not stir the stock while it cooks.

2 Place a colander in a large bowl and pour in the stock. Discard the chicken carcass, vegetables, and seasonings. Strain the stock through a fine wire mesh strainer.

3 Let stand to cool to room temperature. Cover and refrigerate until the fat rises to the top of the stock. Remove and discard the fat. Use the stock at once or refrigerate, covered, for up to 4 days or freeze for up to 6 months.

Each serving (½ cup): 1 g carb, 13 cal, 0 g fat, 0 g sat fat, 3 mg chol, 0 g fib, 2 g pro, 70 mg sod • Carb Choices: 0; Exchanges: None

SLOW-COOKER VERSION: Follow the Leftover Chicken Chicken Stock recipe, at left, using a 6-quart slow cooker. Reduce the water to 7 cups. Cook on high for 8 hours and proceed with steps 2 and 3. Makes 6 cups.

Smoked Turkey Stock

makes 6½ cups

Use this stock for cooking any dish where you want to add some smoky flavor. Try using it for cooking any kind of dried beans, lentils, split peas, or sturdy greens such as kale or mustard. You can also remove the lean meat from the turkey wings after making the stock and add it to a turkey or bean soup.

3 smoked turkey wings
12 cups water
2 large carrots, peeled and cut into 1-inch chunks
2 stalks celery, cut into 1-inch chunks
1 large onion, chopped
4 sprigs Italian parsley
2 garlic cloves, smashed
8 black peppercorns
2 bay leaves

1 Combine all the ingredients in a large pot. Bring just to a simmer over medium heat. Reduce the heat to low and simmer, partially covered, with bubbles gently coming to the surface in the center of the pot, 3 hours. Do not stir the stock while it cooks.

2 Place a colander in a large bowl and pour in the stock. Discard the turkey wings, vegetables, and seasonings. Strain the stock through a fine wire mesh strainer.

3 Let stand to cool to room temperature. Cover and refrigerate until the fat rises to the top of the stock. Remove and discard the fat. Use the stock at once or refrigerate, covered, for up to 4 days or freeze for up to 3 months.

Each serving (½ cup): 1 g carb, 13 cal, 0 g fat, 0 g sat fat, 3 mg chol, 0 g fib, 2 g pro, 112 mg sod • Carb Choices: 0; Exchanges: None

SLOW-COOKER VERSION: Follow the Smoked Turkey Stock recipe, page 150, using a 6-quart slow cooker. Reduce the water to 10 cups. Cook on high for 8 to 10 hours. Makes 8 cups.

Beef Stock

makes 10 cups

Beef stews and soups will taste richer and heartier when made with homemade stock. Browning the bones before making the stock adds a rich caramelized flavor.

4 teaspoons extra virgin olive oil, divided
4 pounds meaty beef bones
12 cups cold water
2 large carrots, peeled and cut into 1-inch chunks
2 stalks celery, cut into 1-inch chunks
1 large onion, chopped
4 sprigs Italian parsley
2 garlic cloves, smashed
8 black peppercorns
2 bay leaves
1 teaspoon kosher salt

1 Heat a large pot over medium-high heat. Add 2 teaspoons of the oil and tilt the pot to coat the bottom evenly.

2 Add half the bones and cook, turning occasionally, until well browned, about 6 minutes. Transfer to a plate. Repeat with the remaining 2 teaspoons oil and the remaining bones. Return all the bones to the pot and add the remaining ingredients.

3 Bring just to a simmer over medium heat. Reduce the heat to low and cook, partially covered, with bubbles gently coming to the surface in the center of the pot, 2 hours. Place a colander in a large bowl and pour in the stock. Discard the bones, vegetables, and seasonings. Strain the stock through a fine wire mesh strainer.

4 Let stand to cool to room temperature. Cover and refrigerate until the fat rises to the top of the stock. Remove and discard the fat. Use the stock at once or refrigerate, covered, for up to 4 days or freeze for up to 6 months.

Each serving (½ cup): 1 g carb, 13 cal, 0 g fat, 0 g sat fat, 3 mg chol, 0 g fib, 2 g pro, 70 mg sod • Carb Choices: 0; Exchanges: None

SLOW-COOKER VERSION: To make the Beef Stock in a slow cooker, prepare the recipe as directed in steps 1 and 2, placing the browned bones in a 6-quart slow cooker. Reduce the water to 10 cups and add the remaining ingredients to the slow cooker. Cook on high for 8 hours and proceed with the recipe. Makes 8 cups.

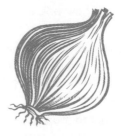

Ham Hock Stock

makes 6½ cups

If you love the slow, simmered porky flavor of Southern dishes like collard greens and black-eyed peas, but don't want the fat and calories from using ham hocks or salt pork, making those dishes with this stock gives you all the flavor without the fat. Be warned, though: this stock is quite high in sodium.

3 pounds smoked ham hocks
12 cups water
2 large carrots, peeled and cut into 1-inch chunks
2 stalks celery, cut into 1-inch chunks
1 large onion, chopped
4 sprigs Italian parsley
2 garlic cloves, smashed
8 black peppercorns
2 bay leaves
1 teaspoon kosher salt

1 Combine all the ingredients in a large pot. Bring just to a simmer over medium heat. Reduce the heat to low and simmer, partially covered, with bubbles gently coming to the surface in the center of the pot, 3 hours. Do not stir the stock while it cooks.

2 Place a colander in a large bowl and pour in the stock. Discard the ham hocks, vegetables, and seasonings. Strain the stock through a fine wire mesh strainer.

3 Let stand to cool to room temperature. Cover and refrigerate until the fat rises to the top of the stock. Remove and discard the fat. Use the stock at once or refrigerate, covered, for up to 4 days or freeze for up to 3 months.

Each serving (½ cup): 2 g carb, 15 cal, 0 g fat, 0 g sat fat, 3 mg chol, 0 g fib, 2 g pro, 105 mg sod • Carb Choices: 0; Exchanges: None

SLOW-COOKER VERSION: Follow the Ham Hock Stock recipe, at left, using a 6-quart slow cooker. Decrease the water to 10 cups and add the remaining ingredients to the slow cooker. Cook on high for 8 to 10 hours and proceed with the recipe. Makes 8 cups.

Shrimp Stock

makes 8 cups

The next time you make a shrimp dish, save the shells and make this stock. Use it anywhere you would use clam juice—in seafood soups or stews—or use as the cooking liquid when you steam clams or mussels.

Shells from 1 pound of shrimp
10 cups cold water
1 large onion, chopped
2 large carrots, peeled and cut into 1-inch chunks
2 stalks celery, cut into 1-inch chunks
4 sprigs Italian parsley
2 garlic cloves, smashed
8 black peppercorns
2 bay leaves
1 teaspoon kosher salt

1 Combine all the ingredients in a large pot. Bring just to a simmer over medium heat. Reduce the heat to low and simmer, partially covered, with bubbles gently coming to the surface in the center of the pot, 45 minutes. Do not stir the stock while it cooks.

2 Place a colander in a large bowl and pour in the stock. Discard the shells, vegetables, and seasonings. Strain the stock through a fine wire mesh strainer.

3 Let stand to cool to room temperature. Use the stock at once or refrigerate, covered, for up to 4 days or freeze for up to 3 months.

Each serving (½ cup): 1 g carb, 19 cal, 0 g fat, 0 g sat fat, 0 mg chol, 0 g fib, 2 g pro, 70 mg sod • Carb Choices: 0; Exchanges: None

Vegetable Soups

Homemade Tomato Soup QUICK

makes 6 servings

Invest a little time to make this soup and you'll wonder why you ever ate canned tomato soup. Even though it's made with canned tomatoes, the soup has pure tomato flavor without the added sugars found in canned versions. You can sprinkle each bowl of soup with a little grated Parmesan or finely shredded sharp Cheddar cheese.

2 teaspoons extra virgin olive oil
1 large onion, chopped
1 carrot, peeled and chopped
1 stalk celery, chopped
2 garlic cloves, minced
2 (28-ounce) cans no-salt-added whole
    tomatoes, undrained
1 cup water
½ teaspoon kosher salt
½ teaspoon dried oregano
½ teaspoon dried basil
¼ teaspoon dried thyme
⅛ teaspoon freshly ground pepper

1 Heat a large pot over medium heat. Add the oil and tilt the pan to coat the bottom evenly. Add the onion, carrot, and celery and cook, stirring often, until softened, 5 minutes. Add the garlic and cook, stirring constantly, until fragrant, 30 seconds.

2 Add the tomatoes with their juice and stir, breaking the tomatoes up with a spoon. Add the water, salt, oregano, basil, thyme, and pepper and bring to a boil over high heat. Cover, reduce the heat to low, and simmer until all the vegetables are very tender, 25 to 30 minutes.

3 Place the vegetable mixture in a in a food processor or blender in batches and process until smooth (add additional water a few tablespoons at a time if necessary to adjust consistency). Return the soup to the pot and reheat over medium heat.

4 Ladle the soup into 6 bowls and serve at once. The soup can be refrigerated, covered, for up to 4 days or frozen for up to 3 months.

Each serving: 13 g carb, 75 cal, 2 g fat, 0 g sat fat, 0 mg chol, 3 g fib, 5 g pro, 309 mg sod • Carb Choices: 1; Exchanges: 3 veg

TWO-TOMATO SOUP QUICK: Follow the Homemade Tomato Soup recipe, at left, adding 8 dry-packed sun-dried tomatoes, chopped, with the canned tomatoes in step 2, and proceed with the recipe.

Each serving: 14 g carb, 82 cal, 2 g fat, 0 g sat fat, 0 mg chol, 3 g fib, 5 g pro, 365 mg sod • Carb Choices: 1; Exchanges: 3 veg

TOMATO AND ROASTED RED PEPPER SOUP QUICK: Follow the Homemade Tomato Soup recipe, at left, adding 1 large red Roasted Bell Pepper (page 21) or 1 cup roasted red peppers from a jar, chopped, with the canned tomatoes in step 2, and proceed with the recipe.

Each serving: 14 g carb, 80 cal, 2 g fat, 0 g sat fat, 0 mg chol, 3 g fib, 5 g pro, 310 mg sod • Carb Choices: 1; Exchanges: 3 veg

Tomato and Fennel Soup

HIGH FIBER

makes 6 servings

Anise-flavored fennel is an ideal partner for tomatoes. This soup has a double dose, using toasted fennel seeds and a fresh fennel bulb. If your fennel bulb still has some of its feathery leaves attached, save some of those to garnish each bowl of soup.

½ teaspoon whole fennel seeds
1 large bulb fennel
2 teaspoons extra virgin olive oil
1 large onion, chopped
1 carrot, peeled and chopped
1 stalk celery, chopped
2 garlic cloves, minced
2 (28-ounce) cans no-salt-added whole
    tomatoes, undrained
1 cup water
½ teaspoon kosher salt
⅛ teaspoon freshly ground pepper

1 Place the fennel seeds in a small dry skillet over medium heat and toast, shaking the pan often, until the fennel seeds are fragrant, about 3 minutes. Transfer to a small plate and allow to cool. Place the fennel seeds in a mortar and crush with a pestle. Alternatively, place the fennel seeds in a small resealable plastic bag. Seal the bag, place on a cutting board, and crush using a meat mallet or the back of a large spoon.

2 Trim the tough outer stalks from the fennel bulb. Cut the fennel bulb in half vertically and cut away and discard the core. Chop the fennel.

3 Heat a large pot over medium heat. Add the oil and tilt the pan to coat the bottom evenly. Add the fennel bulb, onion, carrot, and celery and cook, stirring often, until softened, 5 minutes. Add the garlic and cook, stirring constantly, until fragrant, 30 seconds.

4 Add the tomatoes with their juice and stir, breaking the tomatoes up with a spoon. Add the water, fennel seeds, salt, and pepper and bring to a boil over high heat. Cover, reduce the heat to low, and simmer until all the vegetables are very tender, 25 to 30 minutes.

5 Place the vegetable mixture in a food processor or blender in batches and process until smooth (add additional water a few tablespoons at a time if necessary to adjust consistency). Return the soup to the pot and reheat over medium heat.

6 Ladle the soup into 6 bowls and serve at once. The soup can be refrigerated, covered, for up to 4 days or frozen for up to 3 months.

Each serving: 16 g carb, 87 cal, 2 g fat, 0 g sat fat, 0 mg chol, 4 g fib, 5 g pro, 329 mg sod • Carb Choices: 1; Exchanges: 3 veg

Summer Squash and Tomato Soup QUICK

makes 4 servings

This simple and delicious soup is a healthful way to use abundant summer squash. It's light, brothy, and not too filling, making it the perfect accompaniment to a summer sandwich or salad. Adding the tomato and basil after the soup has cooked keeps them fresh tasting and colorful.

2 teaspoons extra virgin olive oil

1 small onion, chopped

2 garlic cloves, minced

3½ cups Vegetable Stock (page 149) or
low-sodium vegetable broth

2 small summer squash, quartered lengthwise
and sliced

2 small zucchini, quartered lengthwise and
sliced

1 large tomato, chopped

2 tablespoons chopped fresh basil

¼ teaspoon kosher salt

⅛ teaspoon freshly ground pepper

2 tablespoons freshly grated Parmesan

1 Heat a large pot over medium-high heat. Add the oil and tilt the pan to coat the bottom evenly. Add the onion and cook, stirring often, until softened, 5 minutes. Add the garlic and cook, stirring constantly, until fragrant, 30 seconds.

2 Add the stock and bring to a boil over high heat. Add the squash and zucchini and return to a boil. Cover, reduce the heat to low, and simmer until the vegetables are tender, 6 to 8 minutes.

3 Stir in the tomato and return to a boil. Remove from the heat and stir in the basil, salt, and pepper. Ladle the soup into 4 bowls, sprinkle evenly with the Parmesan, and serve at once. The soup can be refrigerated, covered, for up to 4 days.

Each serving: 13 g carb, 89 cal, 4 g fat, 1 g sat fat, 2 mg chol, 3 g fib, 4 g pro, 325 mg sod • Carb Choices: 1; Exchanges: 2 veg

MIX-AND-MATCH CREAMY VEGETABLE SOUPS

Cook any vegetable in the chart below in a large saucepan with 3 cups low-sodium vegetable or chicken broth; 1 (8-ounce) baking potato, peeled and chopped; 1 small onion, chopped; 1 garlic clove, minced; and ½ teaspoon kosher salt until the vegetables are tender. Asparagus, broccoli, zucchini, or yellow squash will take about 10 minutes and cauliflower or fennel will take about 15 minutes.

Puree the mixture in batches in a food processor or blender. Return the soup to the saucepan and gently reheat, thinning with water if necessary. Stir in a fresh herb and 2 teaspoons lemon juice. Ladle the soup into 4 bowls and top evenly with a topping. Each serving has 1 Carb Choice (about 20 grams of carb) and about 100 calories.

Vegetable (4 cups)	Fresh Herb	Topping
Asparagus spears, tough ends trimmed, cut into 1-inch pieces	2 tablespoons chopped fresh Italian parsley	2 tablespoons thinly sliced scallions
Broccoli florets, chopped	2 tablespoons chopped fresh basil	4 tablespoons seeded chopped tomato
Cauliflower florets, chopped	2 teaspoons minced fresh tarragon	2 tablespoons plain low-fat yogurt
Fennel bulb, chopped	1 tablespoon minced fresh chives	1 tablespoon reduced-fat sour cream mixed with 1 tablespoon low-fat milk
Yellow squash, chopped	2 tablespoons chopped fresh chervil	4 tablespoons Homemade Croutons (page 144)
Zucchini, chopped	2 teaspoons minced fresh thyme	2 tablespoons low-fat buttermilk

Root Vegetable Soup HIGH FIBER

makes 6 servings

Lowly rutabagas and celery roots are turned into an earthy soup with robust flavor. Serve it to begin a fall or winter dinner or have it for lunch on a blustery winter day. A little low-fat milk stirred in at the end of cooking gives it extra creaminess.

2 teaspoons extra virgin olive oil

1 medium onion, chopped

2 garlic cloves, minced

3½ cups Vegetable Stock (page 149) or low-sodium vegetable broth

3 small celery roots (about 1 pound), peeled and chopped

1 medium rutabaga (about 1 pound), peeled and chopped

¼ teaspoon kosher salt

⅛ teaspoon freshly ground pepper

2 medium Yukon Gold or red-skinned potatoes (about 1 pound), peeled and chopped

½ cup 1% low-fat milk

Chopped fresh Italian parsley

1 Heat a large pot over medium heat. Add the oil and tilt the pan to coat the bottom evenly. Add the onion and cook, stirring often, until softened, 5 minutes. Add the garlic and cook, stirring constantly, until fragrant, 30 seconds. Add the stock, celery roots, rutabaga, salt, and pepper and bring to a boil over high heat. Cover, reduce the heat to low, and simmer 15 minutes. Add the potatoes, cover, and simmer until all the vegetables are very tender, 15 to 20 minutes longer.

2 Ladle about 2 cups of the vegetable mixture into a medium bowl and mash with a potato masher until smooth. Return the mixture to the pot. Stir in the milk and cook just until heated through, about 1 minute. Ladle the soup into 6 bowls, sprinkle with the parsley, and serve at once. The soup can be refrigerated, covered, for up to 4 days.

Each serving: 29 g carb, 144 cal, 2 g fat, 0 g sat fat, 0 mg chol, 4 g fib, 4 g pro, 277 mg sod • Carb Choices: 2; Exchanges: 1 starch, 3 veg

Roasted Vegetable Soup

HIGH FIBER

makes 8 servings

This big-batch soup is great to take to work and reheat in the microwave or to have on hand for a simple supper. Because of the potatoes, it doesn't freeze well.

2 large carrots, peeled, halved lengthwise, and sliced

2 parsnips, peeled, halved lengthwise, and sliced

1 large red-skinned potato, well scrubbed and cut into ½-inch cubes

4 teaspoons extra virgin olive oil, divided

½ teaspoon kosher salt, divided

¼ teaspoon freshly ground pepper, divided

1 large onion, chopped

1 stalk celery, chopped

1 garlic clove, minced

7 cups Vegetable Stock (page 149) or low-sodium vegetable broth

2 (14½-ounce) cans no-salt added diced tomatoes

¼ cup no-salt-added tomato paste

2 tablespoons chopped fresh Italian parsley

1 Preheat the oven to 425°F.

2 Place the carrots, parsnips, and potato on a large rimmed baking sheet. Drizzle with 2 teaspoons of the oil, and sprinkle with ¼ teaspoon of the salt and ⅛ teaspoon of the pepper. Toss to coat. Arrange the vegetables in a single layer. Bake, turning the vegetables once, until tender and browned, 35 to 40 minutes.

3 Meanwhile, heat a large pot over medium heat. Add the remaining 2 teaspoons oil and tilt the pan to coat the bottom evenly. Add the onion and celery and cook, stirring often, until softened, 5 minutes. Add the garlic and cook, stirring constantly, until fragrant, 30 seconds.

4 Add the stock, tomatoes, tomato paste, remaining ¼ teaspoon salt, and remaining ⅛ teaspoon pepper and bring to a boil over high heat. Cover, reduce the heat to low, and simmer 15 minutes. Add the roasted vegetables, cover, and simmer 10 minutes longer. Remove from the heat and stir in the parsley. Ladle into 8 bowls and serve at once. The soup can be refrigerated, covered, for up to 4 days.

Each serving: 23 g carb, 124 cal, 3 g fat, 0 g sat fat, 0 mg chol, 4 g fib, 3 g pro, 443 mg sod • Carb Choices: 1½; Exchanges: ½ starch, 3 veg

Freezing Soups

Soups are a welcome prize to keep in the freezer for when you need a quick lunch or dinner that requires absolutely no work. When you make soup, make a double batch and freeze half for meals later on. You can keep soup in the freezer for up to 3 months.

Portion soups into family- or individual-size containers (these are perfect to take to work for lunch), leaving some room in the container for the soup to expand when it freezes.

To thaw, leave the soup in the refrigerator overnight. Gently reheat in a saucepan over medium heat. If you forget to thaw in the refrigerator, you can always reheat in the microwave or add a little water or broth when you reheat the soup on the stovetop.

Always taste reheated soup before serving. You'll find most soups need an adjustment in the seasonings to brighten them up—a squeeze of lemon or lime juice or a pinch of salt will do the job.

Almost all soups freeze well. Don't freeze soups that have pasta or noodles, potatoes, or milk. Pasta and noodles become mushy when frozen, potatoes become mealy, and milk curdles.

Roasted Yellow Bell Pepper Soup

makes 6 servings

You can also serve this soup chilled. Hot or cold, its vibrant color and fresh flavor make it perfect for entertaining. It thickens after chilling, so if necessary, stir in a little cold water to adjust the consistency.

1 large leek, halved lengthwise and thinly sliced
2 teaspoons extra virgin olive oil
2 garlic cloves, minced
4 to 4½ cups Vegetable Stock (page 149) or low-sodium vegetable broth
3 large yellow Roasted Bell Peppers (page 21) or 3 cups roasted red or yellow peppers from a jar, chopped
¼ teaspoon kosher salt
⅛ teaspoon freshly ground pepper
¼ cup fresh basil leaves
1 teaspoon sherry vinegar or lemon juice
¾ cup Homemade Croutons (page 144)

1 Submerge the sliced leek in a large bowl of water, lift it out, and drain in a colander. Repeat, using fresh water, until no grit remains in the bottom of the bowl. Drain well.

2 Heat a large pot over medium heat. Add the oil and tilt the pan to coat the bottom evenly. Add the leek and cook, stirring often, until softened, 5 minutes. Add the garlic and cook, stirring constantly, until fragrant, 30 seconds.

3 Add 4 cups of the stock, the roasted peppers, salt, and ground pepper and bring to a boil over high heat. Cover, reduce the heat to low, and simmer until the vegetables are very tender, 15 to 20 minutes.

4 Place the vegetable mixture in a food processor or blender in batches, adding the basil to one of the batches, and process until smooth. Add the remaining ½ cup stock a few tablespoons at a time, if needed, to reach the desired consistency. Return the mixture to the pot and cook over medium heat until just heated through, about 1 minute. Stir in the vinegar. Ladle into 6 bowls, distribute the croutons evenly among the bowls, and serve at once. The soup can be refrigerated, covered, for up to 4 days or frozen for up to 3 months.

Each serving: 13 g carb, 77 cal, 3 g fat, 0 g sat fat, 0 mg chol, 2 g fib, 2 g pro, 265 mg sod • Carb Choices: 1; Exchanges: 2 veg

Easy Vegetable Minestrone HIGH FIBER

makes 6 servings

This homey comforting soup is a forgiving dish. You can change the vegetables depending on what is in the market or in your vegetable bin. Instead of the fennel, use a red or yellow bell pepper or add a chopped yellow squash or zucchini during the last few minutes of cooking. You can use any short whole wheat pasta that you have on hand. Use this recipe as a guide for putting together your own signature soup.

2¼ ounces whole wheat macaroni (about ¾ cup)
1 large bulb fennel
2 teaspoons extra virgin olive oil
1 medium onion, chopped
1 medium carrot, peeled and chopped
1 stalk celery, chopped
1 garlic clove, minced
8 cups Vegetable Stock (page 149) or low-sodium vegetable broth
2 cups coarsely chopped green cabbage
1 (14½-ounce) can no-salt-added diced tomatoes
1 (15-ounce) can no-salt-added red kidney beans, rinsed and drained
¼ cup no-salt-added tomato paste
1 teaspoon dried oregano
½ teaspoon kosher salt
¼ teaspoon freshly ground pepper
3 tablespoons freshly grated Parmesan

1 Cook the macaroni according to the package directions.

2 Meanwhile, trim the tough outer stalks from the fennel. Cut the fennel bulb in half vertically and cut away and discard the core. Chop the fennel.

3 Heat a large pot over medium heat. Add the oil and tilt the pan to coat the bottom evenly. Add the fennel, onion, carrot, and celery and cook, stirring often, until softened, 5 minutes. Add the garlic and cook, stirring constantly, until fragrant, 30 seconds.

4 Add the stock, cabbage, tomatoes, beans, tomato paste, oregano, salt, and pepper and bring to a boil over high heat. Cover, reduce the heat to low, and simmer, stirring occasionally, until the cabbage is almost tender, about 10 minutes. Stir in the macaroni and cook about 1 minute longer. Ladle into 6 bowls, sprinkle evenly with the Parmesan, and serve at once. The soup is best on the day it is made, but it can be refrigerated, covered, for up to 2 days.

Each serving: 37 g carb, 210 cal, 3 g fat, 1 g sat fat, 2 mg chol, 11 g fib, 10 g pro, 405 mg sod • Carb Choices: 2; Exchanges: 1½ starch, 1 veg, 1 plant-based protein

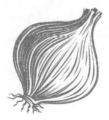

Chile-Spiced Vegetable Soup QUICK

makes 6 servings

2 teaspoons extra virgin olive oil
1 medium onion, diced
1 small red bell pepper, diced
1 small yellow bell pepper, diced
1 jalapeño, seeded and minced
2 garlic cloves, minced
1 tablespoon chili powder
2 teaspoons ground cumin
3 cups Vegetable Stock (page 149) or
**   low-sodium vegetable broth**
3 medium ears corn, kernels cut from the cob
1 large tomato, chopped
2 tablespoons lime juice
Chopped fresh cilantro

1 Heat a large pot over medium heat. Add the oil and tilt the pan to coat the bottom evenly. Add the onion, bell peppers, and jalapeño and cook, stirring often, until the vegetables are softened, 5 minutes. Add the garlic, chili powder, and cumin and cook, stirring, until fragrant, 30 seconds. Add the stock and corn and bring to a boil. Cover, reduce the heat, and simmer until the vegetables are tender, 15 minutes.

2 Remove from the heat and stir in the tomato and lime juice. Ladle into 6 bowls, sprinkle with the cilantro, and serve at once. The soup can be refrigerated, covered, for up to 4 days or frozen for up to 3 months.

Each serving: 17 g carb, 90 cal, 3 g fat, 0 g sat fat, 0 mg chol, 3 g fib, 3 g pro, 160 mg sod • Carb Choices: 1; Exchanges: ½ starch, 2 veg

CHILE-SPICED SHRIMP AND VEGETABLE SOUP: Follow the Chile-Spiced Vegetable Soup recipe, above, adding 8 ounces medium peeled deveined shrimp during the last 2 minutes of cooking.

Each serving: 17 g carb, 119 cal, 3 g fat, 0 g sat fat, 0 mg chol, 3 g fib, 9 g pro, 225 mg sod • Carb Choices: 1; Exchanges: ½ starch, 2 veg, 1 lean protein

Creamy Vegetable Chowder QUICK

makes 4 servings

This creamy soup is a delicious bowl of comfort that you can easily make from pantry ingredients. If you'd like a soup with a more rustic texture, mash the soup a few times with a potato masher to break up some of the vegetables.

2 teaspoons extra virgin olive oil
1 medium onion, chopped
1 garlic clove, minced
2 cups Vegetable Stock (page 149) or
    low-sodium vegetable broth
12 ounces turnips, peeled and chopped
2 carrots, peeled and chopped
1 stalk celery, chopped
⅛ teaspoon dried thyme
½ teaspoon kosher salt
⅛ teaspoon freshly ground pepper
1 cup 1% low-fat milk
1 tablespoon unbleached all-purpose flour
2 tablespoons chopped fresh Italian parsley

1 Heat a large pot over medium heat. Add the oil and tilt the pan to coat the bottom evenly. Add the onion and cook, stirring often, until softened, 5 minutes. Add the garlic and cook, stirring constantly, until fragrant, 30 seconds. Add the stock, turnips, carrots, celery, thyme, salt, and pepper and bring to a boil over high heat. Cover, reduce the heat to low, and simmer until the vegetables are tender, 20 minutes.

2 Whisk together the milk and flour in a small bowl. Add to the soup and return to a simmer. Cook, stirring often, just until slightly thickened, about 3 minutes. Remove from the heat and stir in the parsley. Ladle into 4 bowls and serve at once. The soup can be refrigerated, covered, for up to 4 days.

Each serving: 14 g carb, 98 cal, 3 g fat, 1 g sat fat, 2 mg chol, 3 g fib, 4 g pro, 334 mg sod • Carb Choices: 1; Exchanges: ½ carb, 1 veg, ½ fat

Pumpkin and Roasted Red Pepper Soup QUICK | HIGH FIBER

makes 6 servings

This is a delicious—and much easier—alternative to butternut squash soup. The canned pumpkin makes it a breeze to make. It's perfect for an autumn picnic, a Halloween get-together, or the Thanksgiving table. If you want to dress it up a little, swirl a tablespoon of plain low-fat yogurt into each bowl just before serving.

2 teaspoons extra virgin olive oil
3 large carrots, peeled and chopped
1 large onion, chopped
2 garlic cloves, chopped
½ teaspoon ground cumin
½ teaspoon ground coriander
5 to 5½ cups Vegetable Stock (page 149) or
    low-sodium vegetable broth
1 large red Roasted Bell Pepper (page 21)
    or 1 cup roasted red peppers from a jar,
    chopped
½ teaspoon kosher salt
¼ teaspoon freshly ground pepper
1 (15-ounce) can pumpkin (not pumpkin pie
    filling)
2 tablespoons lemon juice

1 Heat a large pot over medium heat. Add the oil and tilt the pan to coat the bottom evenly. Add the carrots and onion and cook, stirring often, until the vegetables are softened, 5 minutes. Add the garlic, cumin, and coriander and cook, stirring constantly, until fragrant, 30 seconds.

2 Add 5 cups of the stock, the roasted pepper, salt, and ground pepper and bring to a boil over high heat. Cover, reduce the heat to low, and simmer until the vegetables are very tender, 15 to 20 minutes.

3 Place the vegetable mixture in a food processor or blender in batches and process until smooth. Return the soup to the pot and stir in

the pumpkin. Add the remaining ½ cup stock a few tablespoons at a time, if needed, to reach the desired consistency. Cook over medium heat, stirring often, until heated through. Remove from the heat and stir in the lemon juice. Ladle into 6 bowls and serve at once. The soup can be refrigerated, covered, for up to 4 days or frozen for up to 3 months.

Each serving: 16 g carb, 80 cal, 2 g fat, 0 g sat fat, 0 mg chol, 4 g fib, 2 g pro, 324 mg sod • Carb Choices: 1; Exchanges: ½ starch, 2 veg

Curried Cauliflower Apple Soup QUICK

makes 6 servings

Bold curry is a perfect counterpoint to mild-tasting cauliflower in this creamy soup. An apple adds a touch of sweetness and a little half-and-half makes it rich and creamy. It makes an elegant presentation served in fancy coffee cups or teacups, but it's equally at home if you're having lunch at your desk.

2 teaspoons extra virgin olive oil
1 medium onion, chopped
2 garlic cloves, chopped
2 teaspoons curry powder
4 to 4½ cups Chicken Stock (page 149) or
     low-sodium chicken broth
6 cups 2-inch cauliflower florets
1 large apple, peeled, cored, and
     chopped
½ teaspoon kosher salt
¼ cup half-and-half
2 teaspoons lemon juice
6 tablespoons plain low-fat yogurt

1 Heat a large pot over medium heat. Add the oil and tilt the pan to coat the bottom evenly. Add the onion and cook, stirring often, until softened, 5 minutes. Add the garlic and curry powder and cook, stirring constantly, until fragrant, 30 seconds.

2 Add 4 cups of the stock, the cauliflower, apple, and salt and bring to a boil over high heat. Cover, reduce the heat to low, and simmer until the cauliflower is very tender, about 15 minutes.

3 Place the cauliflower mixture in a food processor or blender in batches and process until smooth. Return the soup to the pot and stir in the half-and-half. Add the remaining ½ cup stock a few tablespoons at a time, if needed, to reach the desired consistency. Cook over medium heat, stirring often, until heated through. Remove from the heat and stir in the lemon juice. Ladle into 6 bowls and serve at once. Top each serving with 1 tablespoon of the yogurt. The soup can be refrigerated, covered, for up to 4 days.

Each serving: 13 g carb, 98 cal, 4 g fat, 1 g sat fat, 8 mg chol, 3 g fib, 5 g pro, 127 mg sod • Carb Choices: 1; Exchanges: 2 veg, ½ fat

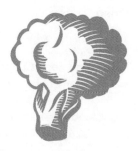

Garden Pea Soup with Dill QUICK | HIGH FIBER

makes 4 servings

You can serve this soup hot or chilled. If you serve it chilled, it's a nice touch to top each bowl with a spoonful of plain low-fat yogurt or cottage cheese. It's excellent when made with fresh peas, and almost as delicious when made with the frozen variety.

2 teaspoons extra virgin olive oil
1 medium onion, chopped
1 garlic clove, minced
2 to 2½ cups water
1 (16-ounce) package frozen green peas or
    3¼ cups shelled fresh peas
¾ teaspoon kosher salt
2 tablespoons chopped fresh dill
1 tablespoon lemon juice

1 Heat a large pot over medium heat. Add the oil and tilt the pan to coat the bottom evenly. Add the onion and cook, stirring often, until the onion is softened, 5 minutes. Add the garlic and cook, stirring constantly, until fragrant, 30 seconds.

2 Add 2 cups of the water, the peas, and salt and bring to a boil over high heat. Cover, reduce the heat to low, and simmer until the peas are tender, 5 minutes. Place the vegetable mixture in a food processor or blender in batches, adding the dill to one of the batches, and process until smooth.

3 Return the soup to the pot and add the remaining ½ cup water a few tablespoons at a time, if needed, to reach the desired consistency. Cook over medium heat, stirring often, until heated through. Remove from the heat and stir in the lemon juice. Ladle into 4 bowls and serve at once. Alternatively, let the soup stand at room temperature until cool. Cover and refrigerate until chilled, at least 4 hours or overnight. The soup can be refrigerated, covered, for up to 4 days or frozen for up to 3 months.

Each serving: 18 g carb, 116 cal, 3 g fat, 0 g sat fat, 0 mg chol, 6 g fib, 6 g pro, 291 mg sod • Carb Choices: 1; Exchanges: 1 starch, 1 veg

Beet Soup with Fennel and Apple HIGH FIBER

makes 6 servings

I make a batch of this soup in the fall when my community-supported agriculture share gives me more beets than I know what to do with. It's a slightly sweet soup that is offset with a splash of red wine vinegar stirred in at the end of cooking. You can serve the soup chilled, too. It thickens when refrigerated, so you may need to stir in a little cold water to adjust the consistency before serving.

1 medium bulb fennel
2 teaspoons extra virgin olive oil
1 medium onion, chopped
1 carrot, peeled and chopped
2 garlic cloves, minced
4 to 4½ cups Vegetable Stock (page 149) or
    low-sodium vegetable broth
1 pound beets, peeled and cubed
1 large apple, peeled, cored, and chopped
½ teaspoon kosher salt
1 tablespoon red wine vinegar
6 tablespoons plain low-fat yogurt
Chopped fresh dill

1 Trim the tough outer stalks from the fennel. Cut the fennel bulb in half vertically and cut away and discard the core. Chop the fennel.

2 Heat a large pot over medium heat. Add the oil and tilt the pan to coat the bottom evenly. Add the fennel, onion, and carrot and cook, stirring often, until softened, 5 minutes. Add the garlic and cook, stirring constantly, until fragrant,

30 seconds. Add 4 cups of the stock, the beets, apple, and salt and bring to a boil over high heat. Cover, reduce the heat to low, and simmer until the vegetables are very tender, 30 to 35 minutes.

3 Place the vegetable mixture in a food processor or blender in batches and process until smooth. Return the soup to the pot and reheat over medium heat. Add the remaining ½ cup stock a few tablespoons at a time, if needed, to reach the desired consistency. Stir in the vinegar. Ladle the soup into 6 bowls, top evenly with the yogurt and dill, and serve at once. The soup can be refrigerated, covered, for up to 4 days or frozen for up to 3 months.

Each serving: 18 g carb, 93 cal, 2 g fat, 0 g sat fat, 1 mg chol, 4 g fib, 3 g pro, 332 mg sod • Carb Choices: 1; Exchanges: ½ carb, 2 veg

Potato-Leek Soup QUICK

makes 6 servings

Incredibly simple, delicious, and comforting—the perfect soup. This pureed version is silky and elegant, but for a chunkier version, skip the food processor and mash the soup slightly with a potato masher.

2 medium leeks, halved lengthwise and thinly sliced

2 teaspoons extra virgin olive oil

1½ pounds Yukon Gold or baking potatoes, peeled and cubed

3½ to 4 cups Chicken Stock (page 149) or low-sodium chicken broth

½ teaspoon kosher salt

½ teaspoon freshly ground pepper

2 tablespoons minced fresh chives (optional)

1 Submerge the sliced leeks in a large bowl of water, lift them out, and drain in a colander. Repeat, using fresh water, until no grit remains in the bottom of the bowl. Drain the leeks well.

2 Heat a large pot over medium heat. Add the oil and tilt the pan to coat the bottom evenly. Add the leeks and cook, stirring often, until softened, 5 minutes. Add the potatoes, 3½ cups of the stock, the salt, and pepper and bring to a boil over high heat. Cover, reduce the heat to low, and simmer until the potatoes are very tender, 15 to 20 minutes.

3 Place the potato mixture in a food processor in batches and pulse just until smooth (do not overprocess). Return the soup to the pot and reheat over medium heat. Add the remaining ½ cup stock a few tablespoons at a time, if needed, to reach the desired consistency. Ladle the soup into 6 bowls, sprinkle evenly with the chives, if using, and serve at once. The soup can be refrigerated, covered, for up to 4 days.

Each serving: 24 g carb, 131 cal, 2 g fat, 1 g sat fat, 3 mg chol, 2 g fib, 5 g pro, 185 mg sod • Carb Choices: 1½; Exchanges: 1½ starch

Sweet Potato–Apple Soup QUICK

makes 6 servings

This is a wonderful starter to Thanksgiving dinner. To dress the soup up for entertaining, thin about ¼ cup of plain low-fat yogurt with a couple teaspoons of low-fat milk and drizzle evenly into each bowl of soup. You can also add a sprinkle of chopped cilantro.

2 teaspoons extra virgin olive oil
1 medium onion, chopped
2 garlic cloves, minced
2½ to 2¾ cups Vegetable Stock (page 149) or low-sodium vegetable broth
1 cup unsweetened apple juice
1½ pounds sweet potatoes, peeled and chopped
½ to 1 teaspoon minced chipotle in adobo sauce
½ teaspoon kosher salt
2 tablespoons lime juice

1 Heat a large saucepan over medium heat. Add the oil and tilt the pan to coat the bottom evenly. Add the onion and cook, stirring often, until softened, 5 minutes. Add the garlic and cook, stirring constantly, until fragrant, 30 seconds. Add 2½ cups of the stock, the apple juice, potatoes, chipotle, and salt and bring to a boil over high heat. Cover, reduce the heat to low, and simmer until the potato is very tender, 15 to 20 minutes.

2 Place the potato mixture in a food processor in batches and process until smooth. Return the soup to the pot reheat over medium heat. Add the remaining ¼ cup stock a few tablespoons at a time, if needed, to reach the desired consistency. Remove from the heat and stir in the lime juice. Ladle the soup into 6 bowls and serve at once. The soup can be refrigerated, covered, for up to 4 days.

Each serving: 23 g carb, 114 cal, 2 g fat, 0 g sat fat, 0 mg chol, 3 g fib, 2 g pro, 247 mg sod • Carb Choices: 1½; Exchanges: 1 starch, ½ carb

Carrot-Ginger Soup QUICK

makes 4 servings

This may seem like a lot of ginger, but the flavor of the ginger in the finished soup is mild. If you can't get your kids to eat carrots, try this soup.

2 teaspoons extra virgin olive oil
1 small onion, chopped
2 garlic cloves, chopped
1 pound carrots, peeled and cut into 1-inch slices
3 to 3½ cups Vegetable Stock (page 149) or low-sodium vegetable broth
1 tablespoon grated fresh ginger
¼ teaspoon kosher salt
2 tablespoons lime juice

1 Heat a large pot over medium heat. Add the oil and tilt the pan to coat the bottom evenly. Add the onion and cook, stirring often, until softened, 5 minutes. Add the garlic and cook, stirring constantly, until fragrant, 30 seconds. Add the carrots, 3 cups of the stock, the ginger, and salt and bring to a boil over high heat. Cover, reduce the heat to low, and simmer until the carrots are very tender, 15 to 20 minutes.

2 Place the carrot mixture in a food processor or blender in batches and process until smooth. Return the soup to the pot and reheat over medium heat. Add the remaining ½ cup stock a few tablespoons at a time, if needed, to reach the desired consistency. Stir in the lime juice. Ladle the soup into 4 bowls and serve at once. The soup can be refrigerated, covered, for up to 4 days or frozen for up to 3 months.

Each serving: 15 g carb, 81 cal, 3 g fat, 0 g sat fat, 0 mg chol, 3 g fib, 1 g pro, 321 mg sod • Carb Choices: 1; Exchanges: 3 veg

Orange-Carrot Soup QUICK

makes 4 servings

Packed with vitamins, this soup will surely ward off a winter cold, or cure the one you catch. I make a double batch of this soup and freeze it in small containers to reheat for an instant and satisfying lunch.

2 teaspoons extra virgin olive oil

1 small onion, chopped

2 garlic cloves, chopped

1 pound carrots, peeled and cut into 1-inch slices

2 to 2½ cups Vegetable Stock (page 149) or low-sodium vegetable broth

1 cup orange juice

¼ teaspoon kosher salt

2 tablespoons lime juice

2 teaspoons grated orange zest

1 Heat a large pot over medium heat. Add the oil and tilt the pan to coat the bottom evenly. Add the onion and cook, stirring often, until softened, 5 minutes. Add the garlic and cook, stirring constantly, until fragrant, 30 seconds. Add the carrots, 2 cups of the stock, the orange juice, and salt and bring to a boil over high heat. Cover, reduce the heat to low, and simmer until the carrots are very tender, 15 to 20 minutes.

2 Place the carrot mixture in a food processor or blender in batches and process until smooth. Return the soup to the pot and reheat over medium heat. Add the remaining ½ cup stock a few tablespoons at a time, if needed, to reach the desired consistency. Stir in the lime juice and orange zest. Ladle the soup into 4 bowls and serve at once. The soup can be refrigerated, covered, for up to 4 days or frozen for up to 3 months.

Each serving: 20 g carb, 106 cal, 3 g fat, 0 g sat fat, 0 mg chol, 3 g fib, 2 g pro, 261 mg sod • Carb Choices: 1; Exchanges: ½ fruit, 3 veg

Butternut Squash Soup HIGH FIBER

makes 6 servings

2 teaspoons extra virgin olive oil

1 medium onion, chopped

2 carrots, peeled and chopped

2 garlic cloves, minced

1 medium butternut squash, peeled, seeded, and chopped (about 5 cups)

3 to 3½ cups Vegetable Stock (page 149) or low-sodium vegetable broth

1 teaspoon kosher salt

1 tablespoon lemon juice

1 Heat a large pot over medium heat. Add the oil and tilt the pan to coat the bottom evenly. Add the onion and carrots and cook, stirring often, until softened, 5 minutes. Add the garlic and cook, stirring constantly, until fragrant, 30 seconds. Add the squash, 3 cups of the stock, and the salt and bring to a boil over high heat. Cover, reduce the heat to low, and simmer until the squash is very tender, 15 to 20 minutes.

2 Place the squash mixture in a food processor or blender in batches and process until smooth. Return the soup to the pot and reheat gently over medium heat. Add the remaining ½ cup stock a few tablespoons at a time, if needed, to reach the desired consistency. Stir in the lemon juice. Ladle the soup into 6 bowls and serve at once. The soup can be refrigerated, covered, for up to 4 days or frozen for up to 3 months.

Each serving: 21 g carb, 95 cal, 2 g fat, 0 g sat fat, 0 mg chol, 4 g fib, 2 g pro, 329 mg sod • Carb Choices: 1½; Exchanges: 1 starch, ½ fruit, 1 veg

BUTTERNUT SQUASH–PEAR SOUP HIGH FIBER: Follow the Butternut Squash Soup recipe, above, adding 2 Bartlett pears, peeled, cored, and chopped, with the squash in step 1.

Each serving: 29 g carb, 128 cal, 2 g fat, 0 g sat fat, 0 mg chol, 4 g fib, 2 g pro, 330 mg sod • Carb Choices: 2; Exchanges: 1 starch, ½ fruit, 1 veg

Butternut Squash Soup with Red Curry and Coconut

makes 6 servings

This is one of my favorite soups for fall and winter. None of the flavors shout at you—there's a hint of ginger, coconut, and curry and they all blend together perfectly in this silky soup. You can make a double batch and freeze the soup for later use. When you reheat it, add another squeeze of fresh lime juice to brighten the flavors.

2 teaspoons extra virgin olive oil

1 medium onion, chopped

2 garlic cloves, minced

1 medium butternut squash, peeled, seeded, and chopped (about 5 cups)

2½ to 3 cups Vegetable Stock (page 149) or low-sodium vegetable broth

½ teaspoon kosher salt

1 teaspoon red curry paste

⅓ cup reduced-fat coconut milk

2 teaspoons lime juice

1 Heat a large saucepan over medium heat. Add the oil and tilt the pan to coat the bottom evenly. Add the onion and cook, stirring often, until softened, 5 minutes. Add the garlic and cook, stirring constantly, until fragrant, 30 seconds. Add the squash, 2½ cups of the stock, and salt and bring to a boil over high heat. Cover, reduce the heat to low, and simmer until the squash is very tender, 15 to 20 minutes.

2 Place the squash mixture in a food processor or blender in batches, adding the curry paste to one of the batches, and process until smooth. Return the soup to the pot, stir in the coconut milk, and reheat gently over medium heat. Stir in the lime juice. Ladle the soup into 6 bowls and serve at once. The soup can be refrigerated, covered, for up to 4 days or frozen for up to 3 months.

Each serving: 19 g carb, 110 cal, 4 g fat, 3 g sat fat, 0 mg chol, 3 g fib, 2 g pro, 216 mg sod • Carb Choices: 1; Exchanges: 1 starch, 1 veg

Celery–Celery Root Soup QUICK

makes 6 servings

If you're never sure what to make with celery root, this soup is a delicious use for it. The elegant silky soup belies the gnarly vegetable it is made from.

2 teaspoons extra virgin olive oil

1 medium onion, chopped

2 stalks celery, including some green leaves, chopped

2 garlic cloves, chopped

2 medium celery roots, peeled and chopped (about 6 cups)

1 medium baking potato, peeled and chopped

4½ to 5 cups Vegetable Stock (page 149) or low-sodium vegetable broth

¾ teaspoons kosher salt

2 teaspoons lemon juice

Chopped fresh chives or dill

1 Heat a large pot over medium heat. Add the oil and tilt the pan to coat the bottom evenly. Add the onion and celery and cook, stirring often, until softened, 5 minutes. Add the garlic and cook, stirring constantly, until fragrant, 30 seconds. Add the celery roots, potato, 4½ cups of the stock, and salt and bring to a boil over high heat. Cover, reduce the heat to low, and simmer until the vegetables are very tender, 25 to 30 minutes.

2 Place the celery root mixture in a food processor or blender in batches and process until smooth. Return the soup to the pot and reheat gently over medium heat. Add the remaining ½ cup stock a few tablespoons at a time, if needed, to reach the desired consistency. Stir in the lemon juice. Ladle the soup into 6 bowls, sprinkle evenly with the chives, and serve at once. The soup can be refrigerated, covered, for up to 4 days.

Each serving: 22 g carb, 127 cal, 2 g fat, 1 g sat fat, 4 mg chol, 3 g fib, 6 g pro, 388 mg sod • Carb Choices: 1½; Exchanges: ½ starch, 3 veg

Parsnip-Pear Soup

QUICK | HIGH FIBER

makes 6 servings

Sweet pears play off the assertively flavored parsnips to make an ideal balance of tastes in this elegant soup. As a garnish, drizzle each bowl with a few drops of extra virgin olive oil or a toasted nut oil such as walnut or hazelnut.

2 teaspoons extra virgin olive oil
1 medium onion, chopped
2 stalks celery, chopped
2 garlic cloves, chopped
4 large parsnips, peeled and cut into 1-inch
  pieces (about 3½ cups)
2 large ripe Bartlett pears, peeled, cored,
  and chopped
4 cups Chicken Stock (page 149) or
  low-sodium chicken broth
¾ teaspoon kosher salt
½ to ¾ cup 1% low-fat milk

1 Heat a large pot over medium heat. Add the oil and tilt the pan to coat the bottom evenly. Add the onion and celery and cook, stirring often, until softened, 5 minutes. Add the garlic and cook, stirring constantly, until fragrant, 30 seconds. Add the parsnips, pears, stock, and salt and bring to a boil over high heat. Cover, reduce the heat to low, and simmer until the parsnips are very tender, 20 to 25 minutes.

2 Place the parsnip mixture in a food processor or blender in batches and process until smooth. Return the soup to the pot, stir in ½ cup of the milk, and reheat gently over medium heat (do not boil). Add the remaining ¼ cup milk a tablespoon at a time, if needed, to reach the desired consistency. Ladle the soup into 6 bowls and serve at once. The soup can be refrigerated, covered, for up to 4 days.

Each serving: 24 g carb, 130 cal, 2 g fat, 1 g sat fat, 4 mg chol, 4 g fib, 5 g pro, 261 mg sod • Carb Choices: 1½; Exchanges: ½ fruit, 3 veg

Spinach Stracciatella QUICK

makes 4 servings

This classic Italian soup featuring eggs and spinach is rich and flavorful. Using Parmigiano-Reggiano in this soup permeates the stock with flavor. With a salad and a slice of crusty bread, it's a delicious meal that feels more special than the work it involves. To easily get the egg into the soup in a slow steady stream, place it in a resealable plastic bag and snip a tiny corner off the bag. Then, hold the bag over the soup and let the egg empty into the pot while you stir the soup.

4 cups Chicken Stock (page 149) or
  low-sodium chicken broth
1 small garlic clove, crushed through a press
½ teaspoon kosher salt
1 large egg, lightly beaten
2 cups thinly sliced fresh spinach
1 ounce freshly grated Parmigiano-Reggiano
  (about ¼ cup)
2 teaspoons lemon juice
Pinch of freshly ground pepper

1 Combine the stock, garlic, and salt in a medium pot and bring to a boil over high heat.

2 Slowly drizzle the egg into the stock mixture, stirring constantly. Turn off the heat and stir in the spinach, Parmigiano-Reggiano, lemon juice, and pepper. Ladle the soup into 4 bowls and serve at once. The soup is best when eaten immediately.

Each serving: 2 g carb, 70 cal, 3 g fat, 2 g sat fat, 62 mg chol, 0 g fib, 8 g pro, 386 mg sod • Carb Choices: 0; Exchanges: ½ lean protein

French Onion Soup with Gruyère Croutons

makes 6 servings

Slowly caramelizing the onions and using two flavorful cheeses are what make this soup wonderful.

1 tablespoon extra virgin olive oil
2 pounds onions, halved lengthwise and thinly sliced
2 garlic cloves, minced
¼ teaspoon kosher salt
2 teaspoons unbleached all-purpose flour
5 cups Beef Stock (page 151) or low-sodium beef broth
½ cup dry red wine
1 sprig fresh thyme
1 bay leaf
¼ teaspoon freshly ground pepper
6 (½-inch) baguette slices, cut on the diagonal, toasted
3 ounces shredded Gruyère or Swiss cheese (about ¾ cup)
3 tablespoons freshly grated Parmesan

1 Heat a large pot over medium heat. Add the oil and tilt the pan to coat the bottom evenly. Add the onions, garlic, and salt and cook, stirring occasionally, until the onions are very soft and lightly browned, 35 to 40 minutes.

2 Sprinkle the onion mixture with the flour and cook, stirring constantly, 2 minutes. Slowly stir in the stock. Add the wine, thyme, bay leaf, and pepper and bring to a boil over high heat. Cover, reduce the heat to low, and simmer 20 minutes.

3 Preheat the broiler.

4 Remove and discard the thyme sprig and bay leaf. Ladle the soup into 6 eight-ounce ovenproof bowls. Sprinkle the baguette slices evenly with the Gruyère, then with the Parmesan. Place one slice on top of each bowl of soup.

5 Arrange the bowls on a large baking sheet and broil until the cheese melts, about 2 minutes. Serve at once. The soup (without the croutons) can be refrigerated, covered, for up to 4 days or frozen for up to 3 months.

Each serving: 26 g carb, 238 cal, 9 g fat, 4 g sat fat, 22 mg chol, 3 g fib, 10 g pro, 590 mg sod • Carb Choices: 2; Exchanges: 1 carb, 2 veg

Hot-and-Sour Soup QUICK

makes 4 servings

I love this soup for lunch and I add or substitute ingredients depending on what's in the refrigerator. Try adding some diced yellow squash or zucchini, snow peas, or cubes of firm tofu. If you have cooked soba noodles or brown rice, add those for a heartier soup.

4 cups Chicken Stock (page 149) or low-sodium chicken broth
½ teaspoon grated fresh ginger
½ teaspoon sugar
4 ounces shiitake mushrooms, stemmed and thinly sliced
2 cups chopped fresh spinach
3 tablespoons reduced-sodium soy sauce
2 tablespoons rice vinegar
1 teaspoon cornstarch
½ to 1 teaspoon chili-garlic paste
¼ teaspoon Asian sesame oil
¼ cup thinly sliced scallions
2 tablespoons chopped fresh cilantro

1 Combine the stock, ginger, and sugar in a large pot and bring to a boil over high heat. Add the mushrooms and return to a boil. Cover, reduce the heat to low, and simmer until the mushrooms are tender, about 8 minutes.

2 Stir in the spinach and cook just until wilted, about 1 minute.

3 Stir together the soy sauce, vinegar, and cornstarch in a small dish. Add the soy sauce mixture to the soup and cook just until slightly thickened,

about 1 minute longer. Remove from the heat and stir in the chili-garlic paste and the oil. Ladle the soup into 4 bowls and sprinkle evenly with the scallions and cilantro. The soup is best when eaten immediately.

Each serving: 5 g carb, 51 cal, 1 g fat, 1 g sat fat, 5 mg chol, 1 g fib, 6 g pro, 609 mg sod • Carb Choices: 0; Exchanges: None

Miso-Vegetable Soup QUICK

makes 6 servings

Light and nourishing, this soup is full of healthful vegetables. You can omit the chili-garlic paste if you prefer a mild soup. Don't boil the soup after adding the miso as it diminishes the aroma and changes the delicate flavor.

2 teaspoons canola oil
2 tablespoons minced fresh ginger
2 garlic cloves, minced
6 cups water
6 ounces shiitake mushrooms, stemmed and thinly sliced
4 ounces snow peas, trimmed and thinly sliced
2 medium carrots, peeled, cut in half lengthwise, and thinly sliced
⅓ cup white miso paste
½ teaspoon chili-garlic paste
½ teaspoon Asian sesame oil
Thinly sliced scallions
Chopped fresh cilantro

1 Heat a large pot over medium heat. Add the canola oil and tilt the pan to coat the bottom evenly. Add the ginger and garlic and cook, stirring constantly, until fragrant, 30 seconds. Add the water and bring to a boil.

2 Add the mushrooms, snow peas, and carrots and return to a boil. Reduce the heat to low and simmer until the vegetables are crisp-tender, about 5 minutes. Ladle about 1 cup of the broth from the soup into a small bowl. Add the miso paste and whisk until the miso dissolves. Stir the miso mixture, chili-garlic paste, and sesame oil into

the soup. Ladle the soup into 6 bowls, top each serving with the scallions and cilantro, and serve at once. The soup is best when eaten immediately.

Each serving: 8 g carb, 66 cal, 2 g fat, 0 g sat fat, 0 mg chol, 2 g fib, 3 g pro, 685 mg sod • Carb Choices: ½; Exchanges: ½ carb

Egg Drop Soup QUICK

makes 4 servings

I had never made egg drop soup until I was developing this recipe. I made it for lunch for the next three days in a row. It's so easy—and so much better than the egg drop soup at the Chinese takeout places in my neighborhood (and probably yours). You can vary this soup in many ways: add cooked noodles, shredded chicken or pork, or baby spinach.

4 cups Chicken Stock (page 149) or low-sodium chicken broth
2 tablespoons reduced-sodium soy sauce
1 (1-inch) piece fresh ginger, thinly sliced
2 garlic cloves, peeled and smashed
2 tablespoons water
2 teaspoons cornstarch
2 large eggs, lightly beaten
2 cups thinly sliced fresh spinach
1 scallion, thinly sliced
¼ teaspoon Asian sesame oil

1 Combine the stock, soy sauce, ginger, and garlic in a large pot and bring to a boil over high heat. Cover, reduce the heat to low, and simmer 5 minutes. Remove and discard the ginger and garlic using a slotted spoon.

2 Stir together the water and cornstarch in a small dish. Add the cornstarch mixture to the stock mixture, stirring constantly. Slowly drizzle the eggs into the stock, stirring constantly. Turn off the heat and stir in the spinach, scallion, and oil. Ladle the soup into 4 bowls and serve at once. The soup is best when eaten immediately.

Each serving: 4 g carb, 77 cal, 3 g fat, 1 g sat fat, 111 mg chol, 0 g fib, 8 g pro, 490 mg sod • Carb Choices: 0; Exchanges: ½ lean protein

Bean Soups

Black Bean Soup   HIGH FIBER

makes 8 servings

This slow-cooking soup tastes authentic—and it is. It starts with dried beans, stock, and a few simple seasonings and then simmers on the stove for a long time. The wait is worth it.

2 teaspoons canola oil
1 large onion, chopped
1 large green bell pepper, chopped
4 garlic cloves, minced
1½ tablespoons ground cumin
2 teaspoons kosher salt
1 teaspoon dried oregano
8 cups Ham Hock Stock (page 152), Smoked Turkey Stock (page 150), or low-sodium chicken broth
1 pound dried black beans, picked over and rinsed
3 tablespoons lime juice
Chopped fresh cilantro, thinly sliced scallions, lime wedges

1 Heat a large pot over medium-high heat. Add the oil and tilt the pot to coat the bottom evenly. Add the onion and bell pepper and cook, stirring often, until the vegetables are softened, 5 minutes. Stir in the garlic, cumin, salt, and oregano and cook, stirring constantly, until fragrant, 30 seconds.

2 Add the stock and beans and bring to a boil over high heat. Cover, reduce the heat to low, and simmer until the beans are tender, 1½ hours. For a thicker soup, transfer 2 cups of the soup to a food processor or blender and process until smooth. Return to the pot and stir in the lime juice. Serve the soup with the cilantro, scallions, and lime wedges. The soup can be refrigerated, covered, for up to 4 days or frozen for up to 3 months.

Each serving: 37 g carb, 215 cal, 2 g fat, 0 g sat fat, 2 mg chol, 13 g fib, 13 g pro, 865 mg sod • Carb Choices: 2; Exchanges: 2 starch, 2 plant-based protein

Quick Black Bean Soup

QUICK | HIGH FIBER

makes 8 servings

When you've no time for cooking bean soup from scratch, this one is full of flavor, satisfying, and best of all, ready in about half an hour. Ancho chile powder is made from ground dried poblano peppers. It has a mild fruity flavor, but you can use regular chili powder.

2 teaspoons canola oil
1 medium onion, chopped
1 small green bell pepper, chopped
2 garlic cloves, minced
1 tablespoon ancho chile powder
2 teaspoons ground coriander
2 teaspoons ground cumin
¼ teaspoon freshly ground pepper
4 cups Chicken Stock (page 149) or low-sodium chicken broth
4 (15-ounce) cans no-salt-added black beans, rinsed and drained
1 (14½-ounce) can no-salt-added diced tomatoes
2 tablespoons lime juice
Chopped fresh cilantro

1 Heat a large pot over medium-high heat. Add the oil and tilt the pot to coat the bottom evenly. Add the onion and bell pepper and cook, stirring often, until the vegetables are softened, 5 minutes. Stir in the garlic, chile powder, coriander, cumin, and ground pepper and cook, stirring constantly, until fragrant, 30 seconds.

2 Add the stock, beans, and tomatoes and bring to a boil over high heat. Cover, reduce the heat to low, and simmer until the vegetables are very tender, about 15 minutes.

3 Transfer 2 cups of the soup to a food processor or blender and process until smooth. Return the soup to the pot. Remove from the heat and stir in the lime juice. Ladle the soup into 8 bowls, sprinkle evenly with the cilantro, and serve at

once. The soup can be refrigerated, covered, for up to 4 days or frozen for up to 3 months.

Each serving: 37 g carb, 244 cal, 4 g fat, 0 g sat fat, 3 mg chol, 12 g fib, 15 g pro, 305 mg sod • Carb Choices: 2; Exchanges: 2 starch, 2 plant-based protein

BLACK BEAN SOUP WITH CHORIZO QUICK HIGH FIBER: Follow the Quick Black Bean Soup recipe, at left, but remove the casings from 4 ounces cured chorizo. Chop the chorizo and cook with the onion and bell pepper in step 1. Proceed with the recipe.

Each serving: 37 g carb, 288 cal, 7 g fat, 2 g sat fat, 12 mg chol, 12 g fib, 17 g pro, 466 mg sod • Carb Choices: 2; Exchanges: 2 starch, ½ high-fat protein, 2 plant-based protein

Pinto Bean Soup HIGH FIBER

makes 8 servings

I grew up with this soup served at least once a week for supper with a crusty pan of cornbread. Nothing could be simpler than this comforting soup. If you prefer not to use the Ham Hock Stock, use Smoked Turkey Stock (page 150), Chicken Stock (page 149), or low-sodium chicken broth. You will need to add 1 teaspoon kosher salt with the beans and broth at the beginning of cooking if you are using anything except the Ham Hock Stock.

1 pound dried pinto beans, picked over and rinsed

8 cups Ham Hock Stock (page 152)

1 Combine the beans and stock in a large pot and bring to a boil over high heat. Cover, reduce the heat to low, and simmer until the beans are tender, about 1 hour 15 minutes.

2 Ladle about 2 cups of the bean mixture into a medium bowl and mash with a potato masher until smooth. Return the beans to the pot. Simmer until the soup is slightly thickened, 15 minutes longer. The soup can be refrigerated, covered, for up to 4 days or frozen for up to 3 months.

Each serving: 35 g carb, 196 cal, 1 g fat, 0 g sat fat, 2 mg chol, 12 g fib, 13 g pro, 581 mg sod • Carb Choices: 2; Exchanges: 2 starch, 2 plant-based protein

Bean and Butternut Squash Mole Soup HIGH FIBER

makes 6 servings

2 teaspoons extra virgin olive oil
1 large onion, chopped
1 large red bell pepper, chopped
2 garlic cloves, minced
2 tablespoons chili powder
2 tablespoons ground cumin
1½ cups Chicken Stock (page 149) or low-sodium chicken broth
1 cup brewed coffee
1 (14½-ounce) can no-salt-added diced tomatoes, undrained
1 (15-ounce) can no-salt-added pinto beans, rinsed and drained
1½ cups chopped butternut squash
2 tablespoons no-salt-added tomato paste
2 tablespoons unsweetened cocoa
½ teaspoon dried oregano
½ teaspoon kosher salt
1 tablespoon lime juice
1 tablespoon honey
¼ cup chopped fresh cilantro

1 Heat a large pot over medium-high heat. Add the oil and tilt the pot to coat the bottom evenly. Add the onion and bell pepper and cook, stirring, until the vegetables are softened, 5 minutes. Stir in the garlic, chili powder, and cumin and cook, stirring until fragrant, 30 seconds.

2 Add the stock, coffee, tomatoes, beans, squash, tomato paste, cocoa, oregano, and salt and bring to a boil. Cover, and simmer until the vegetables are tender, 20 to 25 minutes. Stir in the lime juice and honey. Ladle the soup into 6 bowls and sprinkle evenly with the cilantro. The soup can be refrigerated, covered, for up to 4 days or frozen for up to 3 months.

Each serving: 26 g carb, 151 cal, 3 g fat, 1 g sat fat, 1 mg chol, 7 g fib, 7 g pro, 230 mg sod • Carb Choices: 1½; Exchanges: 1 starch, 2 veg, 1 plant-based protein

Black-eyed Pea and Greens Soup HIGH FIBER

makes 12 servings

Eating black-eyed peas and greens on New Year's Day is a Southern tradition that is said to bring good luck for the coming year. This hearty soup gives you both in one delicious dish.

1 pound dried black-eyed peas, picked over and rinsed

8 cups Ham Hock Stock (page 152), Smoked Turkey Stock (page 150), or low-sodium chicken broth

2 cups water

1 pound fresh collards, kale, or mustard greens, tough stems removed and leaves chopped (about 6 cups)

2 (14½-ounce) cans no-salt-added diced tomatoes

2 stalks celery, diced

1 large onion, chopped

3 dried ancho chiles, seeded and chopped, or ⅛ teaspoon ground cayenne

2 garlic cloves, minced

1 Combine the peas, stock, and water in a large pot and bring to a boil over high heat. (If you are not using Ham Hock Stock, add 1 teaspoon kosher salt.) Cover, reduce the heat to low, and simmer 30 minutes.

2 Meanwhile, submerge the collards in a large bowl of cold water, lift them out, and drain in a colander. Repeat, using fresh water, until no grit remains in the bottom of the bowl. Add the greens and the remaining ingredients to the pot, cover, and simmer until the peas and greens are tender, 30 minutes longer. Ladle the soup into bowls and serve at once. The soup can be refrigerated, covered, for up to 4 days or frozen for up to 3 months.

Each serving: 29 g carb, 165 cal, 1 g fat, 0 g sat fat, 1 mg chol, 9 g fib, 10 g pro, 428 mg sod • Carb Choices: 1½; Exchanges: 1½ starch, 1 veg, 1½ plant-based protein

White Bean Soup

makes 8 servings

It doesn't take much to make a terrific bean soup as you'll see if you try this one. Made from inexpensive pantry staples, it is a winter mainstay.

3 strips center-cut bacon

2 stalks celery, chopped

2 carrots, peeled and chopped

1 large onion, chopped

2 cloves, minced

8 cups Chicken Stock (page 149) or low-sodium chicken broth

1 pound dried cannellini beans or navy beans, picked over and rinsed

1 Cook the bacon in a large pot over medium-high heat until crisp. Drain on paper towels. Drain off and discard all but 2 teaspoons of the bacon drippings. Add the celery, carrots, and onion to the bacon drippings and cook, stirring often, until the vegetables are softened, 5 minutes. Add the garlic and cook, stirring constantly, until fragrant, 30 seconds.

2 Add the stock and beans and bring to a boil over high heat. Finely chop the bacon and add to the soup. Cover, reduce the heat to low, and simmer until the beans are tender, about 1 hour. Ladle the soup into 8 bowls and serve at once. The soup can be refrigerated, covered, for up to 4 days or frozen for up to 3 months.

Each serving: 35 g carb, 219 cal, 2 g fat, 1 g sat fat, 7 mg chol, 11 g fib, 17 g pro, 212 mg sod • Carb Choices: 2; Exchanges: 2 starch, 2 plant-based protein

WHITE BEAN AND ESCAROLE SOUP HIGH FIBER: Follow the White Bean Soup recipe, above, adding 4 cups chopped escarole to the soup during the last 15 minutes of cooking time.

Each serving: 35 g carb, 218 cal, 2 g fat, 1 g sat fat, 7 mg chol, 11 g fib, 17 g pro, 212 mg sod • Carb Choices: 2; Exchanges: 2 starch, 2 plant-based protein

White Bean and Roasted Tomato Soup HIGH FIBER

makes 8 servings

Fresh tomatoes, roasted until they're sweet and caramelized, and a sprinkle of Italian spices elevate white bean soup to something beyond the ordinary. It's a great standby for casual winter entertaining. Add a crisp green salad and crusty rolls and the meal is ready. This soup actually tastes better if you make it a day ahead.

8 plum tomatoes, halved lengthwise

4 teaspoons extra virgin olive oil, divided

¾ teaspoon kosher salt, divided

¼ teaspoon freshly ground pepper

2 stalks celery, chopped

2 carrots, peeled and chopped

1 large onion, chopped

2 garlic cloves, minced

8 cups Chicken Stock (page 149) or low-sodium chicken broth

1 pound dried cannellini beans or navy beans, picked over and rinsed

1 teaspoon dried basil

1 teaspoon dried oregano

1 Preheat the oven to 400°F.

2 Place the tomatoes on a large rimmed baking sheet. Drizzle with 2 teaspoons of the oil and sprinkle with ¼ teaspoon of the salt and ⅛ teaspoon of the pepper and turn to coat. Arrange the tomatoes skin side down in a single layer. Bake until the tomatoes are soft and the bottoms are well browned, 40 to 45 minutes. Let the tomatoes stand until cool enough to handle. Coarsely chop the tomatoes.

3 Meanwhile, heat a large pot over medium-high heat. Add the remaining 2 teaspoons oil and tilt the pot to coat the bottom evenly. Add the celery, carrots, and onion and cook, stirring often, until the vegetables are softened, 5 minutes. Add the garlic and cook, stirring constantly, until fragrant, 30 seconds.

4 Add the stock, beans, basil, oregano, remaining ½ teaspoon salt, and remaining ⅛ teaspoon pepper and bring to a boil over high heat. Cover, reduce the heat to low, and simmer until the beans are tender, about 1 hour. Stir in the tomatoes and cook until heated through, about 2 minutes. Ladle the soup into 8 bowls and serve at once. The soup can be refrigerated, covered, for up to 4 days or frozen for up to 3 months.

Each serving: 31 g carb, 240 cal, 4 g fat, 1 g sat fat, 5 mg chol, 11 g fib, 17 g pro, 272 mg sod • Carb Choices: 2; Exchanges: 2 starch, 2 plant-based protein, ½ fat

Two-Bean Minestrone

HIGH FIBER

makes 8 servings

Any minestrone recipe is just an outline for using what you have in your pantry. Substitute any kind of canned beans for the garbanzo beans, use fresh tomatoes instead of the canned ones, and use any kind of fresh quick-cooking greens for the spinach.

2¼ ounces whole wheat macaroni (about ¾ cup)

2 teaspoons extra virgin olive oil

2 carrots, peeled and chopped

1 stalk celery, chopped

1 medium onion, chopped

2 garlic cloves, minced

6 cups Vegetable Stock (page 149) or low-sodium vegetable broth

1 (14½-ounce) can no-salt-added diced tomatoes

¼ cup no-salt-added tomato paste

½ teaspoon kosher salt

1 teaspoon dried basil

½ teaspoon dried oregano

¼ teaspoon freshly ground pepper

1 (15-ounce) can no-salt-added garbanzo beans, rinsed and drained

1 cup frozen shelled edamame or frozen baby lima beans

1 medium zucchini, cut in half lengthwise and sliced

4 cups chopped fresh spinach

4 tablespoons freshly grated Parmesan

1 Cook the macaroni according to the package directions.

2 Meanwhile, heat a large pot over medium heat. Add the oil and tilt the pot to coat the bottom evenly. Add the carrots, celery, and onion and cook, stirring often, until the vegetables are softened, 5 minutes. Stir in the garlic and cook, stirring constantly, until fragrant, 30 seconds.

3 Add the stock, tomatoes, tomato paste, salt, basil, oregano, and pepper and bring to a boil over high heat. Cover, reduce the heat to low, and simmer until the vegetables are tender, about 20 minutes.

4 Add the garbanzo beans, edamame, and zucchini and cook until the zucchini is crisp-tender, about 5 minutes. Turn off the heat and stir in the spinach and macaroni. Ladle the soup into 8 bowls, sprinkle evenly with the Parmesan, and serve at once. The soup is best on the day it is made, but it can be refrigerated, covered, for up to 2 days.

Each serving: 29 g carb, 180 cal, 3 g fat, 1 g sat fat, 2 mg chol, 6 g fib, 9 g pro, 367 mg sod • Carb Choices: 2; Exchanges: 1 starch, ½ carb, 1 veg, 1 plant-based protein

Curried Lentil Soup   HIGH FIBER

makes 8 servings

Lentils cook quickly and they're one of the very best sources of fiber. This soup makes an easy satisfying weeknight dinner and makes enough for leftovers to take for lunch the next day.

2 teaspoons canola oil

2 large carrots, peeled and chopped

1 medium onion, chopped

1 medium red bell pepper, chopped

2 garlic cloves, minced

2 tablespoons curry powder

7 cups Vegetable Stock (page 149) or low-sodium vegetable broth

1½ cups dried brown lentils, picked over and rinsed

1 (14½-ounce) can no-salt-added diced tomatoes

½ teaspoon kosher salt

4 cups thinly sliced fresh spinach

4 tablespoons plain low-fat yogurt

1 Heat a large pot over medium heat. Add the oil and tilt the pot to coat the bottom evenly. Add the carrots, onion, and bell pepper and cook, stirring often, until the vegetables are

softened, 5 minutes. Stir in the garlic and curry powder and cook, stirring constantly, until fragrant, 30 seconds.

2 Add the stock, lentils, tomatoes, and salt and bring to a boil over high heat. Cover, reduce the heat to low, and simmer until the lentils are tender, about 30 minutes. Stir in the spinach and cook just until wilted, 2 minutes. Ladle the soup into 8 bowls, top evenly with the yogurt, and serve at once. The soup can be refrigerated, covered, for up to 4 days or frozen for up to 3 months.

Each serving: 29 g carb, 194 cal, 2 g fat, 1 g sat fat, 5 mg chol, 11 g fib, 15 g pro, 245 mg sod • Carb Choices: 1½; Exchanges: 1 starch, 1 veg, 2 plant-based protein

Split Pea Soup HIGH FIBER

makes 8 servings

Most people think split peas take hours to cook, but they're ready in about 45 minutes. When you've got a little extra time on a weeknight, make this simple soup. There's enough for leftovers for later in the week when all you have time to do is reheat something. If you prefer a chunky soup, skip the pureeing step.

2 teaspoons extra virgin olive oil

2 carrots, peeled and chopped

2 stalks celery, chopped

1 medium onion, diced

2 garlic cloves, minced

8 cups Chicken Stock (page 149), Ham Hock Stock (page 152), or low-sodium chicken broth

1 pound dried green split peas, picked over and rinsed

1 bay leaf

¾ teaspoon kosher salt

¼ teaspoon freshly ground pepper

1 Heat a large pot over medium-high heat. Add the oil and tilt the pot to coat the bottom evenly. Add the carrots, celery, and onion and cook, stirring often, until the vegetables are softened,

5 minutes. Stir in the garlic and cook, stirring constantly, until fragrant, 30 seconds.

2 Add the stock, peas, bay leaf, salt, and pepper and bring to a boil over high heat. Cover, reduce the heat to low, and simmer until the peas are very tender, about 45 minutes. Remove and discard the bay leaf.

3 Transfer the soup in batches to a food processor or blender and process until smooth. Return the soup to the pot and reheat over medium heat. The soup can be refrigerated, covered, for up to 4 days or frozen for up to 3 months.

Each serving: 34 g carb, 216 cal, 2 g fat, 1 g sat fat, 5 mg chol, 13 g fib, 16 g pro, 269 mg sod • Carb Choices: 2; Exchanges: 2 starch, 2 plant-based protein

Slow-Cooker Split Pea Soup HIGH FIBER

makes 8 servings

When I know it's going to be one of those days when I have no energy left to make dinner, I assemble these few ingredients in a slow cooker in the morning. When I come home, a fragrant, hearty, comforting soup is waiting for me. This is the simplest recipe ever—but so delicious.

6 cups Chicken Stock (page 149) or low-sodium chicken broth

1 pound dried green split peas, picked over and rinsed

2 carrots, peeled and shredded

2 stalks celery, diced

1 large onion, diced

½ teaspoon kosher salt

¼ teaspoon freshly ground pepper

Combine all the ingredients in a 4-quart slow cooker. Cover and cook on low for 8 hours. The soup can be refrigerated, covered, for up to 4 days or frozen for up to 3 months.

Each serving: 27 g carb, 199 cal, 1 g fat, 0 g sat fat, 4 mg chol, 12 g fib, 15 g pro, 197 mg sod • Carb Choices: 2; Exchanges: 2 starch, 2 plant-based protein

Italian Split Pea Soup [HIGH FIBER]

makes 10 servings

This is a gussied-up split pea soup—definitely not for a split pea soup purist. The fennel, tomatoes, and peppers add great depth of flavor, and once the soup is pureed, the red vegetables turn the soup a lovely terra-cotta color.

1 medium bulb fennel
1 tablespoon extra virgin olive oil
1 medium onion, chopped
1 carrot, peeled and chopped
1 stalk celery, chopped
2 garlic cloves, minced
8 cups Chicken Stock (page 149) or
    low-sodium chicken broth
1 pound dried green split peas, picked over
    and rinsed
1 (14½-ounce) can no-salt-added diced tomatoes
1 large red Roasted Bell Pepper (page 21), or
    1 cup roasted red peppers from a jar, chopped
6 dry-packed sun-dried tomatoes, chopped
1 teaspoon dried oregano
½ teaspoon kosher salt
1 teaspoon red wine vinegar

1 Trim the tough outer stalks from the fennel bulb. Cut the bulb in half vertically and discard the core. Chop the fennel.

2 Heat a large pot over medium-high heat. Add the oil and tilt the pot to coat the bottom evenly. Add the onion, carrot, and celery and cook, stirring often, until the vegetables are softened, 5 minutes. Add the garlic and cook, stirring constantly, until fragrant, 30 seconds.

3 Add the stock, peas, diced tomatoes, roasted pepper, sun-dried tomatoes, oregano, and salt and bring to a boil over high heat. Cover, reduce the heat to low, and simmer until the peas and vegetables are very tender, 45 minutes to 1 hour. Add more water or chicken stock, if necessary, during cooking.

4 Transfer the soup to a food processor or blender in batches and process until smooth. Return the soup to the pot and reheat over medium heat. Stir in the vinegar. The soup can be refrigerated, covered, for up to 4 days or frozen for up to 3 months.

Each serving: 31 g carb, 197 cal, 2 g fat, 2 g sat fat, 4 mg chol, 11 g fib, 14 g pro, 232 mg sod • Carb Choices: 2; Exchanges: 2 starch, 2 plant-based protein

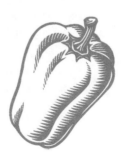

Chicken and Turkey Soups

Classic Chicken Noodle Soup

makes 8 servings

This is traditional chicken soup like your grand-mother used to make. It's easy, but takes quite a lot of time. You can prepare the chicken and broth up to 2 days ahead if you wish.

CHICKEN AND BROTH

1 (4-pound) whole chicken

6 cups cold water

1 large onion, chopped

2 large carrots, peeled and cut in 1-inch chunks

2 stalks celery, cut in 1 inch chunks

4 sprigs Italian parsley

2 garlic cloves, smashed

8 black peppercorns

2 bay leaves

1 teaspoon kosher salt

SOUP

5 cups water

2 stalks celery, chopped

2 large carrots, peeled and chopped

1 medium onion, chopped

8 ounces medium whole wheat egg noodles

¼ cup chopped fresh Italian parsley

1 To make the chicken and broth, remove and discard the giblets and the neck from the chicken. Place the chicken in a large pot. Add the water and remaining ingredients. Bring just to a simmer over medium heat. Reduce the heat to low and simmer, uncovered, with bubbles gently coming to the surface in the center of the pot, 45 minutes. Remove the chicken from the pot and let stand to cool. Remove the meat from the bones and cut into bite-size pieces. Discard the skin and bones. Cover and refrigerate the chicken until you are ready to make the soup.

2 Place a colander in a large bowl and pour in the chicken cooking broth. Discard the vegetables and seasonings. Strain the stock through a fine wire mesh strainer. Let stand to cool to room temperature. Cover and refrigerate until the fat rises to the top of the stock. Remove and discard the fat.

3 To make the soup, combine the prepared broth, the water, celery, carrots, and onion in a large pot and bring to a boil over high heat. Cover, reduce the heat, and simmer until the vegetables are tender, 15 to 20 minutes. Add the cooked chicken and simmer until heated through, about 3 minutes.

4 Meanwhile, cook the egg noodles according to the package directions.

5 Add the noodles and parsley to the soup. Ladle the soup into 8 bowls and serve at once. The soup is best on the day it is made.

Each serving: 23 g carb, 253 cal, 5 g fat, 1 g sat fat, 103 mg chol, 3 g fib, 29 g pro, 261 mg sod • Carb Choices: 1½; Exchanges: 1 starch, 1 veg, 3 lean protein

Quick and Easy Chicken Noodle Soup QUICK | HIGH FIBER

makes 6 servings

Quick-cooking boneless skinless chicken breasts and canned chicken broth make a soup that tastes like it took hours to make. I always like to cook the noodles in a separate pot from the soup, even when I'm in a hurry. Cooking them separately ensures that the broth of the soup will not be cloudy.

4 (4-ounce) boneless skinless chicken breasts
½ teaspoon kosher salt, divided
¼ teaspoon freshly ground pepper, divided
2 teaspoons extra virgin olive oil
8 cups Chicken Stock (page 149) or
    low-sodium chicken broth
2 stalks celery, chopped
2 large carrots, peeled and chopped
1 large onion, chopped
8 ounces medium whole wheat egg noodles
¼ cup chopped fresh Italian parsley

1 Sprinkle the chicken with ¼ teaspoon of the salt and ⅛ teaspoon of the pepper.

2 Heat a skillet over medium heat. Add the oil and tilt the pan to coat the bottom evenly. Add the chicken and cook, turning once, until the juices run clear, about 4 minutes on each side. Transfer the chicken to a cutting board and coarsely chop.

3 Meanwhile, combine the stock, celery, carrots, onion, remaining ¼ teaspoon salt, and remaining ⅛ teaspoon pepper in a large pot and bring to a boil over high heat. Cover, reduce the heat to low, and simmer until the vegetables are tender, 15 to 20 minutes.

4 At the same time, cook the egg noodles according to the package directions.

5 Add the chicken and the noodles to the soup and cook just until heated through, about 1 minute. Stir in the parsley. Ladle the soup into 6 bowls and serve at once. The soup is best on the day it is made.

Each serving: 31 g carb, 270 cal, 6 g fat, 2 g sat fat, 73 mg chol, 4 g fib, 24 g pro, 350 mg sod • Carb Choices: 2; Exchanges: 1½ starch, 1 veg, 2 lean protein

Lemony Chicken Soup with Orzo and Spinach

QUICK | HIGH FIBER

makes 4 servings

When you crave chicken soup but don't feel like all the work involved, this soup is a delicious and quick substitute for the slow-simmered version. The spinach and lemon give the soup vibrant flavor and color to brighten any winter day.

½ cup whole wheat orzo
2 teaspoons extra virgin olive oil
12 ounces boneless skinless chicken breast, cut
    into ½-inch cubes
1 stalk celery, chopped
1 carrot, peeled and chopped
1 small onion, chopped
1 garlic clove, minced
3½ cups Chicken Stock (page 149) or low-
    sodium chicken broth
¼ teaspoon kosher salt
4 cups chopped fresh spinach
1 teaspoon grated lemon zest
1 tablespoon lemon juice
⅛ teaspoon freshly ground pepper

1 Cook the orzo according to the package directions. Set aside.

2 Meanwhile, heat a large saucepan over medium heat. Add the oil and tilt the pan to coat the bottom evenly. Add the chicken, celery, carrot, and

onion and cook, stirring often, until the vegetables are softened, 5 minutes. Add the garlic and cook, stirring constantly, until fragrant, 30 seconds.

3 Add the stock and salt and bring to a boil over high heat. Cover, reduce the heat to low, and simmer until the vegetables are tender, 15 minutes. Stir in the orzo and spinach and cook just until the spinach wilts, about 1 minute. Remove from the heat and stir in the lemon zest, lemon juice, and pepper. Ladle into 4 bowls and serve at once. The soup is best on the day it is made.

Each serving: 20 g carb, 235 cal, 5 g fat, 1 g sat fat, 55 mg chol, 5 g fib, 26 g pro, 278 mg sod • Carb Choices: 1; Exchanges: 1 starch, 1 veg, 3 lean protein, ½ fat

Spring Chicken Soup with Potatoes and Asparagus QUICK

makes 6 servings

On a chilly spring day when the first fresh asparagus appears in the market, this is a comforting soup to serve. If dill is not to your liking, substitute chopped fresh basil or parsley.

4 medium leeks, halved lengthwise and thinly sliced

2 teaspoons extra virgin olive oil

6 cups Chicken Stock (page 149) or low-sodium chicken broth

12 ounces boneless skinless chicken breast, cut into ½-inch cubes

8 ounces baby red-skinned potatoes, well scrubbed and thinly sliced

1 medium carrot, peeled and diced

½ teaspoon kosher salt

⅛ teaspoon freshly ground pepper

8 ounces asparagus, tough ends removed and spears cut into 1-inch pieces

2 tablespoons lemon juice

1 tablespoon chopped fresh dill

1 Submerge the sliced leeks in a large bowl of water, lift them out, and drain in a colander. Repeat, using fresh water, until no grit remains in the bottom of the bowl. Drain well.

2 Heat a large saucepan over medium heat. Add the oil and tilt the pan to coat the bottom evenly. Add the leeks and cook, stirring often, until softened, 8 minutes.

3 Add the stock, chicken, potatoes, carrot, salt, and pepper and bring to a boil over high heat. Cover, reduce the heat to low, and simmer until the potatoes are almost tender, about 5 minutes. Add the asparagus and cook until crisp-tender, 3 minutes longer. Remove from the heat and stir in the lemon juice and dill. Ladle into 6 bowls and serve at once. The soup is best on the day it is made.

Each serving: 19 g carb, 186 cal, 4 g fat, 1 g sat fat, 39 mg chol, 3 g fib, 19 g pro, 284 mg sod • Carb Choices: 1; Exchanges: ½ starch, 2 veg, 2 lean protein

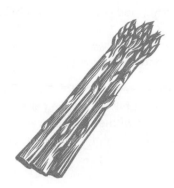

Chicken Tortilla Soup QUICK

makes 6 servings

Lightly spicy and filled with hearty chicken and vegetables, this is a weeknight meal even the kids will eat. Serve it with cornbread muffins and a green salad dressed with Cilantro-Lime Vinaigrette (page 139). If you don't have cooked chicken on hand, cut 1 pound of boneless skinless chicken breasts into cubes and add them with the stock in step 3.

3 (6-inch) corn tortillas, cut in half, then into thin strips

½ teaspoon plus 1 tablespoon chili powder, divided

2 teaspoons canola oil

1 large onion, diced

1 green bell pepper, diced

1 jalapeño, seeded and minced

2 garlic cloves, minced

1 tablespoon ground cumin

3 cups Chicken Stock (page 149) or low-sodium chicken broth

1 (14½ ounce) can no-salt-added diced tomatoes

1 (10-ounce) package frozen corn

½ teaspoon kosher salt

12 ounces chopped cooked chicken breast (about 2 cups)

2 tablespoons lime juice

½ cup chopped fresh cilantro

1 Preheat the oven to 350°F. Place the tortilla strips on a large rimmed baking sheet, sprinkle with ½ teaspoon of the chili powder, and toss to coat. Bake until lightly browned and crisp, 10 minutes.

2 Meanwhile, heat a large saucepan over medium-high heat. Add the oil and tilt the pan to coat the bottom evenly. Add the onion, bell pepper, and jalapeño and cook, stirring often, until the vegetables are softened, 5 minutes. Stir in the garlic, the remaining 1 tablespoon chili powder, and the cumin and cook, stirring constantly, until fragrant, 30 seconds.

3 Stir in the stock, tomatoes, and corn and bring to a boil over high heat. Cover, reduce the heat to low, and simmer until the vegetables are tender, 15 to 20 minutes. Stir in the chicken and cook until heated through. Remove from the heat and stir in the lime juice and cilantro. Ladle into 6 bowls, top evenly with the tortilla strips, and serve at once. The soup (without the tortilla strips) can be refrigerated, covered, for up to 4 days or frozen for up to 3 months.

Each serving: 25 g carb, 225 cal, 4 g fat, 1 g sat fat, 51 mg chol, 3 g fib, 23 g pro, 272 mg sod • Carb Choices: 1½; Exchanges: 1 starch, 2 veg, 2½ lean protein

Coconut Curry Chicken Soup

makes 4 servings

Using curry paste from a jar is an easy way to make authentic-tasting Thai dishes. This simple version of coconut chicken soup tastes as good as the soup in most Thai restaurants, and it's quick and easy to make at home. To my taste, a tablespoon of curry is just right in this soup. If you love spicy foods, add more to your taste, or add a minced jalapeño and some of its seeds with the ginger in step 1.

2 teaspoons canola oil

2 tablespoons minced fresh ginger

2½ cups Chicken Stock (page 149) or low-sodium chicken broth

1 (13½-ounce) can reduced-fat coconut milk

1 tablespoon red curry paste

12 ounces chopped cooked chicken breast (about 2 cups)

1 cup thinly sliced white mushrooms

1 cup snow peas, trimmed and halved

2 tablespoons lime juice

2 cups hot cooked brown basmati rice (page 108)

¼ cup chopped fresh cilantro

1 Heat a large pot over medium heat. Add the oil and tilt the pan to coat the bottom evenly. Add the ginger and cook, stirring constantly, until fragrant, 30 seconds. Add the stock, coconut milk, and curry paste and bring to a boil over high heat.

2 Add the chicken and mushrooms and return to a boil. Cover, reduce the heat to low, and simmer until the mushrooms are tender, about 8 minutes. Add the peas and cook until crisp-tender, about 3 minutes. Remove from the heat and stir in the lime juice.

3 Spoon ½ cup of the rice into each of 4 bowls and ladle the soup over the rice. Sprinkle evenly with the cilantro and serve at once. The soup is best on the day it is made.

Each serving: 17 g carb, 225 cal, 8 g fat, 4 g sat fat, 50 mg chol, 1 g fib, 22 g pro, 165 mg sod • Carb Choices: 1; Exchanges: 1 starch, 2½ lean protein, 1 fat

Italian Turkey Sausage and White Bean Soup

QUICK | HIGH FIBER

makes 8 servings

Italian turkey sausage, tomatoes, and fresh escarole dress up ordinary canned beans to make a hearty winter soup. The spicy Italian sausage infuses every bite with robust flavor.

2 teaspoons extra virgin olive oil

12 ounces hot Italian turkey sausage

2 carrots, peeled and diced

1 large onion, diced

1 stalk celery, diced

2 garlic cloves, minced

3½ cups Chicken Stock (page 149) or low-sodium chicken broth

3 (15-ounce) cans no-salt-added cannellini beans, rinsed and drained

2 (14½-ounce) cans no-salt-added diced tomatoes

½ teaspoon dried thyme

¼ teaspoon freshly ground pepper

4 cups chopped escarole

1 Heat a large pot over medium heat. Add the oil and tilt the pan to coat the bottom evenly. Remove and discard the sausage casings, crumble the sausage, and add to the pot. Add the carrots, onion, and celery, and cook, stirring often, until the vegetables are softened, 5 minutes. Add the garlic and cook, stirring constantly, until fragrant, 30 seconds.

2 Stir in the stock, beans, tomatoes, thyme, and pepper and bring to a boil over high heat. Cover, reduce the heat to low, and simmer until the vegetables are almost tender, about 10 minutes. Stir in the escarole and cook until tender, about 10 minutes. Ladle into 8 bowls and serve at once. The soup can be refrigerated, covered, for up to 4 days or frozen for up to 3 months.

Each serving: 35 g carb, 277 cal, 7 g fat, 0 g sat fat, 28 mg chol, 13 g fib, 17 g pro, 452 mg sod • Carb Choices: 2; Exchanges: 1½ starch, 1 veg, 1 medium-fat protein, 1 plant-based protein

Turkey, Shiitake Mushroom, and Rice Soup

makes 6 servings

2 teaspoons extra virgin olive oil

8 ounces shiitake mushrooms, stemmed and thinly sliced

2 carrots, peeled and chopped

2 stalks celery, chopped

1 medium onion, chopped

2 garlic cloves, minced

6 cups Chicken Stock (page 149) or low-sodium chicken broth

12 ounces chopped cooked turkey breast

1 bay leaf

1 sprig fresh thyme or ¼ teaspoon dried thyme

½ teaspoon kosher salt

¼ teaspoon freshly ground pepper

1¼ cups cooked brown rice (page 108)

1 Heat a large pot over medium-high heat. Add the oil and tilt the pan to coat the bottom evenly. Add the mushrooms, carrots, celery, and onion and cook, stirring often, until the vegetables are softened and most of the liquid has evaporated, 8 minutes. Stir in the garlic and cook, stirring constantly, until fragrant, 30 seconds.

2 Add the stock, turkey, bay leaf, thyme, remaining ½ teaspoon salt, and pepper and bring to a boil over high heat. Cover, reduce the heat, and simmer until the vegetables are tender, 15 to 20 minutes. Remove and discard the bay leaf and thyme sprig. Stir in the rice and cook until heated through. Ladle the soup into 6 bowls and serve at once. The soup can be refrigerated, covered, for up to 4 days.

Each serving: 19 g carb, 221 cal, 5 g fat, 1 g sat fat, 53 mg chol, 2 g fib, 24 g pro, 455 mg sod • Carb Choices: 1; Exchanges: 1 starch, 1 veg, 2½ lean protein

Spicy Turkey and Black Bean Soup QUICK | HIGH FIBER

makes 8 servings

The satisfying spicy flavor of this soup belies how easy it is to make. You can make the soup with lean ground beef or ground skinless chicken instead of the turkey.

2 teaspoons extra virgin olive oil

1 pound ground skinless turkey breast

1 medium onion, chopped

1 red bell pepper, chopped

1 green bell pepper, chopped

2 garlic cloves, minced

2 teaspoons ground cumin

6 cups Chicken Stock (page 149) or low-sodium chicken broth

2 (15-ounce) cans no-salt-added black beans, rinsed and drained

1 (14½-ounce) can no-salt-added diced tomatoes

¼ cup no-salt-added tomato paste

2 teaspoons minced chipotle in adobo sauce

2 tablespoons lime juice

¼ cup chopped fresh cilantro

1 Heat a large pot over medium heat. Add the oil and tilt the pan to coat the bottom evenly. Add the turkey, onion, and bell peppers and cook, stirring often, until the vegetables are softened, 5 minutes. Add the garlic and cumin and cook, stirring constantly, until fragrant, 30 seconds.

2 Add the stock, beans, tomatoes, tomato paste, and chipotle and bring to a boil over high heat. Cover, reduce the heat to low, and simmer until the vegetables are tender, about 15 minutes. Remove from the heat and stir in the lime juice. Ladle into 8 bowls, sprinkle evenly with the cilantro, and serve at once. The soup can be refrigerated, covered, for up to 4 days or frozen for up to 3 months.

Each serving: 23 g carb, 215 cal, 3 g fat, 1 g sat fat, 26 mg chol, 7 g fib, 24 g pro, 259 mg sod • Carb Choices: 1; Exchanges: 1 starch, 1 veg, 2½ lean protein, 1 plant-based protein

Meaty Soups

Vegetable Beef Soup

HIGH FIBER

makes 6 servings

Typically made with beef stew meat that requires long, slow simmering, this quick version of everyone's favorite soup uses tender sirloin. If you'd like to make the broth a little thicker, stir in a couple of tablespoons of no-salt-added tomato paste when you add the stock.

1 pound top sirloin steak, trimmed of all visible fat and cut into ½-inch cubes

¾ teaspoon kosher salt, divided

¼ teaspoon freshly ground pepper, divided

4 teaspoons extra virgin olive oil, divided

4 cups Beef Stock (page 151) or low-sodium beef broth

1 (14½-ounce) can no-salt-added diced tomatoes

2 carrots, peeled and chopped

1 medium onion, chopped

1 stalk celery, chopped

8 ounces red-skinned potatoes, well scrubbed and cut into ½-inch cubes

1 cup 1-inch pieces green beans

½ cup fresh or frozen corn kernels, thawed

½ cup shelled fresh English peas or frozen petite green peas, thawed

¼ cup chopped fresh Italian parsley

1 Sprinkle the steak with ¼ teaspoon of the salt and ⅛ teaspoon of the pepper. Heat a large pot over medium-high heat. Add 2 teaspoons of the oil and tilt the pot to coat the bottom evenly.

2 Add half of the steak and cook, stirring often, until well-browned, about 6 minutes. Transfer to a plate. Repeat with the remaining 2 teaspoons oil and the remaining steak.

3 Add the steak, stock, tomatoes, carrots, onion, celery, remaining ½ teaspoon salt, and remaining ⅛ teaspoon pepper and bring to a boil over high heat. Cover, reduce the heat to low, and simmer 15 minutes. Add the potatoes and cook until the potatoes are almost tender, about 8 minutes. Add the green beans and cook 5 minutes longer. Stir in the corn and peas and cook until heated through, 3 minutes. Remove from the heat and stir in the parsley. Ladle into 6 bowls and serve at once. The soup can be refrigerated, covered, for up to 4 days.

Each serving: 18 g carb, 216 cal, 7 g fat, 2 g sat fat, 31 mg chol, 4 g fib, 21 g pro, 316 mg sod • Carb Choices: 1; Exchanges: 1 starch, 1 veg, 2½ lean protein, ½ fat

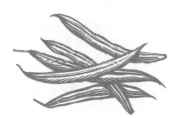

Beef Barley Soup with Mushrooms HIGH FIBER

makes 6 servings

Using tender flank steak makes this classic soup quick to make. Just be sure not to simmer the soup too long after you add the steak or it will become tough.

1½ cups water

½ cup pearl barley

¾ teaspoon kosher salt, divided

12 ounces flank steak, trimmed and cut into ½-inch cubes

⅛ teaspoon freshly ground pepper

4 teaspoons extra virgin olive oil, divided

1 pound cremini mushrooms, sliced

2 carrots, peeled and chopped

1 medium onion, chopped

2 garlic cloves, minced

6 cups Beef Stock (page 151) or low-sodium beef broth

1 bay leaf

1 Combine the water, barley, and ¼ teaspoon of the salt in a medium saucepan and bring to a boil over high heat. Reduce the heat to low, cover, and simmer until the barley is tender, yet firm to the bite, 25 to 30 minutes. Drain and rinse under cold running water.

2 Meanwhile, sprinkle the steak with the remaining ½ teaspoon salt and the pepper. Heat a large pot over medium-high heat. Add 2 teaspoons of the oil and tilt the pot to coat the bottom evenly. Add the steak and cook, stirring often, until well browned on all sides, 3 to 4 minutes. Transfer to a plate.

3 Add the remaining 2 teaspoons oil to the pot and tilt to coat evenly. Add the mushrooms, carrots, and onion and cook, stirring often, until the vegetables are softened and most of the liquid has evaporated, 8 minutes. Add the garlic and cook, stirring constantly, until fragrant, 30 seconds.

4 Add the stock and bay leaf and bring to a boil over high heat. Cover, reduce the heat to low, and simmer until the vegetables are tender, 15 minutes. Remove and discard the bay leaf. Stir in the beef and barley and cook just until heated through, 2 to 3 minutes. Ladle into 6 bowls and serve at once. The soup can be refrigerated, covered, for up to 4 days.

Each serving: 20 g carb, 214 cal, 7 g fat, 2 g sat fat, 22 mg chol, 4 g fib, 17 g pro, 307 mg sod • Carb Choices: 1; Exchanges: 1 starch, 1 veg, 2 lean protein, ½ fat

Italian Meatball Soup HIGH FIBER

makes 4 servings

This soup is a hearty and satisfying one dish meal. The meatballs do take a little time to make and shape, but if you portion the meat using a tablespoon measure, the task goes quickly.

4 teaspoons extra virgin olive oil, divided

12 ounces 95% lean ground beef

3 tablespoons plain dry breadcrumbs

2 tablespoons chopped fresh basil or Italian parsley

1 large egg white

1 garlic clove, minced

½ teaspoon kosher salt, divided

½ teaspoon freshly ground pepper, divided

1 medium onion, chopped

1 carrot, peeled and chopped

1 stalk celery, thinly sliced

3 cups Chicken Stock (page 149) or low-sodium chicken broth

1 (14½-ounce) can no-salt-added diced tomatoes

2 tablespoons no-salt-added tomato paste

½ teaspoon dried oregano

2 cups coarsely chopped escarole

2 tablespoons freshly grated Parmesan

1 Preheat the oven to 400°F. Brush a large rimmed baking sheet with 2 teaspoons of the oil.

2 Combine the beef, breadcrumbs, basil, egg white, garlic, ¼ teaspoon of the salt, and ¼ teaspoon of the pepper in a large bowl and mix well with your hands. Shape the mixture into ½-inch meatballs, using about 1 tablespoon of the mixture for each one. Place the meatballs on the prepared pan and bake until lightly browned, 20 to 25 minutes.

3 Meanwhile, heat a large pot over medium heat. Add the remaining 2 teaspoons oil and tilt the pan to coat the bottom evenly. Add the onion, carrot, and celery and cook, stirring often, until softened, 5 minutes. Add the stock, tomatoes, tomato paste, oregano, remaining ¼ teaspoon salt, and remaining ¼ teaspoon pepper and bring to a boil over high heat.

4 Cover, reduce the heat to low, and simmer, stirring occasionally, until the vegetables are almost tender, about 5 minutes. Stir in the escarole and simmer until tender, about 5 minutes longer. Carefully add the meatballs and simmer 1 to 2 minutes longer. Ladle into 4 bowls, sprinkle evenly with the Parmesan, and serve at once. The soup can be refrigerated, covered, for up to 4 days.

Each serving: 16 g carb, 254 cal, 10 g fat, 3 g sat fat, 55 mg chol, 4 g fib, 24 g pro, 456 mg sod • Carb Choices: 1; Exchanges: 2 veg, 2 lean protein, 1 fat

Lemon-Mint Meatball Soup

makes 8 servings

This is no ho-hum meatball soup. A handful of fresh mint and a generous sprinkling of lemon zest make this an extraordinarily flavorful soup. Moisten your hands with water before you make the meatballs and it will be easier to shape them. Instead of chard, you can use spinach or escarole in this recipe.

4 teaspoons extra virgin olive oil, divided
1 pound 95% lean ground beef
1 large egg
⅓ cup plain dry breadcrumbs
¼ cup chopped fresh mint
¼ cup chopped fresh Italian parsley
2 garlic cloves, minced
1 tablespoon freshly grated lemon zest
¼ teaspoon kosher salt
½ teaspoon freshly ground pepper
2 carrots, peeled and chopped
1 medium onion, chopped
1 stalk celery, chopped
5 cups Chicken Stock (page 149) or
    low-sodium chicken broth
1 (14½-ounce) can no-salt-added diced tomatoes
½ cup whole wheat orzo
8 ounces Swiss chard, tough stems removed
    and leaves chopped
4 tablespoons freshly grated Parmesan

1 Preheat the oven to 400°F. Brush a large rimmed baking sheet with 2 teaspoons of the oil.

2 Combine the beef, egg, breadcrumbs, mint, parsley, garlic, lemon zest, salt, and pepper in a large bowl and mix well with your hands. Shape into ½-inch meatballs. Place on the prepared pan and bake until browned, 20 to 25 minutes.

3 Meanwhile, heat a large pot over medium heat. Add the oil and tilt the pan to coat the bottom. Add the carrots, onion, and celery and cook until softened, 5 minutes. Add the stock and tomatoes and bring to a boil. Stir in the orzo and return to a boil.

4 Cover, reduce the heat to low, and simmer, stirring occasionally, until the orzo is almost tender, about 10 minutes. Carefully add the meatballs and the chard and cook until the chard is tender, about 5 minutes longer. Ladle into 8 bowls, sprinkle evenly with the Parmesan, and serve at once. The soup can be refrigerated, covered, for up to 4 days.

Each serving: 16 g carb, 202 cal, 7 g fat, 2 g sat fat, 65 mg chol, 3 g fib, 18 g pro, 311 mg sod • Carb Choices: 1; Exchanges: 1 starch, 1½ lean protein, ½ fat

Vietnamese Beef Noodle Soup QUICK

makes 4 servings

If you've had this soup in restaurants, but never made it at home, you won't believe how easy it is. There's just one trick: slicing the beef really thin. Be sure to freeze it briefly before slicing. Place the accompaniments in bowls and let people garnish the soup to their individual taste.

12 ounces round steak, trimmed of all visible fat
8 cups Beef Stock (page 151) or low-sodium beef broth
1 onion, thinly sliced
8 thin slices fresh ginger
2 garlic cloves, sliced
1 cinnamon stick
1 star anise
4 ounces rice noodles
Accompaniments: bean sprouts, thinly sliced scallions, thinly sliced jalapeños, fresh mint leaves, fresh basil leaves, lime wedges

1 Place the beef in the freezer for 30 minutes.

2 Combine the stock, onion, ginger, garlic, cinnamon, and anise in a large pot and bring to a boil over high heat. Cover, reduce the heat to low, and simmer 20 minutes. Strain the stock and discard the solids. Return the stock to the pot and bring to a boil over high heat.

3 Meanwhile, prepare the noodles according to the package directions and keep hot.

4 To serve, slice the beef very thinly across the grain. Divide the noodles evenly among 4 bowls. Arrange the beef on top of the noodles. Carefully ladle the boiling broth evenly over the noodles and beef. Arrange the desired accompaniments on a large platter and allow diners to help themselves. Serve at once. The soup is best when eaten immediately.

Each serving: 23 g carb, 228 cal, 3 g fat, 1 g sat fat, 48 mg chol, 0 g fib, 25 g pro, 267 mg sod • Carb Choices: 1½; Exchanges: 1½ starch, 3 lean protein

Pork and Hominy Soup QUICK

makes 6 servings

If you like hominy, you'll love this soup that's really a cross between a soup and a chili. When I make dishes that use ground pork, I like to make my own by pulsing cubed pork chops in a food processor. This way, I know it is lean, since the fat content of supermarket ground pork is not usually on the label.

8 ounces boneless center-cut pork chops, trimmed of all visible fat and cubed
2 teaspoons canola oil
1 medium onion, chopped
1 small green bell pepper, chopped
2 garlic cloves, minced
2 tablespoons chili powder
1 tablespoon ground cumin
¼ teaspoon freshly ground pepper
3 cups Chicken Stock (page 149) or low-sodium chicken broth
1 (14½-ounce) can no-salt-added diced tomatoes
1 (15-ounce) can hominy, rinsed and drained
1 tablespoon fine-grind yellow cornmeal
Chopped fresh cilantro
Lime wedges

1 Place the pork in a food processor in 2 batches and pulse until the meat is finely minced but not ground, 4 to 5 times.

2 Heat a large pot over medium heat. Add the oil and tilt the pan to coat the bottom evenly. Add the pork, onion, and bell pepper and cook, stirring often, until the vegetables are softened, 8 minutes. Add the garlic, chili powder, cumin, and ground pepper and cook, stirring constantly, until fragrant, 30 seconds.

3 Stir in the stock, tomatoes, and hominy and bring to a boil over high heat. Cover, reduce the heat to low, and simmer until the vegetables are tender, about 15 minutes. Sprinkle the cornmeal into the soup, stirring constantly. Simmer until slightly thickened, about 2 minutes. Ladle the

soup into 6 bowls, sprinkle with the cilantro, and serve at once with lime wedges on the side. The soup can be refrigerated, covered, for up to 4 days or frozen for up to 3 months.

Each serving: 16 g carb, 157 cal, 5 g fat, 1 g sat fat, 25 mg chol, 3 g fib, 12 g pro, 275 mg sod • Carb Choices: 1; Exchanges: ½ starch, 1 veg, 1 lean protein

Lentil and Chorizo Soup HIGH FIBER

makes 8 servings

If the spiciness of chorizo is not to your liking, make this soup with mild Italian turkey sausage.

6 ounces fresh chorizo

2 stalks celery, diced

2 carrots, peeled and chopped

1 medium onion, diced

2 garlic cloves, minced

8 cups Chicken Stock (page 149) or low-sodium chicken broth

2 cups dried brown lentils, picked over and rinsed

2 large red Roasted Bell Peppers (page 21) or 2 cups roasted red peppers from a jar, chopped

1 Heat a large pot over medium heat. Remove and discard the sausage casings, crumble the sausage, and add to the pot. Add the celery, carrots, and onion and cook, stirring often, until the vegetables are softened, 5 minutes. Add the garlic and cook, stirring constantly, until fragrant, 30 seconds.

2 Add the stock, lentils, and roasted peppers and bring to a boil over high heat. Cover, reduce the heat, and simmer until the lentils are tender, 30 minutes. Ladle into 8 bowls and serve at once. The soup can be refrigerated, covered, for up to 4 days or frozen for up to 3 months.

Each serving: 35 g carb, 249 cal, 4 g fat, 2 g sat fat, 11 mg chol, 13 g fib, 19 g pro, 296 mg sod • Carb Choices: 2; Exchanges: 1½ starch, 1 veg, 1 medium-fat protein, 1½ plant-based protein, ½ fat

Pork Dumplings in Ginger Broth

makes 4 servings

8 ounces boneless center-cut pork chops, trimmed of all visible fat and cubed

2 tablespoons reduced-sodium soy sauce, divided

2 tablespoons chopped fresh cilantro

3 teaspoons minced fresh ginger, divided

½ teaspoon Asian sesame oil, divided

20 wonton wrappers

7 cups Chicken Stock (page 149) or low-sodium chicken broth

4 cups chopped fresh spinach

¼ cup thinly sliced scallions

1 Place the pork in a food processor in 2 batches and pulse until the meat is finely minced but not ground, 4 to 5 times.

2 Stir together the pork, 1 tablespoon of the soy sauce, cilantro, 1 teaspoon of the ginger, and ¼ teaspoon of the oil in a medium bowl.

3 Working with 1 wonton wrapper at a time, place 1 rounded teaspoon of the pork mixture on each one. Moisten the edge of the wrapper with water, fold one edge over to form a triangle, and pinch the edges together to seal.

4 Combine the stock, remaining 1 tablespoon soy sauce, and remaining 2 teaspoons ginger in a large pot. Bring to a boil over high heat. Reduce the heat to medium-low and add the dumplings a few at a time. Simmer, uncovered, until the dumplings float, about 5 minutes. Transfer the dumplings to 4 bowls using a slotted spoon.

5 Increase the heat to high and return the stock to a boil. Add the spinach and cook just until the spinach wilts, 1 minute. Stir in the scallions and remaining ¼ teaspoon oil. Ladle the stock mixture over the wontons and serve at once. The soup is best when eaten immediately.

Each serving: 25 g carb, 243 cal, 5 g fat, 2 g sat fat, 42 mg chol, 2 g fib, 24 g pro, 797 mg sod • Carb Choices: 1½; Exchanges: 1½ starch, 2½ lean protein

Moroccan Harira HIGH FIBER

makes 6 servings

Usually eaten during the month of Ramadan to break the fast at the end of the day, this Moroccan dish can vary in its ingredients and seasonings, but almost always contains some kind of meat along with beans or lentils stewed together in a fragrant broth. Serve it with whole wheat pita or naan bread.

1 pound boneless leg of lamb, trimmed of all visible fat and cut into ½-inch pieces

¾ teaspoon kosher salt, divided

¼ teaspoon freshly ground pepper, divided

2 teaspoons canola oil

5 cups Chicken Stock (page 149) or low-sodium chicken broth

1 medium onion, chopped

1 stalk celery, chopped

1 medium red bell pepper, chopped

1 (14½-ounce) can no-salt added diced tomatoes

1 cup dried brown lentils, picked over and rinsed

2 garlic cloves, minced

1 tablespoon minced fresh ginger

1 teaspoon ground turmeric

½ teaspoon ground cinnamon

¼ cup chopped fresh cilantro

2 tablespoons lemon juice

1 Sprinkle the lamb with ¼ teaspoon of the salt and ⅛ teaspoon of the ground pepper. Heat a large pot over medium-high heat. Add the oil and tilt the pan to coat the bottom evenly. Add the lamb and cook, stirring often, until well browned, 6 to 8 minutes.

2 Add the stock and bring to a boil over high heat. Cover, reduce the heat to low, and simmer 30 minutes. Add the onion, celery, bell pepper, tomatoes, lentils, garlic, ginger, turmeric, cinnamon, remaining ½ teaspoon salt, and remaining ⅛ teaspoon ground pepper. Cover and simmer until the lentils are tender, about 30 minutes longer. Remove from the heat and stir in the cilantro and lemon juice. Ladle into 6 bowls and serve at once. The soup can be refrigerated, covered, for up to 4 days.

Each serving: 27 g carb, 269 cal, 7 g fat, 2 g sat fat, 50 mg chol, 9 g fib, 27 g pro, 330 mg sod • Carb Choices: 1½; Exchanges: 1 starch, 1 veg, 2 lean protein, 1 plant-based protein

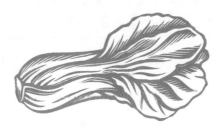

Seafood Soups

New England Clam Chowder QUICK

makes 4 servings

Just two slices of bacon give this creamy soup a complex smoky flavor. Combining the milk and flour before adding them to the soup prevents the milk from curdling.

2 strips center-cut bacon

1 medium onion, chopped

1 stalk celery, chopped

2 cups Shrimp Stock (page 152) or 1 (8-ounce) bottle clam juice plus 1 cup water

12 ounces red-skinned potatoes, well scrubbed and cut into ½-inch cubes

1 bay leaf

¼ teaspoon freshly ground pepper

2 cups 2% low-fat milk

1 tablespoon unbleached all-purpose flour

2 pounds small clams, scrubbed

Chopped fresh Italian parsley (optional)

1 Cook the bacon in a large pot over medium-high heat until crisp. Drain on paper towels and chop. Drain off and discard all but 2 teaspoons of the bacon drippings. Add the onion and celery to the bacon drippings and cook, stirring often, until the vegetables are softened, 5 minutes.

2 Add the stock, potatoes, bay leaf, and pepper and bring to a boil over high heat. Cover, reduce the heat to low, and simmer until the potatoes are almost tender, 6 to 8 minutes.

3 Combine the milk and flour in a medium bowl and whisk until smooth. Add the milk mixture to the pot and bring to a simmer. Add the clams, cover, and simmer until the clams open, about 3 minutes. Discard any unopened clams. Remove and discard the bay leaf. Stir in the bacon. Ladle the soup into 4 bowls and sprinkle with the parsley, if using. Serve at once. The soup is best when eaten immediately.

Each serving: 25 g carb, 226 cal, 6 g fat, 3 g sat fat, 38 mg chol, 2 g fib, 16 g pro, 266 mg sod • Carb Choices: 1½; Exchanges: 1 starch, 1 veg, 1 reduced-fat milk, 1 lean protein, ½ fat

Manhattan Clam Chowder QUICK | HIGH FIBER

makes 4 servings

New Englanders think it's heresy to put tomatoes into clam chowder. Even if you grew up eating only white creamy chowder, you'll find this scarlet soup is a delicious and satisfying one-dish meal.

2 teaspoons extra virgin olive oil
1 medium onion, chopped
1 small green bell pepper, chopped
1 stalk celery, chopped
2 garlic cloves, minced
2 cups Shrimp Stock (page 152) or 1 (8-ounce) bottle clam juice plus 1 cup water
2 (14½-ounce) cans no-salt-added diced tomatoes
½ cup dry white wine
2 tablespoons no-salt-added tomato paste
2 medium red-skinned potatoes, well scrubbed and chopped
½ teaspoon dried thyme
½ teaspoon freshly ground pepper
2 (6½-ounce) cans chopped clams, undrained
2 tablespoons chopped fresh Italian parsley

1 Heat a large pot over medium heat. Add the oil and tilt the pot to coat the bottom evenly. Add the onion, bell pepper, and celery and cook, stirring often, until softened, 5 minutes. Add the garlic and cook, stirring constantly, until fragrant, 30 seconds.

2 Add the stock, tomatoes, wine, tomato paste, potatoes, thyme, and ground pepper. Cover, reduce the heat to low, and simmer until the potatoes are tender, 10 to 12 minutes. Stir in the clams with their juice and cook until heated through, about 2 minutes. Stir in the parsley. Ladle into 4 bowls and serve at once. The soup can be refrigerated, covered, for up to 4 days.

Each serving: 23 g carb, 182 cal, 3 g fat, 0 g sat fat, 16 mg chol, 4 g fib, 10 g pro, 581 mg sod • Carb Choices: 1½; Exchanges: ½ starch, ½ carb, 2 veg, 1 lean protein, ½ fat

CHESAPEAKE BAY CRAB CHOWDER QUICK | HIGH FIBER: Follow the Manhattan Clam Chowder recipe, at left, adding 2 teaspoons crab seasoning with the garlic in step 1. Substitute 12 ounces lump crabmeat for the clams in step 2.

Each serving: 20 g carb, 231 cal, 4 g fat, 1 g sat fat, 86 mg chol, 4 g fib, 21 g pro, 735 mg sod • Carb Choices: 1; Exchanges: ½ starch, ½ carb, 2 veg, 2 lean protein, ½ fat

Cioppino QUICK

makes 6 servings

A few ordinary pantry ingredients along with some fresh seafood combine to make this easy and comforting soup. Use whatever mixture of seafood looks freshest at the market to make this classic soup—crabmeat, sea scallops, swordfish, halibut, or snapper all work well.

1 medium bulb fennel
2 teaspoons extra virgin olive oil
2 stalks celery, diced
1 medium onion, diced
2 garlic cloves, minced
3 cups Chicken Stock (page 149) or low-sodium chicken broth
2 (14½-ounce) cans no-salt-added diced tomatoes
1 (8-ounce) can no-salt-added tomato sauce
½ cup dry white wine
1 teaspoon dried basil
1 teaspoon dried oregano
⅛ teaspoon freshly ground pepper
8 ounces cod or other mild fish fillets, cut into 1-inch cubes
8 ounces medium peeled deveined shrimp
2 tablespoons chopped fresh Italian parsley

1 Trim the tough outer stalks from the fennel. Cut the fennel bulb in half vertically and cut away and discard the core. Chop the fennel.

2 Heat a large pot over medium heat. Add the oil and tilt the pan to coat the bottom evenly. Add the fennel, celery, and onion and cook,

stirring often, until softened, 5 minutes. Add the garlic and cook, stirring constantly, until fragrant, 30 seconds.

3 Stir in the stock, tomatoes, tomato sauce, wine, basil, oregano, and pepper. Cover, reduce the heat to low, and simmer until the vegetables are tender, about 10 minutes. Stir in the cod and shrimp and cook until the shrimp turn pink, about 2 minutes. Remove from the heat and stir in the parsley. Ladle into 6 bowls and serve at once. The soup is best on the day it is made.

Each serving: 13 g carb, 164 cal, 3 g fat, 1 g sat fat, 74 mg chol, 3 g fib, 17 g pro, 228 mg sod • Carb Choices: 1; Exchanges: 2 veg, 2 lean protein

Shrimp Gumbo QUICK

makes 8 servings

I love okra, and I think most everyone else would, too, if it wasn't overcooked. If you don't think you'll convince your family to go for it, the gumbo is delicious, though not authentic, without it. To serve this rich gumbo as a Louisianan would, top each bowl of soup with ¼ cup hot cooked rice.

¼ cup canola oil

½ cup unbleached all-purpose flour

2 stalks celery, chopped

1 green bell pepper, chopped

1 large onion, chopped

2 garlic cloves, minced

4½ cups Shrimp Stock (page 152) or 3½ cups Chicken Stock (page 149) or low-sodium chicken broth plus 1 (8-ounce) bottle clam juice

1 (14½-ounce) can no-salt-added diced tomatoes

1 tablespoon Worcestershire sauce

2 cups sliced fresh okra or 1 (10-ounce) package frozen sliced okra

1 pound medium peeled deveined shrimp

½ teaspoon freshly ground pepper

⅛ teaspoon ground cayenne

1 Heat the oil in a large pot over medium-high heat. Add the flour and cook, stirring constantly, until the flour turns golden brown, 6 to 8 minutes. Add the celery, bell pepper, and onion and cook, stirring often, until the vegetables are softened, 5 minutes. Add the garlic and cook, stirring constantly, until fragrant, 30 seconds.

2 Add the stock, tomatoes, and Worcestershire sauce and bring to a boil over high heat. Cover, reduce the heat to low, and simmer until the vegetables are tender, 15 minutes. Stir in the okra and cook until tender, 5 minutes. Stir in the shrimp, ground pepper, and cayenne and cook until the shrimp turn pink, 2 minutes. Ladle into 8 bowls and serve at once. The soup can be refrigerated, covered, for up to 4 days.

Each serving: 13 g carb, 166 cal, 8 g fat, 1 g sat fat, 85 mg chol, 2 g fib, 12 g pro, 308 mg sod • Carb Choices: 1; Exchanges: 1 carb, 1 lean protein, 1½ fat

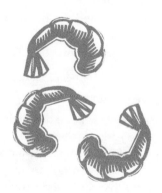

Shrimp and Black Bean Soup with Chile and Lime

QUICK | HIGH FIBER

makes 6 servings

If you're in a hurry, you can skip making the tortilla strips for this soup.

3 (6-inch) corn tortillas, cut in half, then into thin strips

2 teaspoons extra virgin olive oil

1 large onion, diced

1 green bell pepper, diced

1 jalapeño, seeded and minced

2 garlic cloves, minced

1 tablespoon ground cumin

4½ cups Shrimp Stock (page 152) or 3½ cups Chicken Stock (page 149) or low-sodium chicken broth plus 1 (8-ounce) bottle clam juice

1 (14½ ounce) can no-salt-added diced tomatoes

1 (15-ounce) can no-salt-added black beans, rinsed and drained

1 pound medium peeled deveined shrimp

2 tablespoons lime juice

½ cup chopped fresh cilantro

1 Preheat the oven to 350°F. Place the tortilla strips on a baking sheet and bake until crisp, 10 minutes.

2 Meanwhile, heat a large pot over medium heat. Add the oil and tilt the pot to coat the bottom evenly. Add the onion, bell pepper, and jalapeño and cook, stirring often, until softened, 5 minutes. Add the garlic and cumin and cook, stirring constantly, until fragrant, 30 seconds.

3 Add the stock, tomatoes, and beans and bring to a boil. Cover, reduce the heat to low, and simmer until the vegetables are tender, about 15 minutes. Stir in the shrimp and cook until the shrimp turn pink, about 2 minutes. Remove from the heat and stir in the lime juice and cilantro.

Ladle into 6 bowls, top evenly with the tortilla strips, and serve at once. The soup is best on the day it is made.

Each serving: 23 g carb, 193 cal, 3 g fat, 0 g sat fat, 113 mg chol, 6 g fib, 19 g pro, 328 mg sod • Carb Choices: 1½; Exchanges: 1 starch, 1 veg, 1½ lean protein

Coconut Shrimp Soup with Basmati Rice

makes 4 servings

2 teaspoons canola oil

1 small red bell pepper, cut into short, thin strips

1 small onion, halved and sliced

2 tablespoons minced fresh ginger

2 garlic cloves, minced

2½ cups Chicken Stock (page 149) or low-sodium chicken broth

1 (13½-ounce) can reduced-fat coconut milk

1 tablespoon green curry paste

1 pound medium peeled deveined shrimp

2 tablespoons lime juice

2 cups hot cooked brown basmati rice (page 108)

Thinly sliced scallions

Thinly sliced fresh basil leaves

1 Heat a large pot over medium heat. Add the oil and tilt the pot to evenly coat the bottom. Add the bell pepper and onion and cook, stirring often, until the vegetables are softened, 5 minutes. Add the ginger and garlic and cook, stirring constantly, until fragrant, 30 seconds.

2 Add the stock, coconut milk, and curry paste and bring to a boil. Add the shrimp and cook until the shrimp turn pink, 2 minutes. Remove from the heat and stir in the lime juice. Spoon ½ cup of the rice into each of 4 bowls and ladle the soup evenly over the rice. Sprinkle each serving with scallions and basil and serve at once. The soup is best when eaten immediately.

Each serving: 23 g carb, 264 cal, 10 g fat, 6 g sat fat, 171 mg chol, 2 g fib, 24 g pro, 375 mg sod • Carb Choices: 1½; Exchanges: 1 starch, 1 veg, 3 lean protein, 1 fat

Chilled Soups

Chunky Gazpacho

makes 4 servings

If yellow tomatoes are available, they make a colorful substitute for red tomatoes. Serve this soup with a slice of crusty French bread or focaccia. If you like a smooth gazpacho, process the ingredients in batches in a food processor.

2½ cups low-sodium tomato-vegetable juice
2 large tomatoes, chopped
1 small green bell pepper, chopped
1 jalapeño, seeded and minced (optional)
¼ cup diced red onion
¼ cup chopped fresh basil, Italian parsley, or cilantro
1 garlic clove, crushed through a press
1 tablespoon sherry vinegar or white wine vinegar
½ teaspoon kosher salt
⅛ teaspoon freshly ground pepper

Combine all the ingredients in a large bowl. Cover and refrigerate until chilled, 2 hours or up to 2 days. Ladle into 4 bowls and serve.

Each serving: 13 g carb, 59 cal, 0 g fat, 0 g sat fat, 0 mg chol, 3 g fib, 2 g pro, 234 mg sod • Carb Choices: 1; Exchanges: 2 veg

SEAFOOD GAZPACHO: Follow the Chunky Gazpacho recipe, above, but add 8 ounces small cooked chilled peeled deveined shrimp, or 8 ounces chilled crabmeat to the soup just before serving.

Each serving: 13 g carb, 102 cal, 1 g fat, 0 g sat fat, 84 mg chol, 3 g fib, 11 g pro, 330 mg sod • Carb Choices: 1; Exchanges: 2 veg, 1 lean protein

White Gazpacho

makes 4 servings

A classic Spanish soup for the summertime, white gazpacho is made with white grapes, almonds, and cucumbers. It makes a refreshing starter for any spring or summer lunch. Garnish the soup with halved seedless green grapes and a few additional slivers of toasted almonds.

2 slices firm white bread, crusts removed
½ cup cold water
1 large hothouse (English) cucumber, peeled, seeded, and chopped
1 cup seedless green grapes
¼ cup chopped sweet onion
¼ cup slivered almonds, toasted (page 4)
3 tablespoons lemon juice
1 tablespoon extra virgin olive oil
1 small garlic clove, sliced
½ teaspoon ground cumin
½ teaspoon kosher salt

1 Place the bread and water in a shallow dish and let stand until the water is absorbed.

2 Combine the bread and all the remaining ingredients in a food processor or blender and process until smooth. Cover and refrigerate until chilled, at least 2 hours or up to 2 days. Ladle into 4 bowls and serve.

Each serving: 17 g carb, 141 cal, 8 g fat, 1 g sat fat, 0 mg chol, 2 g fib, 3 g pro, 202 mg sod • Carb Choices: 1; Exchanges: ½ starch, ½ fruit, 1 fat

Cucumber-Buttermilk Vichyssoise

makes 4 servings

Similar to a classic potato vichyssoise, this version has the refreshing addition of cucumbers. On a hot summer day, serve it in a drinking glass with a few ice cubes added to make it extra cold.

2 teaspoons extra virgin olive oil
½ large sweet onion, chopped
2 garlic cloves, minced
2 cups Chicken Stock (page 149) or
    low-sodium chicken broth
2 large hothouse (English) cucumbers, peeled,
    seeded, and chopped
1 large baking potato, peeled and chopped
    (about 1½ cups)
½ teaspoon kosher salt
Pinch of white pepper
1 cup low-fat buttermilk
Chopped fresh dill sprigs or thinly sliced fresh
    basil leaves

1 Heat a large pot over medium heat. Add the oil and tilt the pan to coat the bottom evenly. Add the onion and cook, stirring often, until softened, 5 minutes. Add the garlic and cook, stirring constantly, until fragrant, 30 seconds. Add the stock, cucumbers, potato, salt, and pepper and bring to a boil over high heat. Reduce the heat to low, cover, and simmer until the vegetables are very tender, 15 to 20 minutes.

2 Place the vegetable mixture in a food processor or blender in batches and process until smooth. Transfer to a large bowl and let cool to room temperature. Stir in the buttermilk, cover, and refrigerate until chilled, at least 2 hours or up to 2 days. Ladle into 4 bowls, sprinkle with the dill, and serve.

Each serving: 25 g carb, 153 cal, 3 g fat, 1 g sat fat, 6 mg chol, 3 g fib, 7 g pro, 284 mg sod • Carb Choices: 1½; Exchanges: 1 starch, ½ carb, ½ fat

Chilled Cucumber-Mint Soup

makes 4 servings

I like to call this my cucumber smoothie. Though it's delicious enough to serve to the finickiest of guests, I like to keep it in a pitcher in the refrigerator and drink it for an afternoon snack. If you like a chunkier soup, you can shred the cucumbers and mince the scallion, garlic, and mint instead of pureeing them in the food processor.

2 hothouse (English) cucumbers, peeled,
    seeded, and sliced
1 small scallion, thinly sliced
1 small garlic clove, chopped
6 fresh mint leaves
1 cup low-fat buttermilk
2 cups plain low-fat yogurt
2 tablespoons lemon juice
½ teaspoon kosher salt
Pinch of ground white pepper

1 Combine the cucumbers, scallion, garlic, mint, and buttermilk in a food processor or blender and process until smooth.

2 Transfer to a large bowl and stir in the yogurt, lemon juice, salt, and pepper. Cover and refrigerate until chilled, 2 hours or up to 2 days. Ladle into 4 bowls and serve.

Each serving: 16 g carb, 121 cal, 3 g fat, 2 g sat fat, 11 mg chol, 1 g fib, 10 g pro, 294 mg sod • Carb Choices: 1; Exchanges: 1 veg, 1 reduced-fat milk

Chilled Zucchini-Dill Soup

makes 4 servings

This is one of the easiest and tastiest dishes to make when you have too much zucchini. Don't make the soup too far ahead. After about 4 hours in the refrigerator, the vibrant green color of the soup turns to drab olive.

2 teaspoons extra virgin olive oil
½ large sweet onion, chopped
2 garlic cloves, minced
2 cups water
2 medium zucchini (about 1 pound), chopped
¾ teaspoon kosher salt
½ teaspoon grated lemon zest
2½ tablespoons lemon juice
2 tablespoons chopped fresh dill
Pinch of white pepper

1 Heat a large pot over medium heat. Add the oil and tilt the pan to coat the bottom evenly. Add the onion and cook, stirring often, until softened, 5 minutes. Add the garlic and cook, stirring constantly, until fragrant, 30 seconds.

2 Add the water, zucchini, and salt and bring to a boil over high heat. Cover, reduce the heat to low, and simmer until the vegetables are very tender, 12 to 15 minutes (do not overcook, or the zucchini will lose its vibrant green color). Stir in the lemon zest, lemon juice, dill, and pepper.

3 Let the vegetable mixture cool slightly, then place in a food processor or blender in batches and process until smooth. Transfer to a large bowl. Cover and refrigerate until chilled, 2 hours or up to 4 hours. Ladle into 4 bowls and serve.

Each serving: 8 g carb, 56 cal, 3 g fat, 0 g sat fat, 0 mg chol, 2 g fib, 2 g pro, 228 mg sod • Carb Choices: ½; Exchanges: 1 veg, ½ fat

Chilled Avocado-Lime Soup   HIGH FIBER

makes 6 servings

When you need a quick no-cook starter for a summer party, this is a tart and refreshing option. Serve it in pretty stemmed glasses and garnish each one with a swirl of plain yogurt.

2 avocados, pitted and peeled
2½ cups Chicken Stock (page 149) or low-sodium chicken broth, divided
1 cup low-fat buttermilk
½ cup plain fat-free yogurt
2 tablespoons lime juice
¼ cup thinly sliced scallions
½ teaspoon ground cumin
½ teaspoon kosher salt

1 Combine the avocados, 1 cup of the stock, the buttermilk, yogurt, lime juice, scallions, cumin, and salt in a in a food processor or blender and process until smooth.

2 Transfer to a large bowl and stir in the remaining 1½ cups stock. Cover and refrigerate until chilled, 2 hours or up to 1 day. Ladle into 6 bowls and serve.

Each serving: 10 g carb, 139 cal, 10 g fat, 2 g sat fat, 5 mg chol, 4 g fib, 6 g pro, 218 mg sod • Carb Choices: ½; Exchanges: ½ carb, 1½ fat

Chilled Tomatillo Soup

makes 4 servings

Tart tomatillos and cool cucumbers pair up to make the perfect soup to accentuate any summertime Tex-Mex menu you're serving. If you make this soup more than a few hours ahead, taste it before serving and add an additional teaspoon or two of lime juice if you think the flavor needs brightening.

2 teaspoons canola oil

1 medium onion, chopped

1 jalapeño, seeded and chopped

2 garlic cloves, chopped

2 cups Chicken Stock (page 149) or low-sodium chicken broth

12 ounces tomatillos, husks removed, quartered

1 large hothouse (English) cucumber, peeled, seeded, and chopped

¼ teaspoon kosher salt

½ cup whole fresh cilantro leaves

⅓ cup plain low-fat yogurt

2 tablespoons lime juice

1 Heat a large pot over medium heat. Add the oil and tilt the pot to coat the bottom evenly. Add the onion and jalapeño and cook, stirring often, until softened, 5 minutes. Add the garlic and cook, stirring constantly, until fragrant, 30 seconds. Add the stock, tomatillos, cucumber, and salt and bring to a boil over high heat. Cover, reduce the heat to low, and simmer until the vegetables are very tender, 15 to 20 minutes.

2 Let the vegetable mixture cool slightly, then place in a food processor or blender in batches and process until smooth, adding the cilantro to one of the batches. Transfer to a large bowl and whisk in the yogurt and lime juice. Cover and refrigerate until chilled, 2 hours or up to 2 days. Ladle into 4 bowls and serve.

Each serving: 12 g carb, 97 cal, 4 g fat, 1 g sat fat, 4 mg chol, 3 g fib, 5 g pro, 158 mg sod • Carb Choices: 1; Exchanges: 2 veg, ½ fat

Icy Cold Melon-Mint Soup

makes 6 servings

This soup works equally well as a starter or as a dessert. If you serve it as a starter, slivers of prosciutto ham make a nice garnish. If you're serving it as a dessert, float a few blueberries or raspberries on top of each serving.

1 large cantaloupe, seeded, peeled, and chopped (about 8 cups)

1 cup unsweetened apple juice

¼ cup chopped fresh mint

¼ cup lime juice

Pinch of kosher salt

Combine all the ingredients in a food processor or blender and process until smooth. Cover and refrigerate until chilled, 2 hours or up to 8 hours. Ladle into 6 bowls and serve.

Each serving: 23 g carb, 95 cal, 0 g fat, 0 g sat fat, 0 mg chol, 2 g fib, 2 g pro, 48 mg sod • Carb Choices: 1½; Exchanges: 1½ fruit

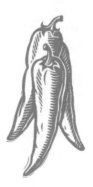

Poultry Main Dishes

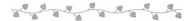

Whole Chicken

Lemon-Herb Roasted Chicken with Pan Sauce

Roast Chicken with Vegetables

Cilantro-Ginger Roasted Chicken

Wine and Garlic Marinated Grilled Whole Chicken

Chicken Pot-au-Feu

Colombian Sancocho

Quick Sautés and Stir-Fries

Herb-Crusted Sautéed Chicken

Sautéed Chicken with Texas Spice Rub

Chicken with Lemon-Caper Sauce

Basil-Crusted Chicken with Tomato-Olive Sauce

Chicken with Fresh Cranberry-Chile Sauce

Chicken with Brandied Mushrooms

Chicken with Green Curry Sauce

Peanut-Crusted Chicken with Honey-Sesame Sauce

Chicken Stir-Fry with Broccoli

Lemon Chicken and Snow Pea Stir-Fry

Thai Chicken and Basil Stir-Fry

Peanut Chicken with Green Beans

Stir-Fried Chicken and Vegetables with Black Bean Sauce

Chicken Pad Thai

Braises and One-Pot Meals

Chicken and Dumplings

Chicken Pot Pie

Chicken, Mushroom, and Spinach Lasagna

Coq au Vin

Braised Chicken with Orange-Caper Sauce

Chicken Simmered with Fennel and Tomatoes

Moroccan Chicken with Dried Apricots and Olives

Spanish Braised Chicken with Tomatoes and Peppers

Chicken with Potatoes, Lemon, and Sage

New Orleans Chicken Stew

Chicken and Pasta with Goat Cheese Sauce

Creamy Chicken Fettuccini

Chicken Biryani

Quick Cassoulet

Chicken, Chorizo, and Rice
Casserole

Curried Chicken and Winter
Vegetable Stew

Chicken and Peanut Stew

Chicken and White Bean
Stew with Bacon and
Arugula

Chicken from the Oven

Oven-Fried Chicken with
Creamy Gravy

Lemon-Garlic Baked
Chicken Breasts

Orange-Soy Baked Chicken

Baked Chicken with
Artichokes and Tomatoes

Baked Chicken with Dried
Plums and Balsamic Vinegar

Lemongrass-Ginger Baked
Chicken

Crispy Oven-Baked Chicken
Breasts

Pesto-Crusted Oven-Baked
Chicken Breasts

Chicken Parmesan

Panko-Crusted Chicken

Spinach and Feta–Stuffed
Chicken

Swiss Chard and Raisin–
Stuffed Chicken

Moroccan-Spiced Chicken
with Feta Tomatoes

Chicken with Tahini Sauce

Tandoori-Style Chicken

Chicken and Vegetables
en Papillote

Grilled Chicken

Grilled BBQ Chicken

Cumin and Lime Grilled
Chicken

Sesame and Lime Grilled
Chicken

Rosemary and Orange
Grilled Chicken

Mustard-Molasses Grilled
Chicken

Grilled Lemon-Curry Chicken

Grilled Chicken with
Cilantro-Jalapeño Sauce

Lager and Lime Marinated
Grilled Chicken

Asian Barbecued Chicken

Grilled Caribbean Chicken

Grilled Cilantro Chicken
with Coconut-Peanut Sauce

Grilled Chicken Yakitori

Grilled Chicken and
Clementine Kebabs

Moroccan-Spiced Chicken
and Vegetable Kebabs

Turkey

Herb Roasted Turkey with Sage Gravy

Lemon-Spice Roasted Turkey

Rosemary Roasted Turkey Breast with Gravy

Chile-Rubbed Roast Turkey Breast

Sage-Rubbed Roasted Boneless Turkey Breast

Turkey Breast Stuffed with Greens and Bacon

Osso Buco–Style Turkey Drumsticks

Sautéed Turkey Cutlets with Raisin Chutney

Grilled Turkey Cutlets with Apple Salsa

Indian-Spiced Turkey Cutlets with Sautéed Peaches

Ground Poultry and Poultry Sausage

Juicy Turkey Burgers

Asian Turkey Burgers

Cheddar-Stuffed Turkey Burgers

Italian Turkey Meatloaf

Salsa Turkey Meatloaf

Turkey Mole Chili

Chicken Sausage Stew with Beans and Escarole

Beer-Braised Chicken Sausages with Fennel and Peppers

Pasta with Turkey Sausage, Peppers, and Kale

Turkey Sausage with Braised Red Cabbage and Apples

Pasta, Turkey Sausage, and White Beans in Garlicky Tomato Sauce

Grilled Italian Turkey Sausage with Peppers and Tomatoes

Other Birds

Spice-Rubbed Roasted Cornish Hens

Citrus-Glazed Cornish Hens

Duck Breast with Dried Cherry–Port Sauce

Duck Breast with Black Currant Vinaigrette

Chicken—especially boneless skinless chicken breast—is the go-to entrée for almost anyone trying to eat more healthfully. When prepared with little added fat, generously seasoned, and served without the skin, chicken makes a healthful and satisfying meal.

As with other foods, portion control is primary when buying and preparing chicken. But chicken breeders have made buying and serving practical portions—especially the breasts—difficult and confusing. Because the white meat is America's favorite part of the bird, poultry companies have bred chickens to have enormous breasts. If you've assumed that half a chicken breast is one serving, you could be eating enough for four. Some boneless skinless chicken breast halves weigh more than a pound.

To keep portions where they should be, look for preportioned chicken breasts that come in 4½- to 5-ounce servings. They cost a little more, but offer a time-saving convenience. Another option for smaller portions is to buy organic chicken. These are always quite a bit smaller than conventional chicken.

If you buy boneless skinless chicken breasts in money-saving family-size packages, these tend to be large chicken breast halves that weigh about 1 pound each. To turn one chicken breast half into four servings, lay a chicken breast half on a cutting board and cut it horizontally in half. You now want to make two portions from each of the two pieces of chicken that you have. Since one end of the chicken is thicker than the other, cut each piece in two, making the piece cut from the thicker end smaller so that the portions will be of equal weight.

Whole bone-in skin-on chicken breasts are another smart option for easy low-fat meals. Meat cooked on the bone always has more flavor and cooking chicken breasts with the skin on (remove it before eating) keeps the chicken moist. The disadvantage of these is that they tend to come in portions large enough for two servings. Look for bone-in skin-on chicken breasts that are about 6 ounces each. If you can't find these, then buy the larger ones, add about 10 minutes to the cooking times given in the recipes here, and share a single breast between two people.

A whole roasted chicken is one of the easiest hands-off meals you can make. Once the chicken is seasoned and in the oven, you can make a quick vegetable side dish and a salad, and still have some time to relax for a few minutes before dinner. When you roast a chicken, it's a good idea to roast two and use the leftovers for meals throughout the week. See 10 Things to Make with Leftover Roasted Chicken (page 204) for some appetizing ideas.

When preparing a whole roasted chicken or turkey, bone-in skin-on chicken breasts, or a whole turkey breast, leave the skin on while the meat cooks and then remove it before eating. The skin keeps the moisture in, but only a negligible amount of the fat from the skin is absorbed into the meat.

Ground turkey is a healthful alternative to ground beef, but extra-lean turkey made from ground turkey breast is so dry I find it acceptable only for moist dishes such as soups, stews, or sauces. For burgers and meatloaf, I prefer regular lean turkey, which is about 7% fat (about the same as lean ground beef).

Chicken and turkey sausages are another good healthy-eating option and they are available in a broad array of flavors to fit into any menu. Look for them in well-stocked supermarkets or gourmet stores. The only caveat is that most sausages are very high in sodium. When you do enjoy a meal made with sausages, limit your sodium intake in other meals throughout the day.

Cornish hens and duck breasts are two more options for healthful and delicious meals. Both make impressive dinners for entertaining and they're much easier to cook than you think.

Poultry is inexpensive, versatile, easy to cook, and a perfect fit for a healthy diet. You'll see slimmed-down versions of many of your favorite dishes in this chapter as well as fresh new flavors to incorporate into appetizing and wholesome menus for your family.

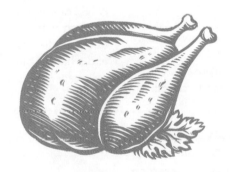

Whole Chicken

Lemon-Herb Roasted Chicken with Pan Sauce

makes 6 servings

This is a timeless roast chicken recipe with an accompanying sauce made right in the roasting pan, so all the browned bits on the bottom of the pan become part of the wonderful sauce. It makes a perfect Sunday supper. Instead of the fresh herb sprigs, you can use 2 teaspoons of dried sage or tarragon to rub under the skin of the chicken. In the sauce, substitute ¼ teaspoon of the dried herb for the fresh.

1 whole chicken (about 3¼ pounds)

2 garlic cloves, minced

2 teaspoons grated lemon zest

½ teaspoon kosher salt

¼ teaspoon plus ⅛ teaspoon freshly ground
   pepper, divided

3 sprigs fresh sage or tarragon

1 medium lemon, halved

1 cup Chicken Stock (page 149) or low-sodium
   chicken broth

2 tablespoons unbleached all-purpose flour

1 teaspoon chopped fresh sage or tarragon

1 Preheat the oven to 400°F.

2 Remove and discard the neck and giblets from the cavity of the chicken. Loosen the skin from the breast and drumsticks by inserting your fingers and gently separating the skin from the meat. Rub the garlic, lemon zest, salt, and ¼ teaspoon of the pepper over the breast and drumsticks underneath the skin. Place 2 of the sage sprigs underneath the loosened skin of the chicken breast. Place the remaining sage sprig and the halved lemon inside the cavity.

3 Place the chicken in a large roasting pan. Bake until an instant-read thermometer inserted into a thigh reads 165°F, 1 hour to 1 hour 15 minutes. Transfer the chicken to a platter, cover loosely with foil, and let stand 10 minutes before carving.

4 Meanwhile, to make the sauce, pour the pan drippings into a fat separator or a 2-cup glass measuring cup. Pour off and discard the fat. Add enough of the chicken stock to make 1¼ cups. Pour the stock mixture into the roasting pan. Add the flour and whisk until smooth. Set the roasting pan over two burners and cook over medium-high heat, whisking constantly, until the sauce comes to a boil and thickens, about 3 minutes. Stir in the chopped sage and the remaining ⅛ teaspoon pepper. Carve the chicken, divide among 6 plates, and drizzle evenly with the sauce. Remove the skin from the chicken before eating.

Each serving: 2 g carb, 165 cal, 4 g fat, 1 g sat fat, 89 mg chol, 0 g fib, 28 g pro, 218 mg sod • Carb Choices: 0; Exchanges: 4 lean protein

TANGERINE-ROSEMARY ROASTED CHICKEN WITH PAN SAUCE: Follow the Lemon-Herb Roasted Chicken with Pan Sauce recipe, at left, substituting grated tangerine zest for the lemon zest and a halved tangerine for the whole lemon. Use rosemary sprigs to place underneath the skin of the breast and use minced fresh rosemary instead of the sage or tarragon for the pan sauce.

Each serving: 2 g carb, 165 cal, 4 g fat, 1 g sat fat, 89 mg chol, 0 g fib, 28 g pro, 218 mg sod • Carb Choices: 0; Exchanges: 4 lean protein

Roast Chicken with Vegetables HIGH FIBER

makes 6 servings

1 whole chicken (about 3¼ pounds)
2 garlic cloves, minced
¾ teaspoon kosher salt, divided
½ teaspoon freshly ground pepper, divided
12 ounces green beans, trimmed
8 ounces baby potatoes, well scrubbed and quartered
8 ounces carrots, peeled and cut into ½-inch-thick sticks
2 teaspoons extra virgin olive oil

1 Preheat the oven to 400°F.

2 Remove and discard the neck and giblets from the cavity of the chicken. Loosen the skin from the breast and drumsticks by inserting your fingers and gently separating the skin from the meat. Rub the garlic, ½ teaspoon of the salt, and ¼ teaspoon of the pepper over the breast and drumsticks underneath the skin.

3 Place the chicken in a large roasting pan. Bake 15 minutes.

4 Meanwhile, combine the green beans, pota-toes, carrots, oil, remaining ¼ teaspoon salt, and remaining ¼ teaspoon pepper in a large bowl and toss to coat. Arrange the vegetables around the chicken. Continue roasting, stirring the veg-etables once, until an instant-read thermometer inserted into a thigh reads 165°F, 45 minutes to 1 hour.

5 Transfer the chicken to a platter, cover loosely with foil, and let stand 10 minutes before carving.

6 Carve the chicken and divide the chicken and vegetables evenly among 6 plates. Remove the skin from the chicken before eating.

Each serving: 14 g carb, 213 cal, 5 g fat, 1 g sat fat, 81 mg chol, 4 g fib, 28 g pro, 263 mg sod • Carb Choices: 1; Exchanges: ½ starch, 1 veg, 4 lean protein

Cilantro-Ginger Roasted Chicken

makes 6 servings

For more pronounced flavor, place the cilantro mixture under the skin of the chicken, then cover and refrigerate for up to 4 hours before roasting. If you're short on time, this Asian-inspired roasted chicken is still delicious going straight into the oven without marinating.

1 cup fresh cilantro leaves
¼ cup chopped fresh ginger
2 tablespoons thinly sliced scallions
2 tablespoons reduced-sodium soy sauce
2 garlic cloves
1 jalapeño, seeded and chopped
1 whole chicken (about 3¼ pounds)

1 Preheat the oven to 400°F.

2 Place the cilantro, ginger, scallions, soy sauce, garlic, and jalapeño in a food processor and pulse until the mixture is finely minced.

3 Remove and discard the neck and giblets from the cavity of the chicken. Loosen the skin from the breast and drumsticks by inserting your fingers and gently separating the skin from the meat. Rub the cilantro mixture over the breast and drumsticks underneath the skin.

4 Place the chicken in a large roasting pan. Bake until an instant-read thermometer inserted into a thigh reads 165°F, 1 hour to 1 hour 15 minutes. Transfer the chicken to a platter, cover loosely with foil, and let stand 10 minutes before carving.

5 Carve the chicken and divide evenly among 6 plates. Remove the skin before eating.

Each serving: 2 g carb, 149 cal, 3 g fat, 1 g sat fat, 81 mg chol, 0 g fib, 26 g pro, 298 mg sod • Carb Choices: 0; Exchanges: 4 lean protein

10 Things to Make with Leftover Roasted Chicken

When you prepare any roast chicken recipe, it's a good idea to roast two chickens at the same time so you can quickly make almost effortless weeknight meals with the leftovers.

Season the chicken with salt and pepper and roast according to the recipe instructions. Let the chicken stand until it is cool enough to handle. Remove and discard the skin, take the meat off the bones, cover, and refrigerate for up to 4 days. Use the chicken for one of the tasty meal ideas below. You can use the chicken carcass to make Leftover-Chicken Chicken Stock (page 150).

1 **FRESH AND SPICY CHICKEN SALAD SANDWICH**   Stir together equal parts mayonnaise and plain low-fat yogurt. Stir in chili-garlic paste to taste and toss with chopped chicken. Layer the chicken inside a whole wheat baguette with thinly sliced cucumber, grated carrot, and fresh cilantro leaves.

2 **GRILLED CHICKEN SANDWICHES WITH TAPENADE**   Spread a thin layer of Tapenade (page 598) or purchased tapenade on thinly sliced whole grain bread. Top with sliced chicken, roasted red peppers, and thinly sliced provolone. Top with another bread slice. Brush the bread lightly with olive oil and grill the sandwiches in a skillet.

3 **CHICKEN AND GOAT CHEESE QUESA-DILLAS**   Spread a thin layer of goat cheese on whole wheat tortillas. Toss shredded chicken with prepared pesto and arrange on top of the tortillas. Sprinkle with chopped roasted red bell peppers and thinly sliced scallions. Fold the quesadillas in half and grill in a skillet.

4 **CHICKEN AND MUSHROOM ENCHILADAS**   Sauté sliced mushrooms and chopped onion in olive oil until tender. Add the chopped chicken and cook until heated through. Spoon the chicken mixture inside whole wheat flour tortillas and arrange in a baking dish. Spoon prepared salsa over the enchiladas, sprinkle with shredded reduced-fat Monterey Jack cheese, and bake at 400°F until the cheese melts.

5 **MISO CHICKEN–VEGETABLE SOUP**   Simmer thinly sliced snow peas, carrots, and mushrooms in water until almost tender. Add chopped chicken and cook until heated through. Remove about ½ cup of the broth from the soup and whisk in white miso (about 1 tablespoon for each cup of water used in the soup). Stir the miso mixture back into the soup. Top with thinly sliced scallions and chopped fresh cilantro.

6 **CHICKEN AND RICE SOUP WITH SPINACH**   Simmer chopped onion, carrot, and celery in chicken broth until tender. Add chopped chicken, cooked brown rice, and chopped fresh spinach and cook until heated through.

7 **LEMON CHICKEN AND VEGETABLE SOUP WITH PESTO** Simmer chopped onion, carrot, celery, and red-skinned potato in chicken broth until tender. Add chopped chicken and grated lemon zest and cook until heated through. Spoon into bowls and top each serving with a bit of prepared pesto.

8 **CHICKEN AND POTATO HASH** Cook onion and cubed red-skinned potato in olive oil in a nonstick skillet until the potato is almost tender. Add cubed chicken and chopped roasted red pepper and cook until heated through. Sprinkle with chopped parsley.

9 **GREEK CHICKEN SALAD** Toss romaine lettuce, sliced cucumbers, red bell peppers, red onion, and pepperoncini peppers with vinaigrette dressing. Top the salad with sliced chicken and sprinkle with feta cheese.

10 **FRUITED CHICKEN SALAD** Toss together chopped chicken, sliced Granny Smith apple, and golden raisins. Drizzle with vinaigrette and a touch of honey and toss to coat. Serve over fresh baby spinach and sprinkle with toasted almonds.

Wine and Garlic Marinated Grilled Whole Chicken

makes 6 servings

Removing the backbone of a chicken makes it lie flat so it cooks more evenly on the grill.

¼ cup dry white wine
2 teaspoons grated lemon zest
2 tablespoons lemon juice
2½ teaspoons extra virgin olive oil, divided
4 garlic cloves, minced
1 scallion, thinly sliced
1 whole chicken (about 3¼ pounds)
½ teaspoon kosher salt
¼ teaspoon freshly ground pepper

1 Combine the wine, lemon zest, lemon juice, 2 teaspoons of the oil, the garlic, and scallion in a large shallow glass dish.

2 Remove and discard the neck and giblets from the cavity of the chicken. Place the chicken breast side down on a cutting board. Cut along both sides of the backbone using poultry shears or a sharp knife. Discard the backbone. Press the chicken flat using your palms.

3 Place the chicken in the dish and turn to coat with the marinade. Cover and refrigerate 8 to 12 hours, turning the chicken occasionally.

4 Preheat the grill to medium heat.

5 Remove the chicken from the marinade and discard the marinade. Pat the chicken dry with paper towels. Loosen the skin from the breast and drumsticks by inserting your fingers and gently separating the skin from the meat. Rub the salt and pepper over the breast and drumsticks underneath the skin.

6 Brush the grill rack with the remaining ½ teaspoon oil. Place the chicken on the grill skin side down. Cover and grill, turning once, until an instant-read thermometer inserted into a thigh reads 165°F, 50 to 60 minutes.

7 Carve the chicken and divide evenly among 6 plates. Remove the skin before eating.

Each serving: 0 g carb, 155 cal, 5 g fat, 1 g sat fat, 81 mg chol, 0 g fib, 26 g pro, 187 mg sod • Carb Choices: 0; Exchanges: 4 lean protein

Chicken Pot-au-Feu HIGH FIBER

makes 6 servings

When you want a simple bowl of comfort food for dinner, this is it. The zucchini isn't strictly traditional for this dish, but it adds some carb-free color and fresh flavor. You could use yellow squash or thin green beans, too.

1 whole chicken (about 3¼ pounds), skinned
6 cups Chicken Stock (page 149) or low-sodium chicken broth
1 small sprig fresh thyme or ¼ teaspoon dried thyme
1 bay leaf
¼ teaspoon kosher salt
¼ teaspoon freshly ground pepper
1 medium leek, halved lengthwise and thinly sliced
8 ounces baby potatoes, well scrubbed
8 ounces baby carrots
2 parsnips, peeled and cut into 1-inch slices
2 small zucchini, halved lengthwise and sliced
¼ cup chopped fresh Italian parsley

1 Place the chicken in a large pot. Add the stock, thyme, bay leaf, salt, and pepper. Bring to a boil over high heat, cover, reduce the heat to low, and simmer 20 minutes.

2 Meanwhile, submerge the sliced leek in a bowl of water, lift it out, and drain in a colander. Repeat, using fresh water, until no grit remains in the bowl. Drain the leek well.

3 Add the leek, potatoes, carrots, and parsnips to the pot. Return to a simmer and cook until the vegetables are tender and the juices of the chicken run clear, 25 minutes longer. Add the zucchini and simmer until crisp-tender, 2 to 3 minutes. Remove and discard the thyme sprig and bay leaf.

4 Transfer the chicken to a cutting board and carve. Stir the parsley into the stock mixture. Divide the chicken, vegetables, and broth evenly among 6 large shallow bowls.

Each serving: 23 g carb, 257 cal, 4 g fat, 1 g sat fat, 86 mg chol, 5 g fib, 32 g pro, 319 mg sod • Carb Choices: 1½; Exchanges: 1 starch, 1 veg, 4 lean protein

Colombian Sancocho

makes 6 servings

This is not authentic sancocho, which usually has starchy vegetables including yucca, plantain, and winter squash. Most recipes also contain a high-sodium seasoning blend called Sazón. This version cuts back on the starchy vegetables and uses cumin, jalapeño, and lots of garlic to stand in for the Sazón.

1 whole chicken (about 3¼ pounds), skinned
6 cups Chicken Stock (page 149) or low-sodium chicken broth
4 garlic cloves, chopped
1 large onion, halved lengthwise and sliced
1 jalapeño, seeded and minced
1 teaspoon ground cumin
¼ teaspoon kosher salt
¼ teaspoon freshly ground pepper
8 ounces red-skinned potatoes, well scrubbed and halved or quartered if large
2 small ears corn, cut in half
2 large carrots, peeled and cut into 1-inch pieces
½ cup chopped fresh cilantro

1 Place the chicken in a large pot. Add the stock, garlic, onion, jalapeno, cumin, salt, and pepper. Bring to a boil over high heat, cover, reduce the heat to low, and simmer 20 minutes.

2 Add the potatoes, corn, and carrots. Return to a simmer and cook until the juices of the chicken run clear, 25 minutes longer.

3 Transfer the chicken to a cutting board and carve. Stir the cilantro into the stock mixture. Divide the chicken, vegetables, and broth evenly among 6 large shallow bowls.

Each serving: 18 g carb, 225 cal, 5 g fat, 1 g sat fat, 82 mg chol, 3 g fib, 29 g pro, 173 mg sod • Carb Choices: 1; Exchanges: 1 starch, 4 lean protein

Quick Sautés and Stir-Fries

Herb-Crusted Sautéed Chicken QUICK

makes 4 servings

When a home-cooked dinner seems an impossibility, sautéed chicken breasts come to the rescue. Ready in just minutes, they taste better—and are better for you—than fast food or a frozen dinner. Serve these with Kalamata Olive Couscous (page 420) and Two-Minute Microwave Broccoli with Lemon Butter (page 449) for a complete meal that you can prepare in about 15 minutes.

4 (4-ounce) boneless skinless chicken breasts
½ teaspoon kosher salt
⅛ teaspoon freshly ground pepper
2 tablespoons chopped fresh basil, dill, or cilantro, or a mix
2 teaspoons extra virgin olive oil

1 Sprinkle the chicken with the salt and pepper, then with the herbs, pressing to adhere herbs.

2 Heat a large skillet over medium heat. Add the oil and tilt the pan to coat the bottom evenly. Add the chicken and cook, turning once, until the juices run clear, about 4 minutes on each side. Divide the chicken among 4 plates and serve at once.

Each serving: 0 g carb, 143 cal, 5 g fat, 1 g sat fat, 63 mg chol, 0 g fib, 23 g pro, 195 mg sod • Carb Choices: 0; Exchanges: 3 lean protein, ½ fat

Sautéed Chicken with Texas Spice Rub QUICK

makes 4 servings

Pair these with Polenta with Cheddar and Roasted Poblano (page 423) and steamed green beans for meal that tastes like you've spent hours in the kitchen. I like to turn these into soft tacos, too. Slice the cooked chicken breasts into thin strips and put them into warm corn tortillas topped with shredded lettuce and salsa.

½ teaspoon kosher salt
½ teaspoon chili powder
¼ teaspoon ground cumin
⅛ teaspoon freshly ground pepper
4 (4-ounce) boneless skinless chicken breasts
2 teaspoons extra virgin olive oil
Lime wedges

1 Stir together the salt, chili powder, cumin, and pepper in a small bowl. Sprinkle the chicken with the spice mixture.

2 Heat a large skillet over medium heat. Add the oil and tilt the pan to coat the bottom evenly. Add the chicken and cook, turning once, until the juices run clear, about 4 minutes on each side. Divide the chicken among 4 plates and serve at once with the lime wedges.

Each serving (chicken only): 0 g carb, 145 cal, 5 g fat, 1 g sat fat, 63 mg chol, 0 g fib, 23 g pro, 202 mg sod • Carb Choices: 0; Exchanges: 3 lean protein, ½ fat

Chicken with Lemon-Caper Sauce QUICK

makes 4 servings

Wine and lemon juice flecked with salty capers makes a tasty low-fat sauce for chicken in this version of chicken piccata. Serve it with a side of quick-cooking fresh whole wheat pasta for an easy weeknight dinner.

4 (4-ounce) boneless skinless chicken breasts
¼ teaspoon kosher salt
⅛ teaspoon plus pinch of freshly ground pepper, divided
2 tablespoons unbleached all-purpose flour
2 teaspoons extra virgin olive oil
½ cup dry white wine
3 tablespoons lemon juice
2 tablespoons capers, rinsed and drained
1 garlic clove, minced
1 tablespoon chopped fresh Italian parsley

1 Sprinkle the chicken with the salt and ⅛ teaspoon of the pepper, then with the flour.

2 Heat a large skillet over medium heat. Add the oil and tilt the pan to coat the bottom evenly. Add the chicken and cook, turning once, until the juices run clear, about 4 minutes on each side. Transfer to a plate and cover to keep warm.

3 Increase the heat to medium-high. Add the wine, lemon juice, capers, garlic, and the remaining pinch of pepper and bring to a boil, stirring to scrape up the browned bits from the bottom of the skillet. Cook until the sauce is slightly thickened, about 3 minutes. Remove from the heat and stir in the parsley. Add any accumulated juices from the chicken to the skillet. Divide the chicken among 4 plates, drizzle evenly with the sauce, and serve at once.

Each serving: 5 g carb, 185 cal, 5 g fat, 1 g sat fat, 63 mg chol, 0 g fib, 24 g pro, 253 mg sod • Carb Choices: 0; Exchanges: 3 lean protein

Basil-Crusted Chicken with Tomato-Olive Sauce

QUICK

makes 4 servings

Depending on how juicy your tomatoes are, you may need to adjust the cooking time on the sauce for this recipe. In colder months I sometimes substitute plum tomatoes, which tend to be less juicy, for the regular tomatoes. Fresh basil and Kalamata olives ensure great flavor, no matter the pedigree of your tomatoes.

4 (4-ounce) boneless skinless chicken breasts
½ teaspoon kosher salt
⅛ teaspoon plus pinch of freshly ground pepper, divided
4 tablespoons chopped fresh basil, divided
4 teaspoons extra virgin olive oil, divided
¼ cup diced onion
1 garlic clove, minced
½ cup dry white wine
2 large tomatoes, chopped
¼ cup Kalamata olives, pitted and halved

1 Sprinkle the chicken with the salt and ⅛ teaspoon of the pepper, then with 2 tablespoons of the basil, pressing to adhere.

2 Heat a large skillet over medium heat. Add 2 teaspoons of the oil and tilt the pan to coat the bottom evenly. Add the chicken and cook, turning once, until the juices run clear, about 4 minutes on each side. Transfer to a plate and cover to keep warm.

3 Increase the heat to medium-high. Add the remaining 2 teaspoons oil and tilt the pan to coat the bottom evenly. Add the onion and cook, stirring often, just until softened, 3 minutes. Add the garlic and cook, stirring constantly, until fragrant, 30 seconds. Add the wine, tomatoes, olives, and the remaining pinch of pepper. Bring to a boil and cook, stirring occasionally, until the sauce is slightly thickened, about 4 minutes. Add any accumulated juices from the chicken to the skillet. Remove from the heat and stir in the remaining 2 tablespoons basil. Divide the chicken among 4 plates. Spoon the sauce evenly over the chicken and serve at once.

Each serving: 6 g carb, 226 cal, 9 g fat, 2 g sat fat, 63 mg chol, 1 g fib, 24 g pro, 291 mg sod • Carb Choices: ½; Exchanges: 1 veg, 3 lean protein

Chicken with Fresh Cranberry-Chile Sauce

QUICK

makes 4 servings

If you ever get a craving for turkey and cranberry sauce, but you don't want to spend all day cooking, this is a delightful dish with a quick-cooking spicy-sweet cranberry sauce. I'd serve it to company any day.

4 (4-ounce) boneless skinless chicken breasts

½ teaspoon plus ⅛ teaspoon kosher salt

½ teaspoon plus ⅛ teaspoon ground cumin, divided

⅛ teaspoon freshly ground pepper

3 tablespoons chopped fresh cilantro, divided

4 teaspoons extra virgin olive oil, divided

¼ cup diced onion

1 jalapeño, seeded and minced

1 cup fresh cranberries or thawed frozen cranberries

½ cup Chicken Stock (page 149) or low-sodium chicken broth

2 tablespoons honey

1 Sprinkle the chicken with ½ teaspoon of the salt, ½ teaspoon of the cumin, and the pepper, then with 2 tablespoons of the cilantro, pressing to adhere.

2 Heat a large skillet over medium heat. Add 2 teaspoons of the oil and tilt the pan to coat the bottom evenly. Add the chicken and cook, turning once, until the juices run clear, about 4 minutes on each side. Transfer to a plate and cover to keep warm.

3 Increase the heat to medium-high. Add the remaining 2 teaspoons oil and tilt the pan to coat the bottom evenly. Add the onion and jalapeño and cook, stirring often, just until softened, 3 minutes. Add the cranberries, stock, remaining ⅛ teaspoon cumin, and remaining ⅛ teaspoon salt and bring to a boil. Cook, stirring occasionally, until the cranberries pop and the sauce is slightly thickened, about 3 minutes. Remove from the heat and stir in the honey and the remaining 1 tablespoon cilantro. Divide the chicken among 4 plates. Spoon the sauce evenly over the chicken and serve at once.

Each serving: 13 g carb, 216 cal, 8 g fat, 1 g sat fat, 63 mg chol, 2 g fib, 24 g pro, 249 mg sod • Carb Choices: 1; Exchanges: 1 carb, 3 lean protein

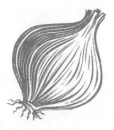

Chicken with Brandied Mushrooms QUICK

makes 4 servings

The mushrooms make this dish. Saturated with mellowed brandy and seasoned with garlic and thyme, they are irresistible, even when you use plain old white mushrooms. They're also delicious with grilled or broiled steaks.

4 (4-ounce) boneless skinless chicken breasts

½ teaspoon plus ⅛ teaspoon kosher salt, divided

⅛ teaspoon plus pinch of freshly ground pepper

1½ teaspoons chopped fresh thyme, divided

4 teaspoons extra virgin olive oil, divided

¼ cup diced onion

2 garlic cloves, minced

8 ounces cremini or white mushrooms, sliced

½ cup Chicken Stock (page 149) or low-sodium chicken broth

¼ cup brandy

1 Sprinkle the chicken with ½ teaspoon of the salt, and ⅛ teaspoon of the pepper, then with 1 teaspoon of the thyme, pressing to adhere.

2 Heat a large skillet over medium heat. Add 2 teaspoons of the oil and tilt the pan to coat the bottom evenly. Add the chicken and cook, turning once, until the juices run clear, about 4 minutes on each side. Transfer to a plate and cover to keep warm.

3 Increase the heat to medium-high. Add the remaining 2 teaspoons oil and tilt the pan to coat the bottom evenly. Add the onion and cook, stirring often, just until softened, 3 minutes. Add the garlic and cook, stirring constantly, until fragrant, 30 seconds. Add the mushrooms, stock, and brandy and bring to a boil. Cook, stirring often, until the mushrooms are tender and most of

the liquid has evaporated, 5 minutes. Stir in the remaining ½ teaspoon thyme, ⅛ teaspoon salt, and pinch of pepper. Add any accumulated juices from the chicken to the skillet. Divide the chicken among 4 plates. Spoon the mushrooms evenly over the chicken and serve at once.

Each serving: 4 g carb, 218 cal, 7 g fat, 1 g sat fat, 63 mg chol, 0 g fib, 25 g pro, 252 mg sod • Carb Choices: 0; Exchanges: 3 lean protein, 1 fat

Chicken with Green Curry Sauce QUICK

makes 4 servings

Basmati or brown rice is a must for serving with this dish to soak up the generous—and delicious—sauce. Add a side dish of steamed or stir-fried vegetables and dinner is done.

¾ cup reduced-fat coconut milk

1 teaspoon green curry paste

1 teaspoon cornstarch

4 (4-ounce) boneless skinless chicken breasts

½ teaspoon kosher salt

4 tablespoons chopped fresh cilantro, divided

4 teaspoons canola oil, divided

2 teaspoons minced fresh ginger

¼ cup thinly sliced scallions

1 tablespoon lime juice

2 teaspoons Asian fish sauce

1 Whisk together the coconut milk, curry paste, and cornstarch in a small bowl until smooth. Set aside.

2 Sprinkle the chicken with the salt, then with 2 tablespoons of the cilantro, pressing to adhere.

3 Heat a large skillet over medium heat. Add 2 teaspoons of the oil and tilt the pan to coat the bottom evenly. Add the chicken and cook, turning once, until the juices run clear, about 4 minutes on each side. Transfer to a plate and cover to keep warm.

4 Increase the heat to medium-high. Add the remaining 2 teaspoons oil and tilt the pan to coat the bottom evenly. Add the ginger and cook, stirring constantly, until fragrant, 30 seconds. Add the coconut milk mixture and the scallions and bring to a boil. Cook, stirring constantly, until the sauce is slightly thickened, about 1 minute. Remove from the heat and stir in the remaining 2 tablespoons cilantro, the lime juice, and fish sauce. Add any accumulated juices from the chicken to the skillet. Divide the chicken among 4 plates. Spoon the sauce evenly over the chicken and serve at once.

Each serving: 4 g carb, 197 cal, 10 g fat, 3 g sat fat, 63 mg chol, 0 g fib, 24 g pro, 462 mg sod • Carb Choices: 0; Exchanges: 3 lean protein, 1½ fat

Peanut-Crusted Chicken with Honey-Sesame Sauce

QUICK

makes 4 servings

With a crunchy peanut crust and a sauce sweetened with honey, you might actually get youngsters to eat this healthful chicken dish. Serve it with rice or soba noodles to soak up all the scrumptious sauce.

⅓ cup unsalted dry-roasted peanuts

4 (4-ounce) boneless skinless chicken breasts

½ teaspoon kosher salt

⅛ teaspoon freshly ground pepper

4 teaspoons canola oil, divided

2 garlic cloves, minced

2 teaspoons minced fresh ginger

½ cup dry sherry

2 tablespoons reduced-sodium soy sauce

2 tablespoons rice vinegar

2 tablespoons honey

1 tablespoon chopped fresh cilantro

¼ teaspoon Asian sesame oil

1 Place the peanuts in a food processor and pulse until coarsely chopped.

2 Sprinkle the chicken with the salt and pepper, then with the peanuts, pressing to adhere.

3 Heat a large skillet over medium heat. Add 2 teaspoons of the canola oil and tilt the pan to coat the bottom evenly. Add the chicken and cook, turning once, until the juices run clear, about 4 minutes on each side. Transfer to a plate and cover to keep warm.

4 Increase the heat to medium-high. Add the remaining 2 teaspoons canola oil and tilt the pan to coat the bottom evenly. Add the garlic and ginger and cook, stirring constantly, until fragrant, 30 seconds. Add the sherry, soy sauce, vinegar, and honey and bring to a boil. Cook, stirring often until the sauce is slightly thickened, about 4 minutes. Remove from the heat and stir in the cilantro and sesame oil. Add any accumulated juices from the chicken to the skillet. Divide the chicken among 4 plates. Spoon the sauce evenly over the chicken and serve at once.

Each serving: 4 g carb, 265 cal, 14 g fat, 2 g sat fat, 63 mg chol, 1 g fib, 26 g pro, 431 mg sod • Carb Choices: 0; Exchanges: 3 lean protein, 2 fat

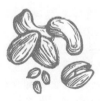

Chicken Stir-Fry with Broccoli QUICK

makes 4 servings

In this stir-fry, and other stir-fry recipes in this book, you can substitute thinly sliced boneless skinless chicken thighs; thinly sliced top sirloin, pork tenderloin, cut into thin strips; or medium peeled and deveined shrimp. Let your pantry and your preferences be your guide.

⅓ cup Chicken Stock (page 149) or low-sodium chicken broth

2 tablespoons reduced-sodium soy sauce

2 tablespoons dry sherry

2 teaspoons cornstarch

¼ teaspoon Asian sesame oil

4 teaspoons canola oil, divided

1 pound boneless skinless chicken breast, cut into thin strips

2 garlic cloves, minced

4 cups broccoli florets, cut into 1-inch pieces

1 small red bell pepper, thinly sliced

2 scallions, thinly sliced

1 Combine the stock, soy sauce, sherry, cornstarch, and sesame oil in a small bowl and stir until the cornstarch dissolves.

2 Heat a large wok or nonstick skillet over medium-high heat. Add 2 teaspoons of the canola oil and tilt the pan to coat the bottom evenly. Add the chicken and cook, stirring constantly, until lightly browned, 2 to 3 minutes. Transfer the chicken to a plate and wipe out the wok with paper towels.

3 Add the remaining 2 teaspoons canola oil to the wok over medium-high heat. Add the garlic and cook, stirring constantly, until fragrant, 30 seconds. Add the broccoli and bell pepper and cook, stirring constantly, until crisp-tender, 3 minutes. Stir in the chicken and the stock mixture and cook until the sauce is thickened,

30 seconds. Remove from the heat and stir in the scallions. Divide evenly among 4 plates and serve at once.

Each serving: 8 g carb, 215 cal, 8 g fat, 1 g sat fat, 63 mg chol, 3 g fib, 26 g pro, 391 mg sod • Carb Choices: ½; Exchanges: 1 veg, 3 lean protein, 1 fat

GINGER CHICKEN AND ASPARAGUS STIR-FRY QUICK : Follow the Chicken Stir-Fry with Broccoli recipe, at left, adding 1 tablespoon minced fresh ginger with the garlic in step 3. Substitute 1 pound asparagus, tough ends removed, cut into 1-inch pieces, for the broccoli.

Each serving: 7 g carb, 211 cal, 8 g fat, 1 g sat fat, 63 mg chol, 2 g fib, 26 g pro, 373 mg sod • Carb Choices: ½; Exchanges: 1 veg, 3 lean protein

Lemon Chicken and Snow Pea Stir-Fry QUICK

makes 4 servings

This stir-fry relies more on zesty lemon than on soy sauce to give it a punch of flavor. Always use a vegetable brush to thoroughly scrub any citrus fruit before grating the zest.

½ cup Chicken Stock (page 149) or low-sodium chicken broth

2 tablespoons reduced-sodium soy sauce

2 teaspoons grated lemon zest

2 tablespoons lemon juice

2 teaspoons cornstarch

1 teaspoon sugar

4 teaspoons canola oil, divided

1 pound boneless skinless chicken breast, cut into thin strips

2 garlic cloves, minced

4 cups snow peas, trimmed and cut in half on the diagonal

2 scallions, thinly sliced

1 Combine the stock, soy sauce, lemon zest, lemon juice, cornstarch, and sugar in a small bowl and stir until the cornstarch and sugar dissolve.

2 Heat a large wok or nonstick skillet over medium-high heat. Add 2 teaspoons of the oil and tilt the pan to coat the bottom evenly. Add the chicken and cook, stirring constantly, until lightly browned, 2 to 3 minutes. Transfer the chicken to a plate and wipe out the wok with paper towels.

3 Add the remaining 2 teaspoons oil to the wok over medium-high heat. Add the garlic and cook, stirring constantly, until fragrant, 30 seconds. Add the snow peas and cook, stirring constantly, until crisp-tender, 3 minutes. Stir in the chicken and the stock mixture and cook until the sauce is thickened, 30 seconds. Remove from the heat and stir in the scallions. Divide evenly among 4 plates and serve at once.

Each serving: 8 g carb, 207 cal, 7 g fat, 1 g sat fat, 63 mg chol, 1 g fib, 25 g pro, 381 mg sod • Carb Choices: ½; Exchanges: 1 veg, 3 lean protein, 1 fat

Thai Chicken and Basil Stir-Fry QUICK

makes 4 servings

As good as most Thai takeout, this stir-fry takes just a few minutes to make. I love the big handful of basil thrown into this dish, but I also usually add about ½ teaspoon of chili-garlic paste with the chicken stock mixture for just a hint of heat.

⅓ cup Chicken Stock (page 149) or low-sodium chicken broth
2 tablespoons dry sherry
1 tablespoon reduced-sodium soy sauce
1 tablespoon Asian fish sauce
2 teaspoons cornstarch
1 teaspoon sugar
¼ teaspoon Asian sesame oil
4 teaspoons canola oil, divided
1 pound boneless skinless chicken breast, cut into thin strips

2 garlic cloves, minced
1 large yellow bell pepper, cut into thin strips
1 medium red onion, halved lengthwise and thinly sliced
1 jalapeño, seeded and minced
⅓ cup thinly sliced fresh basil leaves
1 tablespoon lime juice

1 Combine the stock, sherry, soy sauce, fish sauce, cornstarch, sugar, and sesame oil in a small bowl and stir until the cornstarch and sugar dissolve.

2 Heat a large wok or nonstick skillet over medium-high heat. Add 2 teaspoons of the canola oil and tilt the pan to coat the bottom evenly. Add the chicken and cook, stirring constantly, until lightly browned, 2 to 3 minutes. Transfer the chicken to a plate and wipe out the wok with paper towels.

3 Add the remaining 2 teaspoons canola oil to the wok over medium-high heat. Add the garlic and cook, stirring constantly, until fragrant, 30 seconds. Add the bell pepper, onion, and jalapeño and cook, stirring constantly, until crisp-tender, 3 minutes. Stir in the chicken and the stock mixture and cook until the sauce is thickened, 30 seconds. Remove from the heat and stir in the basil and lime juice. Divide evenly among 4 plates and serve at once.

Each serving: 10 g carb, 217 cal, 8 g fat, 1 g sat fat, 63 mg chol, 2 g fib, 25 g pro, 569 mg sod • Carb Choices: ½; Exchanges: 1 veg, 3 lean protein, 1 fat

Peanut Chicken with Green Beans QUICK

makes 4 servings

This recipe takes what might be a ho-hum dinner—chicken and green beans—and turns it into an unusual and tasty meal. It is also especially good made with shrimp instead of chicken.

8 ounces trimmed green beans
¼ cup natural creamy peanut butter
2 tablespoons reduced-sodium soy sauce
2 tablespoons rice vinegar
1 tablespoon water
4 teaspoons canola oil, divided
1 pound boneless skinless chicken breast, cut into thin strips
2 garlic cloves, minced
1 small red bell pepper, thinly sliced
2 scallions, thinly sliced
¼ cup chopped fresh cilantro

1 Fill a medium saucepan half full with water and bring to a boil over high heat. Add the green beans, return to a boil, and cook just until crisp-tender, about 3 minutes. Drain, let cool slightly, and pat dry with paper towels.

2 Whisk together the peanut butter, soy sauce, vinegar, and water in a small bowl until smooth.

3 Heat a large wok or nonstick skillet over medium-high heat. Add 2 teaspoons of the oil and tilt the pan to coat the bottom evenly. Add the chicken and cook, stirring constantly, until lightly browned, 2 to 3 minutes. Transfer the chicken to a plate and wipe out the wok with paper towels.

4 Add the remaining 2 teaspoons oil to the wok over medium-high heat. Add the garlic and cook, stirring constantly, until fragrant, 30 seconds. Add the green beans, bell pepper, and scallions and cook, stirring constantly, until crisp-tender, 3 minutes. Stir in the chicken and the peanut butter mixture and cook until the sauce is thickened, 30 seconds. Remove from the heat and stir in the cilantro. Divide evenly among 4 plates and serve at once.

Each serving: 10 g carb, 294 cal, 15 g fat, 2 g sat fat, 63 mg chol, 3 g fib, 28 g pro, 422 mg sod • Carb Choices: ½; Exchanges: 2 veg, 3 lean protein, 2½ fat

Stir-Fried Chicken and Vegetables with Black Bean Sauce QUICK

makes 4 servings

Black bean sauce is made from fermented Chinese black beans, garlic, soy sauce, and spices. A small amount adds a pungent salty flavor to a stir-fry. Look for it in the Asian foods section of the supermarket. It will last for months in the refrigerator and you'll love adding it to any basic stir-fry for instant flavor.

⅓ cup Chicken Stock (page 149) or low-sodium chicken broth
2 tablespoons dry sherry
1 tablespoon black bean sauce
2 teaspoons cornstarch
¼ teaspoon Asian sesame oil
4 teaspoons canola oil, divided
1 pound boneless skinless chicken breast, cut into thin strips
2 garlic cloves, minced
2 cups broccoli florets, cut into 1-inch pieces
1 cup fresh sugar snap peas, trimmed
1 large carrot, peeled and cut into short, thin strips
1 small red bell pepper, thinly sliced
¼ cup chopped fresh cilantro

1 Combine the stock, sherry, black bean sauce, cornstarch, and sesame oil in a small bowl and stir until the cornstarch dissolves.

2 Heat a large wok or nonstick skillet over medium-high heat. Add 2 teaspoons of the canola oil and tilt the pan to coat the bottom evenly. Add the chicken and cook, stirring constantly, until lightly browned, 2 to 3 minutes. Transfer the chicken to a plate and wipe out the wok with paper towels.

3 Add the remaining 2 teaspoons canola oil to the wok over medium-high heat. Add the garlic and cook, stirring constantly, until fragrant, 30 seconds. Add the broccoli, peas, carrot, and bell pepper and cook, stirring constantly, until crisp-tender, 3 minutes. Stir in the chicken and the stock mixture and cook until the sauce is thickened, 30 seconds. Remove from the heat and stir in the cilantro. Divide evenly among 4 plates and serve at once.

Each serving: 11 g carb, 226 cal, 8 g fat, 1 g sat fat, 63 mg chol, 3 g fib, 26 g pro, 374 mg sod • Carb Choices: 1; Exchanges: 2 veg, 3 lean protein, 1½ fat

Chicken Pad Thai QUICK

makes 4 servings

If this is one of your restaurant favorites, try this vegetable-packed version at home. It's easy to make and comes together quickly once the vegetables are prepared. When you have all the ingredients in the skillet at the end of cooking, use tongs to toss everything together—the tongs make it easier to grab on to the noodles.

3 ounces wide rice noodles
¼ cup no-salt-added tomato sauce
2 tablespoons sugar
2 tablespoons Asian fish sauce
1 teaspoon chili-garlic paste
6 teaspoons canola oil, divided
8 ounces boneless skinless chicken breast, cut into thin strips

1 cup snow peas, trimmed and cut in half on the diagonal
1 small red bell pepper, thinly sliced
2 large eggs, lightly beaten
2 cups bean sprouts
4 scallions, thinly sliced on the diagonal
4 tablespoons chopped fresh cilantro
2 tablespoons chopped dry-roasted peanuts
Lime wedges

1 Cook the noodles according to the package directions.

2 Meanwhile, stir together the tomato sauce, sugar, fish sauce, and chili-garlic paste in a small bowl, stirring until the sugar dissolves.

3 Heat a large wok or nonstick skillet over medium-high heat. Add 2 teaspoons of the oil and tilt the pan to coat the bottom evenly. Add the chicken and cook, stirring constantly, until lightly browned, 2 to 3 minutes. Transfer the chicken to a plate and wipe out the wok with paper towels.

4 Add 2 teaspoons of the remaining oil to the wok over medium-high heat. Add the peas and bell pepper and cook, stirring constantly, until crisp-tender, 3 minutes. Transfer the vegetables to the plate with the chicken and wipe out the wok with paper towels.

5 Add the remaining 2 teaspoons oil to the wok over medium-high heat. Add the eggs and cook, stirring constantly, until almost firm. Add the chicken and vegetables, the noodles, tomato sauce mixture, bean sprouts, and scallions and cook, tossing constantly, until heated through, about 3 minutes. Spoon onto 4 plates, sprinkle evenly with the cilantro and peanuts, and serve at once with the lime wedges.

Each serving: 33 g carb, 312 cal, 12 g fat, 2 g sat fat, 84 mg chol, 3 g fib, 18 g pro, 758 mg sod • Carb Choices: 2; Exchanges: 1 starch, ½ carb, 1 veg, 2 lean protein, 2 fat

Braises and One-Pot Meals

Chicken and Dumplings

HIGH FIBER

makes 6 servings

This version of dumplings is almost like steamed biscuits that cook on top of the richly flavored soup. Cooking the chicken in chicken broth boosts the flavor of the broth and the chicken. You can double this recipe if it's a favorite for family get-togethers. Use a large Dutch oven instead of a saucepan if you double the recipe.

SOUP

1¼ pounds bone-in chicken breast halves, skinned

4 cups Chicken Stock (page 149) or low-sodium chicken broth

2 carrots, peeled and chopped

2 stalks celery, chopped

1 medium onion, chopped

¼ teaspoon dried thyme

2 tablespoons chopped fresh Italian parsley

DUMPLINGS

1 cup white whole wheat flour or unbleached all-purpose flour

1 teaspoon baking powder

½ teaspoon baking soda

¼ teaspoon salt

2 tablespoons unsalted butter

½ cup low-fat buttermilk

1 To make the soup, place the chicken in a large saucepan. Add the stock and bring just to a simmer over medium heat. Cover, reduce the heat to low, and simmer until the juices run clear, 15 to 20 minutes. Transfer the chicken to a plate to cool. Remove the meat from the bones and cut into bite-size pieces. Discard the skin and bones.

2 Add the carrots, celery, onion, and thyme to the stock remaining in the saucepan. Cover, return to a simmer over low heat, and cook until the vegetables are tender, 15 to 20 minutes. Stir in the chicken and parsley.

3 Meanwhile, to make the dumplings, combine the flour, baking powder, baking soda, salt, and butter in a medium bowl. Cut the butter into the dry ingredients using a pastry blender until the mixture resembles coarse meal. Stir in the buttermilk.

4 Drop the dough by rounded tablespoonfuls into the simmering soup. Cover and simmer until the dumplings are puffed and cooked through, about 20 minutes (do not allow to boil or the dumplings will fall apart). Ladle the soup and dumplings evenly into 6 bowls and serve at once.

Each serving: 22 g carb, 227 cal, 6 g fat, 3 g sat fat, 54 mg chol, 4 g fib, 21 g pro, 445 mg sod • Carb Choices: 1½; Exchanges: 1 carb, 1 veg, 3 lean protein, ½ fat

Chicken Pot Pie

makes 6 servings

Phyllo dough makes a light and crispy low-carb crust for this homey one-dish meal. It's great for weekend entertaining. Serve it with a salad and a classic dessert such as Apple-Walnut Crisp (page 538) or Lemon Pound Cake (page 568) to round out the meal.

7 teaspoons extra virgin olive oil, divided

1½ pounds boneless skinless chicken breast, cut into 1-inch pieces

¾ teaspoon kosher salt, divided

½ teaspoon freshly ground pepper, divided

1 medium onion, chopped

1 stalk celery, chopped

⅓ cup unbleached all-purpose flour

2 garlic cloves, minced

2 cups Chicken Stock (page 149) or low-sodium chicken broth

1½ cups 1% low-fat milk

8 ounces small red-skinned potatoes, well scrubbed and chopped

2 carrots, peeled and chopped

½ pound green beans, trimmed and cut into 1-inch pieces

¼ cup chopped fresh Italian parsley

1 tablespoon chopped fresh sage or 1 teaspoon crumbled dried sage

4 sheets frozen phyllo, thawed

4 tablespoons freshly grated Parmesan

1 Preheat the oven to 350°F. Brush a 2-quart baking dish with 1 teaspoon of the oil.

2 Sprinkle the chicken with ½ teaspoon of the salt and ¼ teaspoon of the pepper. Heat a large nonstick skillet over medium-high heat. Add 2 teaspoons of the remaining oil and tilt the pan to coat the bottom evenly. Add the chicken and cook, stirring often, until well browned, about 8 minutes. Transfer to the prepared baking dish.

3 Add 2 teaspoons of the remaining oil to the skillet. Add the onion and celery and cook, stirring often, until softened, 5 minutes. Add the flour and garlic and cook, stirring constantly, 1 minute. Gradually whisk in the stock and milk and cook, whisking constantly, until the mixture comes to a boil.

4 Add the potatoes, carrots, green beans, remaining ¼ teaspoon salt, and remaining ¼ teaspoon pepper. Cover, reduce the heat, and simmer until the potato is almost tender, about 6 minutes. Stir in the parsley and sage. Carefully pour the vegetable mixture over the chicken in the baking dish.

5 Unroll the phyllo and place one sheet on top of the chicken mixture. Brush the phyllo lightly with some of the remaining 2 teaspoons oil. Sprinkle with 1 tablespoon of the Parmesan. Repeat the layering with remaining phyllo, oil, and Parmesan, ending with the Parmesan. Tuck the overhanging edges of the phyllo inside the baking dish.

6 Place the baking dish on a large baking sheet and bake until the filling is bubbly and the phyllo is lightly browned, 30 minutes. Divide the pot pie evenly among 6 plates and serve at once.

Each serving: 28 g carb, 347 cal, 11 g fat, 3 g sat fat, 75 mg chol, 3 g fib, 33 g pro, 409 mg sod • Carb Choices: 2; Exchanges: 1½ starch, 1 veg, 4 lean protein, 1 fat

Chicken, Mushroom, and Spinach Lasagna [HIGH FIBER]

makes 6 servings

Using no-boil noodles and frozen spinach saves time, making usually labor-intensive lasagna easy enough to enjoy on a weeknight. Children—and spouses—of all ages will love this dish.

5 teaspoons extra virgin olive oil, divided
8 ounces boneless skinless chicken breast
¼ teaspoon kosher salt
¼ teaspoon freshly ground pepper, divided
8 ounces cremini or white mushrooms, sliced
1 small onion, diced
2 garlic cloves, minced
1 (14½-ounce) can no-salt-added diced tomatoes
1 (8-ounce) can no-salt-added tomato sauce
2 tablespoons chopped fresh basil
1 cup part-skim ricotta
4 ounces shredded part-skim mozzarella (about 1 cup)
1 (10-ounce) package frozen chopped spinach, thawed and squeezed dry
9 no-boil lasagna noodles
1 ounce freshly grated Parmesan (about ¼ cup)

1 Preheat the oven to 375°F. Brush an 11 x 7-inch glass baking dish with 1 teaspoon of the oil.

2 Sprinkle the chicken with the salt and ⅛ teaspoon of the pepper. Heat a large nonstick skillet over medium-high heat. Add 2 teaspoons of the remaining oil and tilt the pan to coat the bottom evenly. Add the chicken and cook, turning often, until well browned, about 8 minutes. Transfer to a cutting board and finely chop.

3 Add the remaining 2 teaspoons oil to the skillet. Add the mushrooms and onion and cook, stirring often, until the mushrooms are tender and most of the liquid has evaporated, about 8 minutes. Add the garlic and cook, stirring constantly, until fragrant, 30 seconds. Add the chicken, tomatoes, tomato sauce, and remaining ⅛ teaspoon pepper and bring to a boil. Cook, stirring often, until the sauce is slightly thickened, about 5 minutes. Stir in the basil.

4 Combine the ricotta, mozzarella, and spinach in a medium bowl and stir until well mixed.

5 Spread 1 cup of the sauce in the bottom of the baking dish. Place 3 noodles over the sauce, breaking them as needed to fit the dish. Top the noodles with 1 cup of the cheese mixture and 1 cup of the sauce. Repeat the layering, ending with the noodles. Spread the remaining sauce over the top layer of noodles.

6 Cover the baking dish with foil and place the dish on a large rimmed baking sheet. Bake until the noodles are tender, 30 minutes. Uncover the dish, sprinkle with the Parmesan, and bake, uncovered, until the Parmesan melts, 5 minutes. Let stand 10 minutes before serving. Cut the lasagna into 6 pieces and serve at once.

Each serving: 32 g carb, 326 cal, 11 g fat, 4 g sat fat, 44 mg chol, 4 g fib, 24 g pro, 386 mg sod • Carb Choices: 2; Exchanges: 1½ starch, 1 veg, 2 medium-fat protein, 1 lean protein, 1 fat

Coq au Vin

makes 6 servings

This classic French chicken and wine stew is usually laden with bacon. In this light and healthful version, you brown the chicken in the drippings of just two strips of cooked bacon, then stir the chopped bacon into the dish just before serving. It's just enough to make a rich, intensely flavored dish that will satisfy any Francophile.

2 strips center-cut bacon

2½ pounds bone-in chicken pieces, skinned

½ teaspoon kosher salt, divided

½ teaspoon freshly ground pepper, divided

2 tablespoons unbleached all-purpose flour

8 ounces cremini or white mushrooms, sliced

2 stalks celery, chopped

2 carrots, peeled and chopped

1 medium onion, chopped

1½ cups dry red wine

½ cup Chicken Stock (page 149) or low-sodium chicken broth

1 tablespoon no-salt-added tomato paste

1 sprig fresh thyme or ½ teaspoon dried thyme

3 tablespoons chopped fresh Italian parsley

1 Cook the bacon in a large, deep-sided skillet over medium-high heat until crisp. Drain on paper towels and chop. Pour off and discard all but 2 teaspoons of the drippings.

2 Sprinkle the chicken with ¼ teaspoon of the salt and ¼ teaspoon of the pepper. Sprinkle evenly with the flour. Add the chicken to the skillet and cook, turning often, until well browned on all sides, about 8 minutes. Transfer to a plate.

3 Add the mushrooms, celery, carrots, and onion to the skillet and cook, stirring often, until softened, 5 minutes. Add the wine, stock, tomato paste, thyme, the remaining ¼ teaspoon salt and ¼ teaspoon pepper and bring to a boil. Return the chicken to the skillet. Cover, reduce the heat to low, and simmer until the juices of the chicken run clear, about 30 minutes. Stir in the parsley and the bacon. Divide the chicken evenly among 6 plates, top evenly with the vegetables and sauce, and serve at once.

Each serving: 10 g carb, 206 cal, 4 g fat, 1 g sat fat, 65 mg chol, 2 g fib, 22 g pro, 254 mg sod • Carb Choices: ½; Exchanges: 1 veg, 3 lean protein

Braised Chicken with Orange-Caper Sauce

makes 6 servings

Salty capers and sweet oranges make a vibrant sauce for chicken. You can make this with skinned bone-in chicken thighs if your family prefers dark meat.

4 large oranges

2½ pounds bone-in chicken pieces, skinned

1½ teaspoons ground cumin, divided

½ teaspoon kosher salt, divided

¼ teaspoon freshly ground pepper

2 teaspoons extra virgin olive oil

1 small onion, halved lengthwise and thinly sliced

1 cup Chicken Stock (page 149) or low-sodium chicken broth

1 tablespoon capers, rinsed and drained

3 tablespoons chopped fresh Italian parsley

1 Grate 1 tablespoon zest and squeeze 1 cup juice from the oranges and set aside.

2 Sprinkle the chicken with 1 teaspoon of the cumin, ¼ teaspoon of the salt, and the pepper. Heat a large nonstick skillet over medium-high heat. Add the oil and tilt the pan to coat the bottom evenly. Add the chicken and cook, turning often, until well browned on all sides, about 8 minutes. Transfer to a plate.

3 Add the onion to the skillet and cook, stirring often, until softened, 5 minutes. Add the stock, capers, orange juice, the remaining ½ teaspoon cumin, and the remaining ¼ teaspoon salt and bring to a boil. Return the chicken to the skillet. Cover, reduce the heat to low, and simmer until the juices of the chicken run clear and the sauce is slightly thickened, about 30 minutes. Stir in the parsley. Divide the chicken evenly among 6 plates. Spoon the sauce evenly over the chicken and serve at once.

Each serving: 6 g carb, 153 cal, 5 g fat, 1 g sat fat, 63 mg chol, 1 g fib, 21 g pro, 234 mg sod • Carb Choices: ½; Exchanges: ½ carb, 4 lean protein, ½ fat

Chicken Simmered with Fennel and Tomatoes

makes 4 servings

A spoonful of Dijon infuses the sauce of this dish with mild mustard flavor. Serve it with whole wheat orzo or brown basmati rice so you can enjoy every last drop.

4 (6-ounce) bone-in chicken breast halves, skinned

½ teaspoon kosher salt, divided

¼ teaspoon freshly ground pepper, divided

2 tablespoons unbleached all-purpose flour

4 teaspoons extra virgin olive oil, divided

1 medium fennel bulb, tough outer leaves removed, cored and thinly sliced

1 small onion, halved lengthwise and thinly sliced

1 garlic clove, minced

1½ cups Chicken Stock (page 149) or low-sodium chicken broth

1 tablespoon Dijon mustard

1 cup cherry tomatoes, halved

2 tablespoons chopped fresh Italian parsley

1 Sprinkle the chicken with ¼ teaspoon of the salt and ⅛ teaspoon of the pepper, then with the flour. Heat a large deep skillet over medium heat. Add 2 teaspoons of the oil and tilt the pan to coat the bottom evenly. Add the chicken and cook, turning often, until well browned on both sides, about 8 minutes. Transfer to a plate.

2 Add the remaining 2 teaspoons oil to the skillet and tilt the pan to coat the bottom evenly. Add the fennel and onion to the skillet and cook, stirring often, until softened, 5 minutes. Add the garlic and cook, stirring constantly until fragrant, 30 seconds. Add the stock, mustard, remaining ¼ teaspoon salt, and remaining ⅛ teaspoon pepper and stir to combine. Return the chicken to the skillet and bring to a boil. Cover, reduce the heat to low, and simmer until the juices of the chicken run clear, about 30 minutes. Add the tomatoes and cook just until heated through, 1 minute. Stir in the parsley. Divide the chicken among 4 plates. Spoon the vegetables and cooking liquid over the chicken and serve at once.

Each serving: 11 g carb, 240 cal, 8 g fat, 2 g sat fat, 72 mg chol, 3 g fib, 30 g pro, 374 mg sod • Carb Choices: 1; Exchanges: ½ starch, 2 veg, 3 lean protein, 1 fat

Moroccan Chicken with Dried Apricots and Olives

QUICK

makes 4 servings

Sweet dried apricots and salty olives flavor this exotically spiced chicken. Serve it with whole wheat couscous and steamed green beans for a superb weeknight meal.

¾ teaspoon ground cumin

½ teaspoon kosher salt

½ teaspoon ground ginger

¼ teaspoon ground cinnamon

⅛ teaspoon ground cayenne

4 (4-ounce) skinless boneless chicken thighs

4 teaspoons extra virgin olive oil, divided

1 medium onion, halved lengthwise and thinly sliced

½ cup dry white wine

½ cup Chicken Stock (page 149) or low-sodium chicken broth

6 dried apricots, quartered

8 green olives, pitted and halved

2 tablespoons chopped fresh Italian parsley

1 teaspoon sherry vinegar or white wine vinegar

1 Stir together the cumin, salt, ginger, cinnamon, and cayenne in a small bowl. Sprinkle the chicken with 1½ teaspoons of the spice mixture. Heat a large deep skillet over medium-high heat. Add 2 teaspoons of the oil and tilt the pan to coat the bottom evenly. Add the chicken and cook until well browned, about 3 minutes on each side. Transfer to a plate.

2 Add the remaining 2 teaspoons oil to the skillet and tilt the pan to coat the bottom evenly. Add the onion and cook, stirring often, until softened, 5 minutes. Add the wine and stock and bring to a boil. Return the chicken to the skillet. Add the apricots, olives, and remaining spice mixture and cook until the sauce is slightly thickened, 6 to 8 minutes. Stir in the parsley and vinegar. Divide the chicken among 4 plates. Spoon the sauce evenly over the chicken and serve at once.

Each serving: 11 g carb, 285 cal, 14 g fat, 3 g sat fat, 76 mg chol, 1 g fib, 22 g pro, 335 mg sod • Carb Choices: 1; Exchanges: 1 carb, 3 lean protein, 1 fat

Spanish Braised Chicken with Tomatoes and Peppers

makes 4 servings

Smoked paprika gives this dish a slight smoky flavor, but if you don't have any on hand, it is still delicious with regular paprika. The dish simmers just long enough for you to cook some couscous and toss a salad to make the meal complete.

4 (6-ounce) chicken thighs, skinned
2 teaspoons smoked paprika, divided
½ teaspoon kosher salt
2 teaspoons extra virgin olive oil
1 red or yellow bell pepper, thinly sliced
1 small onion, halved lengthwise and thinly sliced
2 garlic cloves, minced

1 (14½-ounce) can no-salt-added diced tomatoes
⅔ cup dry sherry
½ cup Chicken Stock (page 149) or low-sodium chicken broth
1 tablespoon no-salt-added tomato paste
2 tablespoons chopped fresh Italian parsley
1 teaspoon sherry vinegar or white wine vinegar

1 Sprinkle the chicken with 1 teaspoon of the paprika and the salt. Heat a large deep skillet over medium-high heat. Add the oil and tilt the pan to coat the bottom evenly. Add the chicken and cook until well browned, about 3 minutes on each side. Transfer to a plate.

2 Add the bell pepper and onion to the skillet and cook, stirring often, until softened, 5 minutes. Add the garlic and cook, stirring constantly, until fragrant, 30 seconds. Add the tomatoes, sherry, stock, tomato paste, and remaining 1 teaspoon paprika and bring to a boil. Return the chicken to the skillet, reduce the heat to low, cover, and simmer 20 minutes. Uncover and cook until the sauce is slightly thickened, about 10 minutes. Stir in the parsley and vinegar. Divide the chicken among 4 plates. Spoon the sauce evenly over the chicken and serve at once.

Each serving: 11 g carb, 211 cal, 6 g fat, 1 g sat fat, 81 mg chol, 3 g fib, 21 g pro, 292 mg sod • Carb Choices: 1; Exchanges: 2 veg, 3 lean protein, ½ fat

Chicken with Potatoes, Lemon, and Sage

makes 4 servings

Because they are higher in fat than chicken breasts, thighs are perfect for braising. They stay moist and tender and soak up the flavors of the braising liquid. The lemon slices soften and almost fall apart by the time the chicken is done, infusing their flavor throughout the dish.

4 (6-ounce) chicken thighs, skinned
½ teaspoon kosher salt, divided
¼ teaspoon freshly ground pepper, divided
4 teaspoons extra virgin olive oil, divided
4 lemon slices, about ¼ inch thick and seeded
1 small onion, thinly sliced
2 garlic cloves, minced
1½ cups Chicken Stock (page 149) or low-
**   sodium chicken broth**
1 tablespoon chopped fresh sage or 1 teaspoon
**   crumbled dried sage**
1 pound fingerling or baby potatoes, well
**   scrubbed and halved**

1 Preheat the oven to 350°F.

2 Sprinkle the chicken with ¼ teaspoon of the salt and ⅛ teaspoon of the pepper. Heat a large nonstick skillet over medium-high heat. Add 2 teaspoons of the oil and tilt the pan to coat. Add the chicken and cook until well browned, 3 minutes on each side. Transfer to a large baking dish.

3 Add the lemon slices to the skillet and cook until lightly browned, about 1 minute on each side. Transfer to the baking dish with the chicken.

4 Add the remaining 2 teaspoons oil to the skillet and tilt the pan to coat. Add the onion and cook, stirring often, until tender, 5 minutes. Add the garlic and cook, stirring constantly, until fragrant, 30 seconds. Add the stock, sage, remaining ¼ teaspoon salt, and remaining ⅛ teaspoon pepper and stir, scraping the bottom of the pan to release the browned bits. Bring to a boil. Carefully pour the stock mixture over the chicken. Add the potatoes to the baking dish.

5 Cover with foil and bake until the potatoes are tender, 40 to 45 minutes. Divide the chicken, potatoes, and lemon slices among 4 large shallow bowls. Spoon the cooking juices evenly over each serving.

Each serving: 23 g carb, 266 cal, 9 g fat, 2 g sat fat, 82 mg chol, 3 g fib, 23 g pro, 284 mg sod • Carb Choices: 1½; Exchanges: 1½ starch, 3 lean protein, 1 fat

New Orleans Chicken Stew QUICK | HIGH FIBER

makes 4 servings

This easy dish is a satisfying example of "less-is-more" cooking. Cubes of chicken, ordinary vegetables, and pantry-staple spices combine to make a family-pleasing dinner. You can omit or decrease the hot sauce, depending on your taste. Serve the stew over brown rice.

1 pound boneless skinless chicken thighs, cut
**   into 1-inch pieces**
1 teaspoon paprika
¼ teaspoon freshly ground pepper
¾ teaspoon kosher salt, divided
2 teaspoons extra virgin olive oil
1 medium onion, chopped
1 small green bell pepper, chopped
1 small red bell pepper, chopped
1 stalk celery, chopped
2 garlic cloves, minced
2 (14½-ounce) cans no-salt-added diced tomatoes
½ teaspoon dried oregano
½ to 1 teaspoon hot sauce

1 Place the chicken in a medium bowl, add the paprika, ground pepper, and ½ teaspoon of the salt, and toss to coat. Heat a large deep skillet over medium-high heat. Add the oil and tilt the pan to coat the bottom evenly. Add the chicken and cook, stirring often, until well browned, about 5 minutes.

2 Add the onion, bell peppers, and celery and cook, stirring often, until the vegetables begin to soften, 3 minutes. Add the garlic and cook, stirring constantly, until fragrant, 30 seconds. Add the tomatoes, oregano, and remaining ¼ teaspoon salt and bring to a boil. Reduce the heat to low, cover, and simmer until the chicken and vegetables are very tender, about 20 minutes. Uncover and cook until the sauce is slightly thickened, about 10 minutes. Stir in the hot sauce. Divide the stew evenly among 4 shallow bowls and serve at once.

Each serving: 15 g carb, 251 cal, 11 g fat, 3 g sat fat, 74 mg chol, 5 g fib, 23 g pro, 387 mg sod • Carb Choices: 1; Exchanges: 3 veg, 3 lean protein, ½ fat

Chicken and Pasta with Goat Cheese Sauce

QUICK | HIGH FIBER

makes 4 servings

Omit the chicken and this dish makes a hearty vegetarian entrée. You can also serve smaller portions without the chicken as a side dish with simply prepared fish fillets or shrimp.

4 ounces whole wheat penne or other short pasta (about 1½ cups)

2 (4-ounce) skinless boneless chicken breasts

½ teaspoon kosher salt, divided

¼ teaspoon freshly ground pepper, divided

4 teaspoons extra virgin olive oil, divided

1 medium zucchini, halved lengthwise and thinly sliced

1 medium yellow squash, halved lengthwise and thinly sliced

1 red or yellow bell pepper, thinly sliced

3 ounces crumbled goat cheese (about ¾ cup), at room temperature

1 cup cherry tomatoes, halved

3 tablespoons chopped fresh basil or Italian parsley

1 Cook the pasta according to the package directions. Drain in a colander, reserving ½ cup of the cooking water.

2 Meanwhile, sprinkle the chicken with ¼ teaspoon of the salt and ⅛ teaspoon of the ground pepper. Heat a large nonstick skillet over medium heat. Add 2 teaspoons of the oil and tilt the pan to coat the bottom evenly. Add the chicken and cook, turning once, until the juices run clear, about 4 minutes on each side. Transfer to a plate.

3 Increase the heat to medium-high. Add the remaining 2 teaspoons oil to the skillet and tilt the pan to coat the bottom evenly. Add the zucchini, yellow squash, and bell pepper and cook, stirring often, until crisp-tender, about 3 minutes.

4 Transfer the squash mixture to a large bowl. Thinly slice the chicken breasts and add to the bowl. Add the pasta and goat cheese and toss to combine, adding the reserved pasta cooking water 1 tablespoon at a time, as needed to make a smooth sauce. Stir in the tomatoes, basil, remaining ¼ teaspoon salt, and remaining ⅛ teaspoon ground pepper. Divide evenly among 4 serving plates and serve at once.

Each serving: 28 g carb, 307 cal, 13 g fat, 6 g sat fat, 48 mg chol, 4 g fib, 22 g pro, 288 mg sod • Carb Choices: 2; Exchanges: 1½ starch, 1 veg, 1 medium-fat protein, 2 lean protein, 1 fat

Creamy Chicken Fettuccini QUICK | HIGH FIBER

makes 4 servings

Loaded with fresh vegetables, this pasta satisfies the craving for a creamy rich-tasting sauce without a lot of fat and calories.

4 ounces whole wheat fettuccini
2 (4-ounce) skinless boneless chicken breasts
½ teaspoon kosher salt, divided
¼ teaspoon freshly ground pepper, divided
4 teaspoons extra virgin olive oil, divided
1 medium red bell pepper, thinly sliced
1 medium yellow bell pepper, thinly sliced
1 small zucchini, halved lengthwise and sliced
1 small red onion, halved lengthwise and thinly sliced
2 garlic cloves, minced
2½ ounces reduced-fat cream cheese (about ⅓ cup), at room temperature, cut into small pieces
3 tablespoons chopped fresh Italian parsley
2 teaspoons grated lemon zest

1 Cook the pasta according to the package directions. Drain in a colander, reserving ½ cup of the cooking water.

2 Meanwhile, sprinkle the chicken with ¼ teaspoon of the salt and ⅛ teaspoon of the ground pepper. Heat a large nonstick skillet over medium heat. Add 2 teaspoons of the oil and tilt the pan to coat the bottom evenly. Add the chicken and cook, turning once, until the juices run clear, about 4 minutes on each side. Transfer to a plate.

3 Increase the heat to medium-high. Add the remaining 2 teaspoons oil to the skillet and tilt the pan to coat the bottom evenly. Add the bell peppers, zucchini, and onion and cook, stirring often, until crisp-tender, about 3 minutes. Add the garlic and cook, stirring constantly, until fragrant, 30 seconds.

4 Thinly slice the chicken breasts and add to the skillet. Remove from the heat and add the pasta and cream cheese and toss to combine, adding the reserved pasta cooking water 1 tablespoon at a time, as need to make a smooth sauce. Stir in the remaining ¼ teaspoon salt, remaining ⅛ teaspoon ground pepper, the parsley, and lemon zest. Divide evenly among 4 serving plates and serve at once.

Each serving: 28 g carb, 274 cal, 10 g fat, 4 g sat fat, 44 mg chol, 6 g fib, 19 g pro, 253 mg sod • Carb Choices: 2; Exchanges: 1½ starch, 1 veg, 2 lean protein, 1 fat

Chicken Biryani

makes 4 servings

The rice cooks along with the other ingredients in classic biryani, but because brown rice takes so much longer to cook than the typical white rice used in this dish, I've used cooked brown rice and stirred it in toward the end of cooking. The short cooking time keeps the flavors of the jalapeño, ginger, and fresh tomato vibrant and lively.

1½ teaspoons garam masala
1 teaspoon ground cumin
½ teaspoon kosher salt
¼ teaspoon ground cinnamon
1 pound boneless skinless chicken thighs, cut into 1-inch pieces
2 teaspoons canola oil
1 small onion, chopped
1 jalapeño, seeded and minced
1 tablespoon minced fresh ginger
2 garlic cloves, minced
½ cup Chicken Stock (page 149) or low-sodium chicken broth
1⅓ cups cooked brown basmati rice (page 108)
1 large tomato, chopped
¼ cup golden raisins
¼ cup chopped fresh cilantro
2 tablespoons sliced almonds
Lime wedges

1 Stir together the garam masala, cumin, salt, and cinnamon in a small dish. Sprinkle the chicken with half of the spice mixture. Heat a large nonstick skillet over medium-high heat. Add the oil and tilt the pan to coat the bottom evenly. Add the chicken and cook, stirring often, until well browned, about 6 minutes. Add the onion and jalapeño and cook, stirring often, until softened, 3 minutes. Stir in the ginger, garlic, and remaining spice mixture and cook, stirring constantly, until fragrant, 30 seconds.

2 Add the stock, rice, tomato, and raisins and bring to a boil. Cover, reduce the heat to low, and simmer until heated through, 3 minutes. Stir in the cilantro. Spoon into 4 bowls, sprinkle evenly with the almonds, and serve with the lime wedges.

Each serving: 28 g carb, 329 cal, 13 g fat, 3 g sat fat, 76 mg chol, 3 g fib, 25 g pro, 231 mg sod • Carb Choices: 2; Exchanges: 1 starch, ½ fruit, 1 veg, 3 lean protein, ½ fat

Quick Cassoulet HIGH FIBER

makes 6 servings

Making a traditional, hearty meat and bean cassoulet can be a days-long production. Canned beans, chicken thighs, and turkey kielbasa make this recipe an expeditious and satisfying—though not authentically French—weeknight meal.

1 pound boneless skinless chicken thighs, cut into 1-inch pieces
½ teaspoon kosher salt, divided
½ teaspoon freshly ground pepper, divided
4 teaspoons extra virgin olive oil, divided
4 ounces turkey kielbasa, cut into ½-inch slices
2 carrots, peeled and chopped
1 medium onion, chopped
1 stalk celery, chopped
2 garlic cloves, minced
1¼ cups Chicken Stock (page 149) or low-sodium chicken broth

1 (14½-ounce) can no-salt-added diced tomatoes
2 (15-ounce) cans no-salt-added cannellini beans, rinsed and drained
1 tablespoon no-salt-added tomato paste
½ teaspoon dried thyme
¼ cup chopped fresh Italian parsley
½ cup fresh whole wheat breadcrumbs
1 ounce freshly grated Parmesan (about ¼ cup)

1 Preheat the oven to 350°F.

2 Sprinkle the chicken with ¼ teaspoon of the salt and ¼ teaspoon of the pepper. Heat a large nonstick skillet over medium-high heat. Add 2 teaspoons of the oil and tilt the pan to coat the bottom evenly. Add the chicken and cook, stirring often, until well browned, about 6 minutes. Transfer to a large baking dish.

3 Add the sausage to the skillet and cook, turning often, until well browned, 4 minutes. Transfer to the baking dish with the chicken.

4 Add the carrots, onion, and celery to the skillet and cook, stirring often, until softened, 5 minutes. Add the garlic and cook, stirring constantly, until fragrant, 30 seconds. Add the stock and bring to a boil, stirring to scrape up the browned bits from the bottom of the skillet. Stir in the tomatoes, beans, tomato paste, thyme, remaining ¼ teaspoon salt, and remaining ¼ teaspoon pepper and bring to a boil. Stir in the parsley. Carefully pour the bean mixture over the chicken and sausage in the baking dish.

5 Stir together the breadcrumbs, Parmesan, and the remaining 2 teaspoons of oil in a small bowl and sprinkle evenly over the chicken mixture. Bake, uncovered, until the crumbs are browned, 20 to 25 minutes. Spoon the cassoulet evenly into 6 shallow bowls and serve at once.

Each serving: 28 g carb, 336 cal, 13 g fat, 3 g sat fat, 67 mg chol, 7 g fib, 27 g pro, 486 mg sod • Carb Choices: 1½; Exchanges: 1 starch, 1 veg, 2 lean protein, 1 plant-based protein, 1 fat

Chicken, Chorizo, and Rice Casserole HIGH FIBER

makes 4 servings

The key to baking long-cooking brown rice dishes is to have the cooking liquid at a boil when you pour it over the rice and then bake it at once. This is not a dish you can assemble ahead and bake later.

3 teaspoons canola oil, divided

½ cup long-grain brown rice

12 ounces boneless skinless chicken thighs, cut into 1-inch pieces

¼ teaspoon kosher salt

½ teaspoon paprika

¼ teaspoon freshly ground pepper

2 ounces cured chorizo, casings removed, chopped

1 small onion, chopped

1 small red bell pepper, chopped

1 stalk celery, chopped

2 garlic cloves, minced

¾ cup Chicken Stock (page 149) or low-sodium chicken broth

1 (14½-ounce) can no-salt-added diced tomatoes

1 Preheat the oven to 375°F. Brush an 11 x 7-inch baking dish with 1 teaspoon of the oil. Spread the rice in the prepared dish.

2 Sprinkle the chicken with the salt, paprika, and ground pepper. Heat a large nonstick skillet over medium-high heat. Add the remaining 2 teaspoons oil and tilt the pan to coat the bottom evenly. Add the chicken and cook, stirring often, until well browned, about 6 minutes. Transfer to the baking dish with the rice.

3 Add the sausage to the skillet and cook, turning often, until well browned, 4 minutes. Transfer to the baking dish with the chicken. Drain off and discard most of the drippings in the skillet, leaving the skillet just lightly coated.

4 Add the onion, bell pepper, and celery to the skillet and cook, stirring often, until softened, 5 minutes. Add the garlic and cook, stirring constantly, until fragrant, 30 seconds. Add the stock and tomatoes and bring to a boil, stirring to scrape up the browned bits from the bottom of the skillet. Carefully pour the vegetable mixture over the chicken and sausage in the baking dish. Cover the dish tightly with foil and bake 1 hour. Let stand, covered, for 15 minutes before serving. Spoon evenly into 4 plates and serve at once.

Each serving: 28 g carb, 348 cal, 16 g fat, 4 g sat fat, 70 mg chol, 4 g fib, 23 g pro, 371 mg sod • Carb Choices: 2; Exchanges: 1½ starch, 1 veg, 3 lean protein, 2 fat

Curried Chicken and Winter Vegetable Stew

HIGH FIBER

makes 4 servings

Stirring fresh spinach into this stew during the last few minutes of cooking adds fresh color and flavor to the finished dish. You can also use chopped fresh kale or escarole, but you'll need to simmer the stew about 5 minutes longer for these sturdier greens.

4 teaspoons canola oil, divided

1 pound boneless skinless chicken breast, cut into ½-inch cubes

1 medium onion, chopped

2 garlic cloves, minced

1 tablespoon curry powder

3½ cups Chicken Stock (page 149) or low-sodium chicken broth

1 (14½-ounce) can no-added-salt diced tomatoes

¼ cup no-added-salt tomato paste

2 carrots, peeled, halved lengthwise, and cut into 1-inch slices

1 medium parsnip, peeled, halved lengthwise,
    and cut into 1-inch slices
1 medium turnip, peeled and chopped
¼ cup golden raisins
8 ounces fresh spinach, trimmed and chopped

1 Heat a large saucepan over medium-high heat.
Add 2 teaspoons of the oil and tilt the pan to
coat the bottom evenly. Add the chicken and
cook, stirring often, until well browned, about
8 minutes. Transfer to a plate.

2 Add the remaining 2 teaspoons oil and tilt the
pan to coat the bottom evenly. Add the onion
and cook, stirring often, until softened, 5 minutes. Add the garlic and curry powder and cook,
stirring constantly, until fragrant, 30 seconds.
Add the stock, tomatoes, tomato paste, carrots, parsnip, turnip, raisins, and the chicken and
bring to a boil.

3 Cover, reduce the heat to low, and simmer until
the vegetables are tender, about 20 minutes.
Stir in the spinach and cook just until wilted,
2 minutes. Ladle the stew evenly into 4 bowls
and serve at once. The stew can be refrigerated,
covered, for up to 4 days.

Each serving: 32 g carb, 325 cal, 8 g fat, 2 g sat fat, 67 mg chol, 7 g fib,
31 g pro, 315 mg sod • Carb Choices: 2; Exchanges: ½ starch, ½ carb,
3 veg, 3 lean protein, 1 fat

Chicken and Peanut Stew

HIGH FIBER

makes 6 servings

This unusual stew is flavored with peanut butter,
which also slightly thickens the broth.

1 pound boneless skinless chicken thighs, cut
    into ½-inch pieces
½ teaspoon kosher salt
2 teaspoons extra virgin olive oil
2 tablespoons minced fresh ginger
2 garlic cloves, minced
3 cups Chicken Stock (page 149) or low-sodium
    chicken broth
2 medium sweet potatoes (about 1 pound),
    peeled and chopped
2 carrots, peeled and chopped
1 (14½-ounce) can no-salt added diced tomatoes
1 jalapeño pepper, chopped
⅛ teaspoon ground cayenne
¼ cup natural creamy peanut butter
4 cups chopped fresh spinach
2 tablespoons lime juice

1 Sprinkle the chicken with the salt. Heat a large
saucepan over medium-high heat. Add the oil and
tilt the pan to coat the bottom evenly. Add the
chicken and cook, stirring often, until well browned,
about 8 minutes. Add the ginger and garlic and
cook, stirring constantly, until fragrant, 30 seconds.

2 Add the stock, sweet potatoes, carrots, tomatoes, jalapeño, and cayenne and bring to a boil.
Cover, reduce the heat to low, and simmer until
the vegetables are tender, about 25 minutes. Add
the peanut butter and cook, stirring often, until
smooth. Stir in the spinach and cook just until
wilted, 2 minutes. Stir in the lime juice. Ladle the
stew evenly into 6 bowls and serve at once. The
stew can be refrigerated, covered, for up to 4 days.

Each serving: 20 g carb, 283 cal, 13 g fat, 3 g sat fat, 53 mg chol, 4 g fib,
21 g pro, 333 mg sod • Carb Choices: 1; Exchanges: 1 starch, 1 veg,
2 lean protein, 1½ fat

Chicken and White Bean Stew with Bacon and Arugula QUICK | HIGH FIBER

makes 4 servings

Just two strips of bacon imbue this stew with smoky flavor. Adding a few tablespoons of tomato paste to a soup or stew like this one is a great way to slightly thicken the broth and add another layer of tomato flavor to the finished dish.

2 strips smoked center-cut bacon

12 ounces boneless skinless chicken breast, cut into ½-inch cubes

1 small onion, chopped

1 large carrot, peeled and chopped

1 stalk celery, chopped

1 garlic clove, minced

3 cups Chicken Stock (page 149) or low-sodium chicken broth

1 (15-ounce) can no-salt-added cannellini beans, rinsed and drained

1 (14½-ounce) can no-salt-added diced tomatoes

3 tablespoons no-salt-added tomato paste

½ teaspoon dried oregano

¼ teaspoon freshly ground pepper

2 cups coarsely chopped arugula

2 tablespoons freshly grated Parmesan

1 Cook the bacon in a large saucepan over medium-high heat until crisp. Drain on paper towels. Drain the drippings into a small bowl and return 2 teaspoons of the bacon drippings to the saucepan. Add the chicken to the pan and cook, stirring often, until well browned, about 8 minutes. Transfer to a plate.

2 Add 2 teaspoons of the reserved bacon drippings to the saucepan (discard any remaining drippings). Add the onion, carrot, and celery and cook, stirring often, until softened, 5 minutes. Add the garlic and cook, stirring constantly, until fragrant, 30 seconds. Add the stock, beans, tomatoes, tomato paste, oregano, and pepper and bring to a boil.

3 Cover, reduce the heat to low, and simmer until the vegetables are tender, about 15 minutes. Chop the bacon. Stir in the bacon and arugula and cook just until the arugula is wilted, 2 minutes. Ladle the stew evenly into 4 bowls, sprinkle evenly with the Parmesan and serve at once. The stew can be refrigerated, covered, for up to 4 days.

Each serving: 26 g carb, 312 cal, 10 g fat, 4 g sat fat, 60 mg chol, 7 g fib, 30 g pro, 362 mg sod • Carb Choices: 1½; Exchanges: 1 starch, 2 veg, 3 lean protein, 1 fat

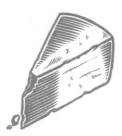

Chicken from the Oven

Oven-Fried Chicken with Creamy Gravy

makes 6 servings

An American classic, this baked "fried" chicken is almost as crispy as the fat-laden variety, thanks to the delightful crunchiness of ground Melba toast crumbs.

CHICKEN

½ teaspoon plus 1 tablespoon extra virgin olive oil, divided

15 whole wheat or white Melba toasts, crumbled

¼ cup unbleached all-purpose flour

1 large egg white

1 tablespoon water

2½ pounds bone-in chicken pieces, skinned

1 teaspoon kosher salt

⅛ teaspoon ground cayenne

GRAVY

1 tablespoon unsalted butter

3 tablespoons unbleached all-purpose flour

¾ cup Chicken Stock (page 149) or low-sodium chicken broth

¾ cup 1% low-fat milk

⅛ teaspoon dried sage

Pinch of freshly ground pepper

1 To make the chicken, position an oven rack in the top third of the oven. Preheat the oven to 375°F. Line a large rimmed baking pan with foil. Place a wire rack in the dish and brush the rack with ½ teaspoon of the oil.

2 Place the Melba toasts in a food processor and process until fine crumbs form. Place the Melba toast crumbs and the remaining 1 tablespoon oil in a shallow dish. Using your fingers, blend the oil evenly into the crumb mixture. Place the flour in another shallow dish. Place the egg white and water in another shallow dish and beat lightly with a fork.

3 Sprinkle the chicken pieces with the salt and cayenne. Dip the chicken, one piece at a time, into the flour, then into the egg white mixture, then into the Melba toast crumb mixture, pressing to adhere the crumbs.

4 Arrange the chicken in a single layer on the rack in the prepared pan. Bake until golden brown and the juices of the chicken run clear, about 45 minutes (do not turn).

5 Meanwhile, to make the gravy, melt the butter in a medium saucepan over medium heat. Add the flour and cook, stirring constantly, for 1 minute. Gradually whisk in the stock and milk.

6 Add the sage and pepper and cook, whisking constantly, until the mixture comes to a boil and thickens, about 2 minutes. Divide the chicken evenly among 6 plates, drizzle evenly with the gravy, and serve at once.

Each serving: 17 g carb, 239 cal, 8 g fat, 3 g sat fat, 70 mg chol, 1 g fib, 24 g pro, 404 mg sod • Carb Choices: 1; Exchanges: 1 carb, 3 lean protein, 1 fat

Lemon-Garlic Baked Chicken Breasts

makes 4 servings

This chicken dish sounds ordinary, but if you love lemon and chicken, it's really delicious. The mashed garlic thickens the sauce, as well as infusing it with flavor. You can use fresh basil or tarragon instead of the parsley if you prefer. Keeping the skin on the chicken while it bakes preserves moisture, but remove it before eating to cut calories and fat.

4 (6-ounce) bone-in skin-on chicken breasts
½ teaspoon kosher salt
⅛ teaspoon freshly ground pepper
2 teaspoons extra virgin olive oil
1 cup Chicken Stock (page 149) or low-sodium chicken broth
1 large lemon, thinly sliced and seeded
4 garlic cloves, crushed
2 tablespoons chopped fresh Italian parsley

1 Preheat the oven to 375°F.

2 Gently loosen but do not detach the skin from the chicken breasts. Rub the salt and pepper over the breast underneath the skin. Heat a large ovenproof skillet over medium-high heat. Add the oil, tilt the pan to coat the bottom evenly. Place the chicken in the skillet skin side down and cook, turning once, until both sides are well browned, about 6 minutes.

3 Add the stock to the skillet. Place the lemon slices and garlic cloves around the chicken. Transfer the skillet to the oven and bake until the juices of the chicken run clear, about 30 minutes.

4 Transfer the chicken to a large plate and cover loosely with foil to keep warm. Set the skillet over medium-high heat and bring the juices to a boil. Using a fork, mash the garlic into small bits. Boil the sauce until slightly thickened, about 3 minutes. Stir in the parsley. Divide the chicken and lemon slices evenly among 4 plates. Spoon the sauce evenly over the chicken and serve at once. Remove the skin before eating.

Each serving: 4 g carb, 176 cal, 5 g fat, 1 g sat fat, 72 mg chol, 1 g fib, 28 g pro, 235 mg sod • Carb Choices: 0; Exchanges: 4 lean protein, ½ fat

Orange-Soy Baked Chicken

makes 4 servings

I love making dishes such as this one where you do a few minutes of prep and then finish it in the oven. It gives you time to make a salad and a vegetable side dish and to have a glass of wine before dinner.

4 (6-ounce) bone-in skin-on chicken breasts
⅛ teaspoon freshly ground pepper
2 teaspoons extra virgin olive oil
¾ cup orange juice
2 tablespoons reduced-sodium soy sauce
½ teaspoon Asian sesame oil
¼ cup thinly sliced scallions

1 Preheat the oven to 375°F.

2 Gently loosen but do not detach the skin from the chicken breasts. Rub the pepper over the breast underneath the skin. Heat a large ovenproof skillet over medium-high heat. Add the olive oil and tilt the pan to coat the bottom evenly. Place the chicken in the skillet skin side down and cook, turning once, until both sides are well browned, about 6 minutes.

3 Stir together the orange juice, soy sauce, and sesame oil in a small bowl. Pour the orange juice mixture over the chicken. Transfer the skillet to the oven and bake until the juices of the chicken run clear, about 30 minutes.

4 Transfer the chicken to 4 plates and drizzle evenly with the pan juices. Sprinkle evenly with the scallions. Remove the skin before eating.

Each serving: 7 g carb, 200 cal, 6 g fat, 1 g sat fat, 71 mg chol, 0 g fib, 28 g pro, 362 mg sod • Carb Choices: ½; Exchanges: ½ fruit, 4 lean protein, ½ fat

Baked Chicken with Artichokes and Tomatoes

makes 4 servings

Plum tomatoes add a bright note to this one-dish meal with another of my favorite go-to ingredients—canned artichokes. If you're having a craving for something salty, throw a few Kalamata olives in with the tomatoes.

4 (6-ounce) bone-in skin-on chicken breasts
¼ teaspoon kosher salt
⅛ teaspoon freshly ground pepper
2 teaspoons extra virgin olive oil
1 cup Chicken Stock (page 149) or low-sodium chicken broth
1 (14-ounce) can artichoke hearts, drained
4 small plum tomatoes, halved
2 garlic cloves, minced
2 tablespoons chopped fresh Italian parsley

1 Preheat the oven to 375°F.

2 Gently loosen but do not detach the skin from the chicken breasts. Rub the salt and pepper over the breast underneath the skin. Heat a large ovenproof skillet over medium-high heat. Add the oil and tilt the pan to coat the bottom evenly. Place the chicken in the skillet, skin side down and cook, turning once, until both sides are well browned, about 6 minutes.

3 Add the stock to the skillet. Place the artichokes, tomatoes, and garlic around the chicken. Transfer the skillet to the oven and bake until the juices of the chicken run clear, about 30 minutes.

4 Transfer the chicken to 4 plates. Stir the parsley into the vegetables in the skillet. Divide the vegetables evenly among the plates. Remove the skin before eating.

Each serving: 9 g carb, 213 cal, 5 g fat, 1 g sat fat, 72 mg chol, 1 g fib, 30 g pro, 386 mg sod • Carb Choices: ½; Exchanges: 2 veg, 4 lean protein, ½ fat

Baked Chicken with Dried Plums and Balsamic Vinegar

makes 4 servings

This sweet-and-sour dish makes its own thickened sauce as it bakes because the dried plums (aka prunes) almost fall apart as they cook.

4 (6-ounce) bone-in skin-on chicken breasts
½ teaspoon plus ⅛ teaspoon kosher salt, divided
¼ teaspoon freshly ground pepper, divided
2 teaspoons extra virgin olive oil
1¼ cups Chicken Stock (page 149) or low-sodium chicken broth
¼ cup balsamic vinegar
½ cup pitted dried plums, quartered
2 garlic cloves, minced
2 tablespoons chopped fresh Italian parsley
1 teaspoon honey

1 Preheat the oven to 375°F.

2 Gently loosen but do not detach the skin from the chicken breasts. Rub ½ teaspoon of the salt and ⅛ teaspoon of the pepper over the breast underneath the skin. Heat a large ovenproof skillet over medium-high heat. Add the oil and tilt the pan to coat the bottom evenly. Place the chicken in the skillet skin side down and cook until both sides are well browned, about 6 minutes.

3 Add the stock and vinegar to the skillet. Place the plums and garlic around the chicken. Transfer the skillet to the oven and bake until the juices of the chicken run clear, about 30 minutes.

4 Transfer the chicken to 4 plates. Stir the parsley, honey, remaining ⅛ teaspoon salt, and remaining ⅛ teaspoon pepper into the sauce in the skillet. Spoon the sauce evenly over the chicken. Remove the skin before eating.

Each serving: 19 g carb, 240 cal, 5 g fat, 1 g sat fat, 72 mg chol, 2 g fib, 28 g pro, 274 mg sod • Carb Choices: 1; Exchanges: 1 carb, 4 lean protein, ½ fat

Lemongrass-Ginger Baked Chicken

makes 4 servings

Ordinary chicken is elevated to a fantastic meal with this intensely flavored rub. It's one of my favorites and is also terrific to rub onto shrimp before baking or grilling. Lemongrass can be very tough, so this is a great use for it, since all the ingredients are ground to a paste in the food processor.

1 teaspoon canola oil
1 cup cilantro leaves
¼ cup chopped fresh ginger
3 tablespoons thinly sliced lemongrass
2 tablespoons reduced-sodium soy sauce
2 garlic cloves, chopped
1 jalapeño, seeded and chopped
4 (6-ounce) bone-in skin-on chicken breasts
Lime wedges

1 Preheat the oven to 375°F. Brush a medium roasting pan with the oil.

2 Combine the cilantro, ginger, lemongrass, soy sauce, garlic, and jalapeño in a food processor and process until the mixture forms a finely minced paste (add a tablespoon or two of water, if necessary, to achieve the desired consistency).

3 Gently loosen but do not detach the skin from the chicken breasts. Rub the cilantro paste over the breast underneath the skin. Arrange the chicken skin side up in the prepared pan. Bake until the juices of the chicken run clear, 30 to 35 minutes. Divide the chicken among 4 plates and serve at once with the lime wedges. Remove the skin before eating.

Each serving: 3 g carb, 159 cal, 4 g fat, 1 g sat fat, 68 mg chol, 0 g fib, 26 g pro, 365 mg sod • Carb Choices: 0; Exchanges: 4 lean protein

Crispy Oven-Baked Chicken Breasts QUICK

makes 4 servings

Melba toasts are the secret ingredient that gives this chicken its fantastic crunch. If you make this dish often, as you are likely to do if you have "fried" chicken lovers at your house, grind up a whole box of Melba toasts at once and store them in an airtight container to make this recipe even faster.

½ teaspoon plus 1 tablespoon extra virgin olive oil, divided
10 whole wheat or white Melba toasts, crumbled
3 tablespoons unbleached all-purpose flour
1 large egg white
1 tablespoon water
1 teaspoon hot sauce
1 garlic clove, crushed through a press
4 (4-ounce) boneless skinless chicken breasts
¼ teaspoon dried oregano
¼ teaspoon dried basil
½ teaspoon kosher salt
⅛ teaspoon freshly ground pepper

1 Position an oven rack in the top third of the oven. Preheat the oven to 375°F. Brush a medium rimmed baking sheet with ½ teaspoon of the oil.

2 Place the Melba toasts in a food processor and process until fine crumbs form. Place the Melba toast crumbs and the remaining 1 tablespoon oil in a shallow dish. Using your fingers, blend the oil evenly into the crumb mixture.

3 Place the flour in a shallow dish. Place the egg white, water, hot sauce, and garlic in another shallow dish and beat lightly with a fork.

4 Sprinkle the chicken with the oregano, basil, salt, and pepper. Dip the chicken, one piece at a time into the flour, then into the egg white mixture, then into the crumb mixture, pressing to adhere the crumbs.

5 Arrange the chicken in a single layer on the prepared pan. Bake until the juices of the chicken run clear, 20 minutes (do not turn). Divide the chicken among 4 plates and serve at once.

Each serving: 14 g carb, 230 cal, 7 g fat, 1 g sat fat, 63 mg chol, 1 g fib, 26 g pro, 317 mg sod • Carb Choices: 1; Exchanges: 1 starch, 3 lean protein, ½ fat

PARMESAN-CRUSTED OVEN-BAKED CHICKEN BREASTS QUICK : Follow the Crispy Oven-Baked Chicken Breasts recipe, at left, reducing the Melba toasts to 7 and adding ⅓ cup freshly grated Parmesan to the crumb mixture in step 2. Proceed with the recipe.

Each serving: 11 g carb, 245 cal, 9 g fat, 3 g sat fat, 69 mg chol, 1 g fib, 28 g pro, 388 mg sod • Carb Choices: 1; Exchanges: 1 starch, 3 lean protein, 1 fat

How to Keep Chicken Breast Moist

The best cooking tip for moist and delicious boneless skinless chicken breast is not to overcook it. The recipes here all call for a 4-ounce portion, which will cook in about 8 minutes in a skillet, on the grill, or under the broiler. Always set a timer when you cook chicken, especially if you are distracted with making vegetables or a salad while the chicken cooks.

If the chicken pieces are thicker on one end than the other, place them between two pieces of plastic wrap and pound them to even thickness with a mallet or a rolling pin so each piece will cook uniformly.

To test for doneness, make a small slit in a piece of the chicken—if it is no longer pink, it's done. Once the chicken is done, transfer it immediately to plates or a serving platter. If left in a hot pan, the chicken will continue to cook and dry out.

Pesto-Crusted Oven-Baked Chicken Breasts QUICK

makes 4 servings

If you keep pesto on hand, this will become a favorite weeknight chicken dish. The pesto adds the fresh flavor of basil and helps the crunchy crumbs stick to the chicken. Try it with purchased sun-dried tomato pesto, too.

½ teaspoon plus 1 tablespoon extra virgin olive oil, divided
10 whole wheat or white Melba toasts, crumbled
4 (4-ounce) boneless skinless chicken breasts
½ teaspoon kosher salt
⅛ teaspoon freshly ground pepper
3 tablespoons Basil Pesto (page 597) or purchased pesto

1 Position an oven rack in the top third of the oven. Preheat the oven to 375°F. Brush a medium rimmed baking sheet with ½ teaspoon of the oil.

2 Place the Melba toasts in a food processor and process until fine crumbs form. Place the Melba toast crumbs and the remaining 1 tablespoon oil in a shallow dish. Using your fingers, blend the oil evenly into the crumb mixture.

3 Place the chicken in a shallow dish. Sprinkle with the salt and pepper. Add the pesto and turn to coat the chicken evenly. Dip the chicken, one piece at a time, into the crumb mixture, pressing to adhere the crumbs.

4 Arrange the chicken in a single layer on the prepared pan. Bake until golden brown and the juices of the chicken run clear, 20 minutes (do not turn). Divide the chicken among 4 plates and serve at once.

Each serving: 15 g carb, 280 cal, 12 g fat, 2 g sat fat, 66 mg chol, 1 g fib, 26 g pro, 299 mg sod • Carb Choices: 1; Exchanges: 1 starch, 3 lean protein, 2 fat

Chicken Parmesan

makes 4 servings

As delicious as the classic dish, this version contains less than half the fat and calories, and all the great taste of the original. This recipe has several parts, but it comes together quickly if you make the sauce while the chicken bakes.

1 recipe Parmesan-Crusted Oven-Baked
    Chicken Breasts (page 233)
2 cups Marinara Sauce (page 593)
1 teaspoon extra virgin olive oil
2 ounces shredded part-skim mozzarella
    (about ½ cup)
2 tablespoons freshly grated Parmesan

1 Prepare the Parmesan-Crusted Oven-Baked Chicken Breasts, maintaining the oven temperature at 375°F after baking the chicken. Heat the sauce over medium-high heat, if cool. Brush a 13 x 9-inch glass baking dish with the oil.

2 Spoon 1 cup of the sauce into the prepared baking dish. Place the chicken on top of the sauce. Spoon ¼ cup of sauce on top of each chicken breast. Sprinkle the chicken evenly with the mozzarella and sprinkle with the Parmesan.

3 Bake, uncovered, until the sauce is bubbly and the cheese melts, 15 minutes. Divide the chicken and sauce evenly among 4 plates and serve at once.

Each serving: 19 g carb, 349 cal, 15 g fat, 5 g sat fat, 78 mg chol, 3 g fib, 33 g pro, 595 mg sod • Carb Choices: 1; Exchanges: 1 starch, 4 lean protein, 2½ fat

Panko-Crusted Chicken `QUICK`

makes 4 servings

My friend Julia Rutland, the mother of two young children, shared this recipe. The flavor is simple enough to appeal to the pickiest child, yet the touch of mustard and the crispy panko breading make it delicious enough to add to your weeknight dinner rotation—even if you don't have kids. Julia sautés this dish, but I've adapted it to bake in the oven to cut back on fat and calories.

½ teaspoon plus 2 teaspoons extra virgin olive
    oil, divided
3 tablespoons unbleached all-purpose flour
1 large egg white
1 tablespoon Dijon mustard
1 tablespoon water
¾ cup panko crumbs
1 ounce freshly grated Parmesan (about ¼ cup)
4 (4-ounce) boneless skinless chicken breasts
½ teaspoon kosher salt
⅛ teaspoon freshly ground pepper

1 Position an oven rack in the top third of the oven. Preheat the oven to 375°F. Brush a medium rimmed baking sheet with ½ teaspoon of the oil.

2 Place the flour in a shallow dish. Place the egg white, mustard, and water in another shallow dish and beat lightly with a fork. Combine the panko crumbs, Parmesan, and the remaining 2 teaspoons oil in another shallow dish. Using your fingers, blend the oil evenly into the crumbs.

3 Sprinkle the chicken with the salt and pepper. Dip the chicken, one piece at a time into the flour, then into the egg white mixture, then into the crumb mixture, pressing to adhere the crumbs.

4 Arrange the chicken in a single layer on the prepared baking sheet. Bake until the juices of the chicken run clear, 20 minutes (do not turn). Turn on the broiler and broil the chicken until the crust is lightly browned, 1 to 2 minutes. Divide the chicken among 4 plates and serve at once.

Each serving: 14 g carb, 236 cal, 7 g fat, 2 g sat fat, 67 mg chol, 0 g fib, 28 g pro, 400 mg sod • Carb Choices: 1; Exchanges: 1 starch, 3 lean protein, 1 fat

Spinach and Feta–Stuffed Chicken

makes 4 servings

Buy slightly larger chicken breasts for this recipe—about 6 ounces each. The smaller ones are too small to stuff.

4 teaspoons extra virgin olive oil, divided
2 garlic cloves, minced
8 ounces fresh spinach, trimmed and chopped
¼ teaspoon freshly ground pepper, divided
4 (6-ounce) boneless skinless chicken breasts
2 ounces crumbled feta cheese (about ½ cup)
¼ teaspoon kosher salt

1 Preheat the oven to 350°F.

2 Heat a large ovenproof skillet over medium heat. Add 2 teaspoons of the oil and tilt the pan to coat the bottom evenly. Add the garlic and cook, stirring constantly, until fragrant, 30 seconds. Add the spinach and cook, turning with tongs, until the spinach is wilted and most of the liquid evaporates, about 2 minutes. Stir in ⅛ teaspoon of the pepper. Transfer to a plate to cool. Wipe out the skillet with paper towels.

3 Cut a horizontal slit at the thicker side of each chicken breast to form a pocket. Stuff about 2 tablespoons of the feta into each pocket, then stuff in about 2 tablespoons of the spinach mixture. Seal each pocket using two wooden toothpicks. Sprinkle the chicken with the salt and remaining ⅛ teaspoon pepper.

4 Heat the skillet over medium-high heat. Add the remaining 2 teaspoons oil and tilt the pan to coat the bottom evenly. Add the chicken and cook, turning once, until browned, about 4 minutes. Transfer the skillet to the oven and bake until the juices of the chicken run clear, about 8 minutes. Divide the chicken among 4 plates and serve at once.

Each serving: 3 g carb, 272 cal, 11 g fat, 3 g sat fat, 102 mg chol, 1 g fib, 38 g pro, 321 mg sod • Carb Choices: 0; Exchanges: 5 lean protein, 1½ fat

Swiss Chard and Raisin–Stuffed Chicken

makes 4 servings

Earthy-tasting Swiss chard and sweet raisins make an unusually flavorful filling for chicken breasts.

¼ cup golden raisins
½ cup Chicken Stock (page 149) or low-sodium chicken broth, divided
4 teaspoons extra virgin olive oil, divided
2 garlic cloves, minced
8 ounces Swiss chard, tough stems removed and leaves chopped
¼ teaspoon freshly ground pepper, divided
4 (6-ounce) boneless skinless chicken breasts
½ teaspoon kosher salt
½ teaspoon ground cumin

1 Preheat the oven to 350°F.

2 Combine the raisins and ¼ cup of the stock in a small saucepan. Set over medium heat until hot. Cover and let stand 15 minutes. Drain.

3 Meanwhile, heat a large ovenproof skillet over medium heat. Add 2 teaspoons of the oil and tilt the pan to coat the bottom evenly. Add the garlic and cook, stirring constantly, until fragrant, 30 seconds. Add the Swiss chard and the remaining ¼ cup stock and cook, stirring often, until the chard is tender and most of the liquid evaporates, about 6 minutes. Stir in ⅛ teaspoon of the pepper. Transfer to a plate to cool. Wipe out the skillet with paper towels.

4 Cut a horizontal slit at the thicker side of each chicken breast to form a pocket. Stuff about 2 tablespoons of the raisins into each pocket, then stuff in about 2 tablespoons of the chard mixture. Seal each pocket using two wooden toothpicks. Sprinkle the chicken with the salt, cumin, and remaining ⅛ teaspoon pepper.

5 Heat the skillet over medium-high heat. Add the remaining 2 teaspoons oil and tilt the pan to coat the bottom. Add the chicken and cook, turning once, until browned, 4 minutes. Transfer the skillet to the oven and bake until the juices of the chicken run clear, 8 minutes. Divide the chicken among 4 plates and serve at once.

Each serving: 10 g carb, 266 cal, 9 g fat, 2 g sat fat, 94 mg chol, 1 g fib, 36 g pro, 343 mg sod • Carb Choices: ½; Exchanges: ½ fruit, 5 lean protein, 1 fat

Moroccan-Spiced Chicken with Feta and Tomatoes

QUICK

makes 4 servings

If you've forgotten to marinate, rub the chicken with the cumin, ginger, cinnamon, and salt, omitting the lemon juice and oil, and broil. The flavor won't be as intense, but it will still be a great weeknight meal that's ready in 20 minutes or less.

1 tablespoon lemon juice
2½ teaspoons extra virgin olive oil, divided
½ teaspoon ground cumin
¼ teaspoon ground ginger
⅛ teaspoon ground cinnamon
Pinch of ground cayenne
4 (4-ounce) boneless skinless chicken breasts
¾ teaspoon kosher salt
4 large plum tomatoes, halved lengthwise
1 ounce finely crumbled feta cheese (about ¼ cup)

1 Combine the lemon juice, 2 teaspoons of the oil, cumin, ginger, cinnamon, and cayenne in a large resealable plastic bag. Add the chicken, seal the bag, and refrigerate 2 to 4 hours.

2 Preheat the broiler. Brush a broiler rack with the remaining ½ teaspoon oil.

3 Remove the chicken from the marinade and discard the marinade. Sprinkle the chicken with the salt and place on the broiler rack. Broil 4 minutes. Remove the broiler pan from the oven and turn the chicken. Place the tomatoes on the rack, cut side up. Sprinkle the tomatoes evenly with the feta. Broil until the juices of the chicken run clear and the tomatoes are slightly softened, about 4 minutes longer. Divide the chicken and tomatoes evenly among 4 plates and serve at once.

Each serving: 3 g carb, 186 cal, 8 g fat, 3 g sat fat, 71 mg chol, 1 g fib, 25 g pro, 373 mg sod • Carb Choices: 0; Exchanges: 3 lean protein, 1 fat

Chicken with Tahini Sauce

makes 4 servings

You can use the sauce as a dip for vegetables or grilled salmon or thin it with a little low-fat milk for a salad dressing.

CHICKEN

½ cup plain low-fat yogurt
2 tablespoons minced fresh ginger
1 tablespoon lemon juice
2 garlic cloves, minced
⅛ teaspoon ground cayenne
4 (4-ounce) boneless skinless chicken breasts
½ teaspoon canola oil
½ teaspoon kosher salt

TAHINI SAUCE

¼ cup plain low-fat yogurt
2 tablespoons tahini (sesame paste)
1 tablespoon chopped fresh Italian parsley
½ teaspoon grated lemon zest
2 teaspoons lemon juice
⅛ teaspoon kosher salt
Pinch of ground cayenne

1 To make the chicken, combine the yogurt, ginger, lemon juice, garlic, and cayenne in a large resealable plastic bag. Add the chicken, seal the bag, and refrigerate 2 to 4 hours.

2 Preheat the broiler. Brush a broiler rack with the oil.

3 Remove the chicken from the marinade and discard the marinade. Sprinkle the chicken with the salt and place on the broiler rack. Broil, turning once, until the juices of the chicken run clear, about 8 minutes.

4 Meanwhile, to make the sauce, combine all the ingredients in a small bowl and stir to mix well. Divide the chicken among 4 plates, drizzle evenly with the sauce, and serve at once.

Each serving: 5 g carb, 194 cal, 8 g fat, 2 g sat fat, 64 mg chol, 0 g fib, 26 g pro, 255 mg sod • Carb Choices: 0; Exchanges: 3 lean protein, 1 fat

Tandoori-Style Chicken

makes 6 servings

The long soak in spicy yogurt is what makes this dish great.

½ cup plain low-fat yogurt
2 garlic cloves, minced
1 tablespoon lemon juice
1 tablespoon minced fresh ginger
1 teaspoon ground coriander
1 teaspoon ground cumin
½ teaspoon paprika
⅛ teaspoon ground cayenne
2½ pounds bone-in chicken pieces, skinned
½ teaspoon canola oil
½ teaspoon kosher salt

1 Combine the yogurt, garlic, lemon juice, ginger, coriander, cumin, paprika, and cayenne in a large resealable plastic bag. Add the chicken, turn to coat, and refrigerate 8 to 12 hours.

2 Preheat the oven to 400°F. Line a rimmed baking sheet with foil and brush foil with the oil.

3 Remove the chicken from the marinade and discard the marinade. Sprinkle the chicken with the salt and transfer to the prepared baking sheet. Bake 20 minutes. Turn and bake until the juices run clear, 20 to 25 minutes longer. Divide the chicken among 6 plates and serve at once.

Each serving: 1 g carb, 120 cal, 3 g fat, 1 g sat fat, 63 mg chol, 0 g fib, 20 g pro, 173 mg sod • Carb Choices: 0; Exchanges: 3 lean protein

Chicken and Vegetables en Papillote QUICK

makes 4 servings

If folding the parchment is intimidating, use foil instead. Instead of chicken, try this recipe with skinless salmon fillets, decreasing the baking time to 15 minutes.

4 small plum tomatoes, quartered
1 small zucchini, halved lengthwise and thinly sliced
1 small yellow squash, halved lengthwise and thinly sliced
¼ cup thinly sliced red onion
2 tablespoons chopped fresh basil
2 teaspoons extra virgin olive oil
¾ teaspoon kosher salt, divided
¼ teaspoon freshly ground pepper, divided
4 (4-ounce) boneless skinless chicken breasts
2 teaspoons grated lemon zest

1 Preheat the oven to 425°F.

2 Place the tomatoes, zucchini, yellow squash, onion, basil, oil, ¼ teaspoon of the salt, and ⅛ teaspoon of the pepper in a large bowl and toss to combine. Sprinkle the chicken with the lemon zest, remaining ½ teaspoon kosher salt, and remaining ⅛ teaspoon pepper.

3 Tear off four 24 x 12-inch pieces of parchment paper. Fold each piece in half crosswise and cut each one to make a rounded heart shape. Open a parchment "heart" and arrange one-quarter of the vegetable mixture in the middle of one side. Top with a chicken breast.

4 Beginning at the bottom end of each "heart" fold the edges of the parchment in overlapping 1-inch segments, crimping as you go, to form a tight seal. (You can also use aluminum foil to make the packets.)

5 Place the packages on a large rimmed baking sheet and bake until the juices of the chicken run clear, 20 minutes. Place the packets on 4 plates and serve at once. Use caution when opening the packets, avoiding the steam that escapes.

Each serving: 6 g carb, 168 cal, 5 g fat, 1 g sat fat, 63 mg chol, 2 g fib, 24 g pro, 274 mg sod • Carb Choices: ½; Exchanges: 1 veg, 3 lean protein, ½ fat

Grilled Chicken

Grilled BBQ Chicken

makes 6 servings

Almost like chili-flavored chicken, this recipe is right at home for casual summer meals. Grill some fresh ears of corn alongside the chicken to make a classic hot weather dinner.

2½ teaspoons canola oil, divided
1 medium onion, diced
2 garlic cloves, minced
2 (8-ounce) cans no-salt-added tomato sauce
2 tablespoons apple cider vinegar
2 tablespoons no-salt-added tomato paste
2 tablespoons light brown sugar
2 teaspoons chili powder
1 teaspoon ground cumin
2½ pounds bone-in chicken pieces, skinned
¾ teaspoon kosher salt
¼ teaspoon freshly ground pepper

1 Heat a medium skillet over medium heat. Add 2 teaspoons of the oil and tilt the pan to coat the bottom evenly. Add the onion and cook, stirring often, until softened, 5 minutes. Add the garlic and cook, stirring constantly, until fragrant, 30 seconds. Add the tomato sauce, vinegar, tomato paste, sugar, chili powder, and cumin and bring to a boil. Reduce the heat to low and simmer, stirring occasionally, until the sauce is thickened, about 10 minutes. Set aside half of the sauce for serving.

2 Preheat the grill to medium heat.

3 Sprinkle the chicken with the salt and pepper.

4 Brush the grill rack with the remaining ½ teaspoon oil. Place the chicken on the grill, cover, and grill, turning once, for 15 minutes. Brush with the sauce, turn, and grill until the juices of the chicken run clear, basting two more times, 10 to 15 minutes longer. Divide the chicken among 6 plates and serve with the reserved sauce.

Each serving: 14 g carb, 192 cal, 5 g fat, 1 g sat fat, 63 mg chol, 2 g fib, 21 g pro, 250 mg sod • Carb Choices: ½; Exchanges: ½ carb, 3 lean protein

Note: To make the chicken in the oven, preheat the oven to 375°F. Brush the rack of a broiler pan with ½ teaspoon canola oil. Place the chicken on the rack and bake 30 minutes. Brush with the sauce, turn, and bake until the juices of the chicken run clear, basting two more times, 20 to 25 minutes longer.

Cumin and Lime Grilled Chicken

makes 6 servings

This simple marinade made from kitchen staples adds vivid flavor to chicken. Use the marinade for boneless skinless chicken breasts, too, but reduce the marinating time to 2 to 4 hours.

¼ cup lime juice
2½ teaspoons canola oil, divided
1 teaspoon ground cumin
1 jalapeño, seeded and chopped
2 garlic cloves, minced
2½ pounds bone-in chicken pieces, skinned
¾ teaspoon kosher salt
Lime wedges

1 Combine the lime juice, 2 teaspoons of the oil, the cumin, jalapeño, and garlic in a large resealable plastic bag. Add the chicken, turn to coat, and refrigerate 8 to 12 hours.

2 Preheat the grill to medium heat.

3 Remove the chicken from the marinade and discard the marinade. Pat the chicken dry with paper towels and sprinkle with the salt.

4 Brush the grill rack with the remaining ½ teaspoon oil. Place the chicken on the grill, cover, and grill, turning occasionally, until the juices of the chicken run clear, 25 to 30 minutes. Divide the chicken among 6 plates and serve at once with the lime wedges.

Each serving: 1 g carb, 119 cal, 4 g fat, 1 g sat fat, 63 mg chol, 0 g fib, 20 g pro, 213 mg sod • Carb Choices: 0; Exchanges: 3 lean protein

Sesame and Lime Grilled Chicken

makes 6 servings

When you need a simple Asian-flavored chicken dish for the grill, this is a crowd-pleasing recipe. Toss sliced summer squash or asparagus spears with canola oil and grill alongside the chicken for a healthful summer meal.

¼ cup lime juice
2 tablespoons reduced-sodium soy sauce
2 tablespoons fresh minced ginger
2 teaspoons honey
½ teaspoon Asian sesame oil
1 garlic clove, minced
2½ pounds bone-in chicken pieces, skinned
½ teaspoon canola oil
Lime wedges

1 Combine the lime juice, soy sauce, ginger, honey, sesame oil, and garlic in a large resealable plastic bag. Add the chicken, turn to coat, and refrigerate 8 to 12 hours.

2 Preheat the grill to medium heat.

3 Remove the chicken from the marinade and discard the marinade. Pat the chicken dry with paper towels.

4 Brush the grill rack with the canola oil. Place the chicken on the grill, cover, and grill, turning occasionally, until the juices of the chicken run clear, 25 to 30 minutes. Divide the chicken among 6 plates and serve at once with the lime wedges.

Each serving: 2 g carb, 125 cal, 4 g fat, 1 g sat fat, 63 mg chol, 0 g fib, 20 g pro, 173 mg sod • Carb Choices: 0; Exchanges: 3 lean protein

Rosemary and Orange Grilled Chicken

makes 6 servings

The combination of rosemary and orange is one of my favorites and this is a great marinade that infuses the chicken with concentrated flavor. I like to serve it in the late fall, when oranges are just starting to get juicy and there's still a little rosemary to be had at the farmers' market.

2 teaspoons grated orange zest
¼ cup orange juice
2½ teaspoons canola oil, divided
2 garlic cloves, minced
2 teaspoons minced fresh rosemary
2½ pounds bone-in chicken pieces, skinned
¾ teaspoon kosher salt
¼ teaspoon freshly ground pepper

1 Combine the orange zest, orange juice, 2 teaspoons of the oil, the garlic, and rosemary in a large resealable plastic bag. Add the chicken, turn to coat, and refrigerate 8 to 12 hours.

2 Preheat the grill to medium heat.

3 Remove the chicken from the marinade and discard the marinade. Pat the chicken dry with paper towels and sprinkle with the salt and pepper.

4 Brush the grill rack with the remaining ½ teaspoon oil. Place the chicken on the grill, cover, and grill, turning occasionally, until the juices of the chicken run clear, 25 to 30 minutes. Divide the chicken among 6 plates and serve at once.

Each serving: 1 g carb, 120 cal, 4 g fat, 1 g sat fat, 63 mg chol, 0 g fib, 20 g pro, 212 mg sod • Carb Choices: 0; Exchanges: 3 lean protein

Mustard-Molasses Grilled Chicken QUICK

makes 4 servings

This recipe is from my good friend Rebecca Reed, a brilliant no-nonsense cook who knows her way around a grill. Here, she takes sweet Southern molasses and pairs it with pungent salty mustard for a simple, perfectly balanced marinade for grilled chicken.

1 tablespoon molasses
1 tablespoon whole grain mustard
4 (4-ounce) boneless skinless chicken breasts
½ teaspoon canola oil
½ teaspoon kosher salt

1 Preheat the grill to medium-high heat.

2 Stir together the molasses and mustard in a shallow dish. Add the chicken and turn to coat. Let stand at room temperature for 15 minutes.

3 Brush the grill rack with the oil. Sprinkle the chicken with the salt, place on the grill, and grill, turning often, until the juices of the chicken run clear, 8 to 10 minutes. Divide the chicken among 4 plates and serve at once.

Each serving: 4 g carb, 144 cal, 4 g fat, 1 g sat fat, 63 mg chol, 0 g fib, 23 g pro, 274 mg sod • Carb Choices: 0; Exchanges: 3 lean protein

Grilled Lemon-Curry Chicken

makes 4 servings

Make a double batch of this chicken when you grill to use for salads or sandwiches later in the week.

2 tablespoons lemon juice
2 teaspoons curry powder
2½ teaspoons canola oil, divided
1 garlic clove, minced
4 (4-ounce) boneless skinless chicken breasts
½ teaspoon kosher salt
2 tablespoons chopped fresh cilantro
Lemon wedges

1 Combine the lemon juice, the curry powder, 2 teaspoons of the oil, and the garlic in a large resealable plastic bag. Add the chicken, turn to coat, and refrigerate 2 to 4 hours.

2 Preheat the grill to medium-high heat.

3 Remove the chicken from the marinade and discard the marinade. Pat the chicken dry with paper towels and sprinkle with the salt.

4 Brush the grill rack with the remaining ½ teaspoon oil. Place the chicken on the grill and grill, turning often, until the juices of the chicken run clear, 8 to 10 minutes. Divide the chicken among 4 plates, sprinkle with the cilantro, and serve with the lemon wedges.

Each serving: 1 g carb, 140 cal, 4 g fat, 1 g sat fat, 63 mg chol, 0 g fib, 23 g pro, 195 mg sod • Carb Choices: 0; Exchanges: 3 lean protein

Grilled Chicken with Cilantro-Jalapeño Sauce QUICK

makes 4 servings

Quickly grilled chicken breasts and a fantastically flavored sauce make this an impressive but easy dish for entertaining. You can easily double the recipe and you can make the sauce up to 4 hours ahead and store it in the refrigerator. If you have spicy food lovers in your midst, a nice presentation for this dish is to grill whole jalapeños while you grill the chicken and garnish each plate with one.

SAUCE
1 cup packed whole fresh cilantro leaves
¼ cup slivered almonds, toasted (page 4)
1 ounce freshly grated Parmesan (about ¼ cup)
3 tablespoons cold water
2 tablespoons thinly sliced scallion,
    green tops only
2 tablespoons extra virgin olive oil
1 tablespoon lime juice
1 garlic clove, chopped
½ small jalapeño, seeded and chopped
¼ teaspoon ground cumin
⅛ teaspoon kosher salt

CHICKEN

½ teaspoon canola oil

4 (4-ounce) boneless skinless chicken breasts

½ teaspoon ground cumin

½ teaspoon kosher salt

¼ teaspoon paprika

¼ teaspoon ground coriander

1 Preheat the grill to medium-high heat.

2 To make the sauce, combine all the ingredients in a food processor and process until the mixture is finely chopped.

3 To make the chicken, brush the grill rack with the oil. Sprinkle the chicken with the cumin, salt, paprika, and coriander.

4 Place the chicken on the grill and grill, turning often, until the juices of the chicken run clear, 8 to 10 minutes. Divide the chicken among 4 plates and serve at once with the sauce.

Each serving: 1 g carb, 217 cal, 12 g fat, 3 g sat fat, 67 mg chol, 0 g fib, 25 g pro, 309 mg sod • Carb Choices: 0; Exchanges: 4 lean protein, 1½ fat

Lager and Lime Marinated Grilled Chicken

makes 4 servings

Beer and fresh lime make an unusual and very flavorful marinade for chicken. Use any light-colored beer that you have on hand for the marinade, as a dark beer will color the chicken.

1 cup lager beer

2 teaspoons grated lime zest

2 tablespoons lime juice

2½ teaspoons canola oil, divided

1 garlic clove, minced

¼ cup chopped fresh cilantro

4 (4-ounce) boneless skinless chicken breasts

½ teaspoon kosher salt

½ teaspoon ground cumin

Lime wedges

1 Combine the beer, lime zest, lime juice, 2 teaspoons of the oil, the garlic, and cilantro in a large resealable plastic bag. Add the chicken, turn to coat, and refrigerate 2 to 4 hours.

2 Preheat the grill to medium-high heat.

3 Remove the chicken from the marinade and discard the marinade. Pat the chicken dry with paper towels and sprinkle with the salt and cumin.

4 Brush the grill rack with the remaining ½ teaspoon oil. Place the chicken on the grill and grill, turning often, until the juices of the chicken run clear, 8 to 10 minutes. Divide the chicken among 4 plates and serve at once with the lime wedges.

Each serving: 1 g carb, 142 cal, 4 g fat, 1 g sat fat, 63 mg chol, 0 g fib, 23 g pro, 196 mg sod • Carb Choices: 0; Exchanges: 3 lean protein

Asian Barbecued Chicken

makes 4 servings

Sweet, tart, and spicy, this chicken is bursting with Asian-inspired flavors. To make a dipping sauce, double the marinade ingredients and store half in an airtight container in the refrigerator until ready to serve.

2 tablespoons light brown sugar

2 tablespoons reduced-sodium soy sauce

1 tablespoon rice vinegar

2½ teaspoons canola oil, divided

2 garlic cloves, minced

1 teaspoon grated fresh ginger

1 teaspoon five-spice powder

½ teaspoon Asian sesame oil

4 (4-ounce) boneless skinless chicken breasts

Lime wedges

1 Combine the sugar, soy sauce, vinegar, 2 teaspoons of the canola oil, the garlic, ginger, five-spice powder, and sesame oil in a large resealable plastic bag. Add the chicken, turn to coat, and refrigerate 2 to 4 hours.

continues on next page

2 Preheat the grill to medium-high heat.

3 Remove the chicken from the marinade and discard the marinade. Pat the chicken dry with paper towels.

4 Brush the grill rack with the remaining ½ teaspoon canola oil. Place the chicken on the grill and grill, turning often, until the juices of the chicken run clear, 8 to 10 minutes. Divide the chicken among 6 plates and serve at once with the lime wedges.

Each serving: 4 g carb, 157 cal, 5 g fat, 1 g sat fat, 63 mg chol, 0 g fib, 23 g pro, 207 mg sod • Carb Choices: 0; Exchanges: 3 lean protein

Grilled Caribbean Chicken

makes 4 servings

Reminiscent of jerk seasoning, this marinade adds mysteriously complex flavor to chicken. Rum and allspice are the unexpected ingredients.

¼ cup chopped fresh cilantro
1 jalapeño, including some of the seeds, minced
3 garlic cloves, minced
1 scallion, thinly sliced
2 tablespoons lime juice
2 tablespoons light rum
2½ teaspoons canola oil, divided
½ teaspoon ground allspice
4 (4-ounce) boneless skinless chicken breasts
½ teaspoon kosher salt

1 Combine the cilantro, jalapeño, garlic, scallion, lime juice, rum, 2 teaspoons of the oil, and the allspice in a large resealable plastic bag. Add the chicken, turn to coat, and refrigerate 2 to 4 hours.

2 Preheat the grill to medium-high heat.

3 Remove the chicken from the marinade and discard the marinade. Pat the chicken dry with paper towels and sprinkle with the salt.

4 Brush the grill rack with the remaining ½ teaspoon oil. Place the chicken on the grill and grill, turning often, until the juices of the chicken run clear, 8 to 10 minutes. Divide the chicken among 4 plates and serve at once.

Each serving: 1 g carb, 148 cal, 4 g fat, 1 g sat fat, 63 mg chol, 0 g fib, 23 g pro, 195 mg sod • Carb Choices: 0; Exchanges: 3 lean protein

Grilled Cilantro Chicken with Coconut-Peanut Sauce

makes 4 servings

Coconut and peanuts are both high in fat and calories, so it's good that a little of this flavorful sauce goes a long way. You can serve it on grilled shrimp or grilled vegetables, too.

4 tablespoons chopped fresh cilantro, divided
2 tablespoons plus ½ teaspoon lime juice, divided
2½ teaspoons canola oil, divided
1 jalapeño pepper, seeded and minced
4 (4-ounce) boneless skinless chicken breasts
¼ cup reduced-fat coconut milk
1 tablespoon natural creamy peanut butter
⅛ teaspoon plus ½ teaspoon kosher salt, divided
Pinch of ground cayenne

1 Combine 3 tablespoons of the cilantro, 2 tablespoons of the lime juice, 2 teaspoons of the oil, and the jalapeño in a large resealable plastic bag. Add the chicken, turn to coat, and refrigerate 2 to 4 hours.

2 Meanwhile, to make the sauce, whisk together the coconut milk, peanut butter, the remaining 1 tablespoon cilantro, remaining ½ teaspoon lime juice, ⅛ teaspoon of the salt, and the cayenne in a small bowl. Cover and refrigerate until ready to serve.

3 Preheat the grill to medium-high heat.

4 Remove the chicken from the marinade and discard the marinade. Pat the chicken dry with paper towels and sprinkle with the remaining ½ teaspoon salt.

5 Brush the grill rack with the remaining ½ teaspoon oil. Place the chicken on the grill and grill, turning often, until the juices of the chicken run clear, 8 to 10 minutes. Divide the chicken among 4 plates and serve at once with the sauce.

Each serving: 2 g carb, 172 cal, 7 g fat, 2 g sat fat, 63 mg chol, 0 g fib, 24 g pro, 251 mg sod • Carb Choices: 0; Exchanges: 3 lean protein, 1 fat

Grilled Chicken Yakitori

makes 4 servings

Yakitori is a Japanese version of chicken skewers.

¼ cup reduced-sodium soy sauce
3 tablespoons mirin
1 tablespoon grated fresh ginger
2 garlic cloves, crushed through a press
½ teaspoon Asian sesame oil
1 pound boneless skinless chicken breasts, cut into 1-inch pieces
4 scallions, cut into 1-inch pieces
1 large red bell pepper, cut into 1-inch pieces
1 large green bell pepper, cut into 1-inch pieces
½ teaspoon canola oil
2 tablespoons chopped fresh cilantro

1 Whisk together the soy sauce, mirin, ginger, garlic, and sesame oil in a small bowl. Transfer half of the mixture to a large resealable plastic bag. Cover and refrigerate the remaining mixture until ready to serve. Add the chicken to the marinade in the plastic bag, turn to coat, and refrigerate 2 to 4 hours.

2 Remove the chicken from the marinade and discard the marinade. Pat the chicken dry with paper towels. Thread the chicken, scallions, and bell peppers onto eight 8- to 10-inch metal skewers.

3 Prepare the grill or heat a large grill pan over medium-high heat.

4 Brush the grill rack or grill pan with the canola oil. Place the kebabs on the grill rack or in the grill pan and grill, turning often, until the juices of the chicken run clear, 8 to 10 minutes.

5 To serve, divide the kebabs among 4 plates. Stir the cilantro into the reserved soy sauce mixture and drizzle over the kebabs. Serve at once.

Each serving: 7 g carb, 170 cal, 4 g fat, 1 g sat fat, 63 mg chol, 2 g fib, 25 g pro, 513 mg sod • Carb Choices: ½; Exchanges: 1 veg, 3 lean protein

Grilled Chicken and Clementine Kebabs QUICK

makes 4 servings

When you want to wow guests with hardly any work, this dish makes a stunning presentation. The skin on the clementines soften on the grill, making them completely edible.

1 pound boneless skinless chicken breasts, cut into 1-inch pieces
2 clementines, unpeeled, each cut into 8 wedges
1 large red onion, cut into 1-inch pieces
1 red bell pepper, cut into 1-inch pieces
2 tablespoons chopped fresh mint
2½ teaspoons extra virgin olive oil
1 teaspoon ground coriander
½ teaspoon kosher salt
¼ teaspoon freshly ground pepper

1 Prepare the grill or heat a large grill pan over medium-high heat.

2 Combine the chicken, clementines, onion, bell pepper, mint, 2 teaspoons of the oil, the coriander, salt, and ground pepper in a large bowl and toss to coat. Thread the chicken, clementines, onion, and bell pepper onto eight 8- to 10-inch metal skewers.

3 Brush the grill rack or grill pan with the remaining ½ teaspoon oil. Place the kebabs on the grill rack or in the grill pan and grill, turning often, until the juices of the chicken run clear, 8 to 10 minutes. Divide the kebabs among 4 plates and serve at once.

Each serving: 9 g carb, 185 cal, 6 g fat, 1 g sat fat, 63 mg chol, 2 g fib, 24 g pro, 197 mg sod • Carb Choices: ½; Exchanges: ½ fruit, 1 veg, 3 lean protein, ½ fat

Moroccan-Spiced Chicken and Vegetable Kebabs QUICK

makes 4 servings

If you're grilling these outside, make enough for the neighbors. The fragrance of the spices as these kebabs cook intoxicating. Serve them with whole wheat couscous and a simple green salad.

1 pound boneless skinless chicken breasts, cut into 1-inch pieces
1 small red bell pepper, cut into 1-inch pieces
1 small yellow squash, cut into 1-inch pieces
8 large cherry tomatoes
8 small white mushrooms
2 garlic cloves, minced
2½ teaspoons extra virgin olive oil, divided
1 teaspoon ground cumin
1 teaspoon paprika
1 teaspoon ground coriander
1 teaspoon grated fresh ginger
½ teaspoon kosher salt
¼ teaspoon freshly ground pepper
Lemon wedges

1 Prepare the grill or heat a large grill pan over medium-high heat.

2 Combine the chicken, bell pepper, squash, tomatoes, mushrooms, garlic, 2 teaspoons of the oil, the cumin, paprika, coriander, ginger, salt, and ground pepper in a large bowl and toss to coat. Thread the chicken and vegetables onto eight 8- to 10-inch metal skewers.

3 Brush the grill rack or grill pan with the remaining ½ teaspoon oil. Place the kebabs on the grill rack or in the grill pan and grill, turning often, until the juices of the chicken run clear, 8 to 10 minutes. Divide the kebabs among 4 plates and serve at once with the lemon wedges.

Each serving: 6 g carb, 175 cal, 6 g fat, 1 g sat fat, 63 mg chol, 1 g fib, 24 g pro, 200 mg sod • Carb Choices: ½; Exchanges: 1 veg, 3 lean protein, ½ fat

Grilled Chicken Kebabs

There's something about serving food on a skewer that adds a festive note to any outdoor party. They're just so fun to eat!

You can turn any of the grilled chicken recipes in this section into colorful chicken and vegetable kebabs for entertaining or just for family. For any of the recipes, use either boneless skinless chicken breasts or boneless skinless chicken thighs, cutting them into 1-inch pieces. For adapting the Grilled BBQ Chicken (page 238) and Cumin and Lime Grilled Chicken (page 238), use 1½ pounds of either boneless skinless chicken thighs or breasts.

Follow instructions in each recipe for marinating, if required, then discard the marinade and thread the chicken onto skewers with 1-inch pieces of vegetables. The kebabs will cook in about the same time as larger pieces of chicken, but to test for doneness, check a piece of chicken in the center of each kebab to make sure it is no longer pink.

Choose quick-cooking vegetables for the skewers and cut them into the same size pieces as the chicken. Try yellow squash, zucchini, bell peppers, fennel, small white mushrooms, cherry tomatoes, sweet or red onion wedges, or scallions.

Arrange the skewers on couscous, whole wheat orzo, brown rice, barley, or a mixed green salad and let the fun begin. (Note that metal skewers will be very hot after being on the grill, so it is best to slide food off the skewers before eating.)

Turkey

Herb Roasted Turkey with Sage Gravy

makes 12 servings, plus leftovers

This is a simple crowd-pleasing turkey that will be a welcome centerpiece of any holiday celebration. Pair the turkey with one of the stuffings that begin on page 530. Baking the stuffing outside the turkey is not only safer (the turkey juices can drip into the stuffing and if the stuffing does not reach 165°F, bacteria can grow), but baked in a dish, the stuffing is never soggy and it develops an irresistible crispness around the edge of the dish.

TURKEY

2 tablespoons minced fresh sage or 2 teaspoons crumbled dried sage

1 tablespoon minced fresh thyme or 1 teaspoon dried thyme

2 teaspoons kosher salt

½ teaspoon freshly ground pepper

1 (12-pound) whole turkey

1 medium onion, peeled and quartered

1 stalk celery, cut into 1-inch pieces

1 large carrot, peeled and cut into 1-inch pieces

½ teaspoon canola oil

GRAVY

3 cups Chicken Stock (page 149) or low-sodium chicken broth

¼ cup unbleached all-purpose flour

1 tablespoon chopped fresh sage or 2 teaspoons crumbled dried sage

½ teaspoon kosher salt

¼ teaspoon freshly ground pepper

1 Preheat the oven to 325°F.

2 To make the turkey, combine the sage, thyme, salt, and pepper in a small bowl. Remove and discard the neck and giblets from the cavity of the turkey. Loosen the skin from the breast and drumsticks by inserting your fingers and gently separating the skin from the meat. Rub the herb mixture over the breast and drumsticks underneath the skin.

3 Place the onion, celery, and carrot inside the cavity. Tuck the wing tips underneath the turkey and tie the legs together with kitchen string.

4 Brush a wire roasting rack with the oil. Place the turkey on the rack into a large roasting pan. Cover the turkey breast with foil and bake 1½ hours. Remove the foil and bake until a thermometer inserted into a thigh registers 165°F, 1 hour to 1 hour 15 minutes. Transfer to a serving platter and cover loosely with foil while preparing the gravy. Discard the onion, celery, and carrot.

5 To make the gravy, remove the rack from the roasting pan. Pour the pan drippings into a fat separator or a glass measuring cup. Pour off and discard the fat. Add enough of the stock to make 3¼ cups. Pour the stock mixture back into the roasting pan. Add the flour and whisk until smooth. Set the roasting pan over two burners and cook over medium-high heat, whisking constantly, until the gravy comes to a boil and thickens, about 8 minutes. Stir in the sage, salt, and pepper. Carve the turkey and serve with the gravy. Remove the skin from the turkey before eating.

Each serving (3 ounces mixed white and dark meat with 2 tablespoons gravy): 1 g carb, 179 cal, 3 g fat, 1 g sat fat, 112 mg chol, 0 g fib, 34 g pro, 210 mg sod • Carb Choices: 0; Exchanges: 5 lean protein

Lemon-Spice Roasted Turkey

makes 12 servings, plus leftovers

Warm cumin and coriander paired with fragrant lemon zest take this turkey in a decidedly non-traditional direction. The turkey roasts with lemons inside the cavity to infuse the meat with citrus flavor. The lemony gravy is great on ordinary mashed potatoes, but it's terrific on Rutabaga-Apple Puree (page 485).

TURKEY

2 garlic cloves, minced

2 tablespoons grated lemon zest

2 teaspoons ground cumin

2 teaspoons kosher salt

1 teaspoon ground coriander

½ teaspoon freshly ground pepper

1 (12-pound) whole turkey

2 large lemons, quartered

½ teaspoon canola oil

GRAVY

3 cups Chicken Stock (page 149) or low-sodium chicken broth

¼ cup unbleached all-purpose flour

3 tablespoons chopped fresh Italian parsley

1 teaspoon grated lemon zest

½ teaspoon kosher salt

¼ teaspoon freshly ground pepper

1 To make the turkey, preheat the oven to 325°F.

2 Combine the garlic, lemon zest, cumin, salt, coriander, and pepper in a small bowl. Remove and discard the neck and giblets from the cavity of the turkey. Loosen the skin from the breast and drumsticks by inserting your fingers and gently separating the skin from the meat. Rub the garlic mixture over the breast and drumsticks underneath the skin.

3 Place the lemons inside the cavity. Tuck the wing tips underneath the turkey and tie the legs together with kitchen string.

4 Brush a wire roasting rack with the oil. Place the turkey on the rack in a large roasting pan. Cover the turkey breast with foil and bake 1½ hours. Remove the foil and bake until a thermometer inserted into a thigh registers 165°F, 1 hour to 1 hour 15 minutes. Transfer to a serving platter and cover loosely with foil while preparing the gravy. Discard the lemons.

5 To make the gravy, remove the rack from the roasting pan. Pour the pan drippings into a fat separator or a glass measuring cup. Pour off and discard the fat. Add enough of the stock to make 3¼ cups. Pour the stock mixture into the roasting pan. Add the flour and whisk until smooth. Set the roasting pan over two burners and cook over medium-high heat, whisking constantly, until the gravy comes to a boil and thickens, about 8 minutes. Stir in the parsley, lemon zest, salt, and pepper. Carve the turkey and serve with the gravy. Remove the skin from the turkey before eating.

Each serving (3 ounces mixed white and dark meat with 2 tablespoons gravy): 1 g carb, 180 cal, 3 g fat, 1 g sat fat, 112 mg chol, 0 g fib, 34 g pro, 211 mg sod • Carb Choices: 0; Exchanges: 5 lean protein

Rosemary Roasted Turkey Breast with Gravy

makes 18 servings

Most people never think about turkey until Thanksgiving, but this versatile recipe will be right at home for any fall or winter get together. Or, make it for your family and enjoy the leftovers in sandwiches, salads, and soups.

2 tablespoons chopped fresh rosemary

4 garlic cloves, minced

1¼ teaspoons kosher salt, divided

¼ teaspoon plus ⅛ teaspoon freshly ground pepper, divided

1 (6-pound) whole bone-in turkey breast

½ teaspoon canola oil

2¾ cups Chicken Stock (page 149) or low-sodium chicken broth

¼ cup unbleached all-purpose flour

1 Preheat the oven to 400°F.

2 Combine the rosemary, garlic, 1 teaspoon of the salt, and ¼ teaspoon of the pepper in a small bowl. Loosen the skin of the turkey breast by inserting your fingers and gently separating the skin from the meat. Rub the seasoning mixture under the loosened skin.

3 Brush a wire roasting rack with the oil. Place the turkey breast on the rack in a large roasting pan. Bake until a thermometer inserted into the center of the breast registers 165°F, about 1 hour and 30 minutes. Transfer to a serving platter and cover loosely with foil while preparing the gravy.

4 Remove the rack from the roasting pan. Pour the pan drippings into a fat separator or a glass measuring cup. Pour off and discard the fat. Add enough of the stock to make 3¼ cups. Pour the stock mixture into the roasting pan. Add the flour and whisk until smooth. Set the roasting pan over two burners and cook over medium-high heat, whisking constantly, until the gravy comes to a boil and thickens, about 8 minutes. Stir in the remaining ¼ teaspoon salt and remaining ⅛ teaspoon pepper. Cut the turkey into thin slices and serve with the gravy. Remove the skin from the turkey before eating.

Each serving: 2 g carb, 139 cal, 1 g fat, 0 g sat fat, 79 mg chol, 0 g fib, 29 g pro, 148 mg sod • Carb Choices: 0; Exchanges: 4 lean protein

Chile-Rubbed Roasted Turkey Breast

Serves 18

A chile-seasoned flavoring paste tucked under the skin gives this turkey breast complex flavor without being too spicy. Turn the leftovers into delicious tacos or enchiladas.

2½ teaspoons plus 1 tablespoon extra virgin olive oil, divided

¼ cup diced onion

2 dried New Mexico chiles, seeded and crumbled

2 garlic cloves, chopped

1 teaspoon ground cumin

1 cup Chicken Stock (page 149) or low-sodium chicken broth

1 teaspoon lime juice

1 teaspoon light brown sugar

1 teaspoon kosher salt

1 (6-pound) bone-in turkey breast

1 Heat a medium saucepan over medium-high heat. Add 2 teaspoons of the oil and tilt the pan to coat the bottom evenly. Add the onion and cook, stirring occasionally, until the onion is tender, 5 minutes. Add the chiles, garlic, and cumin and cook, stirring constantly, until fragrant, 30 seconds.

2 Add the stock and bring to a boil over high heat. Reduce the heat to low and simmer, uncovered, until the chiles are softened and most of the liquid is evaporated, about 15 minutes.

3 Meanwhile, preheat the oven to 400°F.

4 Let the chile mixture cool slightly and place in a food processor. Add 1 tablespoon of the oil, the lime juice, sugar, and salt. Process until smooth.

5 Loosen the skin of the turkey breast by inserting your fingers and gently separating the skin from the meat. Rub the seasoning mixture under the loosened skin.

6 Brush a wire roasting rack with the remaining ½ teaspoon oil. Place the turkey on the rack in a large roasting pan. Bake until a thermometer inserted into the center of the breast registers 165°F, about 1 hour 30 minutes. Transfer to a serving platter, cover loosely with foil, and let stand 10 minutes before carving. Cut the turkey into thin slices and serve. Remove the skin from the turkey before eating.

Each serving: 1 g carb, 149 cal, 2 g fat, 0 g sat fat, 79 mg chol, 0 g fib, 29 g pro, 120 mg sod • Carb Choices: 0; Exchanges: 4 lean protein

Sage-Rubbed Roasted Boneless Turkey Breast

makes 10 servings

Boneless turkey breast roast is worth seeking out for convenience and flavor. Basically, the roast is a half of a boneless turkey breast that is either tied with string or tucked inside a cotton net. Keep the roast tied, or in the net, when you brown the chicken and roast it to help it keep its shape and remove the string or net before serving. These roasts are perfect for small families because you get an exceptional dinner as well as plenty of leftovers from one roast. And the best part: no carving required.

1 (3-pound) boneless skinless turkey breast
1 teaspoon kosher salt
¼ teaspoon freshly ground pepper
2 teaspoons extra virgin olive oil
1 tablespoon minced fresh sage

1 Preheat the oven to 325°F.

2 Sprinkle the turkey with the salt and pepper. Heat a large ovenproof skillet over medium-high heat. Add the oil and tilt the pan to coat the bottom evenly. Add the turkey and cook, turning often, until well browned on all sides, about 6 minutes. Remove the skillet from the heat and sprinkle the turkey with the sage.

3 Transfer the skillet to the oven and bake until a thermometer inserted into the center of the turkey registers 165°F, 1 hour 15 minutes to 1 hour 30 minutes.

4 Transfer to a serving platter, cover loosely with foil, and let stand 10 minutes before slicing. Cut the turkey into thin slices and serve.

Each serving: 0 g carb, 154 cal, 2 g fat, 0 g sat fat, 89 mg chol, 0 g fib, 32 g pro, 168 mg sod • Carb Choices: 0; Exchanges: 4 lean protein

Turkey Breast Stuffed with Greens and Bacon

makes 10 servings

Any stuffed entrée is sure to impress guests. This turkey's uptown looks are tempered by the homespun stuffing ingredients and a sauce that you may as well call gravy. Serve it with Buttermilk Mashed Potatoes (page 482).

2 strips smoked center-cut bacon
1 small onion, chopped
2 garlic cloves, minced
1¼ cups Chicken Stock (page 149) or low-sodium chicken broth, divided
12 ounces kale, tough stems removed and leaves thinly sliced
¼ cup plain dry breadcrumbs
1 teaspoon kosher salt, divided
½ teaspoon freshly ground pepper, divided
1 (3-pound) boneless skinless turkey breast
1 teaspoon canola oil
1 tablespoon unbleached all-purpose flour

1 Cook the bacon in a large skillet over medium-high heat until crisp. Drain on paper towels. Drain off and discard all but 2 teaspoons of the bacon drippings. Add the onion to the bacon drippings in the pan and cook, stirring often, until softened, 5 minutes. Add the garlic and cook, stirring constantly, until fragrant, 30 seconds. Add ½ cup of the stock and the kale. Cook, stirring often, until the kale is tender and most of the liquid has evaporated, 6 to 8 minutes. Remove from the heat. Finely chop the bacon and add to the kale. Stir in the breadcrumbs, ½ teaspoon of the salt, and ¼ teaspoon of the pepper.

2 Preheat the oven to 400°F.

3 Place the turkey on a sheet of plastic wrap. Make a cut lengthwise down one side of the

turkey, cutting to, but not through, the other side. Open the butterflied portions, laying the turkey flat. Place plastic wrap over the turkey and flatten to a ½-inch thickness using a meat mallet or rolling pin.

4 Sprinkle both sides of the turkey with the remaining ½ teaspoon salt and ⅛ teaspoon of the remaining pepper. Spoon the kale mixture evenly over the turkey and roll up, jellyroll fashion, starting with the long side. Secure the roll with kitchen string at 3-inch intervals.

5 Brush a large roasting pan with the oil. Place the turkey seam side down in the pan. Bake until a thermometer inserted in the center of the turkey registers 165°F, about 1 hour. Transfer to a serving platter, cover loosely with foil, and let stand 10 minutes before carving.

6 To make the sauce, pour the pan drippings into a fat separator or a glass measuring cup. Pour off and discard the fat. Add enough of the remaining stock to make 1 cup. Pour the stock mixture into the roasting pan. Add the flour and whisk until smooth. Set the roasting pan over two burners and cook over medium-high heat, whisking constantly, until the sauce comes to a boil and thickens, about 3 minutes. Stir in the remaining ⅛ teaspoon pepper. Cut the turkey into thin slices and serve with the sauce.

Each serving: 5 g carb, 186 cal, 2 g fat, 1 g sat fat, 91 mg chol, 1 g fib, 35 g pro, 255 mg sod • Carb Choices: 0; Exchanges: 5 lean protein

Osso Buco–Style Turkey Drumsticks

makes 6 servings

Before you begin this recipe, dig out your largest roasting pan. Though they are mostly bone—which adds wonderful flavor—turkey drumsticks are huge. I like to make this dish on a cold snowy day and serve it for a comforting dinner with mashed potatoes or egg noodles.

6 (10- to 12-ounce) turkey drumsticks, skinned
½ teaspoon kosher salt
½ teaspoon freshly ground pepper
4 teaspoons extra virgin olive oil, divided
2 carrots, peeled and chopped
2 stalks celery, chopped
1 medium onion, chopped
2 garlic cloves, minced
¾ cup dry white wine
1¾ cups Chicken Stock (page 149) or low-sodium chicken broth
1 (14½-ounce) can no-salt-added diced tomatoes
3 tablespoons no-salt-added tomato paste
1 bay leaf

1 Preheat the oven to 325°F.

2 Sprinkle the drumsticks with the salt and pepper. Heat a large skillet over medium-high heat. Add 2 teaspoons of the oil and tilt the pan to coat the bottom evenly. Add the drumsticks and cook, turning often, until well browned on all sides, about 10 minutes. Transfer to a large roasting pan.

3 Add the remaining 2 teaspoons oil and tilt the pan to coat the bottom evenly. Add the carrots, celery, and onion to the skillet and cook, stirring often, until the vegetables soften and begin to brown, 8 minutes. Add the garlic and cook, stirring constantly, until fragrant, 30 seconds. Add the wine and bring to a boil, stirring to scrape up the browned bits from the bottom of the skillet. Cook until most of the liquid evaporates, 2 minutes. Stir in the stock, tomatoes, tomato paste, and bay leaf and bring to a boil. Carefully pour the mixture over the turkey. Cover tightly with foil and bake until the turkey is very tender, about 2 hours. Remove and discard the bay leaf.

4 Transfer the turkey to 6 deep bowls and spoon the sauce and vegetables evenly over the turkey.

Each serving: 9 g carb, 318 cal, 9 g fat, 2 g sat fat, 168 mg chol, 2 g fib, 43 g pro, 269 mg sod • Carb Choices: ½; Exchanges: 1 veg, 6 lean protein, ½ fat

Sautéed Turkey Cutlets with Raisin Chutney QUICK

makes 4 servings

The combination of sweet raisins and salty capers makes a flavorful accompaniment to plain turkey breast cutlets. You can substitute dried thyme for the fresh. Use ½ teaspoon for seasoning the turkey and ⅛ teaspoon in the chutney.

4 (4-ounce) turkey breast cutlets
1½ teaspoons chopped fresh thyme, divided
½ teaspoon kosher salt
¼ teaspoon freshly ground pepper
3 teaspoons extra virgin olive oil, divided
¼ cup diced onion
1 garlic clove, minced
½ cup Chicken Stock (page 149) or low-sodium chicken broth
½ cup golden raisins
2 teaspoons capers, rinsed and drained
2 teaspoons apple cider vinegar
1 tablespoon orange marmalade

1 Sprinkle the turkey with 1 teaspoon of the thyme, the salt, and pepper. Heat a large skillet over medium heat. Add 2 teaspoons of the oil and tilt the pan to coat the bottom evenly. Add the turkey and cook, turning once, until the juices run clear, about 4 minutes on each side. Transfer to a plate and cover with foil to keep warm.

2 Increase the heat to medium-high. Add the remaining 1 teaspoon oil to the skillet and tilt the pan to coat the bottom evenly. Add the onion and cook, stirring often, until just softened, about 3 minutes. Add the garlic and cook, stirring constantly, until fragrant, 30 seconds. Add the stock, raisins, capers, and vinegar and cook, stirring occasionally, until most of the liquid is absorbed, about 3 minutes. Remove from the heat and stir in the marmalade and remaining

½ teaspoon thyme. Divide the turkey among 4 plates and serve with the chutney.

Each serving: 19 g carb, 198 cal, 4 g fat, 1 g sat fat, 34 mg chol, 1 g fib, 22 g pro, 278 mg sod • Carb Choices: 1; Exchanges: 1 carb, 3 lean protein, ½ fat

Grilled Turkey Cutlets with Apple Salsa

makes 4 servings

Apple and mint give turkey a light fresh flavor. Enjoy this recipe in the spring and summer for an unexpected take on turkey.

TURKEY

¼ cup unsweetened apple juice
2 tablespoons chopped fresh mint
2 garlic cloves, minced
1½ teaspoons extra virgin olive oil, divided
1 teaspoon grated lime zest
4 (4-ounce) turkey breast cutlets
½ teaspoon kosher salt

SALSA

2 medium Granny Smith apples, cored and chopped
2 tablespoons diced red onion
1 small jalapeño, seeded and minced
1 tablespoon chopped fresh mint
1 tablespoon lime juice
1 teaspoon extra virgin olive oil
⅛ teaspoon kosher salt

1 To make the turkey, combine the apple juice, mint, garlic, 1 teaspoon of the oil, and the lime zest in a large resealable plastic bag. Add the turkey, turn to coat, and refrigerate 2 to 4 hours.

2 Preheat the grill to medium-high heat.

3 Remove the turkey from the marinade and discard the marinade. Pat the turkey dry with paper towels and sprinkle with the salt.

4 Brush the grill rack with the remaining ½ teaspoon oil. Place the turkey on the grill and grill, turning often, until no longer pink, 8 to 10 minutes.

5 Meanwhile, to make the salsa, combine all the ingredients in a medium bowl and stir to combine. Divide the turkey among 4 plates and serve with the salsa.

Each serving: 13 g carb, 153 cal, 2 g fat, 0 g sat fat, 34 mg chol, 2 g fib, 21 g pro, 252 mg sod • Carb Choices: 1; Exchanges: 1 fruit, 3 lean protein

Indian-Spiced Turkey Cutlets with Sautéed Peaches QUICK

makes 4 servings

Serve this light and lean turkey with Quinoa, Zucchini, and Mint Salad (page 113) for a refreshing summer meal. You can use 2 nectarines or 4 apricots instead of the peaches if you wish.

4 (4-ounce) turkey breast cutlets
3 teaspoons minced fresh ginger, divided
¾ teaspoon ground cumin, divided
¾ teaspoon ground coriander, divided
½ teaspoon kosher salt
4 teaspoons canola oil, divided
2 large ripe peaches, pitted and sliced
1 scallion, thinly sliced
2 tablespoons chopped fresh cilantro
1 tablespoon lime juice
Lime wedges

1 Sprinkle the turkey with 2 teaspoons of the ginger, ½ teaspoon of the cumin, ½ teaspoon of the coriander, and the salt. Heat a large nonstick skillet over medium heat. Add 2 teaspoons of the oil and tilt the pan to coat the bottom evenly. Add the turkey and cook, turning once, until the juices run clear, about 4 minutes on each side. Transfer to a plate.

2 Increase the heat to medium-high. Add the remaining 2 teaspoons oil to the skillet and tilt the pan to coat the bottom evenly. Add the peaches and scallion, then add the remaining 1 teaspoon ginger, ¼ teaspoon cumin, and ¼ teaspoon coriander. Cook, stirring often, until the peaches are warmed through and the scallion is crisp-tender, about 3 minutes. Remove from the heat and stir in the cilantro and lime juice. Divide the turkey among 4 plates. Top evenly with the peach mixture and serve with the lime wedges.

Each serving: 9 g carb, 169 cal, 5 g fat, 0 g sat fat, 34 mg chol, 2 g fib, 22 g pro, 217 mg sod • Carb Choices: ½; Exchanges: ½ fruit, 3 lean protein, 1 fat

Ground Poultry and Poultry Sausage

Juicy Turkey Burgers

QUICK | HIGH FIBER

makes 4 servings

Finely chopped mushrooms are the secret to these juicy burgers. Be creative with the bread you use. Instead of a kaiser roll, serve the burgers inside whole wheat pita bread or serve them open-face on a slice of toasted whole grain bread.

4 ounces white mushrooms
1 pound ground lean turkey
¼ cup plain dry breadcrumbs
1 large egg white
1 garlic clove, minced
¼ teaspoon kosher salt
¼ teaspoon freshly ground pepper
2 teaspoons canola oil
4 whole wheat kaiser rolls, split and toasted
Lettuce leaves

1 Place the mushrooms in a food processor and pulse until finely chopped.

2 Combine the mushrooms, turkey, breadcrumbs, egg white, garlic, salt, and pepper in a medium bowl and mix thoroughly with your hands. Shape into 4 patties.

3 Heat a large nonstick skillet over medium-high heat. Add the oil and tilt the pan to coat the bottom evenly. Add the burgers and cook, turning once, until no longer pink, 5 minutes on each side. Serve the burgers in the rolls, topped with the lettuce.

Each serving: 30 g carb, 292 cal, 10 g fat, 2 g sat fat, 49 mg chol, 4 g fib, 23 g pro, 405 mg sod • Carb Choices: 2; Exchanges: 2 starch, 2 lean protein, ½ fat

TURKEY BACON BURGERS QUICK HIGH FIBER : Follow the Juicy Turkey Burgers recipe, at left, but before preparing the burgers, cook 2 strips center-cut bacon until crisp, drain on paper towels, and chop. Add the bacon to the turkey mixture, shape into patties, and cook as directed.

Each serving: 29 g carb, 307 cal, 11 g fat, 2 g sat fat, 52 mg chol, 4 g fib, 24 g pro, 469 mg sod • Carb Choices: 2; Exchanges: 2 starch, 3 lean protein, 1 fat

GOAT CHEESE AND HERB TURKEY BURGERS QUICK HIGH FIBER : Follow the Juicy Turkey Burgers recipe, at left, adding 2 tablespoons chopped fresh basil to the turkey mixture. Cook as directed, topping each burger with 1 tablespoon crumbled goat cheese during the last 2 minutes of cooking.

Each serving: 29 g carb, 318 cal, 12 g fat, 4 g sat fat, 54 mg chol, 4 g fib, 25 g pro, 442 mg sod • Carb Choices: 2; Exchanges: 2 starch, 3 lean protein, 1 fat

Asian Turkey Burgers

QUICK | HIGH FIBER

makes 4 servings

Sweet and spicy hoisin sauce and fresh minced ginger flavor these outstanding burgers. If you love the taste of hoisin sauce, spread a little more on the rolls. Cucumber and cabbage stand in for lettuce and tomato, giving these burgers superior crunch.

1 large egg white
1 tablespoon hoisin sauce
1 tablespoon reduced-sodium soy sauce
4 ounces white mushrooms
1 pound ground lean turkey
¼ cup plain dry breadcrumbs
2 tablespoons chopped fresh cilantro
1 tablespoon minced fresh ginger
1 garlic clove, minced
2 teaspoons canola oil
4 whole wheat kaiser rolls, split and toasted
½ hothouse (English) cucumber, thinly sliced
1 cup thinly sliced cabbage

1 Whisk together the egg white, hoisin sauce, and soy sauce in a large bowl.

2 Place the mushrooms in a food processor and pulse until finely chopped. Add the mushrooms, turkey, breadcrumbs, cilantro, ginger, and garlic to the egg white mixture and mix thoroughly with your hands. Shape into 4 patties.

3 Heat a large nonstick skillet over medium-high heat. Add the oil and tilt the pan to coat the bottom evenly. Add the burgers and cook, turning once, until no longer pink, 5 minutes on each side. Serve the burgers in the rolls, topped with the cucumber and cabbage.

Each serving: 32 g carb, 300 cal, 10 g fat, 2 g sat fat, 49 mg chol, 5 g fib, 24 g pro, 554 mg sod • Carb Choices: 2; Exchanges: 2 starch, 2 lean protein, ½ fat

Cheddar-Stuffed Turkey Burgers QUICK | HIGH FIBER

makes 4 servings

Biting into the cheese inside these burgers is a delicious surprise. Extra-sharp Cheddar cheese is one of my favorite ingredients for salads and sandwiches. If it's finely shredded, a tiny amount can flavor a whole dish. It's definitely a must-have refrigerator staple.

4 ounces white mushrooms
1 pound ground lean turkey
¼ cup plain dry breadcrumbs
1 large egg white
1 garlic clove, minced
2 teaspoons chili powder
½ teaspoon cumin
¼ teaspoon kosher salt
¼ teaspoon freshly ground pepper
1 ounce finely shredded reduced-fat extra-
    sharp Cheddar cheese (about ¼ cup)
2 teaspoons canola oil
4 whole wheat kaiser rolls, split and toasted
4 large leaves leaf lettuce
¾ cup Fresh Tomato Salsa (page 41) or
    purchased tomato salsa

1 Place the mushrooms in a food processor and pulse until finely chopped.

2 Combine the mushrooms, turkey, breadcrumbs, egg white, garlic, chili powder, cumin, salt, and pepper in a medium bowl and mix thoroughly with your hands. Shape into 8 patties. Place 1 tablespoon of the Cheddar on top of each of 4 of the patties. Top with the remaining 4 patties and pinch the edges to seal.

3 Heat a large nonstick skillet over medium-high heat. Add the oil and tilt the pan to coat the bottom evenly. Add the burgers and cook, turning once, until no longer pink, 5 minutes on each side. Serve the burgers in the rolls, topped with the lettuce and salsa.

Each serving: 30 g carb, 319 cal, 12 g fat, 3 g sat fat, 54 mg chol, 4 g fib, 25 g pro, 468 mg sod • Carb Choices: 2; Exchanges: 2 starch, 3 lean protein, 1 fat

Italian Turkey Meatloaf

makes 6 servings

Your family may never ask for beef meatloaf again after trying this one made from a flavorful mixture of ground turkey and turkey sausage. Chopped fresh mushrooms add flavor as well as moisture. Any leftovers reheat beautifully in the microwave, or make great cold meatloaf sandwiches.

8 ounces white mushrooms
2 teaspoons extra virgin olive oil
½ cup finely diced onion
1 garlic clove, minced
½ teaspoon kosher salt
½ teaspoon dried oregano
½ teaspoon dried basil
¼ teaspoon freshly ground pepper
1 pound ground lean turkey
8 ounces Italian turkey sausage, casings removed
¾ cup no-salt-added tomato sauce, divided
½ cup plain dry breadcrumbs
⅓ cup 1% low-fat milk
1 large egg, lightly beaten
¼ cup chopped fresh Italian parsley

1 Preheat the oven to 350°F.

2 Place the mushrooms in a food processor and pulse until finely chopped.

3 Heat a medium nonstick skillet over medium-high heat. Add the oil and tilt the pan to coat the bottom evenly. Add the mushrooms and onion and cook, stirring often, until the vegetables are softened and most of the liquid has evaporated, 8 minutes. Add the garlic, salt, oregano, basil, and pepper and cook, stirring constantly, until fragrant, 30 seconds. Transfer to a plate and let cool slightly.

4 Combine the turkey, turkey sausage, ¼ cup of the tomato sauce, the breadcrumbs, milk, egg, parsley, and the mushroom mixture in a large bowl. Mix thoroughly with your hands. Place the mixture in a large shallow baking dish and shape into a 10 x 4-inch loaf.

5 Spread the remaining ½ cup tomato sauce over the loaf and bake 1 hour. Let stand 5 minutes before slicing. Cut the meatloaf into 6 slices and serve at once.

Each serving: 13 g carb, 218 cal, 10 g fat, 2 g sat fat, 85 mg chol, 1 g fib, 20 g pro, 411 mg sod • Carb Choices: 1; Exchanges: ½ starch, 1 veg, 2 lean protein, 1 fat

Salsa Turkey Meatloaf

makes 6 servings

If you're trying to get your family out of the weekly taco night rut, this spicy meatloaf offers up the same flavors, but with a different twist. Serve the meatloaf with Buttermilk Mashed Potatoes (page 482).

8 ounces white mushrooms
2 teaspoons extra virgin olive oil
½ cup finely diced onion
1 jalapeño, seeded and minced
1 garlic clove, minced
1½ teaspoons ground cumin
½ teaspoon kosher salt
¼ teaspoon freshly ground pepper
1½ pounds ground lean turkey
1 (14½-ounce) can no-salt added diced
    tomatoes, drained
½ cup plain dry breadcrumbs
⅓ cup 1% low-fat milk
1 large egg, lightly beaten
¼ cup chopped fresh cilantro

1 Preheat the oven to 350°F.

2 Place the mushrooms in a food processor and pulse until finely chopped.

3 Heat a medium nonstick skillet over medium-high heat. Add the oil and tilt the pan to coat the bottom evenly. Add the mushrooms, onion, and jalapeño and cook, stirring often, until the vegetables are softened and most of the liquid has evaporated, 8 minutes. Add the garlic, cumin, salt, and pepper and cook, stirring constantly, until fragrant, 30 seconds. Transfer to a plate and let cool slightly.

4 Combine the turkey, tomatoes, breadcrumbs, milk, egg, cilantro, and the mushroom mixture in a large bowl. Mix thoroughly with your hands. Place the mixture in a large shallow baking dish and shape into a 10 x 4-inch loaf. Bake 1 hour. Let stand 5 minutes before slicing. Cut the meatloaf into 6 slices and serve at once.

Each serving: 12 g carb, 208 cal, 8 g fat, 2 g sat fat, 85 mg chol, 1 g fib, 21 g pro, 263 mg sod • Carb Choices: 1; Exchanges: ½ starch, 1 veg, 3 lean protein

Turkey Mole Chili HIGH FIBER

makes 6 servings

This unusual chili has layers of flavor from spices, cocoa powder, and honey. The touch of honey rounds out the slightly bitter flavor from the coffee and cocoa powder.

2 teaspoons extra virgin olive oil
1 pound ground extra-lean turkey
1 large onion, chopped
1 large red bell pepper, chopped
2 garlic cloves, minced
2 tablespoons chili powder
2 tablespoons ground cumin
½ teaspoon dried oregano
1 cup brewed coffee
2 cups Chicken Stock (page 149) or low-sodium chicken broth
1 (15-ounce) can no-salt-added black beans, rinsed and drained
1 (14½-ounce) can no-salt-added diced tomatoes
2 tablespoons no-salt-added tomato paste
2 tablespoons unsweetened cocoa
¼ teaspoon kosher salt
2 tablespoons lime juice
1 tablespoon honey
Thinly sliced scallions
Chopped fresh cilantro

1 Heat a large saucepan over medium-high heat. Add the oil and tilt the pan to coat the bottom evenly. Add the turkey, onion, and bell pepper and cook, stirring often, until the turkey is no longer pink, 8 minutes. Add the garlic, chili powder, cumin, and oregano and cook, stirring constantly, until fragrant, 30 seconds.

2 Add the coffee, stock, beans, tomatoes, tomato paste, cocoa, and salt and bring to a boil. Reduce the heat to low, cover, and simmer 25 to 30 minutes. Remove from the heat and stir in the lime juice and honey. Divide the chili among 6 bowls and sprinkle each serving with scallions and cilantro. The chili can be refrigerated, covered, for up to 4 days or frozen for up to 3 months.

Each serving: 24 g carb, 214 cal, 4 g fat, 1 g sat fat, 24 mg chol, 7 g fib, 22 g pro, 282 mg sod • Carb Choices: 1½; Exchanges: 1 starch, 1 veg, 3 lean protein

Chicken Sausage Stew with Beans and Escarole

QUICK | HIGH FIBER

makes 4 servings

Chicken sausage comes in so many delicious flavors, it's hard to choose which ones to try. For this dish, select one flavored with sun-dried tomatoes, fennel, or roasted garlic.

2 teaspoons extra virgin olive oil
8 ounces chicken sausage, cut into ½-inch slices
1 small onion, chopped
1 carrot, chopped
1 stalk celery, chopped
1 garlic clove, minced
3 cups Chicken Stock (page 149) or low-sodium chicken broth
1 (14-ounce) can no-salt-added navy or cannellini beans, rinsed and drained
1 (14½-ounce) can no-salt-added diced tomatoes
3 tablespoons no-salt-added tomato paste
½ teaspoon dried oregano
¼ teaspoon freshly ground pepper
3 cups coarsely chopped escarole
2 tablespoons freshly grated Parmesan

1 Heat a large saucepan over medium-high heat. Add the oil and tilt the pan to coat the bottom evenly. Add the sausage and cook, turning often, until lightly browned, about 6 minutes. Transfer to a plate. Add the onion, carrot, and celery and cook, stirring often, until softened, 5 minutes. Add the garlic and cook, stirring constantly, until fragrant, 30 seconds. Add the stock, beans, tomatoes, tomato paste, oregano, pepper, and sausage and bring to a boil.

2 Reduce the heat to low, cover, and simmer for 10 minutes. Stir in the escarole and cook until the escarole is tender, about 5 minutes. Ladle the stew into 4 bowls, sprinkle evenly with the Parmesan, and serve at once. The stew can be refrigerated, covered, for up to 4 days.

Each serving: 27 g carb, 288 cal, 11 g fat, 3 g sat fat, 64 mg chol, 8 g fib, 20 g pro, 680 mg sod • Carb Choices: 1½; Exchanges: 1 starch, 1 veg, 2 medium-fat protein, ½ fat

Beer-Braised Chicken Sausages with Fennel and Peppers QUICK | HIGH FIBER

makes 4 servings

Fennel-, mushroom-, or roasted pepper–flavored chicken sausage would work well with this recipe. You can also make this with plain turkey kielbasa with delicious results.

1 medium bulb fennel
4 teaspoons extra virgin olive oil, divided
4 links chicken sausage (about 1 pound), halved lengthwise
1 yellow bell pepper, cut into strips
1 medium onion, halved lengthwise and thinly sliced
2 garlic cloves, minced
1 cup lager beer
1 tablespoon light brown sugar
¼ cup chopped fresh Italian parsley

1 Trim the tough outer stalks from the fennel. Cut the fennel bulb in half vertically and cut away and discard the core. Cut each half lengthwise into ¼-inch slices.

2 Heat a large nonstick skillet over medium-high heat. Add 2 teaspoons of the oil and tilt the pan to coat the bottom evenly. Add the sausages and cook until well browned on both sides, 4 to 6 minutes. Transfer to a plate.

3 Add the remaining 2 teaspoons oil and tilt the pan to coat the bottom evenly. Add the fennel, bell pepper, and onion and cook, stirring often, until softened, 5 minutes. Add the garlic and cook, stirring constantly, until fragrant, 30 seconds. Place

the sausages on top of the vegetables. Pour the beer over the sausages and bring to a boil.

4 Reduce the heat to low, cover, and simmer, stirring occasionally, until the vegetables are tender, about 10 minutes. Uncover and stir in the sugar. Increase the heat to medium-high and cook, stirring often, until most of the liquid is evaporated, about 3 minutes. Transfer the sausages to 4 plates. Stir the parsley into the vegetable mixture and serve with the sausages.

Each serving: 19 g carb, 274 cal, 14 g fat, 3 g sat fat, 75 mg chol, 4 g fib, 16 g pro, 708 mg sod • Carb Choices: 1; Exchanges: ½ carb, 2 veg, 2 medium-fat protein, 1 fat

Pasta with Turkey Sausage, Peppers, and Kale

QUICK | HIGH FIBER

makes 4 servings

Boldly flavored sausage and kale make this dish a family favorite. Sometimes I use turkey kielbasa instead of the turkey sausage, and if I find mild yellow banana peppers, they make a flavorful substitute for the bell pepper.

4 ounces whole wheat penne or other short pasta (about 1½ cups)

4 cups chopped fresh kale

2 teaspoons extra virgin olive oil

1 pound Italian turkey sausage, cut into 1½-inch pieces

1 medium red bell pepper, thinly sliced

1 medium onion, halved lengthwise and thinly sliced

2 garlic cloves, minced

1 (14½-ounce) can no-salt-added diced tomatoes

½ teaspoon dried oregano

½ teaspoon dried basil

¼ teaspoon freshly ground pepper

2 tablespoons freshly grated Parmesan

1 Cook the pasta according to the package directions, adding the kale during the last 5 minutes of cooking. Drain.

2 Meanwhile, heat a large nonstick skillet over medium heat. Add the oil and tilt the pan to coat the bottom evenly. Add the sausage and cook, turning often, until well browned, about 6 minutes. Transfer to a plate.

3 Add the bell pepper and onion and cook, stirring often, until softened, 5 minutes. Add the garlic and cook, stirring constantly, until fragrant, 30 seconds.

4 Add the turkey, tomatoes, oregano, basil, and ground pepper and bring to a boil. Reduce the heat to low, cover, and simmer, stirring occasionally, until the vegetables are tender, about 5 minutes. Add the pasta mixture and stir to combine. Spoon the pasta mixture evenly onto 4 plates, sprinkle evenly with the Parmesan, and serve at once.

Each serving: 37 g carb, 346 cal, 13 g fat, 1 g sat fat, 53 mg chol, 6 g fib, 23 g pro, 656 mg sod • Carb Choices: 2½; Exchanges: 1½ starch, 3 veg, 2 medium-fat protein, ½ fat

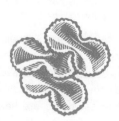

Turkey Sausage with Braised Red Cabbage and Apples QUICK

makes 4 servings

This easy, comforting, and inexpensive meal is one of those dishes that tastes better than you think it could from the simple ingredient list.

2 teaspoons extra virgin olive oil
4 links Italian turkey sausage (about 1 pound), halved lengthwise
1 small onion, halved lengthwise and thinly sliced
4 cups thinly sliced red cabbage
1 large Granny Smith apple, peeled, cored, and chopped
1¼ cups Chicken Stock (page 149) or low-sodium chicken broth, divided
¼ teaspoon caraway seeds
⅛ teaspoon freshly ground pepper
1 tablespoon red wine vinegar

1 Heat a large nonstick skillet over medium-high heat. Add the oil and tilt the pan to coat the bottom evenly. Add the sausage and cook until well browned on both sides, 4 to 6 minutes. Transfer to a plate.

2 Add the onion and cook, stirring often, until softened, 5 minutes. Stir in the cabbage, apple, 1 cup of the stock, the caraway seeds, and pepper. Bring to a boil.

3 Reduce the heat to low, cover, and simmer, stirring occasionally, until the cabbage is tender, about 15 minutes. Return the sausages to the skillet, add the remaining ¼ cup stock, cover, and simmer until the sausages are heated through, about 3 minutes. Transfer the sausages to 4 plates, stir the vinegar into the cabbage mixture, and serve with the sausages.

Each serving: 12 g carb, 215 cal, 12 g fat, 1 g sat fat, 52 mg chol, 3 g fib, 17 g pro, 604 mg sod • Carb Choices: 1; Exchanges: ½ fruit, 1 veg, 2 medium-fat protein, ½ fat

Pasta, Turkey Sausage, and White Beans in Garlicky Tomato Sauce QUICK | HIGH FIBER

makes 6 servings

This is an easy skillet meal with simple flavors everyone will enjoy for a weeknight dinner. Add a green salad made with what's on hand in the refrigerator and you've got a satisfying supper.

4 ounces whole wheat penne or other short pasta (about 1½ cups)
4 teaspoons extra virgin olive oil, divided
8 ounces Italian turkey sausage, cut into 1½-inch slices
1 medium onion, chopped
4 garlic cloves, minced
1 (28-ounce) can no-salt-added whole tomatoes, undrained and chopped
1 (15-ounce) can no-salt-added cannellini beans, rinsed and drained
⅛ teaspoon freshly ground pepper
2 tablespoons chopped fresh Italian parsley
3 tablespoons freshly grated Parmesan

1 Cook the pasta according to the package directions.

2 Meanwhile, heat a large nonstick skillet over medium heat. Add 2 teaspoons of the oil and tilt the pan to coat the bottom evenly. Add the sausage and cook, turning often, until well browned, about 6 minutes. Transfer to a plate.

3 Add the remaining 2 teaspoons oil and tilt the pan to coat the bottom evenly. Add the onion and cook, stirring occasionally, until softened, 5 minutes. Add the garlic and cook, stirring constantly, until fragrant, 30 seconds.

4 Stir in the tomatoes and their juices, the beans, pepper, and the sausage and bring to a boil. Reduce the heat to low, cover, and simmer

15 minutes. Add the pasta and parsley and stir to combine. Spoon the pasta mixture evenly onto 6 plates, sprinkle evenly with the Parmesan, and serve at once.

Each serving: 32 g carb, 242 cal, 8 g fat, 1 g sat fat, 19 mg chol, 6 g fib, 13 g pro, 264 mg sod • Carb Choices: 2; Exchanges: 1½ starch, 1 veg, 1 medium-fat protein, 1 lean protein, ½ fat

Grilled Italian Turkey Sausage with Peppers and Tomatoes QUICK

makes 4 servings

Nothing could be simpler than this dish of grilled sausages and vegetables. The tangy vinaigrette drizzled over the dish gives it great flavor with no fuss. It's a lovely dish to enjoy in late fall before storing the grill for the season.

4 plum tomatoes, halved lengthwise
1 large red onion, cut into 8 wedges
1 green bell pepper, cut into 1-inch slices
1 red or yellow bell pepper, cut into 1-inch slices
2 tablespoons plus 2½ teaspoons extra-virgin olive oil, divided
1 pound hot or mild Italian turkey sausage links
2 tablespoons red wine vinegar
½ teaspoon Dijon mustard
1 garlic clove, crushed through a press
¼ teaspoon kosher salt
¼ teaspoon dried oregano
¼ teaspoon dried basil
¼ teaspoon freshly ground pepper

1 Prepare the grill or heat a large grill pan over medium-high heat.

2 Combine the tomatoes, onion, and bell peppers in a large bowl. Drizzle with 2 teaspoons of the oil and toss to coat.

3 Brush the grill rack or grill pan with ½ teaspoon of the remaining oil. Pierce the sausages several times using the point of a small knife. Place the sausages, onion, and bell peppers on the grill and grill, turning often, until the juices of the sausages run clear and the vegetables are crisp-tender, about 10 minutes. Place the tomatoes on the grill during the last 3 to 4 minutes of cooking time and grill, turning once, just until heated through.

4 Meanwhile, whisk together the remaining 2 tablespoons oil, the vinegar, mustard, garlic, salt, oregano, basil, and ground pepper in a small bowl. To serve, divide the sausages and vegetables among 4 plates and drizzle evenly with the dressing.

Each serving: 10 g carb, 264 cal, 17 g fat, 3 g sat fat, 64 mg chol, 3 g fib, 18 g pro, 587 mg sod • Carb Choices: ½; Exchanges: 1 veg, 2 lean protein, 1½ fat

Other Birds

Spice-Rubbed Roasted Cornish Hens

makes 4 servings

Cornish hens are so easy to make and they take less than an hour to bake. For a side dish that bakes in the same amount of time as the hens, serve these with Butternut Squash and Gruyère Gratin (page 494).

½ teaspoon coriander seeds
½ teaspoon cumin seeds
4 whole black peppercorns
½ teaspoon kosher salt
2 (1½-pound) Cornish hens, skinned

1 Preheat the oven to 350°F.

2 Place the coriander, cumin, and peppercorns in a small dry skillet over medium heat and toast, shaking the pan often, until the spices are fragrant, 3 minutes. Transfer to a small plate and allow to cool. Place the spices in a mortar and crush with a pestle. Alternatively, place them in a small resealable plastic bag. Seal the bag, place on a cutting board, and crush using a meat mallet or the back of a large spoon. Add the salt to the spice mixture and rub over the hens.

3 Place the hens in a roasting pan. Bake until an instant-read thermometer inserted into a thigh reads 165°F, about 45 minutes. Transfer the hens to a platter, cover loosely, and let stand 10 minutes before serving. Cut each hen in half. Divide the halved hens among 4 plates and serve at once.

Each serving: 0 g carb, 187 cal, 5 g fat, 1 g sat fat, 146 mg chol, 0 g fib, 32 g pro, 227 mg sod • Carb Choices: 0; Exchanges: 5 lean protein

Citrus-Glazed Cornish Hens

makes 4 servings

The sugars in the orange juice leave the hens lightly glazed with citrus flavor. These are versatile enough to serve year-round. Enjoy them with a pasta or grain salad alongside in the summer and with mashed sweet potatoes in the fall and winter.

1 cup orange juice
¼ cup lemon juice
1 small onion, chopped
2 garlic cloves, chopped
2 (1½-pound) Cornish hens, cut in half lengthwise and skinned
½ teaspoon kosher salt
¼ teaspoon freshly ground pepper

1 Combine the orange juice, lemon juice, onion, and garlic in a food processor and process until smooth. Transfer the mixture to a large resealable plastic bag. Add the hens, turn to coat, and refrigerate 8 to 12 hours.

2 Preheat the oven to 400°F.

3 Remove the hens from the marinade and discard the marinade. Pat dry with paper towels. Sprinkle the hens with the salt and pepper. Place the hens in a roasting pan. Bake until an instant-read thermometer inserted into a thigh reads 165°F, 35 to 40 minutes. Transfer the hens to a platter, cover loosely with foil, and let stand 10 minutes before serving. Cut each hen in half. Divide halved hens among 4 plates and serve at once.

Each serving: 2 g carb, 194 cal, 5 g fat, 1 g sat fat, 146 mg chol, 0 g fib, 32 g pro, 227 mg sod • Carb Choices: 0; Exchanges: 5 lean protein

Duck Breast with Dried Cherry–Port Sauce [QUICK]

makes 4 servings

Duck breast is an easy yet luxurious main course for entertaining. Take care not to overcook it, as it can quickly become dry and chewy.

4 (6-ounce) duck breast halves, skinned
½ teaspoon kosher salt
⅛ teaspoon freshly ground pepper
2 teaspoons extra virgin olive oil
1 shallot, minced
½ cup tawny port
⅓ cup dried cherries
1 teaspoon honey

1 Sprinkle the duck with the salt and pepper. Heat a large skillet over medium-high heat. Add the oil and tilt the pan to coat the bottom evenly. Add the duck and cook, turning once, 3 minutes on each side for medium-rare, or to the desired degree of doneness. Transfer to a plate and cover loosely with foil to keep warm.

2 Add the shallot to the skillet and cook, stirring often, until softened, 3 minutes. Add the port and cherries and bring to a boil, stirring to scrape up the browned bits from the bottom of the skillet. Cook until the sauce is slightly thickened, about 3 minutes. Remove from the heat and stir in the honey.

3 Transfer the duck to a cutting board and cut into thin slices. Arrange the duck on 4 plates and spoon the sauce evenly over each serving. Serve at once.

Each serving: 12 g carb, 271 cal, 6 g fat, 1 g sat fat, 182 mg chol, 0 g fib, 36 g pro, 275 mg sod • Carb Choices: 1; Exchanges: ½ carb, ½ fruit, 5 lean protein, ½ fat

Duck Breast with Black Currant Vinaigrette [QUICK]

makes 4 servings

You can make the vinaigrette well ahead of time, but don't store it in the refrigerator. It should be at room temperature when you drizzle it over the duck.

2 tablespoons black currant preserves
1 tablespoon sherry vinegar or rice vinegar
1 tablespoon plus 2 teaspoons extra virgin olive oil, divided
¼ teaspoon Dijon mustard
½ teaspoon kosher salt, divided
⅛ teaspoon plus ¼ teaspoon freshly ground pepper, divided
4 (6-ounce) duck breast halves, skinned

1 Whisk together the preserves, vinegar, 1 tablespoon of the oil, the mustard, ¼ teaspoon of the salt, and ⅛ teaspoon of the pepper in a small bowl.

2 Sprinkle the duck with the remaining ¼ teaspoon salt and remaining ¼ teaspoon pepper. Heat a large skillet over medium-high heat. Add the remaining 2 teaspoons oil and tilt the pan to coat the bottom evenly. Add the duck and cook, turning once, 3 minutes on each side for medium-rare, or to the desired degree of doneness.

3 Transfer the duck to a cutting board and cut into thin slices. Arrange the duck on 4 plates and drizzle evenly with the vinaigrette. Serve at once.

Each serving: 1 g carb, 195 cal, 4 g fat, 1 g sat fat, 182 mg chol, 0 g fib, 35 g pro, 167 mg sod • Carb Choices: 0; Exchanges: 5 lean protein

BEEF, PORK, AND LAMB MAIN DISHES

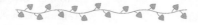

Steaks and Stir-Fries

Grilled T-Bone with Green Peppercorn–Garlic Crust

Steak with Quick Mushroom-Rosemary Sauce

Pan-Seared Steak with Avocado-Olive Relish

Ginger-Lime Grilled Steak with Pineapple Salsa

Spinach-Stuffed Steak Roll

Steak Tacos with Salsa Salad

Filets Mignons with Cabernet-Butter Sauce

Steak with Balsamic Banana Peppers

London Broil with Sherry Mushrooms

Beef, Artichoke, and Pepper Kebabs with Olive Vinaigrette

Beef and Pineapple Kebabs with Soy Dipping Sauce

Merlot-Marinated Beef Kebabs

Beef and Broccoli Stir-Fry

Beef, Green Bean, and Basil Stir-Fry

Beef Roasts

Perfect-Every-Time Beef Tenderloin

Eye of Round with Roasted Garlic–Horseradish Sauce

Garlic and Lime Beef Roast with Cilantro Pesto

Brined Eye of Round Roast

Beef Braises and One-Pot Meals

Classic Beef Pot Roast

Beef Pot Roast with Root Vegetables

Beef Pot Roast with Port and Coriander

Asian Beef Pot Roast

Beer-Braised Beef Brisket

Slow-Cooker Beef Brisket with Onion Gravy

Ropa Vieja Tacos

Chile-Braised Beef

Beef Carbonnade

Beef Bourguignon

Wine and Red Pepper– Braised Beef Stew

Beef and Red Bean Chili

Beef Stroganoff

Ground Beef

Moist and Lean Burgers

Blue Cheese Burgers with Caramelized Onions

Beef, Cheddar, and Black Bean Burgers

Open-Face Greek Burgers

Ginger-Sesame Burgers with
Grilled Scallions

Greek Beef and Orzo Pilaf

Asian Beef Lettuce Wraps

Old-Fashioned Meatloaf

Chile Pepper Meatloaf

Beef Kefta with
Yogurt Sauce

Swedish Meatballs

Spaghetti and Meatballs

Pasta with Beef and
Mushroom Bolognese Sauce

Weeknight Beef and
Spinach Lasagna

Beef and Barley Chili

Beef, Black Bean, and
Beer Chili

Three-Way Cincinnati Chili

Beef and Vegetable–Stuffed
Bell Peppers

Beef and Bean Enchiladas
with Ancho Chile Sauce

Pork Chops

Skillet Pork Chops

Pork Chops with
Sautéed Apples

Pork Chops with White
Beans and Sage

Pork Chops with
Apricot-Walnut Sauce

Pork Chops with Mango
Chutney Sauce

Oven-Fried Pork Chops
with Cream Gravy

Five-Spice Pork Chops with
Hoisin Onions

Grilled Orange and Sage–
Brined Pork Chops

Grilled Smoky BBQ
Pork Chops

Pork Tenderloins
and Roasts

Rosemary Roasted
Pork Tenderloin

Roasted Pork Tenderloin
with Pears and Sage

Apricot-Mustard-Glazed
Pork Tenderloin

Soy-Maple-Glazed
Pork Tenderloin

Lime-Marinated Grilled
Pork Tenderloin

Pork Medallions with
Fennel and Onion

Pork Stir-Fry with
Peas and Ginger

Pork Stir-Fry with Broccoli,
Scallions, and Hoisin Sauce

Pork Stir-Fry with
Red Curry Sauce

Garlic-Studded Rosemary-
Fennel Pork Roast

Thyme-Crusted Pork Loin
with Roasted Peaches

Maple-Brined
Pork Loin Roast

Sausage and Swiss Chard–
Stuffed Pork Loin Roast

Pork Braises and One-Pot Meals

Cider-Braised Pork Roast with Onions

Pork Braised with Peppers and Paprika

Hoisin-Braised Pork Stew

Pork, Butternut Squash, and Kale Stew

Red Chile Pork and Hominy Stew

Pork and Butternut Squash Tagine

Pork and Apple Stew with Sage

Lamb Chops

Pan-Seared Lamb Chops with Mint Pesto

Grilled Marinated Lamb Chops with Orange-Mint Relish

Lamb Chops with Blackberry-Thyme Sauce

Lamb Roasts

Rosemary-Garlic Roasted Rack of Lamb

Black Olive–Crusted Rack of Lamb

Roasted Leg of Lamb with Potatoes and Olives

Boneless Leg of Lamb with Mint Tapenade

Lamb Braises and One-Pot Meals

Lamb Tagine

Lamb Shanks Braised in Roasted Poblano Sauce

Braised Lamb with Parsnips and Dried Plums

Irish Lamb Stew

Beef, pork, and lamb can easily fit into any well-balanced healthy diet. Buying the leanest cuts of meat, trimming away any visible fat, choosing the best cooking method for each cut of meat, and paying attention to portion size are fundamental to enjoying meats in a healthy diet.

Beef is America's favorite meat and it's possible to enjoy many cuts and preparations of beef even if you're watching your waistline and limiting your fat intake. See Beef Basics (page 267) for the leanest cuts to buy and the best way to prepare each one. All your favorites are there—steaks, roasts, beef for braising, and ground beef.

When buying pork, look for the word "loin" on the label. Center-cut (these are from the leanest part) pork loin chops are quick-cooking solutions for weeknight suppers. They are delicious when pan-seared, grilled, or baked. For a quick juicy roast (done in about 30 minutes), you can't beat pork tenderloin. Tenderloins can also be sliced and quickly pan seared, just like a pork chop. Because it is the tenderest cut of pork, use tenderloin for stir-fries, too. For special dinners or a Sunday supper, a pork loin roast takes longer to cook than the smaller tenderloin, but it is just as moist and delicious. See Cooking Lean Pork (page 301) for tips for making the most of the leanest cuts.

Lamb chops and rack of lamb are the exact same cut of lamb. Cut the rack between the bones into separate pieces and you have lamb chops. Both are lean and delicious and are perfect for any celebration dinner. A leg of lamb is just the thing for a large gathering or for a small family when you want to have leftovers. For a lamb stew or braise, precut stew meat can be too fatty. Buy lamb shoulder (you could use a leg of lamb, though it is pricier) and cut it into pieces yourself to ensure that you are getting the leanest meat. Braised Lamb with Parsnips and Dried Plums (page 323) is one of my favorite recipes for transforming an inexpensive cut into what tastes like a gourmet meal.

Recognizing a sensible portion size is one of the most difficult skills for people who are new to adopting healthy eating habits. Contrary to what your favorite restaurant serves, a portion of meat (or chicken, turkey, fish, or shrimp) is 3 ounces of cooked meat—about 4 ounces before cooking. In other words, the entrées most restaurants serve are enough for 3 or 4 people! To "eyeball" a portion of beef (or any meat, poultry, or fish), remember that a 3-ounce serving is about the size of a deck of cards. Fill the rest of your plate with a whole grain side dish and plenty of vegetables and you have a satisfying and nutritious meal.

Steaks and Stir-Fries

Grilled T-Bone with Green Peppercorn–Garlic Crust

makes 4 servings

A great steak doesn't need much added to it, but green peppercorns are a simple yet flavorful seasoning. They are actually immature black peppercorns and they are not quite as spicy as black peppercorns and their flavor is cleaner and fresher.

1 (1¼-pound) T-bone steak, trimmed of all visible fat
1 teaspoon extra virgin olive oil, divided
1½ teaspoons whole green peppercorns
4 garlic cloves, minced
½ teaspoon kosher salt

1 Place the steak in a shallow dish and lightly coat with ½ teaspoon of the oil, the peppercorns, and garlic. Cover and refrigerate at least 6 hours or up to 12 hours.

2 Prepare the grill or heat a large grill pan over medium-high heat.

3 Sprinkle the steak with the salt. Brush the grill rack or grill pan with the remaining ½ teaspoon oil. Place the steak on the grill rack or in the grill pan and grill, turning once, 3 minutes on each side for medium-rare, or to the desired degree of doneness.

4 Transfer the steak to a cutting board, cover loosely with foil, and let stand 5 minutes. Cut the steak into thin slices, divide evenly among 4 plates, and serve at once.

Each serving: 1 g carb, 157 cal, 8 g fat, 2 g sat fat, 41 mg chol, 0 g fib, 20 g pro, 219 mg sod • Carb Choices: 0; Exchanges: 3 lean protein, 1½ fat

Steak with Quick Mushroom-Rosemary Sauce QUICK

makes 4 servings

This is a versatile weeknight entrée that you can vary according to what you have on hand. You can use any kind of tender steak—or even boneless skinless chicken breasts (substitute white wine for the red if you use chicken). Make the dish with whatever mushrooms are available and use sage or thyme instead of the rosemary.

1 (1-pound) strip, top sirloin, tri-tip, flank, or ranch steak, trimmed of all visible fat
¾ teaspoon kosher salt, divided
¼ teaspoon plus ⅛ teaspoon freshly ground pepper, divided
4 teaspoons extra virgin olive oil, divided
2 garlic cloves, minced
8 ounces cremini or white mushrooms, thinly sliced
1 large tomato, chopped
½ cup dry red wine
2 teaspoons chopped fresh rosemary or ½ teaspoon dried rosemary, crumbled

1 Sprinkle the steak with ½ teaspoon of the salt and ¼ teaspoon of the pepper. Heat a large heavy-bottomed skillet over medium-high heat. Add 2 teaspoons of the oil and tilt the pan to coat the bottom evenly. Add the steak and cook, turning once, 4 minutes on each side, or to the desired degree of doneness. Transfer the steak to a cutting board, cover loosely with foil, and let stand while you make the sauce.

2 Add the remaining 2 teaspoons oil to the skillet and tilt the pan to coat the bottom evenly. Add the garlic and cook, stirring constantly, until fragrant, 30 seconds. Add the mushrooms,

tomato, wine, and rosemary and cook, stirring often, until the mushrooms are tender and most of the liquid has evaporated, 6 to 8 minutes. Stir in the remaining ¼ teaspoon salt and remaining ⅛ teaspoon pepper.

3 Cut the steak across the grain into thin slices and divide among 4 plates. Top with the mushroom sauce and serve at once.

Each serving: 4 g carb, 228 cal, 9 g fat, 2 g sat fat, 42 mg chol, 0 g fib, 26 g pro, 266 mg sod • Carb Choices: 0; Exchanges: 3 lean protein, 1 fat

Beef Basics

Beef is a delicious and satisfying option for healthful eating—as long as you choose the leanest cuts and enjoy a sensible portion. To buy the leanest cuts and choose the best method for cooking them, follow the guidelines below.

STEAKS TO BROIL, PAN SEAR, OR GRILL

Steaks to Cook without Marinating

T-bone, tenderloin (filet mignon), top loin (strip steak), top sirloin, tri-tip, flank, and ranch steak

Steaks to Marinate, Then Cook

Round tip, eye of round, bottom round, top round, sirloin tip, and chuck shoulder steak

BEEF TO ROAST

Beef tenderloin, eye of round roast, round tip roast, and sirloin tip center roast

BEEF TO BRAISE IN LIQUID

Flat half brisket, beef chuck shoulder roast, and bottom round roast

GROUND BEEF

Always choose 95% lean ground beef

Pan-Seared Steak with Avocado-Olive Relish

makes 4 servings

Creamy, rich avocados, salty olives, and acidic tomatoes combine to make this distinctively flavored relish that pairs perfectly with a steak.

1 (1-pound) strip, top sirloin, tri-tip, flank, or
ranch steak, trimmed of all visible fat
4 teaspoons extra virgin olive oil, divided
1 garlic clove, minced
2 teaspoons grated lemon zest
½ teaspoon ground coriander
⅛ teaspoon freshly ground pepper
1 small avocado, pitted, peeled, and chopped
1 cup grape tomatoes, halved
¼ cup Kalamata olives, pitted and chopped
2 tablespoons diced red onion
2 tablespoons chopped fresh Italian parsley
1 tablespoon lemon juice
½ teaspoon kosher salt

1 Place the steak in a shallow dish, rub with 2 teaspoons of the oil, the garlic, lemon zest, coriander, and pepper. Cover and refrigerate at least 6 hours or up to 12 hours.

2 To make the relish, combine the avocado, tomatoes, olives, onion, parsley, and lemon juice in a medium bowl and stir to mix well.

3 Sprinkle the steak with the salt. Heat a large heavy-bottomed skillet over medium-high heat. Add the remaining 2 teaspoons oil and tilt the pan to coat the bottom evenly. Add the steak and cook, turning once, 4 minutes on each side for medium-rare, or to the desired degree of doneness.

4 Transfer the steak to a cutting board, cover loosely with foil, and let stand 5 minutes. Cut across the grain into thin slices. Divide the steak and relish evenly among 4 plates and serve at once.

Each serving: 5 g carb, 383 cal, 19 g fat, 3 g sat fat, 42 mg chol, 2 g fib, 26 g pro, 342 mg sod • Carb Choices: 0; Exchanges: ½ carb, 3 lean protein, 3 fat

Ginger-Lime Grilled Steak with Pineapple Salsa

makes 4 servings

This ginger-lime marinade gives any steak a fantastic flavor.

1 (1-pound) strip, top sirloin, tri-tip, flank, or ranch steak, trimmed of all visible fat

2½ teaspoons canola oil, divided

3 teaspoons grated lime zest, divided

3 teaspoons grated fresh ginger, divided

⅛ teaspoon ground cayenne

2 cups diced fresh pineapple

¼ cup diced red bell pepper

2 tablespoons chopped fresh cilantro

1 tablespoon lime juice

1 jalapeño, seeded and minced

¾ teaspoon kosher salt

1 Place the steak in a shallow dish, rub with 2 teaspoons of the oil, 2 teaspoons of the lime zest, 1 teaspoon of the ginger, and the cayenne. Cover and refrigerate at least 6 hours or up to 12 hours.

2 To make the salsa, combine the pineapple, bell pepper, cilantro, lime juice, jalapeño, remaining 1 teaspoon lime zest, and remaining 1 teaspoon ginger in a medium bowl and stir to mix well.

3 Prepare the grill or heat a large grill pan over medium-high heat.

4 Sprinkle the steak with the salt. Brush the grill rack or grill pan with the remaining ½ teaspoon oil. Place the steak on the grill rack or in the grill pan and grill, turning once, 3 minutes on each side for medium-rare, or to the desired degree of doneness.

5 Transfer the steak to a cutting board, cover loosely with foil, and let stand 5 minutes. Cut across the grain into thin slices. Divide the steak and salsa evenly among 4 plates and serve at once.

Each serving: 11 g carb, 212 cal, 7 g fat, 2 g sat fat, 42 mg chol, 2 g fib, 25 g pro, 263 mg sod • Carb Choices: 1; Exchanges: ½ fruit, 3 lean protein, ½ fat

Spinach-Stuffed Steak Roll

makes 6 servings

Anything stuffed gives a special touch to dinner, but most people don't realize how easy it is to do. This steak is stuffed with ingredients that require no preparation, but they pay off as a flavorful filling for this impressive main course.

1 teaspoon canola oil

1 (1½-pound) flank steak, trimmed of all visible fat

½ teaspoon kosher salt

½ teaspoon freshly ground pepper

1 (10-ounce) package frozen chopped spinach, thawed and squeezed dry

½ cup red Roasted Bell Peppers (page 21) or roasted red peppers from a jar, chopped

2 ounces shredded Gruyère (about ½ cup)

1 Preheat the oven to 400°F. Brush a medium roasting pan with the oil.

2 Place the steak on a sheet of plastic wrap. Cut horizontally through the center of the steak, cutting to, but not through, the other side. Open the butterflied portions, laying the steak flat. Place plastic wrap over the steak and flatten to an even thickness using a meat mallet or rolling pin. Sprinkle both sides of the steak with the salt and ground pepper.

3 Place the spinach, roasted peppers, and Gruyère evenly over the steak and roll up, jelly-roll fashion, starting with the long side. Secure the roll with kitchen string at 3-inch intervals.

4 Place the steak seam side down in the prepared pan. Bake 20 to 25 minutes or to desired degree of doneness. Transfer to a serving platter, cover loosely with foil, and let stand 10 minutes before slicing. Cut the steak roll into ½-inch slices and serve at once.

Each serving: 2 g carb, 233 cal, 12 g fat, 5 g sat fat, 53 mg chol, 1 g fib, 27 g pro, 259 mg sod • Carb Choices: 0; Exchanges: 3 lean protein, ½ fat

Steak Tacos with Salsa Salad HIGH FIBER

makes 4 servings

With lean sliced steak and loads of vegetables all wrapped in whole grain tortillas, these tacos are a complete healthy handheld meal. If you don't have time to marinate, use a flank steak and season it with the chili powder and cumin before cooking.

¼ cup plus 1 tablespoon lime juice, divided

4 garlic cloves, minced

2 teaspoons chili powder

1 teaspoon ground cumin

1 (1-pound) round tip, eye round, bottom round, sirloin tip, or chuck shoulder steak, trimmed of all visible fat

¾ teaspoon kosher salt, divided

4 teaspoons canola oil, divided

2 cups thinly sliced romaine lettuce

1 large tomato, coarsely chopped

½ cup fresh cilantro leaves

1 jalapeño, seeded and minced

8 (6-inch) whole wheat flour tortillas, warmed

1 Combine ¼ cup of the lime juice, the garlic, chili powder, and cumin in a large resealable plastic bag. Add the steak, turn to coat, and refrigerate 8 to 12 hours.

2 Remove the steak from the marinade and discard the marinade. Pat dry with paper towels. Sprinkle the steak with ½ teaspoon of the salt. Heat a large heavy-bottomed skillet over medium-high heat. Add 2 teaspoons of the oil and tilt the pan to coat the bottom evenly. Add the steak and cook, turning once, 3 minutes on each side for medium-rare, or to the desired degree of doneness. Transfer the steak to a cutting board, cover loosely with foil, and let stand 5 minutes before slicing.

3 Meanwhile, make the salad. Combine the remaining 1 tablespoon lime juice, remaining 2 teaspoons oil, and remaining ¼ teaspoon salt in a large bowl and whisk to mix well. Add the lettuce, tomato, cilantro, and jalapeño and toss to coat. Cut the steak across the grain into slices and divide among the tortillas. Top the steak with ½ cup of the salad and serve at once.

Each serving: 28 g carb, 321 cal, 14 g fat, 2 g sat fat, 75 mg chol, 17 g fib, 29 g pro, 725 mg sod • Carb Choices: 1; Exchanges: 1 starch, 1 veg, 3 lean protein, 2 fat

Filets Mignons with Cabernet-Butter Sauce QUICK

makes 4 servings

Though there is only a tablespoon of butter in this recipe, it's enough to give the sauce a rich flavor and silky texture.

4 (4-ounce) filets mignons, trimmed of all visible fat

½ teaspoon kosher salt

⅛ teaspoon freshly ground pepper

½ cup Beef Stock (page 151) or low-sodium beef broth

½ cup Cabernet Sauvignon

1 tablespoon chilled unsalted butter

½ teaspoon chopped fresh thyme or ⅛ teaspoon dried thyme

1 Sprinkle the steaks with the salt and pepper. Heat a large heavy-bottomed skillet over medium-high heat. Add the steaks to the dry skillet and cook, turning once, 2 minutes on each side for medium-rare, or to the desired degree of doneness. Transfer to a plate and cover loosely with foil to keep warm.

2 Add the stock and wine to the skillet, bring to a boil, and cook until reduced to 3 tablespoons, about 5 minutes. Remove from the heat and whisk in the butter and thyme. Divide the steaks among 4 plates, drizzle evenly with the sauce, and serve at once.

Each serving: 1 g carb, 194 cal, 8 g fat, 4 g sat fat, 60 mg chol, 0 g fib, 23 g pro, 243 mg sod • Carb Choices: 0; Exchanges: 3 lean protein, ½ fat

Steak with Balsamic Banana Peppers QUICK

makes 4 servings

In this recipe, steak is simply seasoned and seared in a skillet, then served with banana peppers that are just lightly browned and flavored with balsamic vinegar and garlic. It's perfect for a weeknight dinner. If you can't find banana peppers, try poblano peppers or red or yellow bell peppers.

1 (1-pound) strip, top sirloin, tri-tip, flank, or ranch steak, trimmed of all visible fat
¾ teaspoon kosher salt, divided
¼ teaspoon cracked black pepper
4 teaspoons extra virgin olive oil, divided
6 large mild yellow banana peppers, sliced lengthwise
3 tablespoons balsamic vinegar
2 garlic cloves, minced

1 Sprinkle the steak with ½ teaspoon of the salt and the cracked pepper. Heat a large heavy-bottomed skillet over medium-high heat. Add 2 teaspoons of the oil and tilt the pan to coat the bottom evenly. Add the steak and cook, turning once, 3 minutes on each side for medium-rare, or to the desired degree of doneness. Transfer the steak to a cutting board and cover loosely with foil.

2 Add the remaining 2 teaspoons oil to the skillet and tilt to coat. Add the banana peppers and the remaining ¼ teaspoon salt and cook, stirring often, until lightly browned and crisp-tender, about 5 minutes. Stir in the vinegar and garlic and cook, stirring often, until most of the vinegar evaporates, 2 minutes. Cut the steak across the grain into thin slices and divide evenly among 4 plates. Top the steak evenly with the peppers and serve at once.

Each serving: 6 g carb, 216 cal, 9 g fat, 2 g sat fat, 42 mg chol, 2 g fib, 26 g pro, 273 mg sod • Carb Choices: ½; Exchanges: 1 veg, 3 lean protein, 1 fat

London Broil with Sherry Mushrooms

makes 4 servings

Dry sherry adds a nutty complex flavor to the mushrooms in this dish. Use dry sherry, not cooking sherry, which tastes salty and artificial. If you don't have sherry on hand, use dry white wine in this recipe.

¾ cup Beef Stock (page 151) or low-sodium beef broth, divided
2 tablespoons sherry vinegar
2 teaspoons Dijon mustard
4½ teaspoons extra virgin olive oil, divided
¼ teaspoon plus pinch freshly ground pepper, divided
1 sprig fresh thyme or rosemary
1 (1-pound) top round London broil, trimmed of all visible fat
¾ teaspoon kosher salt, divided
8 ounces mixed mushrooms (such as shiitake, cremini, or oyster), sliced
¼ cup diced onion
2 garlic cloves, minced
2 teaspoons chopped fresh thyme or rosemary
¼ cup dry sherry
1 tablespoon cold water
2 teaspoons cornstarch

1 Combine ¼ cup of the stock, the vinegar, mustard, 2 teaspoons of the oil, ¼ teaspoon of the pepper, and the thyme sprig in a shallow dish and stir to mix well. Add the steak, turn to coat, cover, and refrigerate at least 6 hours or up to 12 hours.

2 Preheat the broiler. Brush the rack of a broiler pan with ½ teaspoon of the remaining oil.

3 Remove the steak from the marinade and discard the marinade. Sprinkle the steak with ½ teaspoon of the salt and place on the broiler

rack. Broil 4 to 6 minutes on each side for medium-rare or to the desired degree of doneness. Transfer the steak to a cutting board, cover loosely with foil, and let stand 5 minutes.

4 Meanwhile, heat a large nonstick skillet over medium-high heat. Add the remaining 2 teaspoons oil and tilt the pan to coat the bottom evenly. Add the mushrooms, onion, garlic, thyme, and remaining ¼ teaspoon salt and cook, stirring often, until the mushrooms are tender and most of the liquid has evaporated, 6 to 8 minutes. Add the sherry and cook, stirring often until most of the liquid has evaporated, 2 minutes. Stir in the remaining ½ cup stock and bring to a boil. Stir the water and cornstarch together in a small bowl and stir into the mushroom mixture. Cook, stirring constantly, until the sauce is thickened, 1 minute. Stir in the remaining pinch of pepper.

5 Cut the steak across the grain into thin slices, divide evenly among 4 plates, and top evenly with the mushrooms.

Each serving: 6 g carb, 203 cal, 5 g fat, 2 g sat fat, 51 mg chol, 0 g fib, 29 g pro, 411 mg sod • Carb Choices: ½; Exchanges: 1 veg, 4 lean protein

Beef, Artichoke, and Pepper Kebabs with Olive Vinaigrette QUICK

makes 4 servings

These pretty kebabs with vibrant colors and flavors make a delicious centerpiece for a summer cookout. You can double the recipe if necessary. Serve these with whole wheat orzo or whole wheat couscous.

2 tablespoons red wine vinegar

1 tablespoon, plus 2½ teaspoons extra virgin olive oil, divided

½ teaspoon Dijon mustard

¼ teaspoon freshly ground pepper, divided

¼ cup pitted green olives, chopped

1 tablespoon minced shallot or sweet onion

¼ cup plus 2 tablespoons chopped fresh basil, divided

4 garlic cloves, minced

½ teaspoon kosher salt

1 pound top sirloin or flank steak, trimmed of all visible fat and cut into 1-inch pieces

1 medium red onion, cut into 8 wedges

1 red bell pepper, cut into 1-inch pieces

1 yellow bell pepper, cut into 1-inch pieces

1 (13-ounce) can artichoke hearts, drained and halved

1 To make the vinaigrette, whisk together the vinegar, 1 tablespoon of the oil, the mustard, and ⅛ teaspoon of the ground pepper in a small bowl. Stir in the olives and the shallot. Set aside.

2 Combine ¼ cup of the basil, the garlic, salt, 2 teaspoons of the remaining oil, and remaining ⅛ teaspoon ground pepper and in a large bowl. Add the steak, onion, bell peppers, and artichoke hearts and toss to coat. Thread onto eight 8- to 10-inch metal skewers.

3 Prepare the grill or heat a large grill pan over medium-high heat.

4 Brush the grill rack or grill pan with the remaining ½ teaspoon oil. Place the kebabs on the grill rack or in the grill pan and grill, turning occasionally, 6 to 8 minutes for medium-rare, or to the desired degree of doneness.

5 Stir the remaining 2 tablespoons basil into the vinaigrette. To serve, arrange the kebabs on a serving platter and drizzle with the vinaigrette.

Each serving: 14 g carb, 285 cal, 12 g fat, 3 g sat fat, 41 mg chol, 2 g fib, 28 g pro, 596 mg sod • Carb Choices: 1; Exchanges: 2 veg, 3½ lean protein, 1½ fat

Beef and Pineapple Kebabs with Soy Dipping Sauce `QUICK`

makes 4 servings

Use fresh pineapple for this recipe. Its sturdier texture will hold up to being skewered and grilled better than canned pineapple chunks.

¼ cup reduced-sodium soy sauce
¼ cup lime juice
1 teaspoon honey
¼ teaspoon Asian sesame oil
⅛ teaspoon ground cayenne
1 pound top sirloin or flank steak, trimmed of all visible fat and cut into 1-inch pieces
4 scallions, cut into 1-inch pieces
1 red bell pepper, cut into 1-inch pieces
1 green bell pepper, cut into 1-inch pieces
½ pineapple, cored and cut into 1-inch cubes
½ teaspoon canola oil

1 Combine the soy sauce, lime juice, honey, sesame oil, and cayenne in a small bowl and whisk to mix well. Set aside.

2 Combine the steak, scallions, bell peppers, and pineapple in a large bowl. Drizzle with 3 table-spoons of the soy sauce mixture and toss to coat. Thread onto eight 8- to 10-inch metal skewers.

3 Prepare the grill or heat a large grill pan over medium-high heat.

4 Brush the grill rack or grill pan with the canola oil. Place the kebabs on the grill rack or in the grill pan and grill, turning occasionally, 6 to 8 min-utes for medium-rare, or to the desired degree of doneness.

5 To serve, arrange the kebabs on a serving platter and serve with the remaining soy sauce mixture.

Each serving: 14 g carb, 213 cal, 5 g fat, 2 g sat fat, 64 mg chol, 2 g fib, 27 g pro, 641 mg sod • Carb Choices: 1; Exchanges: ½ carb, ½ fruit, 3 lean protein

Merlot-Marinated Beef Kebabs

makes 4 servings

Red wine tenderizes and flavors these kebabs, making them a tasty choice for a summer cookout. I love the look the whole mushrooms and whole cherry tomatoes give these kebabs, but you can use whatever vegetables you have on hand.

½ cup Merlot or other dry red wine
1 tablespoon brown sugar
2½ teaspoons extra virgin olive oil, divided
1 teaspoon Dijon mustard
2 garlic cloves, minced
1 pound top sirloin or flank steak, trimmed of all visible fat and cut into 1-inch pieces
8 small whole white or cremini mushrooms
8 cherry tomatoes
1 yellow bell pepper, cut into 1-inch pieces
1 red onion, cut into 8 wedges
½ teaspoon kosher salt
¼ teaspoon freshly ground pepper

1 Combine the wine, sugar, 2 teaspoons of the oil, the mustard, and garlic in a shallow dish and stir until the sugar dissolves. Add the steak, turn to coat, cover, and refrigerate at least 6 hours or up to 12 hours.

2 Preheat the broiler. Brush the rack of a broiler pan with the remaining ½ teaspoon oil.

3 Remove the beef from the marinade and dis-card the marinade. Thread the beef, mushrooms, tomatoes, bell pepper, and onion onto eight 8- to 10-inch metal skewers. Sprinkle with the salt and ground pepper.

4 Place the kebabs on the broiler rack and broil, turning occasionally, 6 to 8 minutes for medium-rare, or to the desired degree of doneness. Divide the kebabs among 4 plates and serve at once.

Each serving: 8 g carb, 208 cal, 7 g fat, 2 g sat fat, 46 mg chol, 1 g fib, 26 g pro, 212 mg sod • Carb Choices: ½; Exchanges: 1 veg, 3 lean protein

Beef and Broccoli Stir-Fry

QUICK

makes 4 servings

Asian sesame oil is a must for adding flavor to stir-fries. A tiny amount infuses the entire dish with toasty sesame flavor. Since you use only a small amount of it in any recipe, a bottle can last a long time. Store it in the refrigerator so it will last longer.

⅓ cup Chicken Stock (page 149) or low-sodium chicken broth
2 tablespoons reduced-sodium soy sauce
1 tablespoon cornstarch
1 teaspoon Asian sesame oil
¼ teaspoon chili-garlic paste
6 teaspoons canola oil, divided
1 pound top sirloin or flank steak, trimmed of all visible fat and cut into ¼-inch-thick slices
2 tablespoons minced fresh ginger
2 garlic cloves, minced
4 cups broccoli florets
1 small red bell pepper, thinly sliced
4 scallions, cut into 2-inch pieces
¼ cup chopped fresh cilantro

1 Combine the stock, soy sauce, cornstarch, sesame oil, and chili-garlic paste in a small bowl and stir until the cornstarch dissolves and set aside.

2 Heat a large wok or nonstick skillet over medium-high heat. Add 2 teaspoons of the canola oil and tilt the pan to coat the bottom evenly. Add half of the beef and cook, stirring constantly, until lightly browned, 2 to 3 minutes. Transfer the beef to a plate. Repeat with 2 teaspoons of the remaining canola oil and the remaining beef.

3 Wipe out the wok with paper towels. Add the remaining 2 teaspoons canola oil to the wok over medium-high heat. Add the ginger and garlic

and cook, stirring constantly, until fragrant, 30 seconds. Add the broccoli, bell pepper, and scallions and cook, stirring constantly, until crisp-tender, 5 minutes. Stir in the beef and the stock mixture and cook, stirring constantly, until the sauce is thickened, 30 seconds. Remove from the heat and stir in the cilantro. Divide evenly among 4 plates and serve at once.

Each serving: 10 g carb, 269 cal, 13 g fat, 3 g sat fat, 46 mg chol, 3 g fib, 28 g pro, 399 mg sod • Carb Choices: ½; Exchanges: 2 veg, 3 lean protein, 1½ fat

BEEF AND ASPARAGUS STIR-FRY WITH PEANUTS QUICK: Follow the Beef and Broccoli Stir-Fry recipe, at left, substituting 1 pound asparagus, tough ends removed, cut into 1-inch pieces for the broccoli in step 3. Omit the cilantro and stir in 2 tablespoons chopped unsalted dry-roasted peanuts.

Each serving: 10 g carb, 291 cal, 15 g fat, 3 g sat fat, 46 mg chol, 3 g fib, 28 g pro, 381 mg sod • Carb Choices: ½; Exchanges: 2 veg, 3 lean protein, 2 fat

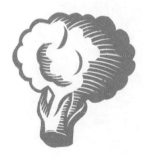

Beef, Green Bean, and Basil Stir-Fry QUICK

makes 4 servings

If you're trying to get the meat lovers in your family to cut back on their portions, stir-fries are a way to nudge them in a healthier direction. With lots of flavorful vegetables and a delicious sauce, carnivores will be happy with less meat. Serve this with brown rice or soba noodles for a generous and filling meal.

8 ounces green beans, trimmed

⅓ cup Chicken Stock (page 149) or low-sodium chicken broth

2 tablespoons reduced-sodium soy sauce

1 tablespoon cornstarch

¼ teaspoon chili-garlic paste

6 teaspoons canola oil, divided

1 pound top sirloin or flank steak, trimmed of all visible fat and cut into ¼-inch-thick slices

2 garlic cloves, minced

1 small yellow bell pepper, thinly sliced

1 small red onion, halved lengthwise and thinly sliced

¼ cup chopped fresh basil

1 Fill a medium saucepan half full with water and bring to a boil over high heat. Add the green beans, return to a boil, and cook just until crisp-tender, about 3 minutes. Drain, let cool slightly, and pat dry with paper towels.

2 Combine the stock, soy sauce, cornstarch, and chili-garlic paste in a small bowl and stir until the cornstarch dissolves.

3 Heat a large wok or nonstick skillet over medium-high heat. Add 2 teaspoons of the oil and tilt the pan to coat the bottom evenly. Add half of the beef and cook, stirring constantly, until lightly browned, 2 to 3 minutes. Transfer the beef to a plate. Repeat with 2 teaspoons of the remaining oil and the remaining beef.

4 Wipe out the wok with paper towels. Add the remaining 2 teaspoons oil to the wok over medium-high heat. Add the garlic and cook, stirring constantly, until fragrant, 30 seconds. Add the green beans, bell pepper, and onion and cook, stirring constantly, until crisp-tender, 5 minutes. Stir in the beef and the stock mixture and cook, stirring constantly, until the sauce is thickened, 30 seconds. Remove from the heat and stir in the basil. Divide evenly among 4 plates and serve at once.

Each serving: 10 g carb, 265 cal, 13 g fat, 2 g sat fat, 46 mg chol, 3 g fib, 27 g pro, 380 mg sod • Carb Choices: ½; Exchanges: 2 veg, 3 lean protein, 1½ fat

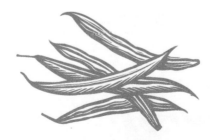

Beef Roasts

Perfect-Every-Time Beef Tenderloin QUICK

makes 8 servings

A beef tenderloin needs little other than salt and pepper to season it. If you want to serve it with a sauce, try Romesco Sauce (page 593) or Chimichurri Sauce (page 594). The cooking method here gives the tenderloin a nice brown crust and perfectly pink center.

1 (2-pound) beef tenderloin, trimmed of all visible fat
1 teaspoon kosher salt
½ teaspoon freshly ground pepper
2 teaspoons extra virgin olive oil

1 Preheat the oven to 400°F.

2 Sprinkle the tenderloin with the salt and pepper. Heat a large heavy-bottomed ovenproof skillet over medium-high heat. Add the oil and tilt the pan to coat the bottom evenly. Add the tenderloin and cook, turning to brown all sides, about 5 minutes.

3 Transfer the skillet to the oven and bake until an instant-read thermometer inserted into the center of the tenderloin reads 145°F about 15 minutes. Transfer the tenderloin to a cutting board, cover loosely with foil, and let stand about 10 minutes. Cut into slices, divide evenly among 8 plates, and serve at once.

Each serving: 0 g carb, 187 cal, 9 g fat, 3 g sat fat, 79 mg chol, 0 g fib, 25 g pro, 190 mg sod • Carb Choices: 0; Exchanges: 3 lean protein

ESPRESSO-RUBBED BEEF TENDERLOIN QUICK: Follow the Perfect-Every-Time Beef Tenderloin recipe, at left, combining the salt, pepper, 2 teaspoons light brown sugar, and 1½ teaspoons finely ground espresso in a small bowl. Rub the mixture over the tenderloin and proceed with the recipe.

Each serving: 1 g carb, 191 cal, 9 g fat, 3 g sat fat, 79 mg chol, 0 g fib, 25 g pro, 191 mg sod • Carb Choices: 0; Exchanges: 3 lean protein

HERB-CRUSTED BEEF TENDERLOIN QUICK: Follow the Perfect-Every-Time Beef Tenderloin recipe, at left, through step 2. Transfer the tenderloin from the skillet to a plate and rub with 2 garlic cloves, minced; 2 teaspoons minced fresh rosemary; and 2 teaspoons minced fresh thyme. Return the tenderloin to the skillet and bake as directed in step 3.

Each serving: 0 g carb, 188 cal, 9 g fat, 3 g sat fat, 79 mg chol, 0 g fib, 25 g pro, 191 mg sod • Carb Choices: 0; Exchanges: 3 lean protein

Eye of Round with Roasted Garlic–Horseradish Sauce

makes 8 servings

Eye of round, also known as poor man's tenderloin, is a deliciously flavorful cut of beef if cooked properly. The three secrets to success with eye of round are to marinate the meat, not to overcook it, and to slice it very thinly.

½ cup dry red wine
¼ cup red wine vinegar
1 small onion, thinly sliced
4 garlic cloves, minced
2 teaspoons whole black peppercorns, crushed
1 (2-pound) eye of round roast, trimmed of all visible fat
1 head garlic
1¼ teaspoons kosher salt, divided
2 teaspoons extra virgin olive oil
½ cup plain low-fat Greek yogurt or strained yogurt (page 11)
2 tablespoons mayonnaise
1 tablespoon prepared horseradish, drained
1 teaspoon lemon juice

1 To make the roast, combine the wine, vinegar, onion, minced garlic, and peppercorns in a large resealable plastic bag. Add the roast, seal the bag, and refrigerate 8 hours and up to 24 hours.

2 Preheat the oven to 325°F.

3 Separate the head of garlic into cloves, but do not peel. Place on a sheet of foil and wrap tightly. Place in a small baking dish.

4 Remove the roast from the marinade and discard the marinade. Pat the roast dry with paper towels. Sprinkle the roast with 1 teaspoon of the salt.

5 Heat a large heavy-bottomed ovenproof skillet over medium-high heat. Add the oil and tilt the pan to coat the bottom evenly. Cook the roast, turning occasionally, until well browned on all sides, about 6 minutes.

6 Place the roast and the prepared head of garlic in the oven. Bake the roast, turning once, until an instant-read thermometer inserted into the center reads 145°F, and the garlic is very soft, 40 to 45 minutes. Cover the roast loosely with foil and let stand about 10 minutes.

7 Meanwhile, to make the sauce, unwrap the garlic and let stand until cool enough to handle. Squeeze the garlic pulp from each clove into a small bowl. Whisk in the yogurt, mayonnaise, horseradish, lemon juice, and the remaining ¼ teaspoon salt. Cut the beef into thin slices and divide evenly among 8 plates. Serve with the sauce.

Each serving: 3 g carb, 197 cal, 8 g fat, 2 g sat fat, 50 mg chol, 0 g fib, 26 g pro, 278 mg sod • Carb Choices: 0; Exchanges: 3 lean protein, ½ fat

Garlic and Lime Beef Roast with Cilantro Pesto

makes 8 servings

This recipe uses an easy technique to infuse maximum flavor into a lean roast. Small slits are cut into the beef, the slits are filled with seasonings, and then the beef is refrigerated overnight. The seasonings infuse the roast with flavor.

4 garlic cloves, minced
1 tablespoon grated lime zest
2 teaspoons ground cumin
¼ teaspoon ground cayenne
¼ teaspoon freshly ground pepper
1 (2-pound) eye of round roast, trimmed of all visible fat
1 teaspoon kosher salt
2 teaspoons extra virgin olive oil
1 recipe Cilantro Pesto (page 597)

1 To make the roast, combine the garlic, lime zest, cumin, cayenne, and pepper in a small bowl and stir to mix well. Using a slender sharp-pointed knife, cut about 16 (½-inch) deep slits into the roast. Insert a pinch of the garlic mixture into each slit. Place the roast in a shallow dish, cover, and refrigerate overnight or up to 24 hours.

2 Preheat the oven to 325°F.

3 Sprinkle the roast with the salt. Heat a large heavy-bottomed ovenproof skillet over medium-high heat. Add the oil and tilt the pan to coat the bottom evenly. Cook the roast, turning occasionally, until well browned on all sides, about 6 minutes. Transfer to the oven and bake, turning once, until an instant-read thermometer inserted into the center of the roast reads 145°F, 40 to 45 minutes. Cover the roast loosely with foil and let stand about 10 minutes. Cut into thin slices and divide evenly among 8 plates. Serve with the pesto.

Each serving: 2 g carb, 246 cal, 14 g fat, 3 g sat fat, 48 mg chol, 1 g fib, 26 g pro, 247 mg sod • Carb Choices: 0; Exchanges: 3 lean protein, 2 fat

Brined Eye of Round Roast

makes 8 servings

If brining helps tenderize and add flavor to pork and poultry, why not try it with beef? It works magic to add flavor and moisture to this super-lean cut of meat.

3 cups Beef Stock (page 151) or low-sodium beef broth
1 cup dry red wine
½ cup kosher salt
½ cup sugar
4 garlic cloves, chopped
2 tablespoons chopped fresh rosemary
2 teaspoons black peppercorns, crushed
1 (2-pound) eye of round roast, trimmed of all visible fat
¼ teaspoon freshly ground pepper
2 teaspoons extra virgin olive oil

1 Combine the stock, wine, salt, and sugar in a medium bowl. Whisk until the salt and sugar dissolve. Pour the mixture into a large heavy-duty resealable plastic bag. Add the garlic, rosemary, and peppercorns. Place the roast in the bag and seal. Refrigerate at least 8 hours and up to 12 hours, turning the bag occasionally.

2 Preheat the oven to 325°F.

3 Remove the roast from the marinade and discard the marinade. Pat the roast dry with paper towels. Sprinkle with the ground pepper.

4 Heat a large heavy-bottomed ovenproof skillet over medium-high heat. Add the oil and tilt the pan to coat the bottom evenly. Cook the roast, turning occasionally, until well browned on all sides, about 6 minutes. Transfer to the oven and bake, turning once, until an instant-read thermometer inserted into the center of the roast reads 145°F, 40 to 45 minutes. Cover the roast loosely with foil and let stand about 10 minutes. Cut into thin slices and divide evenly among 8 plates.

Each serving: 2 g carb, 162 cal, 5 g fat, 2 g sat fat, 46 mg chol, 0 g fib, 25 g pro, 467 mg sod • Carb Choices: 0; Exchanges: 3 lean protein

Beef Braises and One-Pot Meals

Classic Beef Pot Roast

makes 6 servings

This roast is perfect for a cold weather Sunday supper. Take the simpler route and serve the roast with the broth it cooks in or thicken the broth to make gravy. Both options are given in the recipe. Either way, serve the roast with Buttermilk Mashed Potatoes (page 482).

2 pounds beef chuck shoulder roast or bottom round roast, trimmed of all visible fat

1 teaspoon kosher salt

½ teaspoon freshly ground pepper

4 teaspoons extra virgin olive oil, divided

2 carrots, peeled and chopped

2 stalks celery, chopped

1 medium onion, chopped

4 garlic cloves, chopped

½ cup dry red wine

2 to 3 cups Beef Stock (page 151) or low-sodium beef broth, divided

¼ cup no-salt-added tomato paste

2 sprigs fresh thyme or ½ teaspoon dried thyme

2 tablespoons cold water (optional)

1½ tablespoons unbleached all-purpose flour (optional)

1 Preheat the oven to 325°F.

2 Sprinkle the roast with the salt and pepper. Heat a Dutch oven over medium-high heat. Add 2 teaspoons of the oil and tilt the pan to coat the bottom evenly. Add the roast and cook, turning to brown on all sides, 6 to 8 minutes. Transfer the roast to a plate.

3 Add the remaining 2 teaspoons oil to the Dutch oven and tilt to coat. Add the carrots, celery, and onion and cook, stirring often, until the vegetables are softened, 5 minutes. Add the garlic and cook, stirring constantly, until fragrant, 30 seconds. Add the wine and bring to a boil, stirring to scrape up the browned bits from the bottom of the Dutch oven. Return the roast to the Dutch oven. Add 2 cups of the stock, tomato paste, and thyme and bring to a boil. Add the additional stock, if necessary, to almost cover the roast. Cover and bake 3 hours. Remove the roast from the Dutch oven, place on a serving platter, and cover with foil to keep warm.

4 Pour the vegetable mixture through a strainer. You may add the vegetables to the platter with the roast, or discard them (though they are flavorful, some may think they are too overcooked to eat). Pour the strained broth into a medium saucepan and bring to a boil over high heat. Cook, uncovered, until reduced to about 1½ cups, about 8 minutes.

5 You can serve the beef with the broth, or thicken the broth to make a gravy. To make gravy, combine the water and flour in a small bowl and stir until smooth. Slowly whisk the flour mixture into the broth, whisking constantly until thickened, 1 minute. Reduce the heat and simmer 5 minutes. Cut the roast into thick slices and divide evenly among 6 plates. Drizzle evenly with the broth or gravy and serve at once.

Each serving (including the vegetables): 5 g carb, 192 cal, 7 g fat, 2 g sat fat, 49 mg chol, 1 g fib, 22 g pro, 203 mg sod • Carb Choices: 0; Exchanges: 1 veg, 3 lean protein, ½ fat

BALSAMIC BEEF POT ROAST: Follow the Classic Beef Roast recipe, at left, adding ½ cup balsamic vinegar with the stock in step 3, and proceed as directed.

Each serving (including the vegetables): 8 g carb, 201 cal, 7 g fat, 2 g sat fat, 49 mg chol, 1 g fib, 22 g pro, 206 mg sod • Carb Choices: ½; Exchanges: 1 veg, 3 lean protein, ½ fat

Tips for Better Braising

Take the extra step to brown meats before braising. Browning caramelizes the outside of the meat, making it more flavorful. This step also creates browned bits in the bottom of the pan, which add flavor to the cooking liquid.

With lean cuts of beef, pork, and lamb, it is imperative to have the meat almost completely submerged in the cooking liquid. I've tried braising lean meats with various amounts of liquid and found that almost covering the meat with broth, wine, or other liquid makes a significantly more tender, moist stew or pot roast. If you've added all the cooking liquid that a recipe calls for and the meat is not almost covered, add more stock or water. A larger pot will require more liquid to cover the meat.

The lean cuts of meat used in these recipes are low in calories and fat—so lean, in fact that you can skip the step given in most braising recipes to skim off the fat from the drippings. Using lean cuts makes the amount of fat in the drippings miniscule.

The preferred pot for braising is a Dutch oven—a large deep-sided, heavy-bottomed, metal pot with a tight-fitting lid. The deep sides allow the meat to be submerged in the cooking liquid, the heavy bottom allows for an even temperature when browning and braising, and the tight-fitting lid keeps the liquid from evaporating.

Keep the heat low when braising. If you are braising in the oven, 325°F is an ideal temperature that will maintain the dish at a slow simmer. On the stovetop, adjust the heat so that bubbles break the surface of the liquid at the edge of the pot.

Braised dishes almost always taste better if you make them a day ahead. Once the dish is done, let it cool, then cover and refrigerate. When ready to serve, gently reheat on the stovetop, or bake in a 350°F oven until heated through, 30 to 45 minutes, depending on the quantity.

Beef Pot Roast with Root Vegetables HIGH FIBER

makes 6 servings

2 pounds beef chuck shoulder roast or bottom round roast, trimmed of all visible fat

1 teaspoon kosher salt

½ teaspoon freshly ground pepper

4 teaspoons extra virgin olive oil, divided

2 carrots, peeled and chopped

2 stalks celery, chopped

1 medium onion, chopped

4 garlic cloves, chopped

2 to 3 cups Beef Stock (page 151) or low-sodium beef broth, divided

¼ cup no-salt-added tomato paste

1 pound red-skinned potatoes, well scrubbed and cut into 1-inch pieces

8 ounces parsnips, peeled and cut into 1-inch pieces

8 ounces turnips, peeled and cut into 1-inch pieces

1 Preheat the oven to 325°F.

2 Sprinkle the roast with the salt and pepper. Heat a Dutch oven over medium-high heat. Add 2 teaspoons of the oil and tilt the pan to coat the bottom evenly. Add the roast and cook, turning to brown on all sides, 6 to 8 minutes. Transfer the roast to a plate.

3 Add the remaining 2 teaspoons oil to the Dutch oven and tilt to coat. Add the carrots, celery, and onion and cook, stirring often, until the vegetables are softened, 5 minutes. Add the garlic and cook, stirring constantly, 30 seconds. Add 2 cups of the stock and bring to a boil, stirring to scrape up the browned bits from the bottom of the Dutch oven. Return the roast to the Dutch oven. Add the tomato paste and bring to a boil. Add the additional stock, if necessary, to almost cover the roast. Cover and bake 2 hours.

4 Remove the Dutch oven from the oven and arrange the potatoes, parsnips, and turnips around the roast (add additional stock or water, if necessary to almost cover the vegetables). Cover and bake until the roast and the vegetables are very tender, about 1 hour longer.

5 Remove the roast from the Dutch oven, place on a serving platter, and cover with foil.

6 Pour the vegetable mixture through a strainer and transfer the vegetables to the platter with the roast. Pour the strained broth into a medium saucepan and bring to a boil over high heat. Cook, uncovered, until reduced to about 1½ cups, about 8 minutes. Cut the roast into thick slices and divide the roast and vegetables evenly among 6 shallow bowls. Ladle the broth evenly over the beef and vegetables and serve at once.

Each serving: 20 g carb, 255 cal, 8 g fat, 2 g sat fat, 49 mg chol, 4 g fib, 24 g pro, 213 mg sod • Carb Choices: 1; Exchanges: 1 starch, 1 veg, 3 lean protein, ½ fat

Beef Pot Roast with Port and Coriander

makes 6 servings

2 pounds beef chuck shoulder roast or bottom round roast, trimmed of all visible fat

2 teaspoons ground cumin

1 teaspoon kosher salt

½ teaspoon freshly ground pepper

4 teaspoons extra virgin olive oil, divided

2 carrots, peeled and chopped

2 stalks celery, chopped

1 medium onion, chopped

4 garlic cloves, chopped

1 tablespoon ground coriander

1 cup ruby port

2 to 3 cups Beef Stock (page 151) or low-sodium beef broth, divided

¼ cup no-salt-added tomato paste

2 tablespoons cold water

1½ tablespoons unbleached all-purpose flour

1 Preheat the oven to 325°F.

2 Sprinkle the roast with the cumin, salt, and pepper. Heat a Dutch oven over medium-high heat. Add 2 teaspoons of the oil and the roast and cook, turning to brown on all sides, 6 to 8 minutes. Transfer the roast to a plate.

3 Add the remaining 2 teaspoons oil to the Dutch oven. Add the carrots, celery, and onion and cook, until the vegetables are softened, 5 minutes. Add the garlic and coriander and cook, stirring constantly, 30 seconds. Add the port and bring to a boil. Return the roast to the Dutch oven. Add 2 cups of the stock and the tomato paste. Add the additional stock, if necessary, to almost cover the roast. Cover and bake 3 hours. Transfer the roast to a serving platter, and cover with foil.

4 Pour the vegetable mixture through a strainer and discard the vegetables. Pour the strained broth into a medium saucepan and bring to a boil over high heat. Cook, uncovered, until reduced to about 1½ cups, about 8 minutes.

5 Whisk together the water and flour in a small bowl until smooth. Slowly whisk the flour mixture into the broth, whisking constantly, until thickened, 1 minute. Reduce the heat and simmer 5 minutes. Cut the roast into thick slices and divide evenly among 6 plates. Drizzle the sauce evenly over the roast and serve at once.

Each serving (including the vegetables): 7 g carb, 222 cal, 8 g fat, 2 g sat fat, 49 mg chol, 2 g fib, 22 g pro, 204 mg sod • Carb Choices: ½; Exchanges: 1 veg, 3 lean protein, ½ fat

Asian Beef Pot Roast

makes 8 servings

4 teaspoons canola oil, divided
2 pounds beef chuck shoulder roast or bottom round roast, trimmed of all visible fat
2 carrots, peeled and chopped
2 stalks celery, chopped
1 medium onion, chopped

¼ cup minced fresh ginger
4 garlic cloves, chopped
½ cup dry sherry
2 to 3 cups Beef Stock (page 151) or low-sodium beef broth, divided
¼ cup packed dark brown sugar
¼ cup reduced-sodium soy sauce
¼ cup no-salt-added tomato paste
¼ teaspoon Asian sesame oil

1 Preheat the oven to 325°F.

2 Heat a Dutch oven over medium-high heat. Add 2 teaspoons of the canola oil and tilt the pan to coat the bottom evenly. Add the roast and cook, turning to brown on all sides, 6 to 8 minutes. Transfer the roast to a plate.

3 Add the remaining 2 teaspoons canola oil to the Dutch oven and tilt to coat. Add the carrots, celery, and onion and cook, stirring often, until the vegetables are softened, 5 minutes. Add the ginger and garlic and cook, stirring constantly, until fragrant, 30 seconds. Add the sherry and bring to a boil, stirring to scrape up the browned bits from the bottom of the Dutch oven. Add 2 cups of the stock, the sugar, soy sauce, and tomato paste and bring to a boil. Return the roast to the Dutch oven. Add the additional stock, if necessary, to almost cover the roast. Cover and bake until the roast is fork-tender, 3 hours. Remove the roast from the Dutch oven, place on a serving platter, and cover with foil to keep warm.

4 Pour the vegetable mixture through a wire strainer and discard the vegetables. Pour the strained broth into a medium saucepan and bring to a boil over high heat. Cook, uncovered, until reduced to 1½ cups, about 8 minutes. Stir in the sesame oil. Cut the roast into thick slices and divide evenly among 8 plates. Drizzle the sauce evenly over the roast and serve at once.

Each serving: 13 g carb, 228 cal, 8 g fat, 2 g sat fat, 49 mg chol, 1 g fib, 24 g pro, 481 mg sod • Carb Choices: 1; Exchanges: 1 carb, 1 veg, 3 lean protein, ½ fat

Beer-Braised Beef Brisket

makes 12 servings

An abundance of sweet caramelized onions and slightly bitter dark beer combine to make a scrumptious sauce for tender beef brisket.

1 (3-pound) flat half beef brisket, trimmed of all visible fat
1 teaspoon kosher salt, divided
¼ teaspoon freshly ground pepper
4 teaspoons extra virgin olive oil, divided
2 large onions, thinly sliced
2 garlic cloves, minced
1 (12-ounce) bottle dark beer, at room temperature
2 tablespoons no-salt-added tomato paste
1 bay leaf
1 teaspoon balsamic vinegar

1 Preheat the oven to 325°F.

2 Sprinkle the brisket with ¾ teaspoon of the salt and the pepper. Heat a large Dutch oven over medium-high heat. Add 2 teaspoons of the oil and the brisket and cook, turning to brown on both sides, 6 to 8 minutes. Transfer the brisket to a plate.

3 Add the remaining 2 teaspoons oil to the Dutch oven and tilt the pan to coat the bottom evenly. Add the onions and cook, stirring often, until lightly browned, 8 to 10 minutes. Add the garlic and cook, stirring constantly, until fragrant, 30 seconds. Add the beer, tomato paste, bay leaf and remaining ¼ teaspoon salt and cook, stirring to scrape up the browned bits from the bottom of the pot.

4 Return the brisket to the pot. Cover and bake until the roast is very tender, 2½ to 3 hours. Transfer the roast to a cutting board. Stir the vinegar into the onion mixture in the Dutch oven. Remove and discard the bay leaf. Slice the roast across the grain into thick slices and divide evenly among 12 plates. Spoon the onion mixture evenly over the roast and serve at once.

Each serving: 4 g carb, 184 cal, 6 g fat, 2 g sat fat, 48 mg chol, 1 g fib, 24 g pro, 136 mg sod • Carb Choices: 0; Exchanges: 3 lean protein

SLOW-COOKER VERSION: To make this dish in a slow cooker, prepare the recipe as directed in step 2, placing the browned meat in a 6-quart slow cooker. Proceed through step 3. Add the beer and onion mixture to the slow cooker and cook on high for 8 hours.

Slow-Cooker Beef Brisket with Onion Gravy

makes 12 servings

It takes about 15 minutes to get this brisket ready for the slow cooker—time well spent when you come home to a delicious dinner after a long day at work. The onions suffuse the meat with flavor and the slow cooker makes the meat fork-tender.

1 (3-pound) flat half beef brisket, trimmed of all visible fat
1 teaspoon kosher salt, divided
½ teaspoon freshly ground pepper, divided
2 teaspoons extra virgin olive oil
2 medium onions (about 1 pound), halved lengthwise and thinly sliced
1 cup Beef Stock (page 151) or low-sodium beef broth
2 garlic cloves, minced
2 tablespoons cold water
1½ tablespoons unbleached all-purpose flour

1 Sprinkle the brisket with ¾ teaspoon of the salt and ¼ teaspoon of the pepper. Heat a large skillet over medium-high heat. Add the oil and tilt the pan to coat the bottom evenly. Add the brisket and cook, turning to brown on both sides, 6 to 8 minutes.

2 Place the onions, stock, garlic, the remaining ¼ teaspoon salt, and remaining ¼ teaspoon pepper in a 6-quart oval slow cooker. Place the brisket on top of the onion mixture. Cover and cook on low until the brisket is very tender, 8 hours.

3 Transfer the brisket to a cutting board and cover to keep warm. Whisk together the water and flour in a small bowl. Stir the flour mixture into the stock mixture. Cover and cook on high until the gravy is slightly thickened, about 10 minutes. Slice the roast across the grain into thick slices and divide evenly among 12 plates. Spoon the gravy evenly over the roast and serve at once.

Each serving: 4 g carb, 169 cal, 6 g fat, 2 g sat fat, 49 mg chol, 1 g fib, 24 g pro, 169 mg sod • Carb Choices: 0; Exchanges: 3 lean protein

Ropa Vieja Tacos HIGH FIBER

makes 8 servings

Ropa vieja means "old clothes," which is what this rich, flavorful stew looks like with its tender shreds of meat and sliced peppers. Instead of serving it inside flour tortillas, you can serve it over brown rice if you prefer.

2 pounds flank steak, trimmed of all
visible fat

½ teaspoon kosher salt

¼ teaspoon freshly ground pepper

4 teaspoons extra virgin olive oil, divided

1 large onion, thinly sliced

1 large green bell pepper, thinly sliced

1 large red bell pepper, thinly sliced

2 garlic cloves, minced

2 teaspoons chili powder

1 teaspoon ground cumin

1 teaspoon dried oregano

¼ teaspoon ground cayenne

1 (14½-ounce) can no-salt-added diced
tomatoes

¼ cup pimento-stuffed green olives, sliced

2 tablespoons no-salt-added tomato paste

16 (6-inch) whole wheat flour tortillas, warmed

1 cup Winter Tomato Salsa (page 41) or
purchased salsa

Chopped fresh cilantro

Lime wedges

1 Cut the steak crosswise into 3-inch pieces. Sprinkle the steak with the salt and pepper. Heat a Dutch oven over medium-high heat. Add 2 teaspoons of the oil and tilt the pan to coat the bottom evenly. Add half of the steak and cook, turning to brown on both sides, 6 to 8 minutes. Transfer to a plate. Repeat with the remaining steak (additional oil should not be necessary). Return the steak to the pot and add water to cover. Bring to a boil. Reduce the heat to low, cover, and simmer until the steak is very tender, adding additional water, if necessary, to keep the steak almost covered, about 1½ hours.

2 Transfer the steak to a plate. Increase the heat to high and cook the liquid, uncovered, until reduced to 2 cups. Shred the beef using 2 forks and set aside.

3 Meanwhile, heat a large nonstick skillet over medium-high heat. Add the remaining 2 teaspoons oil and tilt the pan to coat the bottom evenly. Add the onion and bell peppers and cook, stirring often, until the vegetables are softened, 8 minutes. Add the garlic, chili powder, cumin, oregano, and cayenne and cook, stirring constantly, until fragrant, 30 seconds. Add the 2 cups of cooking liquid, the shredded beef, tomatoes, olives, and tomato paste and bring to a boil. Reduce the heat to low, cover, and simmer until the peppers are tender, 10 minutes. Uncover and simmer until the stew is thickened, 5 to 10 minutes longer.

4 Serve the stew in the tortillas, topped with the salsa and cilantro with the lime wedges alongside. The stew can be frozen for up to 3 months.

Each serving: 33 g carb, 392 cal, 16 g fat, 4 g sat fat, 48 mg chol, 18 g fib, 27 g pro, 730 mg sod • Carb Choices: 1½; Exchanges: 1 starch, 1 veg, 3 lean protein, 1½ fat

Chile-Braised Beef

makes 8 servings

Use this spicy beef as a filling for Tex-Mex dishes such as tacos, burritos, enchiladas, or tostadas. You can make this with a beef brisket instead of the flank steak. A brisket will take an additional 30 minutes to 1 hour to cook.

2 pounds flank steak, trimmed of all visible fat
1 teaspoon kosher salt
2 teaspoons extra virgin olive oil
4 cups Beef Stock (page 151) or low-sodium beef broth
4 dried ancho chiles, crumbled
1 cup no-salt-added tomato sauce
2 tablespoons no-salt-added tomato paste
1 teaspoon ground cumin

1 Cut the steak crosswise into 3-inch pieces. Sprinkle the beef with the salt. Heat a Dutch oven over medium-high heat. Add the oil and tilt the pan to coat the bottom evenly. Add half of the steak and cook, turning to brown on both sides, 6 to 8 minutes. Transfer to a plate. Repeat with the remaining steak (additional oil should not be necessary). Return the steak to the pot.

2 Add the stock and chiles and bring to a boil. Reduce the heat to low, cover, and simmer until the steak is very tender, adding water, if necessary, to keep the steak almost covered, about 1½ hours.

3 Transfer the meat to a plate and shred using 2 forks. Return the meat to the stock mixture. Add the tomato sauce, tomato paste, and cumin and simmer, uncovered, until almost all the liquid has evaporated, 30 minutes. The beef can be frozen for up to 3 months. Use the beef as a filling for Tex-Mex dishes, or serve as a main dish with rice and beans as accompaniments.

Each serving: 8 g carb, 218 cal, 11 g fat, 4 g sat fat, 48 mg chol, 3 g fib, 22 g pro, 285 mg sod • Carb Choices: ½; Exchanges: 1 veg, 3 lean protein

Beef Carbonnade

makes 8 servings

Serve this comforting stew with whole wheat egg noodles or mashed potatoes to soak up the delicious juices.

2 strips center-cut bacon, coarsely chopped
2 large onions, halved and sliced
2 garlic cloves, minced
2 pounds beef chuck shoulder roast or bottom round roast, trimmed of all visible fat and cut into 1-inch cubes
2 tablespoons unbleached all-purpose flour
1 teaspoon kosher salt
¼ teaspoon freshly ground pepper
2 cups Beef Stock (page 151) or low-sodium beef broth
1 (12-ounce) bottle dark beer
2 tablespoons no-salt-added tomato paste

1 Cook the bacon in a Dutch oven over medium-high heat until crisp. Drain on paper towels and set aside. Pour off all but 2 teaspoons of the drippings into a small bowl. Reserve the drippings.

2 Add the onions to the Dutch oven and reduce the heat to medium. Cook the onions, stirring occasionally, until very soft, about 25 minutes. Add the garlic and cook, stirring constantly, 30 seconds. Transfer the onion mixture to a plate. Do not wash the Dutch oven.

3 Preheat the oven to 325°F.

4 Place the beef in a large bowl. Sprinkle with the flour, salt, and pepper and toss to coat. Increase the heat under the Dutch oven to medium-high. Add 2 teaspoons of the reserved bacon drippings and half of the beef and cook, turning occasionally, until browned, 6 minutes. Transfer the beef to a plate. Repeat with the remaining drippings (use canola oil if there are not enough drippings) and beef.

5 Add the stock, beer, and tomato paste to the Dutch oven and bring to a boil, stirring to scrape

up the browned bits in the bottom of the pot. Return the bacon, onions, and beef to the Dutch oven.

6 Cover and bake until the beef is very tender, about 3 hours. For a slightly thickened broth, uncover the Dutch oven during the last 30 to 45 minutes of baking. Divide the stew evenly among 8 shallow bowls and serve at once.

Each serving: 8 g carb, 211 cal, 8 g fat, 3 g sat fat, 53 mg chol, 1 g fib, 24 g pro, 481 mg sod • Carb Choices: ½; Exchanges: ½ carb, 3 lean protein, ½ fat

SLOW-COOKER VERSION: To make in a slow cooker, prepare the recipe through steps 1 and 2, placing the onions in a 6-quart slow cooker. Proceed through step 4 and 5, using only 1 cup of the beef stock. Add the stock, beer, and bacon to the slow cooker and cook on high for 8 hours.

Beef Bourguignon

makes 8 servings

The deep flavor of this dish comes from a combination of bacon, brandy, and red wine. You can make it in advance—it's actually better when you reheat it the next day.

2 strips center-cut bacon, coarsely chopped

2 pounds beef chuck shoulder roast or bottom round roast, trimmed of all visible fat and cut into 1-inch cubes

2 tablespoons unbleached all-purpose flour

1 teaspoon kosher salt

¼ teaspoon freshly ground pepper

2 teaspoons extra virgin olive oil

1 medium onion, chopped

1 stalk celery, chopped

2 garlic cloves, minced

⅓ cup brandy

2 cups dry red wine

2 tablespoons no-salt-added tomato paste

8 ounces pearl onions or small boiling onions

1 pound small whole white or cremini mushrooms

2 tablespoons chopped fresh Italian parsley

1 Preheat the oven to 325°F.

2 Cook the bacon in a Dutch oven over medium-high heat until crisp. Drain on paper towels and set aside. Pour off all but 2 teaspoons of the drippings into a small bowl. Reserve the drippings.

3 Place the beef in a large bowl. Sprinkle with the flour, salt, and pepper and toss to coat. Add half of the beef to the Dutch oven and cook over medium heat, turning occasionally, until well browned, about 6 minutes. Transfer the beef to a plate. Repeat with the reserved bacon drippings and beef.

4 Add the oil to the Dutch oven and tilt the pot to coat the bottom evenly. Add the onion and celery and cook, stirring often, until softened, about 5 minutes. Add the garlic and cook, stirring constantly, until fragrant, 30 seconds.

5 Add the brandy and bring to a boil, stirring to scrape up the browned bits in the bottom of the pot. Add the bacon, beef, wine, and tomato paste and bring to a boil. Cover and bake 2 hours.

6 Meanwhile, bring a medium saucepan of water to a boil. Add the pearl onions and cook 1 minute. Drain in a colander and rinse with cold running water. Peel the onions, leaving the roots intact (the skins will slip off easily after boiling).

7 Remove the Dutch oven from the oven and stir in the onions and mushrooms. Bake until the beef is very tender, 1 hour longer. Stir in the parsley just before serving. Divide the stew evenly among 8 shallow bowls and serve at once.

Each serving: 10 g carb, 283 cal, 9 g fat, 3 g sat fat, 53 mg chol, 1 g fib, 24 g pro, 238 mg sod • Carb Choices: ½; Exchanges: 1 veg, 3 lean protein, 1 fat

Wine and Red Pepper–Braised Beef Stew

makes 8 servings

Pureed roasted red peppers and anchovies make a complex and richly flavored sauce for this stew. This is one of my very favorite fall and winter meals.

1 large red Roasted Bell Pepper (page 21) or 1 cup roasted red peppers from a jar, chopped

1½ cups Beef Stock (page 151) or low-sodium beef broth, divided

¼ cup no-salt-added tomato paste

2 canned anchovy fillets, drained

2 pounds beef chuck shoulder roast or bottom round roast, trimmed of all visible fat and cut into 1-inch cubes

¾ teaspoon kosher salt, divided

¼ teaspoon freshly ground pepper

¼ cup unbleached all-purpose flour

6 teaspoons extra virgin olive oil, divided

2 carrots, peeled and chopped

2 stalks celery, chopped

1 medium onion, chopped

2 garlic cloves, minced

½ cup dry red wine

Pinch of crushed red pepper

1 Preheat the oven to 325°F.

2 Combine the roasted peppers, ½ cup of the beef stock, tomato paste, and anchovies in a food processor and process until smooth. Set aside.

3 Sprinkle the beef with ¼ teaspoon of the salt and the ground pepper. Place the flour in a shallow dish. Add the beef, a few pieces at a time, and toss to lightly coat.

4 Heat a Dutch oven over medium-high heat. Add 2 teaspoons of the oil and tilt the pot to coat the bottom evenly. Add half of the beef and cook, turning occasionally, until well browned, about 6 minutes. Transfer the beef to a plate. Repeat with 2 teaspoons of the remaining oil and the remaining beef.

5 Add the remaining 2 teaspoons oil to the Dutch oven. Add the carrots, celery, and onion and cook, stirring often, until the vegetables are softened, 5 minutes. Add the garlic and cook, stirring constantly, 30 seconds. Add the wine and bring to a boil. Stir in the beef, red pepper mixture, remaining 1 cup stock, remaining ¼ teaspoon salt, and crushed red pepper and bring to a boil.

6 Cover and bake until the beef is very tender, about 3 hours. Divide the stew evenly among 8 shallow bowls and serve at once. The stew can be frozen for up to 3 months.

Each serving: 9 g carb, 223 cal, 9 g fat, 2 g sat fat, 50 mg chol, 2 g fib, 24 g pro, 290 mg sod • Carb Choices: ½; Exchanges: 1 veg, 3 lean protein, ½ fat

SLOW-COOKER VERSION: To make this dish in a slow cooker, prepare the recipe as directed through step 4, placing the browned meat in a 6-quart slow cooker. Proceed through step 5. Add the stock and vegetable mixture to the slow cooker and cook on high for 8 hours.

Beef and Red Bean Chili HIGH FIBER

makes 8 servings

Cooking the dried beans right along with the beef and all the seasonings make this one of the most flavorful chilis you'll ever try.

2 tablespoons chili powder

2 teaspoons ground cumin

½ teaspoon dried oregano

½ teaspoon freshly ground pepper

½ teaspoon kosher salt

2 pounds beef chuck shoulder roast or bottom round roast, trimmed of all visible fat and cut into ½-inch cubes

6 teaspoons extra virgin olive oil, divided

1 large onion, chopped

1 large red or green bell pepper, chopped

2 garlic cloves, minced

4 cups water

3½ cups Beef Stock (page 151) or low-sodium beef broth

2 (14½-ounce) cans no-added-salt whole tomatoes, undrained and chopped

¼ cup no-salt-added tomato paste

2 cups dried red kidney beans, picked over and rinsed

1 teaspoon minced chipotle in adobo sauce

Thinly sliced scallions

Chopped fresh cilantro

1 Combine the chili powder, cumin, oregano, ground pepper, and salt in a dish. Sprinkle the beef with 1 tablespoon of the spice mixture.

2 Heat a Dutch oven over medium-high heat. Add 2 teaspoons of the oil and half of the beef and cook until well browned, about 6 minutes. Transfer the beef to a plate. Repeat with 2 teaspoons of the remaining oil and the remaining beef.

3 Add the remaining 2 teaspoons oil and the onion and bell pepper and cook, stirring often, until softened, 5 minutes. Add the garlic and the remaining spice mixture and cook, stirring constantly, until fragrant, 30 seconds.

4 Add the beef, water, stock, tomatoes and their juices, tomato paste, beans, and chipotle and bring to a boil. Reduce the heat to low, cover, and simmer until the beef and beans are very tender, about 2½ hours. Stir the chili every 30 minutes and add additional water if necessary. If the chili is too thin when the beans are tender, uncover and simmer until thickened. Spoon into 8 bowls, and top with the scallions and cilantro. The chili can be frozen for up to 3 months.

Each serving: 34 g carb, 356 cal, 9 g fat, 2 g sat fat, 49 mg chol, 11 g fib, 34 g pro, 418 mg sod • Carb Choices: 2; Exchanges: 1½ starch, 1 veg, 3 lean protein, 1 plant-based protein, ½ fat

Beef Stroganoff QUICK

makes 4 servings

1 pound top sirloin steak, trimmed of all visible fat and cut into ¼-inch-thick slices

¾ teaspoon kosher salt, divided

¼ teaspoon freshly ground pepper, divided

6 teaspoons extra virgin olive oil, divided

1 medium onion, halved and sliced

12 ounces sliced cremini or white mushrooms

2 garlic cloves, minced

2 tablespoons unbleached all-purpose flour

2 cups Beef Stock (page 151) or low-sodium beef broth

¼ cup dry sherry

¼ cup reduced-fat sour cream

2 tablespoons chopped fresh Italian parsley

3 cups hot cooked whole wheat egg noodles

1 Sprinkle the steak with ½ teaspoon of the salt and ⅛ teaspoon of the pepper. Heat a large non-stick skillet over medium-high heat. Add 2 teaspoons of the oil and half of the steak, and cook until browned, 6 minutes. Transfer to a plate. Repeat with 2 teaspoons of the remaining oil and the remaining steak.

2 Add the remaining 2 teaspoons oil, the onion, and the mushrooms, and cook until browned, 5 minutes. Add the garlic and flour and cook, stirring constantly, 1 minute. Stir in the beef stock, sherry, remaining ¼ teaspoon salt, and remaining ⅛ teaspoon pepper and bring to boil. Reduce the heat to medium-low, add the beef, and cook until heated through, about 2 minutes. Remove from the heat and stir in the sour cream and parsley. Divide the noodles evenly among 4 plates and top with the stroganoff.

Each serving: 29 g carb, 395 cal, 15 g fat, 4 g sat fat, 74 mg chol, 3 g fib, 33 g pro, 351 mg sod • Carb Choices: 2; Exchanges: 1½ starch, 1 veg, ½ lean protein, 1½ fat

Ground Beef

Moist and Lean Burgers

QUICK | HIGH FIBER

makes 4 servings

The addition of a little yogurt is the secret to keeping these lean and healthy burgers moist. Use the Creamy Herb Dressing (page 141) or Avocado Dressing (page 143) instead of mayonnaise for spreading on the buns.

1 pound 95% lean ground beef
¼ cup plain low-fat yogurt
2 tablespoons shredded sweet onion
1 garlic clove, minced
½ teaspoon kosher salt
⅛ teaspoon freshly ground pepper
4 whole wheat kaiser rolls, split and toasted
4 large leaves leaf lettuce
1 medium tomato, sliced

1 Combine the beef, yogurt, onion, garlic, salt, and pepper in a medium bowl and mix thoroughly with your hands. Shape into 4 patties.

2 Heat a large nonstick skillet over medium-high heat. Add the burgers and cook, turning once, 4 minutes on each side for medium, or to the desired degree of doneness. Serve the burgers in the rolls, topped with the lettuce and tomato.

Each serving: 25 g carb, 275 cal, 7 g fat, 3 g sat fat, 66 mg chol, 4 g fib, 27 g pro, 420 mg sod • Carb Choices: 2½; Exchanges: 1½ starch, 3 lean protein

Blue Cheese Burgers with Caramelized Onions HIGH FIBER

makes 4 servings

These grown-up open-face burgers make a nice lunch with a salad of baby greens served alongside. You can make the onions a day ahead and reheat them in the microwave to save time.

2 teaspoons extra virgin olive oil
1 large onion, halved and thinly sliced
¾ teaspoon kosher salt, divided
1 pound 95% lean ground beef
¼ cup plain low-fat yogurt
2 teaspoons chopped fresh thyme or
    ¼ teaspoon dried thyme
⅛ teaspoon freshly ground pepper
2 tablespoons finely crumbled blue cheese
4 (½-inch) diagonally cut slices whole wheat
    Italian bread, toasted
1 large tomato, sliced

1 Heat a large nonstick skillet over medium heat. Add the oil and tilt the pan to coat the bottom evenly. Add the onion and ¼ teaspoon of the salt and cook, stirring occasionally, until very soft and browned, about 25 minutes.

2 When the onions are almost done, combine the beef, yogurt, thyme, the remaining ½ teaspoon salt, and the pepper in a medium bowl and mix thoroughly with your hands. Shape into 4 patties.

3 Heat a large nonstick skillet over medium-high heat. Add the burgers and cook, turning once, 4 minutes on each side for medium, or to the desired degree of doneness, sprinkling evenly with the blue cheese during the last 2 minutes of cooking.

4 To serve, place one slice of bread on each of 4 plates. Top each with a tomato slice, then with a burger. Top evenly with the onions and serve at once.

Each serving: 20 g carb, 288 cal, 10 g fat, 4 g sat fat, 70 mg chol, 5 g fib, 29 g pro, 479 mg sod • Carb Choices: 1; Exchanges: 1 starch, 1 veg, 3 lean protein, 1 fat

Beef, Cheddar, and Black Bean Burgers QUICK | HIGH FIBER

makes 4 servings

Black beans make a delicious and healthful stand-in for part of the beef in these burgers. Top the burgers with salsa instead of the lettuce and tomato to add even more spice.

1 cup canned no-salt-added black beans, rinsed and drained

12 ounces 95% lean ground beef

2 tablespoons shredded reduced-fat extra-sharp Cheddar cheese

¼ cup plain dry breadcrumbs

¼ cup chopped fresh cilantro

1 jalapeño, seeded and minced

2 teaspoons chili powder

1 teaspoon ground cumin

½ teaspoon kosher salt

⅛ teaspoon freshly ground pepper

2 teaspoons canola oil

4 whole wheat sandwich rolls, toasted

1 medium tomato, sliced

4 large leaves leaf lettuce

1 Place the beans in a large bowl and mash with a potato masher. Add the beef, Cheddar, breadcrumbs, cilantro, jalapeño, chili powder, cumin, salt, and pepper and mix thoroughly with your hands. Shape into 4 patties.

2 Heat a large nonstick skillet over medium heat. Add the oil and tilt the pan to coat the bottom evenly. Add the patties and cook, turning once, 4 minutes on each side for medium, or to the desired degree of doneness. Serve the patties in the rolls, topped with the tomato and lettuce.

Each serving: 38 g carb, 340 cal, 9 g fat, 2 g sat fat, 49 mg chol, 7 g fib, 26 g pro, 532 mg sod • Carb Choices: 2; Exchanges: 1½ starch, ½ carb, 3 lean protein, 1 fat

Open-Face Greek Burgers QUICK

makes 4 servings

The feta cheese infuses these burgers throughout with tart salty flavor. If you want to add a little more spice, finely chop a pickled pepperoncini pepper and add it to the beef mixture.

1 pound 95% lean ground beef

2 ounces finely crumbled feta cheese (about ½ cup)

¼ cup Kalamata olives, pitted and chopped

2 tablespoons chopped fresh mint

⅛ teaspoon freshly ground pepper

2 teaspoons canola oil

4 (4-inch) whole wheat pita breads, warmed

1 medium tomato, sliced

1 cup thinly sliced romaine lettuce

½ hothouse (English) cucumber, sliced

1 Combine the beef, feta, olives, mint, and pepper in a medium bowl and mix thoroughly with your hands. Shape into 4 patties.

2 Heat a large nonstick skillet over medium heat. Add the oil and tilt the pan to coat the bottom evenly. Add the patties and cook, turning once, 4 minutes on each side for medium, or to the desired degree of doneness. Serve the patties in the pita breads, topped with the tomato, lettuce, and cucumber.

Each serving: 20 carb, 310 cal, 13 g fat, 5 g sat fat, 78 mg chol, 3 g fib, 28 g pro, 494 mg sod • Carb Choices: 1¼; Exchanges: 1 starch, ½ carb, 3 lean protein, 1½ fat

Ginger-Sesame Burgers with Grilled Scallions QUICK | HIGH FIBER

makes 4 servings

Fresh ginger and Asian sesame oil give comfort-food burgers an unusual twist. Serve them with Roasted Sweet Potatoes with Ginger and Lime (page 488) and Cilantro-Sesame Slaw (page 91).

1 pound 95% lean ground beef
¼ cup minced scallions
1 garlic clove, crushed through a press
1 tablespoon grated fresh ginger
1 tablespoon reduced-sodium soy sauce
1 teaspoon Asian sesame oil
¼ teaspoon kosher salt
8 scallions, cut into 6-inch lengths
1½ teaspoons canola oil, divided
4 whole wheat kaiser rolls, split

1 Combine the beef, minced scallions, garlic, ginger, soy sauce, sesame oil, and salt in a medium bowl and mix thoroughly with your hands. Shape into 4 patties.

2 Place the whole scallions in a shallow dish, drizzle with 1 teaspoon of the canola oil, and turn to coat.

3 Prepare the grill or heat a large grill pan over medium-high heat.

4 Brush the grill rack or grill pan with the remaining ½ teaspoon canola oil. Grill the burgers, turning once, 4 minutes on each side for medium, or to the desired degree of doneness. Meanwhile, grill the whole scallions, turning occasionally, until lightly charred, 6 to 8 minutes. Grill the rolls cut side down until lightly toasted, about 30 seconds. Serve the patties in the rolls, topped with the grilled scallions.

Each serving: 25 g carb, 298 cal, 10 g fat, 3 g sat fat, 66 mg chol, 4 g fib, 27 g pro, 494 mg sod • Carb Choices: 1½; Exchanges: 1½ starch, 1 veg, 3 lean protein, 1 fat

RED CURRY BURGERS QUICK | HIGH FIBER : Follow the recipe for Ginger-Sesame Burgers with Grilled Scallions, at left, adding 2 teaspoons red curry paste to the meat mixture in step 1. Proceed as directed.

Each serving: 26 g carb, 299 cal, 10 g fat, 3 g sat fat, 66 mg chol, 4 g fib, 27 g pro, 539 mg sod • Carb Choices: 2; Exchanges: 1½ starch, 1 veg, 3 lean protein, 1 fat

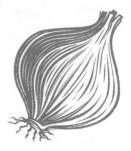

Greek Beef and Orzo Pilaf

QUICK | HIGH FIBER

makes 4 servings

Spices and fresh mint infuse this humble ground beef dish with sophisticated flavor. It's an ideal one-dish weeknight meal that will please adults and children alike. Serve it with Greek Salad (page 84).

12 ounces 95% lean ground beef, crumbled
1 medium onion, diced
1 medium red bell pepper, diced
6 ounces whole wheat orzo (about 1 cup)
2 garlic cloves, minced
1 teaspoon ground cumin
1 teaspoon kosher salt
¼ teaspoon ground cinnamon
2 cups Chicken Stock (page 149) or
    low-sodium chicken broth
1 cup chopped plum tomatoes
3 tablespoons chopped fresh Italian parsley
2 tablespoons chopped fresh mint
1 tablespoon lemon juice

1 Combine the beef, onion, and bell pepper in a large nonstick skillet. Place over medium-high heat and cook, stirring occasionally, until the beef is browned, about 8 minutes.

2 Stir in the orzo, garlic, cumin, salt, and cinnamon and cook, stirring constantly, until fragrant, 1 minute. Add the stock and bring to a boil over high heat. Cover, reduce the heat to low, and simmer, stirring occasionally, until the orzo is tender and most of the liquid is absorbed, 15 minutes.

3 Remove the skillet from the heat. Stir in the tomatoes, parsley, mint, and lemon juice. Cover and let stand 5 minutes. Divide the pilaf evenly among 4 plates and serve at once.

Each serving: 39 g carb, 299 cal, 5 g fat, 2 g sat fat, 51 mg chol, 7 g fib, 27 g pro, 404 mg sod • Carb Choices: 2; Exchanges: 2 starch, 2 lean protein

Asian Beef Lettuce Wraps QUICK

makes 4 servings

If your kids like Asian flavors, this is a dish they will really enjoy. Let them help assemble the "fixings"—the lettuce, cucumber, and bean sprouts—while you make the quick beef filling. They'll think it's fun to assemble their own wraps at the table, too.

1 pound 95% lean ground beef
2 tablespoons minced fresh ginger
3 tablespoons reduced-sodium soy sauce
1 tablespoon lime juice
¼ teaspoon Asian sesame oil
¼ teaspoon chili-garlic paste
½ cup thinly sliced scallions
2 tablespoons chopped fresh mint
2 tablespoons chopped fresh cilantro
1 small head Bibb lettuce, separated into leaves
1 hothouse (English) cucumber, cut into short,
    thin strips
1 cup bean sprouts
Lime wedges

1 Combine the beef and ginger in a medium nonstick skillet. Place over medium-high heat and cook, stirring occasionally, until the beef is browned, about 8 minutes. Stir in the soy sauce, lime juice, oil, and chili-garlic paste and cook, stirring often, until most of the liquid has evaporated, about 2 minutes.

2 To serve, transfer the beef mixture to a serving bowl and stir in the scallions, mint, and cilantro. Arrange the lettuce, cucumber, and bean sprouts on a serving platter. Allow each person to assemble their own rolls, spooning the beef into the lettuce leaves and topping with the cucumber and bean sprouts. Serve with the lime wedges.

Each serving: 7 g carb, 195 cal, 7 g fat, 3 g sat fat, 67 mg chol, 2 g fib, 27 g pro, 535 mg sod • Carb Choices: ½; Exchanges: 1 veg, 3 lean protein

Old-Fashioned Meatloaf

makes 4 servings

The homiest and most comforting of classic American dishes, this healthful meatloaf makes the perfect Sunday supper. You can make great sandwiches from the leftovers, too.

2 teaspoons extra virgin olive oil
⅓ cup finely diced onion
⅓ cup finely diced red bell pepper
1 garlic clove, minced
1 teaspoon kosher salt
¼ teaspoon dried oregano
¼ teaspoon freshly ground pepper
⅛ teaspoon dried thyme
1 pound 95% lean ground beef
½ cup no-salt-added tomato sauce, divided
⅓ cup plain dry breadcrumbs
¼ cup 1% low-fat milk
1 large egg, lightly beaten
2 tablespoons chopped fresh Italian parsley

1 Preheat the oven to 350°F.

2 Heat a medium nonstick skillet over medium-high heat. Add the oil and tilt the pan to coat the bottom evenly. Add the onion and bell pepper and cook, stirring often, until softened, 5 minutes. Add the garlic, salt, oregano, ground pepper, and thyme and cook, stirring constantly, until fragrant, 30 seconds. Transfer to a plate and let cool slightly.

3 Combine the beef, ¼ cup of the tomato sauce, breadcrumbs, milk, egg, parsley, and the onion mixture in a large bowl. Mix thoroughly with your hands. Place the mixture in a shallow baking dish and shape into an 8 x 4-inch loaf.

4 Spread the remaining ¼ cup tomato sauce over the loaf and bake 1 hour. Let stand 5 minutes before slicing. Cut the meatloaf into slices, divide evenly among 4 plates, and serve at once.

Each serving: 12 g carb, 244 cal, 9 g fat, 3 g sat fat, 112 mg chol, 1 g fib, 26 g pro, 426 mg sod • Carb Choices: 1; Exchanges: 1 carb, 3 lean protein, 1 fat

MEATLOAF WITH SUN-DRIED TOMATOES: Follow the Old-Fashioned Meatloaf recipe, at left, adding ½ cup red Roasted Bell Peppers (page 21) or roasted red peppers from a jar, chopped, and ¼ cup dry-packed sun-dried tomatoes, diced in step 2 and proceed with the recipe.

Each serving: 15 g carb, 256 cal, 10 g fat, 3 g sat fat, 112 mg chol, 2 g fib, 27 g pro, 498 mg sod • Carb Choices: 1; Exchanges: 1 carb, 3 lean protein, 1 fat

Chile Pepper Meatloaf

makes 4 servings

The fresh zing of cilantro and pungent chili powder elevates meatloaf to new heights of flavor. Using tomato sauce instead of typical ketchup on top of the meatloaf gives it flavor and moisture, but without the added sugar and salt.

2 teaspoons extra virgin olive oil
⅓ cup finely diced onion
⅓ cup finely diced red bell pepper
1 jalapeño, seeded and minced
1 garlic clove, minced
1½ teaspoons chili powder
1 teaspoon ground cumin
1 teaspoon kosher salt
¼ teaspoon freshly ground pepper
Pinch of ground cayenne
1 pound 95% lean ground beef
½ cup no-salt-added tomato sauce, divided
⅓ cup plain dry breadcrumbs
¼ cup 1% low-fat milk
1 large egg, lightly beaten
2 tablespoons chopped fresh cilantro

1 Preheat the oven to 350°F.

2 Heat a medium nonstick skillet over medium-high heat. Add the oil and tilt the pan to coat the bottom evenly. Add the onion, bell pepper, and jalapeño and cook, stirring often, until softened, 5 minutes. Add the garlic, chili powder, cumin, salt, ground pepper, and cayenne and cook,

stirring constantly, until fragrant, 30 seconds. Transfer to a plate and let cool slightly.

3 Combine the beef, ¼ cup of the tomato sauce, breadcrumbs, milk, egg, cilantro, and the onion mixture in a large bowl. Mix thoroughly with your hands. Place the mixture in a shallow baking dish and shape into an 8 x 4-inch loaf.

4 Spread the remaining ¼ cup tomato sauce over the loaf and bake 1 hour. Let stand 5 minutes before slicing. Cut the meatloaf into slices, divide evenly among 4 plates, and serve at once.

Each serving: 13 g carb, 251 cal, 10 g fat, 3 g sat fat, 112 mg chol, 2 g fib, 26 g pro, 449 mg sod • Carb Choices: 1; Exchanges: 1 carb, 3 lean protein, 1 fat

Beef Kefta with Yogurt Sauce QUICK | HIGH FIBER

makes 4 servings

You can serve the kefta on their own, or turn them into a sandwich by serving them in warmed whole wheat pita bread with shredded lettuce, chopped cucumber, and chopped tomato. You can also shape them into mini meatballs, using about 2 tablespoons of meat mixture for each one, and serve them with the sauce as an appetizer.

¾ cup water

½ cup fine-grind bulgur

¾ cup plain low-fat yogurt

2 tablespoons tahini (sesame paste)

2 tablespoon lemon juice

2 tablespoons plus ¼ cup chopped fresh cilantro, divided

1¼ teaspoons kosher salt, divided

½ teaspoon canola oil

12 ounces 95% lean ground beef

2 tablespoons minced onion

1 garlic clove, crushed through a press

1 teaspoon fresh grated ginger

1 teaspoon ground cumin

¼ teaspoon ground cinnamon

1 Pour the water into a small saucepan and bring to a boil over high heat. Remove from the heat and add the bulgur. Cover and let stand until the water is absorbed, 20 minutes.

2 Combine the yogurt, tahini, lemon juice, 2 tablespoons of the cilantro, and ¼ teaspoon of the salt in a small bowl and whisk until smooth. Cover and refrigerate until ready to serve.

3 Preheat the broiler. Brush a broiler rack with the oil.

4 To make the kefta, place the bulgur in a large bowl. Add the beef, onion, garlic, ginger, cumin, cinnamon, remaining ¼ cup cilantro, and remaining 1 teaspoon salt and mix thoroughly with your hands. Shape the mixture into eight 4-inch-long cylinders, using about ⅓ cup of the mixture for each one.

5 Arrange the kefta on the rack and broil, turning once, until well browned, 8 to 10 minutes. Divide the kefta evenly among 4 plates and serve with the sauce.

Each serving: 20 g carb, 248 cal, 9 g fat, 3 g sat fat, 52 mg chol, 4 g fib, 23 g pro, 436 mg sod • Carb Choices: 1 ; Exchanges: 1 starch, 2 lean protein, 1 fat

Swedish Meatballs QUICK

makes 4 servings

Super-lean beef and yogurt substituted for the usual sour cream make these meatballs far healthier, but no less flavorful, than the traditional version. Serve them with whole wheat egg noodles.

2 slices rye sandwich bread, each cut into 4 pieces
1 pound 95% lean ground beef
2 tablespoons minced onion
2 garlic cloves, minced
1 large egg white
¾ teaspoon kosher salt, divided
¼ teaspoon freshly ground pepper, divided
¼ teaspoon ground nutmeg, divided
2 teaspoons extra virgin olive oil
1½ cups Chicken Stock (page 149) or low-sodium chicken broth
1½ tablespoons unbleached all-purpose flour
½ cup plain low-fat Greek yogurt or strained yogurt (page 11)
2 tablespoons chopped fresh Italian parsley

1 Place the bread in a food processor and process until fine crumbs form (you should have about 1 cup).

2 Combine the breadcrumbs, beef, onion, garlic, egg white, ¼ teaspoon of the salt, ⅛ teaspoon of the pepper, and ⅛ teaspoon of the nutmeg in a large bowl and mix thoroughly with your hands. Shape the mixture into about 32 (1-inch) meatballs.

3 Heat a large nonstick skillet over medium-high heat. Add the oil and tilt the pan to coat the bottom evenly. Add the meatballs in batches and cook, turning often, until no longer pink in the centers, 6 to 8 minutes. Transfer to a plate.

4 Whisk together the broth and flour in a medium bowl until smooth. Add the broth mixture to the pan and cook, whisking often, until the mixture comes to a boil and thickens, about 3 minutes. Stir in the remaining ½ teaspoon salt, ⅛ teaspoon pepper, and ⅛ teaspoon nutmeg.

5 Return the meatballs to the skillet and cook until heated through, about 2 minutes. Reduce the heat to low. Stir in the yogurt and cook, stirring constantly, just until heated through (do not boil). Remove from the heat and stir in the parsley. Divide the meatballs and sauce evenly among 4 shallow bowls and serve at once.

Each serving: 10 g carb, 253 cal, 9 g fat, 4g sat fat, 74 mg chol, 1 g fib, 31 g pro, 455 mg sod • Carb Choices: 1; Exchanges: 1 starch, 3 lean protein, ½ fat

Spaghetti and Meatballs

HIGH FIBER

makes 4 servings

Ground beef and turkey sausage combine in these hearty meatballs. They are baked until lightly browned, then simmered in a classic tomato sauce. This dish is comfort food at its best.

1 recipe Marinara Sauce (page 593)
½ teaspoon canola oil
8 ounces Italian turkey sausage
8 ounces 95% lean ground beef
2 tablespoons minced onion
2 garlic cloves, minced
1 large egg white
2 tablespoons freshly grated Parmesan
¼ cup plain dry breadcrumbs
¼ cup chopped fresh Italian parsley
⅛ teaspoon freshly ground pepper
6 ounces whole wheat spaghetti
2 tablespoons finely shredded Parmesan

1 Warm the sauce over medium heat, if necessary. Preheat the oven to 375°F. Line a large rimmed baking sheet with foil. Place a wire rack in the pan and brush the rack with the oil.

2 To make the meatballs, remove the sausage from the casings and place in a large bowl. Add the beef, onion, garlic, egg white, grated Parmesan, breadcrumbs, parsley, and pepper and mix thoroughly with your hands. Shape the mixture into

about 32 (1-inch) meatballs and place on the prepared rack. Bake until the meatballs are lightly browned, about 20 minutes.

3 Transfer the meatballs to the pan of sauce. Simmer 5 minutes.

4 Meanwhile, cook the spaghetti according to the package directions. Divide the spaghetti evenly among 4 shallow bowls and top evenly with the meatballs and sauce. Sprinkle evenly with the shredded Parmesan and serve at once. You can make a double batch of the meatballs and sauce and freeze half for up to 3 months.

Each serving: 58 g carb, 471 cal, 14 g fat, 3 g sat fat, 61 mg chol, 10 g fib, 33 g pro, 582 mg sod • Carb Choices: 3½; Exchanges: 2½ starch, 2 veg, 1 medium-fat protein, 1½ lean protein, 1 fat

Pasta with Beef and Mushroom Bolognese Sauce HIGH FIBER

makes 6 servings

Meaty mushrooms stand in for part of the beef in this satisfying sauce. You can serve the sauce over Parmesan Polenta (page 422) instead of the pasta.

12 ounces 95% lean ground beef, crumbled

8 ounces cremini or white mushrooms, sliced

1 medium onion, diced

1 carrot, peeled and diced

1 stalk celery, diced

2 garlic cloves, minced

½ cup dry red wine

1 (28-ounce) can no-salt-added whole tomatoes, undrained and chopped

2 tablespoons no-salt-added tomato paste

½ teaspoon kosher salt

¼ teaspoon freshly ground pepper

¼ cup chopped fresh basil

12 ounces whole wheat fettuccini or spaghetti

3 tablespoons freshly grated Parmesan

1 Combine the beef, mushrooms, onion, carrot, celery, and garlic in a large nonstick skillet and cook over medium-high heat, stirring often, until the beef is browned, about 8 minutes.

2 Stir in the wine and cook, stirring often, until almost all the liquid is absorbed, 2 minutes. Add the tomatoes with their juice, tomato paste, salt, and pepper and bring to a boil. Reduce the heat to low and simmer, uncovered, until the vegetables are tender and the sauce is thickened, 15 to 20 minutes. Stir in the basil during the last 5 minutes of cooking.

3 Meanwhile, cook the pasta according to the package directions. Divide the pasta among 6 shallow bowls and top evenly with the sauce. Sprinkle evenly with the Parmesan and serve at once. You can make a double batch of the sauce and freeze half for up to 3 months.

Each serving: 52 g carb, 329 cal, 5 g fat, 2 g sat fat, 37 mg chol, 9 g fib, 24 g pro, 212 mg sod • Carb Choices: 3; Exchanges: 2½ starch, 2 veg, 2 lean protein

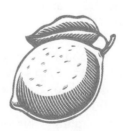

Weeknight Beef and Spinach Lasagna HIGH FIBER

makes 6 servings

No-boil lasagna noodles and frozen spinach make this dish quick to assemble. While the lasagna bakes, make a tossed green salad and dinner is ready.

1 teaspoon extra virgin olive oil

8 ounces 95% lean ground beef, crumbled

1 small onion, diced

2 garlic cloves, minced

1 (14½-ounce) can no-salt-added diced tomatoes

1 (8-ounce) can no-salt-added tomato sauce

½ teaspoon dried basil

½ teaspoon dried oregano

1 cup low-fat cottage cheese

4 ounces shredded part-skim mozzarella (about 1 cup)

1 (10-ounce) package frozen chopped spinach, thawed and squeezed dry

9 no-boil lasagna noodles

2 tablespoons freshly grated Parmesan

1 Preheat the oven to 375°F. Brush an 11 x 7-inch glass baking dish with the oil.

2 Combine the beef and onion in a large nonstick skillet. Place over medium heat and cook, stirring often, until the beef is browned, 5 minutes. Add the garlic and cook, stirring constantly, until fragrant, 30 seconds. Add the tomatoes, tomato sauce, basil, and oregano, and bring to a boil. Cook, stirring often, until the sauce is slightly thickened, about 5 minutes.

3 Combine the cottage cheese, mozzarella, and spinach in a medium bowl and stir until well mixed.

4 Spread ¾ cup of the sauce in the bottom of the prepared baking dish. Place 3 noodles over the sauce, breaking them as needed to fit the dish. Top the noodles with 1½ cups of the cheese mixture and ¾ cup of the sauce. Repeat the layering, ending with the noodles. Spread the remaining sauce over the top layer of noodles.

5 Cover the baking dish with foil and place the dish on a large rimmed baking sheet. Bake until the noodles are tender, 30 minutes. Uncover, sprinkle the lasagna with the Parmesan, and bake, uncovered, until the Parmesan melts, 5 minutes. Let stand 10 minutes before serving. Cut the lasagna into 6 pieces and serve.

Each serving: 30 g carb, 290 cal, 7 g fat, 4 g sat fat, 36 mg chol, 4 g fib, 22 g pro, 452 mg sod • Carb Choices: 2; Exchanges: 1½ starch, 1 veg, 1 medium-fat protein, 2 lean protein

SAUSAGE AND MUSHROOM LASAGNA HIGH FIBER: Follow the Weeknight Beef and Spinach Lasagna recipe, at left, substituting ground Italian turkey sausage for the beef and adding 1 cup chopped cremini or white mushrooms with the onion in step 2. Proceed as directed.

Each serving: 31 g carb, 307 cal, 10 g fat, 3 g sat fat, 35 mg chol, 4 g fib, 21 g pro, 674 mg • Carb Choices: 2; Exchanges: 1½ starch, 2 veg, 3 medium-fat protein

BEEF AND ROASTED RED PEPPER LASAGNA HIGH FIBER: Follow the Weeknight Beef and Spinach Lasagna recipe, at left, substituting 1 large red Roasted Bell Pepper (page 21) or 1 cup roasted red peppers from a jar, chopped, for the spinach in step 3. Proceed as directed.

Each serving: 29 g carb, 278 cal, 7 g fat, 4 g sat fat, 36 mg chol, 4 g fib, 21 g pro, 384 mg sod • Carb Choices: 2; Exchanges: 1½ starch, 1 veg, 1 medium-fat protein, 2 lean protein

Beef and Barley Chili `HIGH FIBER`

makes 6 servings

Instead of the ground beef, you can make this chili with ground turkey or chicken, or with diced boneless skinless chicken breast. The barley adds its own meaty (yet high-fiber) texture to the chili.

12 ounces 95% lean ground beef, crumbled

1 medium onion, chopped

1 medium green bell pepper, chopped

1 jalapeño, seeded and minced

3 garlic cloves, minced

2½ tablespoons chili powder

1 tablespoon ground cumin

2 cups water

1¾ cups Beef Stock (page 151) or low-sodium beef broth

1 (15-ounce) can no-salt-added red kidney beans, rinsed and drained

1 (14½-ounce) can no-salt-added diced tomatoes

½ cup pearl barley

3 tablespoons no-salt-added tomato paste

1 tablespoon lime juice

Chopped fresh cilantro

1 Combine the beef, onion, bell pepper, and jalapeño in a large saucepan. Place over medium heat and cook, stirring often, until the beef is browned, 5 minutes. Add the garlic, chili powder, and cumin and cook, stirring constantly, until fragrant, 30 seconds.

2 Add the water, stock, beans, tomatoes, barley, and tomato paste and bring to a boil. Reduce the heat to low, cover, and simmer until the barley is tender, yet firm to the bite, about 30 minutes. Remove from the heat and stir in the lime juice. Ladle the chili evenly into 6 bowls, sprinkle evenly with the cilantro, and serve at once. The chili can be frozen for up to 3 months.

Each serving: 33 g carb, 262 cal, 6 g fat, 2 g sat fat, 37 mg chol, 10 g fib, 19 g pro, 228 mg sod • Carb Choices: 2; Exchanges: 1½ starch, 1 veg, 1½ lean protein, ½ plant-based protein

Beef, Black Bean, and Beer Chili `QUICK` `HIGH FIBER`

makes 4 servings

Dark beer gives this chili a more complex taste, but you can substitute beef stock if you prefer not to use beer. This recipe employs a trick you can use for adding body and a hint of thickness to any soup or stew: Stir in a tablespoon of yellow cornmeal during the last 5 minutes of cooking.

8 ounces 95% lean ground beef, crumbled

1 medium onion, chopped

1 medium green bell pepper, chopped

2 garlic cloves, minced

2 tablespoons chili powder

2 tablespoons ground cumin

½ teaspoon dried oregano

1¾ cups Beef Stock (page 151) or low-sodium beef broth

1 (12-ounce) bottle dark beer

1 (14½-ounce) can no-salt-added diced tomatoes

1 (15-ounce) can no-salt-added black beans, rinsed and drained

1 tablespoon fine-grind yellow cornmeal

1 tablespoon fresh lime juice

1 Combine the beef, onion, and bell pepper in a large saucepan. Place over medium heat and cook, stirring often, until the beef is browned, 5 minutes. Add the garlic, chili powder, cumin, and oregano and cook, stirring constantly, until fragrant, 30 seconds.

2 Add the stock, beer, tomatoes, and beans and bring to a boil. Reduce the heat to low, cover, and simmer 25 to 30 minutes. Gradually stir the cornmeal into the chili and cook until thickened, 5 minutes longer. Remove from the heat and stir in the lime juice. Ladle the chili evenly into 4 bowls and serve at once. The chili can be frozen for up to 3 months.

Each serving: 31 g carb, 271 cal, 4K g fat, 1 g sat fat, 37 mg chol, 8 g fib, 21 g pro, 366 mg sod • Carb Choices: 2; Exchanges: 1 starch, 1 carb, 2 lean protein, 1 plant-based protein

Three-Way Cincinnati Chili HIGH FIBER

makes 6 servings

You can find restaurants all around Cincinnati and Northern Kentucky that specialize in this chili. This is the basic "three-way," with chili, spaghetti, and Cheddar cheese. You can make a "four-way" by adding kidney beans to the chili and a "five-way" by topping each serving of the chili with chopped onions.

1 pound 95% lean ground beef
4 cups water
1 large onion, diced
2 garlic cloves, minced
1 (6-ounce) can no-salt-added tomato paste
2 tablespoons chili powder
½ teaspoon ground cinnamon
½ teaspoon ground allspice
½ teaspoon ground cumin
½ teaspoon kosher salt
Pinch of ground cayenne
12 ounces whole wheat spaghetti
2 ounces shredded reduced-fat extra-sharp
  Cheddar cheese (about ½ cup)

1 Combine the beef and water in a large saucepan and, using your hands, finely crumble the beef. Add the onion, garlic, tomato paste, chili powder, cinnamon, allspice, cumin, salt, and cayenne and bring to a boil over high heat. Reduce the heat to low and simmer, uncovered, stirring occasionally, until the chili is thickened, 2 to 2½ hours.

2 Cook the spaghetti according to the package directions. Divide the spaghetti among 6 shallow bowls. Ladle the chili evenly over the spaghetti and sprinkle with the Cheddar. The chili can be frozen for up to 3 months.

Each serving: 51 g carb, 369 cal, 7 g fat, 3 g sat fat, 52 mg chol, 9 g fib, 28 g pro, 315 mg sod • Carb Choices: 3; Exchanges: 2½ starch, 2 veg, ½ high-fat protein, 2 lean protein

Beef and Vegetable–Stuffed Bell Peppers HIGH FIBER

makes 4 servings

Roasting the peppers before stuffing them gives them wonderful flavor. And, since they are halved, they're easy to stuff. These reheat beautifully in the microwave, so if you've got a bumper crop of peppers, make a double batch and have the leftovers for lunch.

4 medium red or green bell peppers, halved
  lengthwise and seeded
1 teaspoon canola oil
12 ounces 95% lean ground beef
1 small onion, chopped
1 carrot, peeled and chopped
2 garlic cloves, minced
1 large zucchini, chopped
1 (14½-ounce) can no-salt-added diced
  tomatoes, drained
1 (8-ounce) can no-salt-added tomato sauce
½ teaspoon kosher salt
⅛ teaspoon freshly ground pepper
¼ cup plain dry breadcrumbs
2 tablespoons chopped fresh Italian parsley

1 Preheat the broiler. Line a large roasting pan with foil. Place the bell peppers cut side down in a single layer in the pan. Broil, turning the pan as necessary, until the skins of the peppers are blackened and blistered. Let stand until cool enough to handle. Peel away the skins.

2 Preheat the oven to 375°F. Brush a 13 x 9-inch baking dish with the oil.

3 Combine the beef, onion, carrot, and garlic in a large nonstick skillet. Place over medium heat and cook, stirring often, until the beef is browned and the vegetables are softened, 5 minutes. Stir in the zucchini and cook, stirring often, until softened, about 3 minutes. Add the tomatoes, tomato sauce, salt, and ground pepper and cook, stirring often, until the mixture is thickened, about 5 minutes.

4 Remove from the heat and stir in the bread-crumbs and parsley. Fill each pepper half with about ½ cup of the beef mixture. Arrange the stuffed peppers in a single layer in the prepared baking dish. Bake, uncovered, until the peppers are hot, 25 to 30 minutes. Divide the peppers among 4 plates and serve at once.

Each serving: 28 g carb, 257 cal, 6 g fat, 2 g sat fat, 47 mg chol, 7 g fib, 22 g pro, 308 mg sod • Carb Choices: 1½; Exchanges: 5 veg, 2 lean protein

Beef and Bean Enchiladas with Ancho Chile Sauce HIGH FIBER

makes 5 servings

Ancho chile powder is a convenient way to get the sweet mild flavor of the chiles into foods without having to soak the dried chiles them-selves. If you can't find it, these enchiladas are just as good made with regular chili powder.

SAUCE

1 (14½-ounce) can no-salt-added diced tomatoes
2 teaspoons canola oil, divided
1 small onion, diced
2 garlic cloves, minced
2 teaspoons ancho chile powder
½ teaspoon ground cumin
½ teaspoon kosher salt
2 tablespoons chopped fresh cilantro

ENCHILADAS

12 ounces 95% lean ground beef
1 medium onion, chopped
1 red bell pepper, chopped
3 garlic cloves, minced
1 tablespoon ancho chile powder
2 teaspoons ground cumin
1 (14½-ounce) can no-salt-added diced tomatoes
1 cup canned no-salt-added black beans
¼ cup chopped fresh cilantro
10 (6-inch) corn tortillas, warmed
2 ounces shredded reduced-fat Monterey Jack cheese (about ½ cup)

1 To make the sauce, place the tomatoes in a food processor or blender and process until smooth. Set aside.

2 Heat a medium skillet over medium-high heat. Add 1 teaspoon of the oil and tilt the pan to coat the bottom evenly. Add the onion and cook, stirring often, until softened, 5 minutes. Add the garlic, chile powder, cumin, and salt, and cook, stirring constantly until fragrant, 30 seconds.

3 Stir in the pureed tomatoes and bring to a boil. Reduce the heat to low and simmer, uncov-ered, until the sauce is slightly thickened, about 5 minutes. Stir in the cilantro and set aside.

4 Preheat the oven to 375°F. Brush a 13 x 9-inch baking dish with the remaining 1 teaspoon oil.

5 To make the enchiladas, combine the beef, onion, and bell pepper in a large nonstick skillet. Place over medium heat and cook, stirring often, until the beef is browned, 5 minutes. Add the garlic, chile powder, and cumin and cook, stirring constantly, until fragrant, 30 seconds. Add the tomatoes and beans and bring to a boil. Cook, stirring often, until most of the liquid is evapo-rated, about 5 minutes. Stir in the cilantro.

6 Spoon a generous ⅓ cup of the filling down the center of each tortilla. Roll up and place seam side down in the prepared baking dish. Spoon the sauce over the enchiladas and cover the dish with foil. Place the baking dish on a large rimmed baking sheet and bake until heated through, 20 minutes. Sprinkle with the Monterey Jack and bake, uncovered, until the cheese melts, 5 minutes longer. Let stand 5 minutes before serving. Divide the enchiladas among 5 plates and serve at once.

Each serving: 47 g carb, 370 cal, 10 g fat, 3 g sat fat, 49 mg chol, 10 g fib, 25 g pro, 445 mg sod • Carb Choices: 3; Exchanges: 2 starch, 2 veg, ½ high-fat protein, 2 lean protein

Pork Chops

Skillet Pork Chops QUICK

makes 4 servings

Quick-cooking center-cut pork chops are a change of pace from boneless skinless chicken breasts for weeknight dinners. This recipe is quite basic, but it has wonderful flavor, it goes with any side dish, and you can make it in about 15 minutes.

4 (5-ounce) bone-in center-cut pork loin chops, trimmed of all visible fat

½ teaspoon kosher salt

⅛ teaspoon freshly ground pepper

4 teaspoons extra virgin olive oil, divided

2 tablespoons diced onion

1 garlic clove, minced

½ cup Chicken Stock (page 149) or low-sodium chicken broth

1 tablespoon chopped fresh Italian parsley (optional)

1 Sprinkle the chops with the salt and pepper. Heat a large nonstick skillet over medium heat. Add 2 teaspoons of the oil and tilt the pan to coat the bottom evenly. Add the chops and cook, turning once, until well browned and slightly pink in the center, about 3 minutes on each side. Transfer to a plate and cover loosely with foil to keep warm.

2 Add the remaining 2 teaspoons oil to the skillet and tilt to coat the pan. Add the onion and cook, stirring often, until softened, 3 minutes. Add the garlic and cook, stirring constantly, until fragrant, 30 seconds. Add the stock and bring to a boil, stirring to scrape up the browned bits from the bottom of the pan. Cook until reduced by half. Stir in the parsley, if using. Place the chops on 4 plates and drizzle evenly with the stock mixture.

Each serving: 1 g carb, 177 cal, 9 g fat, 2 g sat fat, 59 mg chol, 0 g fib, 21 g pro, 219 mg sod • Carb Choices: 0; Exchanges: 3 lean protein, 1 fat

Pork Chops with Sautéed Apples QUICK

makes 4 servings

In this dish, the apples are just lightly sautéed, so their texture and color stay intact—it's perfect for experimenting with a couple of varieties in a single recipe. I like to serve this with mustard, kale, or broccoli rabe because the sweet apples offset the slight bitterness of the greens.

4 (5-ounce) bone-in center-cut pork loin chops, trimmed of all visible fat

½ teaspoon plus pinch of kosher salt, divided

¼ teaspoon freshly ground pepper, divided

4 teaspoons extra virgin olive oil, divided

2 Gala apples, peeled, cored, and sliced

½ cup thinly sliced red onion

⅓ cup unsweetened apple juice

1 tablespoon lemon juice

2 teaspoons chopped fresh rosemary

1 Sprinkle the chops with ½ teaspoon of the salt and ⅛ teaspoon of the pepper. Heat a large nonstick skillet over medium heat. Add 2 teaspoons of the oil and tilt the pan to coat the bottom evenly. Add the chops and cook, turning once, until well browned and slightly pink in the center, about 3 minutes on each side. Transfer to a plate and cover loosely with foil to keep warm.

2 Add the remaining 2 teaspoons oil to the skillet and tilt to coat the pan. Add the apples and onion and cook, stirring often, until the apples are slightly softened, 3 minutes. Add the apple juice, remaining pinch of salt, and remaining ⅛ teaspoon pepper and cook, stirring often, until the apples are tender and most of the liquid has evaporated. Stir in the lemon juice and rosemary. Divide the pork chops among 4 plates. Spoon the apples evenly over the chops and serve at once.

Each serving: 15 g carb, 228 cal, 9 g fat, 2 g sat fat, 58 mg chol, 2 g fib, 21 g pro, 221 mg sod • Carb Choices: 1; Exchanges: 1 fruit, 3 lean protein, 1 fat

Pork Chops with White Beans and Sage

QUICK | HIGH FIBER

makes 4 servings

Canned beans taste slow-simmered in this hearty dish. The beans are quickly heated in a broth that incorporates all the flavorful browned bits from cooking the pork chops, and a little sage and lemon make happy partners.

4 (5-ounce) bone-in center-cut pork loin chops, trimmed of all visible fat

¾ teaspoon kosher salt, divided

¼ teaspoon freshly ground pepper, divided

4 teaspoons extra virgin olive oil, divided

¼ cup diced onion

1 garlic clove, minced

1 (15-ounce) can no-salt-added cannellini beans, rinsed and drained

½ cup Chicken Stock (page 149) or low-sodium chicken broth

1 tablespoon lemon juice

2 teaspoons chopped fresh sage or ½ teaspoon crumbled dried sage

1 Sprinkle the chops with ½ teaspoon of the salt and ⅛ teaspoon of the pepper. Heat a large non-stick skillet over medium heat. Add 2 teaspoons of the oil and tilt the pan to coat the bottom evenly. Add the chops and cook, until well browned and slightly pink in the center, about 3 minutes on each side. Transfer to a plate and keep warm.

2 Add the remaining 2 teaspoons oil to the skillet and tilt to coat the pan. Add the onion and cook, stirring often, until softened, 3 minutes. Add the garlic and cook, stirring constantly until fragrant, 30 seconds. Add the beans and stock and bring to a boil. Reduce the heat to low and simmer, uncovered, until the beans are heated through and most of the stock has evaporated, about 3 minutes. Stir in the lemon juice, sage, and remaining ¼ teaspoon salt and ⅛ teaspoon pepper. Divide the pork chops and beans evenly among 4 plates and serve at once.

Each serving: 16 g carb, 266 cal, 10 g fat, 2 g sat fat, 59 mg chol, 5 g fib, 26 g pro, 258 mg sod • Carb Choices: 1; Exchanges: 1 starch, 3 lean protein, 1 plant-based protein, 1 fat

Cooking Lean Pork

Cook pork chops over medium, not medium-high heat. They should quietly sizzle when they go into the skillet, but the heat should not be so high that they brown too quickly before they are cooked on the inside.

To test for doneness in pork chops, cut a small slit in the center of a chop. The meat should be slightly pink and the juices should be clear. For pork roasts, roast until an instant-read thermometer inserted into the center reads 145°F. Overcooking lean pork results in dry tough meat.

Brined pork chops (such as the Grilled Orange and Sage-Brined Pork Chops and Apple-Rosemary-Brined Pork Chops recipes, pages 304–305) and pork loin (such as the Maple-Brined Pork Loin Roast recipe, page 311) are more forgiving at the stove or grill. Marinating in a solution of salt and sugar increases the amount of moisture inside the protein, so it's tender and juicy (and more flavorful than meat that isn't brined) even if you are not a watchful cook.

As with any roasted meat or poultry, always let a pork roast stand for about 10 minutes before slicing to allow the juices to be reabsorbed into the center of the meat.

Pork Chops with Apricot-Walnut Sauce QUICK

makes 4 servings

You've probably got all the ingredients in your pantry to make this impressive dish. Apricots and thyme make harmonious partners for pork chops (but you can make this recipe with bone-less skinless chicken breasts, too) and earthy walnuts lend a lovely crunch.

4 (5-ounce) bone-in center-cut pork loin chops, trimmed of all visible fat

½ teaspoon kosher salt

⅛ teaspoon freshly ground pepper

4 teaspoons extra virgin olive oil, divided

2 tablespoons diced onion

1 garlic clove, minced

½ cup Chicken Stock (page 149) or low-sodium chicken broth

⅓ cup chopped dried apricots

¼ cup orange juice

2 tablespoons walnuts, toasted and chopped (page 4)

2 teaspoons chopped fresh thyme or ½ teaspoon dried thyme

1 Sprinkle the chops with the salt and pepper. Heat a large nonstick skillet over medium heat. Add 2 teaspoons of the oil and tilt the pan to coat the bottom evenly. Add the chops and cook, turning once, until well browned and slightly pink in the center, about 3 minutes on each side. Transfer to a plate and cover loosely with foil to keep warm.

2 Add the remaining 2 teaspoons oil to the skillet and tilt to coat the pan. Add the onion and cook, stirring often, until softened, 3 minutes. Add the garlic and cook, stirring constantly, until fragrant, 30 seconds. Add the stock, apricots, and orange juice and bring to a boil, stirring to scrape up the browned bits from the bottom of the pan. Cook until reduced by half. Stir in the walnuts and thyme. Place the chops on 4 plates and spoon the sauce evenly over the chops.

Each serving: 9 g carb, 236 cal, 12 g fat, 3 g sat fat, 59 mg chol, 1 g fib, 22 g pro, 220 mg sod • Carb Choices: ½; Exchanges: ½ fruit, 3 lean protein, 1½ fat

Pork Chops with Mango Chutney Sauce QUICK

makes 4 servings

A little chutney needs to go a long way in this dish, so if your brand has extra large chunks, chop the chutney before adding it to the dish. A spinach salad and a grain dish such as quinoa or couscous make lovely partners for the pork chops.

4 (5-ounce) bone-in center-cut pork loin chops, trimmed of all visible fat

½ teaspoon curry powder

½ teaspoon kosher salt

4 teaspoons canola oil, divided

2 tablespoons diced onion

1 garlic clove, minced

¼ cup Chicken Stock (page 149) or low-sodium chicken broth

⅓ cup mango chutney

2 tablespoons chopped fresh cilantro

1 tablespoon lime juice

1 Sprinkle the chops with the curry powder and salt. Heat a large nonstick skillet over medium heat. Add 2 teaspoons of the oil and tilt the pan to coat the bottom evenly. Add the chops and cook, turning once, until well browned and slightly pink in the center, about 3 minutes on each side. Transfer to a plate and cover loosely with foil to keep warm.

2 Add the remaining 2 teaspoons oil to the skillet and tilt to coat the pan. Add the onion and cook, stirring often, until softened, 3 minutes. Add the garlic and cook, stirring constantly, until

fragrant, 30 seconds. Add the stock and chutney and bring to a boil, stirring to scrape up the browned bits from the bottom of the pan. Cook until the sauce is slightly thickened, about 3 minutes. Remove from the heat and stir in the cilantro and lime juice. Place the chops on 4 plates and drizzle evenly with the sauce.

Each serving: 15 g carb, 230 cal, 9 g fat, 2 g sat fat, 58 mg chol, 0 g fib, 21 g pro, 264 mg sod • Carb Choices: 1; Exchanges: 1 carb, 3 lean protein, 1 fat

Oven-Fried Pork Chops with Cream Gravy QUICK

makes 4 servings

This was one of my dad's favorite meals when I was growing up. My mom served it with her giant "cat head" biscuits so none of the gravy would go to waste. This version is almost as delicious as hers, but far more healthful. The chops are baked with a cornflake crust to give them crunch without frying and the gravy is made with low-fat milk. You can soak it up with Baking Powder Biscuits (page 519). If you're making your own cornflake crumbs, it takes 2½ cups of cornflakes to make 1 cup of crumbs.

½ teaspoon canola oil

¼ cup plus 3 tablespoons unbleached all-purpose flour, divided

1 large egg white

1 tablespoon water

1 cup cornflake crumbs

4 (4-ounce) boneless center-cut pork loin chops, trimmed of all visible fat

¾ teaspoon kosher salt, divided

⅛ teaspoon ground cayenne

2 tablespoons low-fat buttermilk

½ cup Chicken Stock (page 149) or low-sodium chicken broth

½ cup 1% low-fat milk

2 teaspoons unsalted butter

Pinch of freshly ground pepper

1 Preheat the oven to 375°F. Line a large rimmed baking sheet dish with foil. Place a wire rack in the baking sheet and brush the rack with the oil.

2 Place ¼ cup of the flour in a shallow dish. Place the egg white and water in another shallow dish and beat lightly with a fork. Place the cornflake crumbs in a third shallow dish.

3 Place the pork chops on a plate and sprinkle with ½ teaspoon of the salt and the cayenne. Drizzle with the buttermilk and turn to coat. Dip the chops, one at a time, into the flour, then into the egg white mixture, then into the cornflake crumbs, pressing to adhere. Place the chops on the prepared rack. Bake, without turning, until the crust is golden brown and the chops are slightly pink in the center, 20 to 25 minutes. Transfer the chops to plates using a metal spatula.

4 About 5 minutes before the chops are done, make the gravy. Combine the stock, milk, remaining 3 tablespoons flour, and remaining ¼ teaspoon salt in a small saucepan and whisk until smooth. Cook over medium-high heat, stirring often, until the mixture comes to a boil and thickens, about 3 minutes. Stir in the butter and pepper. Place the chops on 4 plates and spoon the gravy evenly over the chops.

Each serving: 25 g carb, 306 cal, 9 g fat, 4 g sat fat, 72 mg chol, 1 g fib, 29 g pro, 437 mg sod • Carb Choices: 1½; Exchanges: 1 starch, ½ carb, 3 lean protein, ½ fat

Five-Spice Pork Chops with Hoisin Onions

makes 4 servings

Meat and caramelized onions are harmonious partners, but this version takes the traditional pairing in an Asian direction. The mouthwatering flavors of this dish come from premade spice mix and bottled sauce, so it's effortless to make.

2 medium onions (about 1 pound), halved lengthwise and thinly sliced
4 teaspoons canola oil, divided
¾ teaspoon five-spice powder, divided
¾ teaspoon kosher salt, divided
Pinch of ground cayenne
1 tablespoon hoisin sauce
1 tablespoon light brown sugar
4 (4-ounce) boneless center-cut pork loin chops, trimmed of all visible fat

1 Preheat the oven to 400°F.

2 Place the onions on a large rimmed baking sheet. Drizzle with 2 teaspoons of the oil and sprinkle with ¼ teaspoon of the five-spice powder, ¼ teaspoon of the salt, and the cayenne. Toss to coat. Arrange the onions in a single layer. Bake, stirring once, until tender and lightly browned, about 30 minutes. Transfer the onions to a small bowl. Add the hoisin sauce and stir to combine.

3 Meanwhile, about 10 minutes before the onions are done, stir together the sugar, remaining ½ teaspoon five-spice powder, and remaining ½ teaspoon salt in a small bowl. Sprinkle the chops with the sugar mixture.

4 Heat a large nonstick skillet over medium heat. Add the remaining 2 teaspoons oil and tilt the pan to coat the bottom evenly. Add the chops and cook, turning once, until well browned and slightly pink in the center, about 3 minutes on each side. Place the chops on 4 plates and top evenly with the onions.

Each serving: 15 g carb, 265 cal, 11 g fat, 3 g sat fat, 65 mg chol, 2 g fib, 25 g pro, 327 mg sod • Carb Choices: 1; Exchanges: ½ carb, 1 veg, 3 lean protein, 1 fat

Grilled Orange and Sage-Brined Pork Chops

makes 4 servings

These are foolproof moist pork chops, even when you're using the leanest cuts of pork. The only drawback is that you have to remember to marinate them for at least 8 hours—but the time is well spent for these juicy chops.

¾ cup water
¼ cup orange juice
2 tablespoons kosher salt
2 tablespoons sugar
2 garlic cloves, crushed
2 tablespoons chopped fresh sage or 2 teaspoons crumbled dried sage
1 tablespoon grated orange zest
4 (5-ounce) bone-in center-cut pork loin chops, trimmed of all visible fat
¼ teaspoon freshly ground pepper
½ teaspoon canola oil

1 Combine the water, orange juice, salt, and sugar in a medium bowl. Whisk until the salt and sugar dissolve. Pour the mixture into a large heavy-duty resealable plastic bag. Add the

garlic, sage, and orange zest. Place the chops in the bag and seal. Refrigerate at least 8 hours and up to 12 hours, turning the bag occasionally.

2 Prepare the grill or heat a large grill pan over medium-high heat.

3 Remove the chops from the marinade and discard the marinade. Pat the chops dry with paper towels and sprinkle with the pepper.

4 Brush the grill rack or grill pan with the oil. Grill the chops, turning occasionally, until well browned and slightly pink in the center, about 6 minutes. Place the chops on 4 plates and serve at once.

Each serving: 2 g carb, 194 cal, 9 g fat, 3 g sat fat, 69 mg chol, 0 g fib, 25 g pro, 471 mg sod • Carb Choices: 0; Exchanges: 3½ lean protein

APPLE-ROSEMARY-BRINED PORK CHOPS: Follow the recipe for Orange-and-Sage Brined Pork Chops, at left, substituting 1 cup of unsweetened apple juice for the water and orange juice. Substitute 2 tablespoons chopped fresh rosemary or 2 teaspoons dried rosemary for the sage. Omit the orange zest. Proceed with the recipe.

Each serving: 3 g carb, 199 cal, 9 g fat, 3 g sat fat, 69 mg chol, 0 g fib, 25 g pro, 471 mg sod • Carb Choices: 0; Exchanges: 3½ lean protein

Grilled Smoky BBQ Pork Chops QUICK

makes 4 servings

This sauce has a fraction of the sodium of purchased barbecue sauces and a nice balance of sweet-and-sour flavors. This is moderately spicy— if you love spice, add another ¼ teaspoon chipotle.

½ cup no-salt-added tomato sauce
2 tablespoons light brown sugar
2 teaspoons apple cider vinegar
¼ teaspoon minced chipotle in adobo sauce
4 (5-ounce) bone-in center-cut pork loin chops, trimmed of all visible fat
½ teaspoon kosher salt
¼ teaspoon freshly ground pepper
½ teaspoon canola oil

1 Combine the tomato sauce, sugar, vinegar, and chipotles in a small saucepan. Set over medium heat and cook, stirring often, until the sauce comes to a boil. Set aside 4 tablespoons of the sauce for serving.

2 Prepare the grill or heat a large grill pan over medium-high heat.

3 Sprinkle the chops with the salt and pepper. Brush the grill rack or grill pan with the oil. Grill the chops, basting with the remaining sauce and turning occasionally, until well browned and slightly pink in the center, about 6 minutes. Place the chops on 4 plates, drizzle evenly with the reserved sauce, and serve at once.

Each serving: 9 g carb, 215 cal, 8 g fat, 3 g sat fat, 69 mg chol, 0 g fib, 25 g pro, 223 mg sod • Carb Choices: ½; Exchanges: ½ carb, 3½ lean protein

Pork Tenderloins and Roasts

Rosemary Roasted Pork Tenderloin QUICK

makes 4 servings

This is a surefire dish for weeknight entertaining. It's simple yet pleasing flavors pair well with Wilted Spinach–Mushroom Salad (page 86) and Sweet Potato and Pear Puree (page 489). The maple syrup glaze is sticky, so be sure to line the pan with foil.

½ teaspoon canola oil

1 (1-pound) pork tenderloin, trimmed of all visible fat

½ teaspoon kosher salt

¼ teaspoon freshly ground pepper

1 tablespoon real maple syrup

1½ tablespoons chopped fresh rosemary or 1 teaspoon crumbled dried rosemary

1 Preheat the oven to 400°F. Line a rimmed baking sheet with foil and brush the foil with the oil.

2 Sprinkle the tenderloin with the salt and pepper. Brush the maple syrup over the tenderloin. Sprinkle with the rosemary, pressing to adhere to the pork.

3 Place on the prepared baking sheet and bake, turning once, until an instant-read thermometer inserted into the center of the tenderloin reads 145°F, 15 to 20 minutes. Cover loosely with foil and let stand about 10 minutes. Cut the tenderloin into thin slices, divide evenly among 4 plates, and serve at once.

Each serving: 4 g carb, 151 cal, 4 g fat, 1 g sat fat, 63 mg chol, 0 g fib, 23 g pro, 185 mg sod • Carb Choices: 0; Exchanges: 3 lean protein

Roasted Pork Tenderloin with Pears and Sage QUICK

makes 4 servings

The addition of fresh pears and sage upgrades an everyday pork tenderloin to a distinctive autumn meal. I like to double this for a crowd and serve it on a buffet. It's as delicious at room temperature as it is hot.

3 teaspoons extra virgin olive oil, divided

1 (1-pound) pork tenderloin, trimmed of all visible fat

4 teaspoons chopped fresh sage or 2 teaspoons crumbled dried sage

½ teaspoon plus a pinch of kosher salt, divided

¼ teaspoon plus ⅛ teaspoon freshly ground pepper, divided

2 ripe pears, cored and sliced

1 Preheat the oven to 400°F. Brush a large rimmed baking sheet with 1 teaspoon of the oil.

2 Sprinkle the tenderloin with 2 teaspoons of the sage, ½ teaspoon of the salt, and ¼ teaspoon of the pepper. Place the pork on the prepared baking sheet.

3 Combine the pears, the remaining 2 teaspoons oil, 2 teaspoons sage, ⅛ teaspoon pepper, and pinch of salt in a large bowl and toss to coat. Arrange the pears in a single layer around the pork.

4 Bake, turning the pork and the pears once, until an instant-read thermometer inserted into the center of the tenderloin reads 140°F, 15 to 20 minutes. Cover loosely with foil and let stand about 10 minutes. Cut the tenderloin into thin slices, divide the pork and pears evenly among 4 plates, and serve at once.

Each serving: 13 g carb, 211 cal, 7 g fat, 2 g sat fat, 63 mg chol, 3 g fib, 23 g pro, 203 mg sod • Carb Choices: 1; Exchanges: 1 fruit, 3 lean protein, ½ fat

Removing Silver Skin

Pork tenderloin has a shiny white connective tissue called silver skin on one side of the surface of the meat. If left on, it can cause the tenderloin to curl once heated and gives the meat an unpleasant texture. To remove it, place the tenderloin on a cutting board and slide the tip of a knife underneath the silver skin at one end of the tenderloin. Holding the meat from the starting end, slowly slide the knife back and forth, with the blade of the knife pointed upward (to prevent cutting away meat) until the silver skin is removed.

Apricot-Mustard-Glazed Pork Tenderloin QUICK

makes 4 servings

Browning meat before roasting gives it a flavorful caramelized crust.

¼ cup apricot preserves
2 tablespoons whole grain Dijon mustard
1 (1-pound) pork tenderloin, trimmed of all visible fat
½ teaspoon kosher salt
¼ teaspoon freshly ground pepper
½ teaspoon canola oil

1 Preheat the oven to 400°F.

2 Combine the preserves and the mustard in a small bowl and stir to mix well. Sprinkle the tenderloin with the salt and pepper.

3 Heat a large ovenproof skillet over medium-high heat. Add the oil and tilt the pan to coat the bottom evenly. Add the tenderloin and cook, turning often, until browned on all sides, about 5 minutes. Brush the tenderloin with the preserves mixture and bake, turning once, until an instant-read thermometer inserted into the center of the tenderloin reads 145°F, 15 to 20 minutes. Cover loosely with foil and let stand about 10 minutes. Cut the tenderloin into thin slices, divide evenly among 4 plates, and serve at once.

Each serving: 14 g carb, 197 cal, 5 g fat, 1 g sat fat, 63 mg chol, 0 g fib, 23 g pro, 338 mg sod • Carb Choices: 1; Exchanges: 1 carb, 3 lean protein

Soy-Maple-Glazed Pork Tenderloin QUICK

makes 4 servings

The pairing of sweet maple syrup and salty soy sauce makes a delicious glaze for pork.

2 tablespoons real maple syrup
1 tablespoon reduced-sodium soy sauce
1 (1-pound) pork tenderloin, trimmed of all visible fat
¼ teaspoon kosher salt
¼ teaspoon freshly ground pepper
½ teaspoon canola oil

1 Preheat the oven to 400°F.

2 Combine the maple syrup and the soy sauce in a small bowl and stir to mix well. Sprinkle the tenderloin with the salt and pepper.

3 Heat a large ovenproof skillet over medium-high heat. Add the oil and tilt the pan to coat the bottom evenly. Add the tenderloin and cook, turning often, until browned on all sides, about 5 minutes. Brush the tenderloin with the maple syrup mixture and bake, turning once, until an instant-read thermometer inserted into the center of the tenderloin reads 145°F, 15 to 20 minutes. Cover loosely with foil and let stand about 10 minutes. Cut the tenderloin into thin slices, divide evenly among 4 plates, and serve at once.

Each serving: 7 g carb, 165 cal, 4 g fat, 1 g sat fat, 63 mg chol, 0 g fib, 23 g pro, 267 mg sod • Carb Choices: ½; Exchanges: ½ carb, 3 lean protein

Lime-Marinated Grilled Pork Tenderloin

makes 4 servings

The citrus marinade is flavorful, yet the pork is versatile enough that you can serve it with almost any kind of side dish.

3 tablespoons lime juice
1 small onion, thinly sliced
2 garlic cloves, minced
⅛ teaspoon ground cayenne
1 (1-pound) pork tenderloin, trimmed of all visible fat
¾ teaspoon kosher salt
½ teaspoon canola oil

1 Combine the lime juice, onion, garlic, and cayenne in a large resealable plastic bag. Add the pork and turn to coat. Seal the bag and refrigerate 4 hours and up to 8 hours.

2 Remove the pork from the bag and discard the marinade. Pat the pork dry with paper towels and sprinkle with the salt.

3 Preheat the grill. Brush the grill rack with the oil. Grill the pork, turning occasionally, until an instant-read thermometer inserted into the center of the tenderloin reads 145°F, 15 to 20 minutes. Cover loosely with foil and let stand about 10 minutes. Cut the tenderloin into thin slices, divide evenly among 4 plates, and serve at once.

Each serving: 0 g carb, 132 cal, 4 g fat, 1 g sat fat, 63 mg chol, 0 g fib, 23 g pro, 255 mg sod • Carb Choices: 0; Exchanges: 3 lean protein

JERK-MARINATED GRILLED PORK TENDERLOIN: Follow the Lime-Marinated Grilled Pork Tenderloin recipe, above, adding 2 teaspoons jerk seasoning and omitting the cayenne in step 1. Proceed with the recipe.

Each serving: 0 g carb, 132 cal, 4 g fat, 1 g sat fat, 63 mg chol, 0 g fib, 23 g pro, 395 mg sod • Carb Choices: 0; Exchanges: 3 lean protein

Pork Medallions with Fennel and Onion QUICK

makes 4 servings

Cutting a pork tenderloin into slices before cooking gives you tender little pork steaks that cook up in minutes. The mild-flavored fennel and sweet onion make a wonderful accompaniment to the pork.

1 medium bulb fennel
1 (1-pound) pork tenderloin, trimmed of all visible fat and cut into 12 slices
¾ teaspoons kosher salt, divided
¼ teaspoon freshly ground pepper, divided
4 teaspoons extra virgin olive oil, divided
½ large sweet onion, thinly sliced
2 tablespoons chopped fennel fronds or fresh Italian parsley

1 Trim the tough outer stalks from the fennel. Cut the fennel bulb in half vertically and cut away and discard the core. Cut each half lengthwise into ¼-inch slices.

2 Sprinkle the pork with ½ teaspoon of the salt and ⅛ teaspoon of the pepper.

3 Heat a large nonstick skillet over medium-high heat. Add 2 teaspoons of the oil and tilt the pan to coat the bottom evenly. Add the pork and cook, turning once, until well browned, about 3 minutes on each side. Transfer to a plate and cover loosely with foil to keep warm.

4 Add the remaining 2 teaspoons oil to the same skillet. Add the onion, fennel, remaining ¼ teaspoon salt, and remaining ⅛ teaspoon pepper and cook, stirring often, until crisp-tender, about 6 minutes. Stir in the fennel fronds. Cut the tenderloin into thin slices, divide the pork and fennel mixture evenly among 4 plates, and serve at once.

Each serving: 9 g carb, 210 cal, 9 g fat, 2 g sat fat, 63 mg chol, 2 g fib, 24 g pro, 290 mg sod • Carb Choices: ½; Exchanges: 2 veg, 3 lean protein, 1 fat

Pork Stir-Fry with Peas and Ginger QUICK

makes 4 servings

¼ cup Chicken Stock (page 149) or low-sodium chicken broth

2 tablespoons reduced-sodium soy sauce

2 teaspoons rice vinegar

2 teaspoons cornstarch

¼ teaspoon Asian sesame oil

4 teaspoons canola oil, divided

1 pound pork tenderloin, trimmed of all visible fat and cut into thin strips

3 tablespoons minced fresh ginger

2 garlic cloves, minced

4 cups snow peas, trimmed

1 large red bell pepper, thinly sliced

¼ cup chopped fresh cilantro

1 Combine the stock, soy sauce, vinegar, cornstarch, and sesame oil in a small bowl and stir until the cornstarch dissolves.

2 Heat a large wok or nonstick skillet over medium-high heat. Add 2 teaspoons of the canola oil and tilt the pan to coat the bottom evenly. Add the pork and cook, stirring constantly, until lightly browned, 2 to 3 minutes. Transfer the pork to a plate and wipe out the wok with paper towels.

3 Add the remaining 2 teaspoons canola oil to the wok over medium-high heat. Add the ginger and garlic and cook, stirring constantly, until fragrant, 30 seconds. Add the snow peas and bell pepper and cook, stirring constantly, until crisp-tender, 3 minutes. Stir in the pork and the stock mixture and cook until the sauce is thickened, 30 seconds. Remove from heat and stir in the cilantro. Divide evenly among 4 plates and serve at once.

Each serving: 13 g carb, 237 cal, 9 g fat, 2 g sat fat, 68 mg chol, 3 g fib, 25 g pro, 366 mg sod • Carb Choices: 1; Exchanges: 2 veg, 3 lean protein, 1 fat

Pork Stir-Fry with Broccoli, Scallions, and Hoisin Sauce

QUICK

makes 4 servings

¼ cup Chicken Stock (page 149) or low-sodium chicken broth

2 tablespoons reduced-sodium soy sauce

1 tablespoon hoisin sauce

2 teaspoons rice vinegar

2 teaspoons cornstarch

4 teaspoons canola oil, divided

1 pound pork tenderloin, trimmed of all visible fat and cut into thin strips

3 garlic cloves, minced

4 cups small broccoli florets

1 large red bell pepper, thinly sliced

2 scallions, cut into 1-inch pieces

¼ cup chopped fresh cilantro

1 Combine the stock, soy sauce, hoisin sauce, vinegar, and cornstarch in a small bowl and stir until the cornstarch dissolves.

2 Heat a large wok or nonstick skillet over medium-high heat. Add 2 teaspoons of the oil and tilt the pan to coat the bottom evenly. Add the pork and cook, stirring constantly, until lightly browned, 2 to 3 minutes. Transfer the pork to a plate and wipe out the wok with paper towels.

3 Add the remaining 2 teaspoons oil to the wok over medium-high heat. Add the garlic and cook, stirring constantly, until fragrant, 30 seconds. Add the broccoli, bell pepper, and scallions and cook, stirring constantly, until crisp-tender, 3 minutes. Stir in the pork and the stock mixture and cook until the sauce is thickened, 30 seconds. Remove from the heat and stir in the cilantro. Divide evenly among 4 plates and serve at once.

Each serving: 12 g carb, 228 cal, 9 g fat, 2 g sat fat, 68 mg chol, 3 g fib, 26 g pro, 451 mg sod • Carb Choices: 1; Exchanges: 2 veg, 3 lean protein, 1 fat

Pork Stir-Fry with Red Curry Sauce QUICK

makes 4 servings

½ cup reduced-fat coconut milk
2 tablespoons lime juice
1 tablespoon reduced-sodium soy sauce
1 teaspoon red curry paste
1 teaspoon cornstarch
4 teaspoons canola oil, divided
1 pound pork tenderloin, trimmed of all visible fat and cut into thin strips
3 tablespoons minced fresh ginger
2 garlic cloves, minced
2 cups small broccoli florets
1 large carrot, peeled and cut into thin matchstick strips
1 large red bell pepper, thinly sliced
¼ cup chopped fresh basil

1 Combine the coconut milk, lime juice, soy sauce, curry paste, and cornstarch in a small bowl and whisk until smooth.

2 Heat a large wok or nonstick skillet over medium-high heat. Add 2 teaspoons of the oil and tilt the pan to coat the bottom evenly. Add the pork and cook, stirring constantly, until lightly browned, 2 to 3 minutes. Transfer the pork to a plate and wipe out the wok with paper towels.

3 Add the remaining 2 teaspoons oil to the wok over medium-high heat. Add the ginger and garlic and cook, stirring constantly, until fragrant, 30 seconds. Add the broccoli, carrot, and bell pepper and cook, stirring constantly, until crisp-tender, 3 minutes. Stir in the pork and the coconut milk mixture and cook until the sauce is thickened, 30 seconds. Remove from the heat and stir in the basil. Divide evenly among 4 plates and serve at once.

Each serving: 10 g carb, 226 cal, 10 g fat, 3 g sat fat, 68 mg chol, 3 g fib, 24 g pro, 258 mg sod • Carb Choices: 1; Exchanges: 2 veg, 3 lean protein, 1 fat

Garlic-Studded Rosemary-Fennel Pork Roast

makes 8 servings

This is a super-simple yet flavorful roast to make for garlic lovers. Inserting the garlic into the roast, then refrigerating it for up to 4 hours infuses the meat with flavor.

1 (2-pound) boneless pork loin roast, trimmed of all visible fat
4 garlic cloves, peeled and thinly sliced
½ teaspoon fennel seeds
2 teaspoons minced fresh rosemary
¼ teaspoon freshly ground pepper
1 teaspoon kosher salt
2 teaspoons extra virgin olive oil

1 Cut about 20 small slits into the pork using the tip of a small knife. Insert a slice of garlic into each slit (reserve any remaining garlic slices for another use). Place the fennel in a mortar and crush with a pestle. Alternatively, place the spices in a small resealable plastic bag. Seal the bag, place on a cutting board, and crush using a meat mallet or the back of a large spoon. Rub the pork with the fennel, rosemary, and pepper. Place the pork in a shallow dish, cover, and refrigerate at least 1 hour or up to 4 hours.

2 Preheat the oven to 300°F.

3 Sprinkle the pork with the salt. Heat a large ovenproof skillet over medium-high heat. Add the oil and tilt the pan to coat the bottom evenly. Add the pork and cook, turning occasionally, until browned on all sides, about 8 minutes. Transfer the skillet to the oven and bake, turning once, until an instant-read thermometer inserted into the center of the roast reads 145°F, 50 to 55 minutes. Cover loosely with foil and let stand about 10 minutes. Cut into thin slices, divide evenly among 8 plates, and serve at once.

Each serving: 1 g carb, 173 cal, 8 g fat, 3 g sat fat, 63 mg chol, 0 g fib, 22 g pro, 193 mg sod • Carb Choices: 0; Exchanges: 3 lean protein

Thyme-Crusted Pork Loin with Roasted Peaches

makes 8 servings

Peaches and pork are an amazing flavor pairing. I enjoy making this dish in September, when it's finally cool enough that I crave hearty meats and the very last of the peaches are at the farmers' market.

4 teaspoons extra virgin olive oil, divided
1 (2-pound) boneless pork loin roast, trimmed of all visible fat
1 teaspoon kosher salt
½ teaspoon freshly ground pepper
4 teaspoons chopped fresh thyme, divided
4 large peaches, pitted and sliced

1 Preheat the oven to 300°F. Brush a large roasting pan with 1 teaspoon of the oil.

2 Sprinkle the pork with the salt and pepper. Heat a large skillet over medium-high heat. Add 1 teaspoon of the remaining oil and tilt the pan to coat the bottom evenly. Add the pork and cook, turning occasionally, until browned on all sides, about 8 minutes.

3 Transfer the pork to the prepared roasting pan and sprinkle with 2 teaspoons of the thyme. Bake 30 minutes. Combine the peaches, the remaining 2 teaspoons oil and 2 teaspoons thyme and toss to coat. Turn the pork and arrange the peaches in a single layer around the pork. Bake, stirring the peaches once, until an instant-read thermometer inserted into the center of the roast reads 145°F, 20 to 25 minutes longer. Cover loosely with foil and let stand about 10 minutes. Cut the pork into thin slices. Divide the pork and peaches evenly among 8 plates and serve at once

Each serving: 5 g carb, 200 cal, 10 g fat, 3 g sat fat, 63 mg chol, 1 g fib, 23 g pro, 193 mg sod • Carb Choices: 0; Exchanges: 3 lean protein, ½ fat

Maple-Brined Pork Loin Roast

makes 8 servings

2 teaspoons whole black peppercorns, crushed
3 cups apple cider
1 cup water
½ cup real maple syrup
¼ cup kosher salt
4 garlic cloves, minced
1 (2-pound) boneless pork loin roast, trimmed of all visible fat
1 teaspoon freshly ground pepper
2 teaspoons extra virgin olive oil

1 Combine the cider, water, maple syrup, and salt in a medium bowl. Whisk until the salt and sugar dissolve. Pour the mixture into a resealable plastic bag. Add the crushed peppercorns, garlic, and pork and seal the bag. Refrigerate at least 8 hours and up to 12 hours, turning the bag occasionally.

2 Preheat the oven to 300°F.

3 Remove the roast from the marinade and discard the marinade. Pat the roast dry with paper towels. Sprinkle the roast with the ground pepper.

4 Heat a large ovenproof skillet over medium-high heat. Add the oil and tilt the pan to coat the bottom evenly. Add the pork and cook, turning occasionally, until browned on all sides, about 8 minutes. Transfer the skillet to the oven and bake, turning once, until an instant-read thermometer inserted into the center of the roast reads 145°F, 50 to 55 minutes. Cover loosely with foil and let stand about 10 minutes. Cut into thin slices, divide evenly among 8 plates, and serve at once.

Each serving: 3 g carb, 182 cal, 8 g fat, 3 g sat fat, 63 mg chol, 0 g fib, 22 g pro, 264 mg sod • Carb Choices: 0; Exchanges: 3 lean protein

Sausage and Swiss Chard–Stuffed Pork Loin Roast

makes 8 servings

Pounding the roast takes some real muscle, but it's worth the effort for this special occasion entrée. Serve it with Sweet Potato and Pear Puree (page 489).

6 ounces Italian turkey sausage

1 small onion, diced

1 pound Swiss chard, tough stems removed and leaves chopped

2 garlic cloves, minced

1½ cups Chicken Stock (page 149) or low-sodium chicken broth, divided

¼ cup golden raisins

¾ teaspoon kosher salt, divided

½ teaspoon freshly ground pepper, divided

1 (2-pound) boneless pork loin roast, trimmed of all visible fat

2 tablespoons plus 1 teaspoon Dijon mustard, divided

¼ cup dry white wine

1½ tablespoons unbleached all-purpose flour

1 Preheat the oven to 450°F.

2 Remove and discard the sausage casings. Crumble the sausage into a large nonstick skillet. Add the onion and set the skillet over medium heat. Cook, stirring often, until the sausage is lightly browned and the onion is softened, 5 minutes. Stir in the chard and garlic, then add ½ cup of the stock. Cook, stirring often, until the chard is tender, 6 to 8 minutes. Remove from the heat and stir in the raisins, ¼ teaspoon of the salt, and ⅛ teaspoon of the pepper.

3 Make a cut lengthwise down the center of the pork, cutting to, but not through the bottom.

Open the butterflied portions, laying the pork flat. Starting from the center of each half, slice lengthwise down the center of each half, cutting to, but not through, the bottom. Unfold the pork so it lies flat. Place plastic wrap over the pork and flatten to a ¾-inch thickness using a meat mallet or rolling pin.

4 Spread 1 tablespoon of the mustard over the cut side of the pork. Spoon the stuffing mixture evenly over the pork and roll up, jellyroll fashion, starting with the long side. Secure the roll with kitchen string at 3-inch intervals. Sprinkle the pork with the remaining ½ teaspoon of salt and ¼ teaspoon of the remaining pepper. Brush with 1 tablespoon of the remaining mustard. Place the pork seam side down on a rack in a roasting pan.

5 Bake for 20 minutes. Reduce the oven temperature to 350°F. Bake until an instant-read thermometer inserted into the center of the pork reads 145°F, 20 to 25 minutes longer. Transfer the roast to a serving platter, cover loosely with foil, and let stand until the temperature reaches 160°F, about 10 minutes.

6 Meanwhile, remove the rack from the roasting pan and place the roasting pan across two stovetop burners over medium heat. Whisk together the remaining 1 cup chicken stock, the wine, and flour in a medium bowl and whisk into the pan drippings. Cook, whisking constantly, for 5 minutes, until the mixture comes to a boil and thickens. Stir in the remaining 1 teaspoon mustard and remaining ⅛ teaspoon pepper. Pour the sauce through a fine wire mesh strainer. Cut the pork into slices and divide evenly among 8 plates. Drizzle the pork evenly with the sauce and serve at once.

Each serving: 9 g carb, 244 cal, 10 g fat, 4 g sat fat, 82 mg chol, 1 g fib, 28 g pro, 538 mg sod • Carb Choices: ½; Exchanges: ½ carb, ½ medium-fat protein, 3 lean protein

Pork Braises and One-Pot Meals

Cider-Braised Pork Roast with Onions

makes 8 servings

Serve the pork with roasted potatoes or whole wheat egg noodles to soak up the wonderfully flavored cooking liquid. Braising is usually done with a high-fat cut of pork, but the technique works well here with a leaner and healthier cut. To keep the meat from falling apart when you carve it, cut into thick slices as you would with a beef pot roast.

½ teaspoon whole coriander seeds
1 (2-pound) boneless pork roast, trimmed of all
    visible fat
1 teaspoon kosher salt
¼ teaspoon freshly ground pepper
4 teaspoons extra virgin olive oil, divided
1 large onion, halved lengthwise and thinly sliced
1 tablespoon unbleached all-purpose flour
2 garlic cloves, minced
1½ cups hard apple cider
¾ cup Chicken Stock (page 149) or
    low-sodium chicken broth

1 Preheat the oven to 325°F.

2 Place the coriander in a mortar and crush with a pestle. Alternatively, place the coriander in a small resealable plastic bag. Seal the bag, place on a cutting board, and crush using a meat mallet or the back of a large spoon. Rub the pork with the crushed coriander, salt, and pepper.

3 Heat a large Dutch oven over medium-high heat. Add 2 teaspoons of the oil and tilt the pot to coat the bottom evenly. Add the pork and cook, turning occasionally, until browned on all sides, about 8 minutes. Transfer the pork to a plate.

4 Add the remaining 2 teaspoons oil to the Dutch oven and tilt the pot to coat the bottom evenly. Add the onion and cook, stirring often, until lightly browned, 8 to 10 minutes. Stir in the flour and garlic and cook, stirring constantly, about 1 minute. Slowly add the cider and stock, stirring to remove the browned bits from the bottom of the Dutch oven. Return the pork to the Dutch oven and bring to a boil.

5 Cover and bake until the pork is very tender, 2½ to 3 hours. Cut the roast into thick slices and divide evenly among 8 shallow bowls. Spoon the onions and cooking juices evenly over the pork and serve at once.

Each serving: 5 g carb, 215 cal, 10 g fat, 3 g sat fat, 63 mg chol, 0 g fib, 23 g pro, 211 mg sod • Carb Choices: 0; Exchanges: 3 lean protein, ½ fat

SLOW-COOKER VERSION: To make this dish in a slow cooker, prepare the pork as directed through step 3, placing the browned meat in a 6-quart slow cooker. Proceed with step 4, adding the onion mixture to the slow cooker. Cook on high for 8 hours.

Pork Braised with Peppers and Paprika

makes 8 servings

Hungarian paprika gives this dish pungent flavor, but you can make it with regular paprika.

½ teaspoon cumin seeds
3 teaspoons hot Hungarian paprika, divided
1 teaspoon kosher salt
¼ teaspoon freshly ground pepper
2 pounds boneless pork loin, trimmed of all visible fat and cut into 1-inch cubes
4 teaspoons extra virgin olive oil, divided
2 large red bell peppers, cut into 1-inch pieces
1 large onion, chopped
2 garlic cloves, minced
1 cup Chicken Stock (page 149) or low-sodium chicken broth
2 (14½-ounce) cans no-salt-added whole tomatoes, chopped
2 tablespoons no-salt-added tomato paste

1 Preheat the oven to 325°F.

2 Place the cumin seeds in a small dry skillet over medium heat and toast, shaking the pan often, until fragrant, about 3 minutes. Transfer to a small dish and allow to cool. Place the cumin in a mortar and crush with a pestle. Alternatively, place the seeds in a small resealable plastic bag. Seal the bag, place on a cutting board, and crush using a meat mallet or the back of a large spoon. Combine the crushed cumin, 1 teaspoon of the paprika, the salt, and ground pepper in a small dish. Place the pork in a large bowl, sprinkle with the spice mixture, and toss to coat.

3 Heat a Dutch oven over medium-high heat. Add 2 teaspoons of the oil and tilt the pot to coat the bottom evenly. Add half of the pork and cook, turning occasionally, until browned on all sides, about 6 minutes. Transfer the pork to a plate. Repeat with the remaining pork.

4 Add the remaining 2 teaspoons oil to the Dutch oven and tilt the pot to coat the bottom evenly. Add the bell peppers and onion and cook, stirring often, until lightly browned, 8 to 10 minutes. Stir in the garlic and remaining 2 teaspoons paprika and cook, stirring constantly, until fragrant, 30 seconds. Add the stock, stirring to remove the browned bits from the bottom of the skillet. Stir in the pork, tomatoes, and tomato paste and bring to a boil.

5 Cover and bake 2 hours. Uncover and bake until the pork is very tender and the stew is slightly thickened, 30 to 40 minutes longer. Spoon the stew evenly into 8 shallow bowls and serve at once.

Each serving: 9 g carb, 223 cal, 10 g fat, 3 g sat fat, 64 mg chol, 2 g fib, 24 g pro, 230 mg sod • Carb Choices: ½; Exchanges: 2 veg, 3 lean protein

SLOW-COOKER VERSION: To make this dish in a slow cooker, prepare the pork as directed through step 3, placing the browned meat in a 6-quart slow cooker. Proceed with step 4, adding the vegetable mixture to the slow cooker. Cook on high for 8 hours.

Hoisin-Braised Pork Stew

makes 8 servings

When you're bored with making comfort-food stews, try this intriguing Asian-inspired version. It's sweet, spicy, and out of the ordinary. All you need to make it a meal is a side of brown rice.

2 pounds boneless pork loin, trimmed of all visible fat and cut into ½-inch cubes
1 tablespoon five-spice powder
4 teaspoons canola oil, divided

8 ounces white mushrooms, sliced

1 large onion, halved lengthwise and thinly sliced

2 tablespoons minced fresh ginger

2 garlic cloves, minced

2 cups Chicken Stock (page 149) or low-sodium chicken broth

¼ cup hoisin sauce

1 teaspoon chili-garlic paste

1 large red bell pepper, thinly sliced

2 tablespoons cornstarch

1 tablespoon reduced-sodium soy sauce

1 tablespoon water

½ teaspoon Asian sesame oil

Thinly sliced scallions

1 Sprinkle the pork with the five-spice powder. Heat a Dutch oven over medium-high heat. Add 2 teaspoons of the oil and the pork and cook until browned, 8 minutes. Transfer to a plate.

2 Add the remaining 2 teaspoons oil, the mushrooms, and onion and cook, stirring, until softened, 8 minutes. Add the ginger and garlic and cook, stirring constantly, 30 seconds.

3 Return the pork to the pot. Add the stock, hoisin sauce, and chili-garlic paste. Reduce the heat to low, cover, and simmer 30 minutes. Add the bell pepper and cook until tender, 15 minutes.

4 Stir together the cornstarch, soy sauce, water, and sesame oil in a small bowl. Add the cornstarch mixture to the pot and cook, stirring constantly, until the stew is thickened, 2 minutes. Spoon the stew evenly into 8 shallow bowls, sprinkle with the scallions, and serve at once.

Each serving: 10 g carb, 235 cal, 9 g fat, 2 g sat fat, 73 mg chol, 1 g fib, 27 g pro, 243 mg sod • Carb Choices: ½; Exchanges: ½ carb, 3 lean protein, ½ fat

Pork, Butternut Squash, and Kale Stew HIGH FIBER

makes 4 servings

When colorful leaves are skittering down the sidewalk in autumn, this stew will make a warming dinner. Filled with squash, tomatoes, and greens, it's as dazzling as the leaves outside.

1 pound boneless pork tenderloin, trimmed of all visible fat and cut into ½-inch cubes

½ teaspoon kosher salt, divided

¼ teaspoon freshly ground pepper, divided

4 teaspoons extra virgin olive oil, divided

1 medium onion, chopped

1 small butternut squash, peeled, seeded, and cut into ¾-inch cubes (about 4 cups)

1 (14½-ounce) can no-salt-added diced tomatoes

3 cups Chicken Stock (page 149) or low-sodium chicken broth

¼ cup no-salt-added tomato paste

8 ounces kale, tough stems removed and leaves chopped (about 4 cups)

1 Sprinkle the pork with ¼ teaspoon of the salt and ⅛ teaspoon of the pepper. Heat a Dutch oven over medium-high heat. Add 2 teaspoons of the oil and the pork and cook, until browned, 8 minutes. Transfer to a plate.

2 Add the remaining 2 teaspoons oil to the Dutch oven and tilt the pan to coat the bottom evenly. Add the onion and cook, stirring often, until softened, 5 minutes. Return the pork to the pot. Add the squash, tomatoes, stock, tomato paste, remaining ¼ teaspoon salt, and remaining ⅛ teaspoon pepper and bring to a boil. Reduce the heat to low, cover, and simmer 20 minutes. Stir in the kale and cook until the vegetables are tender and the stew is slightly thickened, 20 minutes longer. Spoon the stew evenly into 4 shallow bowls and serve at once.

Each serving: 31 g carb, 322 cal, 9 g fat, 2 g sat fat, 74 mg chol, 9 g fib, 32 g pro, 405 mg sod • Carb Choices: 2; Exchanges: 1 starch, 3 veg, 3 lean protein, 1 fat

Red Chile Pork and Hominy Stew HIGH FIBER

makes 4 servings

This fiery dish will wake up your taste buds on a winter day. It uses ancho chile powder, but regular chili powder will do. And this stew makes great use of hominy, a much-underutilized pantry staple.

1 pound boneless pork tenderloin, trimmed of all visible fat and cut into ½-inch cubes
½ teaspoon kosher salt, divided
¼ teaspoon freshly ground pepper, divided
4 teaspoons extra virgin olive oil, divided
1 medium onion, chopped
1 green bell pepper, chopped
2 garlic cloves, minced
1 tablespoon ancho chile powder or regular chili powder
2 teaspoons ground cumin
3 cups Chicken Stock (page 149) or low-sodium chicken broth
1 (15-ounce) can hominy, rinsed and drained
1 (14½-ounce) can no-salt-added diced tomatoes
¼ cup no-salt-added tomato paste
¼ cup chopped fresh cilantro

1 Sprinkle the pork with ¼ teaspoon of the salt and ⅛ teaspoon of the ground pepper. Heat a Dutch oven over medium-high heat. Add 2 teaspoons of the oil and tilt the pan to coat the bottom evenly. Add the pork and cook, turning occasionally, until well browned, 8 minutes. Transfer to a plate.

2 Add the remaining 2 teaspoons oil to the Dutch oven and tilt the pan to coat the bottom evenly. Add the onion and bell pepper and cook, stirring often, until softened, 5 minutes. Add the garlic, chile powder, and cumin and cook, stirring constantly, until fragrant, 30 seconds.

3 Return the pork to the pot. Add the stock, hominy, tomatoes, tomato paste, remaining ¼ teaspoon salt, and remaining ⅛ teaspoon ground pepper and bring to a boil over high heat. Reduce the heat to low, cover, and simmer 20 minutes. Remove from the heat and stir in the cilantro. Spoon the stew evenly into 4 shallow bowls and serve at once

Each serving: 24 g carb, 316 cal, 10 g fat, 3 g sat fat, 77 mg chol, 5 g fib, 31 g pro, 415 mg sod • Carb Choices: 1½; Exchanges: 1 carb, 2 veg, 3 lean protein, 1 fat

Pork and Butternut Squash Tagine HIGH FIBER

makes 4 servings

Colorful with bell pepper, tomatoes, and butternut squash, this dish is flavored with traditional Moroccan spices. Couscous is the perfect side dish for this stew to soak up all the delicious juices.

1 pound boneless pork tenderloin, trimmed of all visible fat and cut into ½-inch cubes
½ teaspoon kosher salt, divided
¼ teaspoon freshly ground pepper, divided
4 teaspoons extra virgin olive oil, divided
1 medium onion, chopped
1 green bell pepper, chopped
1 jalapeño, seeded and minced
2 garlic cloves, minced
½ teaspoon ground ginger
½ teaspoon ground cumin
½ teaspoon ground allspice
½ teaspoon ground cinnamon
1 small butternut squash, peeled, seeded, and cut into ¾-inch cubes (about 4 cups)
1 (14½-ounce) can no-salt-added diced tomatoes
2 cups Chicken Stock (page 149) or low-sodium chicken broth
¼ cup no-salt-added tomato paste
2 tablespoons chopped fresh cilantro
1 tablespoon lemon juice

1 Preheat the oven to 325°F.

2 Sprinkle the pork with ¼ teaspoon of the salt and ⅛ teaspoon of the ground pepper. Heat a Dutch oven over medium-high heat. Add 2 teaspoons of the oil and tilt the pan to coat the bottom evenly. Add the pork and cook, turning occasionally, until well browned, 8 minutes. Transfer to a plate.

3 Add the remaining 2 teaspoons oil to the Dutch oven and tilt the pan to coat the bottom evenly. Add the onion, bell pepper, and jalapeño and cook, stirring often, until softened, 5 minutes. Add the garlic, ginger, cumin, allspice, and cinnamon and cook, stirring constantly, until fragrant, 30 seconds.

4 Return the pork to the pot. Add the squash, tomatoes, stock, tomato paste, remaining ¼ teaspoon salt, and remaining ⅛ teaspoon ground pepper and bring to a boil. Cover and bake until the pork and vegetables are very tender, 1 hour. Stir in the cilantro and lemon juice. Spoon the tagine evenly into 4 shallow bowls and serve at once.

Each serving: 31 g carb, 311 cal, 9 g fat, 2 g sat fat, 74 mg chol, 9 g fib, 30 g pro, 360 mg sod • Carb Choices: 2; Exchanges: 1 starch, 3 veg, 3 lean protein, 1 fat

Pork and Apple Stew with Sage

makes 4 servings

This unusual dish tastes much better than it sounds—or looks. The apples break apart as the stew cooks, making a thick sauce with a touch of sweetness. It's definitely not a dish for company, but it will warm and comfort your family on a winter night. Serve this homey dish with slices of rye bread.

1 pound boneless pork tenderloin, trimmed of all visible fat and cut into ½-inch cubes
½ teaspoon kosher salt, divided
¼ teaspoon freshly ground pepper, divided
4 teaspoons extra virgin olive oil, divided
1 medium onion, halved and sliced
2 tablespoons unbleached all-purpose flour
3 cups Chicken Stock (page 149) or low-sodium chicken broth
8 ounces small red-skinned potatoes, well scrubbed and quartered
2 large Granny Smith apples, peeled, cored, and cut into 8 wedges
½ teaspoon Dijon mustard
2 teaspoons chopped fresh sage or ½ teaspoon crumbled dried sage

1 Sprinkle the pork with ¼ teaspoon of the salt and ⅛ teaspoon of the pepper. Heat a Dutch oven over medium-high heat. Add 2 teaspoons of the oil and tilt the pot to coat the bottom evenly. Add the pork and cook, turning occasionally, until well browned, 8 minutes. Transfer to a plate.

2 Add the remaining 2 teaspoons oil to the pan and tilt to coat. Add the onion and cook, stirring often, until softened, 5 minutes. Sprinkle the onion with the flour and cook, stirring constantly, 1 minute. Stir in the stock and bring to a boil, stirring constantly. Add the potatoes and pork and return to a boil. Reduce the heat to low, cover, and simmer 10 minutes. Add the apples, mustard, sage, remaining ¼ teaspoon salt, and remaining ⅛ teaspoon pepper and simmer until the apples are tender and begin to fall apart, 6 to 8 minutes longer. Spoon the stew evenly into 4 shallow bowls and serve at once.

Each serving: 23 g carb, 281 cal, 9 g fat, 2 g sat fat, 72 mg chol, 2 g fib, 27 g pro, 317 mg sod • Carb Choices: 1½; Exchanges: 1 starch, ½ fruit, 3 lean protein, ½ fat

Lamb Chops

Pan-Seared Lamb Chops with Mint Pesto QUICK

makes 4 servings

When you want an impressive meal with next to no effort, simple lamb chops paired with a fresh mint pesto (banish the jelly!) are what to serve.

8 (4-ounce) lamb rib chops, trimmed of all
    visible fat
¼ teaspoon kosher salt
¼ teaspoon freshly ground pepper
1 recipe Mint Pesto (page 597)

Heat a large heavy-bottomed skillet over medium-high heat. Sprinkle the lamb chops with the salt and pepper. Cook the lamb 2 minutes on each side for medium-rare, or to the desired degree of doneness. Divide the chops among 4 plates, spoon 2 tablespoons of the pesto onto each plate, and serve at once.

Each serving: 3 g carb, 265 cal, 16 g fat, 5 g sat fat, 95 mg chol, 1 g fib, 26 g pro, 194 mg sod • Carb Choices: 0; Exchanges: 3 lean protein, 2 fat

Grilled Marinated Lamb Chops with Orange-Mint Relish

makes 4 servings

If you don't want to heat up the grill, you can cook the lamb chops in a skillet. Follow the cooking directions for the Pan-Seared Lamb Chops with Mint Pesto (above).

8 (4-ounce) lamb rib chops, trimmed of all
    visible fat
½ cup orange juice
1 garlic clove, crushed through a press
2 tablespoons chopped fresh mint, divided
2 large navel oranges
1 jalapeño, seeded and minced
1 tablespoon minced red onion
1 teaspoon extra virgin olive oil
¼ teaspoon kosher salt
¼ teaspoon freshly ground pepper
½ teaspoon canola oil

1 Combine the lamb, orange juice, garlic, and 1 tablespoon of the mint in a large resealable plastic bag. Seal the bag and refrigerate 4 hours and up to 8 hours, turning the bag occasionally.

2 Cut a thin slice from the top and bottom of the oranges, exposing the flesh. Stand each orange upright, and using a sharp knife, thickly cut off the peel, following the contour of the fruit and removing all the white pith and membrane. Holding the oranges over a bowl, carefully cut along both sides of each section to free it from the membrane. Discard any seeds and let the sections fall into the bowl. Break the sections into small bits using two forks. Stir in the jalapeño, onion, remaining 1 tablespoon mint, and the olive oil.

3 Remove the lamb from the marinade and discard the marinade. Pat the lamb dry with paper towels and sprinkle with the salt and pepper.

4 Prepare the grill or heat a large grill pan over medium-high heat. Brush the grill rack or grill pan with the canola oil. Place the chops on the grill rack or in the grill pan and grill, turning once, 2 minutes on each side for medium-rare, or to the desired degree of doneness. Divide the chops and relish evenly among 4 plates and serve at once.

Each serving: 15 g carb, 239 cal, 9 g fat, 3 g sat fat, 93 mg chol, 3 g fib, 25 g pro, 116 mg sod • Carb Choices: 1; Exchanges: 1 fruit, 3 lean protein

Lamb Chops with Blackberry-Thyme Sauce QUICK

makes 4 servings

This silky wine-infused blackberry sauce adds a touch of elegance to lamb chops. You can make the sauce ahead and reheat it, adding the whole blackberries just before serving.

2 teaspoons extra virgin olive oil

⅓ cup minced shallot

1 garlic clove, minced

½ cup dry red wine

½ cup Beef Stock (page 151) or low-sodium beef broth

2 tablespoons real maple syrup

1 (12-ounce) package unsweetened frozen blackberries, thawed

1 tablespoon cold water

1 teaspoon cornstarch

2 teaspoons chopped fresh thyme, divided

Pinch plus ½ teaspoon kosher salt, divided

Pinch plus ¼ teaspoon freshly ground pepper, divided

8 (4-ounce) lamb rib chops, trimmed of all visible fat

1 Heat a medium skillet over medium heat. Add the oil and tilt the pan to coat the bottom evenly. Add the shallot and cook, stirring often, until softened, about 3 minutes. Add the garlic and cook, stirring constantly, until fragrant, 30 seconds. Add the wine, stock, and maple syrup.

2 Reserve ½ cup of the blackberries and set aside. Add the remaining blackberries to the skillet. Bring to a boil and cook, crushing the berries with the back of a spoon, until the blackberry mixture is slightly thickened, 6 to 8 minutes.

3 Place a fine wire mesh strainer over a small saucepan and pour in the blackberry mixture. Press the mixture through the strainer, discarding the solids. Stir together the water and cornstarch in a small bowl until the cornstarch dissolves. Stir the cornstarch mixture into the sauce.

4 Set the saucepan over medium heat and cook, whisking constantly, until the sauce comes to a boil and thickens, 3 minutes. Stir in the reserved ½ cup blackberries, ½ teaspoon of the thyme, the pinch of salt, and the pinch of pepper and cook until the blackberries are heated through, 30 seconds.

5 Meanwhile, heat a large heavy-bottomed skillet over medium-high heat. Sprinkle the lamb chops with the remaining 1½ teaspoons thyme, ½ teaspoon salt, and ¼ teaspoon pepper. Cook the lamb 2 minutes on each side for medium rare, or to the desired degree of doneness. Divide the chops among 4 plates, drizzle evenly with the sauce, and serve at once.

Each serving: 19 g carb, 286 cal, 10 g fat, 3 g sat fat, 94 mg chol, 0 g fib, 26 g pro, 262 mg sod • Carb Choices: 1; Exchanges: ½ carb, ½ fruit, 3 lean protein, ½ fat

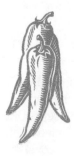

Lamb Roasts

Rosemary-Garlic Roasted Rack of Lamb

makes 8 servings

Rack of lamb makes a beautiful presentation on the plate. Ask the butcher to "french" the lamb, which means that the meat is removed from the bones, giving the finished roast a more elegant look.

3 (1¼-pound) racks of lamb, trimmed
4 garlic cloves, thinly sliced
½ teaspoon freshly ground pepper
3 tablespoons chopped fresh rosemary
1 teaspoon kosher salt

1 Using a knife with a thin pointed blade, pierce 2 small slits between each rib on the underside of each lamb rack. Insert a slice of garlic into each slit (reserve any remaining garlic for another use). Sprinkle the lamb with the pepper, then with the rosemary, pressing to adhere. Place the lamb in a large shallow dish, cover, and refrigerate 8 hours.

2 Preheat the oven to 450°F. Place a rack in a large roasting pan.

3 Sprinkle the lamb evenly with salt and place, meaty side up, on the rack. Bake until an instant-read thermometer inserted into the center registers 145°F, 20 to 25 minutes. Transfer the lamb to a cutting board and cover loosely with foil. Let stand about 10 minutes. Cut the lamb racks into 8 chops. Divide the chops evenly among 8 plates and serve at once.

Each serving: 1 g carb, 156 cal, 6 g fat, 3 g sat fat, 87 mg chol, 0 g fib, 23 g pro, 183 mg sod • Carb Choices: 0; Exchanges: 3 lean protein

Black Olive–Crusted Rack of Lamb

makes 8 servings

A blend of olives, lemon zest, and thyme makes a flavorful crust for rack of lamb.

3 (1¼-pound) racks of lamb, trimmed of all visible fat
½ teaspoon kosher salt
⅛ teaspoon freshly ground pepper
2 teaspoons plus 2 tablespoons extra virgin olive oil, divided
1 cup plain dry breadcrumbs
⅓ cup Kalamata olives, pitted and minced
2 garlic cloves, finely chopped
1 tablespoon grated lemon zest
¼ teaspoon dried thyme
1 tablespoon lemon juice

1 Preheat the oven to 400°F. Place a rack in a large roasting pan.

2 Sprinkle the lamb with the salt and pepper. Heat a large skillet over medium-high heat. Add 2 teaspoons of the oil and the lamb and cook until browned on all sides, 8 minutes. Place the lamb, meaty side up, on the rack.

3 Combine the breadcrumbs, olives, garlic, lemon zest, and thyme in a small bowl. Stir in the remaining 2 tablespoons oil and the lemon juice. Pat the breadcrumb mixture on top of the lamb.

4 Bake until an instant-read thermometer inserted into the center registers 145°F for medium-rare, 15 to 20 minutes. Transfer the lamb to a cutting board and cover loosely with foil. Let stand about 10 minutes. Cut the lamb racks into 8 chops. Divide the chops evenly among 8 plates and serve at once.

Each serving: 11 g carb, 270 cal, 13 g fat, 4 g sat fat, 87 mg chol, 1 g fib, 25 g pro, 313 mg sod • Carb Choices: ½; Exchanges: ½ starch, 3 lean protein, 1½ fat

Roasted Leg of Lamb with Potatoes and Olives

makes 16 servings

This trouble-free one-pan meal makes entertaining easy.

1 tablespoon plus 2 teaspoons extra virgin olive oil, divided
1 tablespoon chopped fresh rosemary
1 tablespoon chopped fresh sage
1 tablespoon chopped fresh thyme
1½ teaspoons kosher salt, divided
¼ teaspoon plus ⅛ teaspoon freshly ground pepper, divided
1 (4-pound) boneless leg of lamb, trimmed of all visible fat
4 garlic cloves, thinly sliced
3¾ pounds baby or fingerling potatoes, well scrubbed and halved
¾ cup Kalamata olives, pitted

1 Preheat the oven to 400°F.

2 Combine 1 tablespoon of the oil, the rosemary, sage, thyme, 1 teaspoon of the salt, and ¼ teaspoon of the pepper in a small bowl. Cut 16 small slits into the lamb; insert a slice of the garlic and a pinch of oil mixture into each slit. Coat the lamb with the remaining oil mixture. Place the lamb in a roasting pan. Bake 1 hour.

3 Combine the potatoes, olives, remaining 2 teaspoons oil, remaining ½ teaspoon salt, and remaining ⅛ teaspoon pepper in a large bowl and toss to coat. Arrange the potatoes around the lamb and bake, stirring the potatoes occasionally, until a thermometer inserted into the center of the lamb registers 145°F, 20 to 25 minutes. Transfer the lamb to a cutting board and cover loosely with foil. Let stand about 10 minutes. Meanwhile, continue baking the potatoes until golden brown, about 10 minutes longer.

Carve the lamb into thin slices and serve with the potatoes and olives.

Each serving: 18 g carb, 308 cal, 16 g fat, 7 g sat fat, 82 mg chol, 2 g fib, 22 g pro, 242 mg sod • Carb Choices: 1; Exchanges: 1 starch, 3 medium-fat protein, ½ fat

Boneless Leg of Lamb with Mint Tapenade

makes 16 servings

1 small onion, cut into wedges
4 garlic cloves
1 tablespoon grated lemon zest
¼ cup fresh lemon juice
1 tablespoon extra virgin olive oil
1 teaspoon kosher salt
½ teaspoon freshly ground pepper
¼ teaspoon ground cayenne
1 (4-pound) boned leg of lamb, trimmed of all visible fat
Double recipe Mint Tapenade (page 598)

1 Combine the onion, garlic, lemon zest, lemon juice, oil, salt, pepper, and cayenne in a food processor and pulse until the mixture forms a paste.

2 Spread the onion mixture onto the lamb. Roll the lamb and tie at 3-inch intervals with string. Place in a dish, cover, and refrigerate 8 hours.

3 Preheat the oven to 450°F.

4 Place the roast on a rack in a roasting pan. Bake 20 minutes. Decrease the oven temperature to 300°F and bake until an instant-read thermometer inserted into the center of the lamb registers 145°F, 25 to 30 minutes. Transfer to a cutting board and cover with foil. Let stand 10 minutes. Remove the string and cut the lamb into thin slices. Serve with the tapenade.

Each serving: 2 g carb, 241 cal, 16 g fat, 6 g sat fat, 83 mg chol, 0 g fib, 21 g pro, 208 mg sod • Carb Choices: 0; Exchanges: 3 medium-fat protein, ½ fat

Lamb Braises and One-Pot Meals

Lamb Tagine HIGH FIBER

makes 4 servings

Lamb pairs quite flavorfully with the spices of this Moroccan-inspired stew. Sweet potato and dried apricots lend some sweetness that is tempered by the acidic tomatoes. Couscous is the traditional accompaniment for a tagine, but it's good with quinoa or rice, as well.

1 pound boneless leg of lamb, trimmed of all
   visible fat and cut into ½-inch cubes
¾ teaspoon kosher salt, divided
2 teaspoons extra virgin olive oil
1 medium onion, chopped
1 red bell pepper, chopped
2 garlic cloves, minced
2 teaspoons chopped fresh ginger
1 teaspoon ground cumin
1 teaspoon ground coriander
¼ teaspoon ground cinnamon
1½ cups Chicken Stock (page 149) or
   low-sodium chicken broth
1 (14½-ounce) can no-salt-added diced tomatoes
¼ cup no-salt-added tomato paste
1 medium sweet potato, peeled and chopped
8 dried apricot halves, chopped
¼ cup chopped fresh cilantro
1 tablespoon lemon juice

1 Preheat the oven to 325°F.

2 Sprinkle the lamb with ¼ teaspoon of the salt. Heat a Dutch oven over medium-high heat. Add the oil and tilt the pan to coat the bottom evenly. Add the lamb and cook, turning occasionally, until well browned, 8 minutes. Transfer to a plate.

3 Add the onion and bell pepper to the Dutch oven and cook, stirring often, until softened,

5 minutes. Add the garlic, ginger, cumin, coriander, and cinnamon and cook, stirring constantly, until fragrant, 30 seconds.

4 Return the lamb to the pot. Add the stock, tomatoes, tomato paste, and remaining ½ teaspoon salt and bring to a boil. Cover and bake 1 hour.

5 Remove the pot from the oven and stir in the potato and apricots. Cover and bake until the vegetables are tender, about 45 minutes longer. Stir in the cilantro and lemon juice. Spoon the tagine evenly into 4 shallow bowls and serve at once.

Each serving: 30 g carb, 312 cal, 9 g fat, 3 g sat fat, 74 mg chol, 5 g fib, 28 g pro, 427 mg sod • Carb Choices: 2; Exchanges: ½ starch, ½ fruit, 2 veg, 3 lean protein, ½ fat

Lamb Shanks Braised in Roasted Poblano Sauce

makes 6 servings

I can't wait for the weather to get cool so I can make this dish every year in late September. The poblanos are a must for the sauce—seek them out at a Latino market if your supermarket doesn't stock them. They are what give the sauce its complex smoky flavor. Serve this dish with polenta or whole wheat orzo to soak up every drop.

6 (¾-pound) lamb shanks, trimmed of all visible fat
½ teaspoon kosher salt
½ teaspoon freshly ground pepper
2 teaspoons extra virgin olive oil
2 carrots, peeled and diced
2 stalks celery, diced
1 medium onion, diced
2 garlic cloves, minced
¾ cup dry red wine
1¾ cups Beef Stock (page 151) or low-sodium
   beef broth
1 (14½-ounce) can no-salt-added diced tomatoes
4 poblano chiles, roasted (page 21) and
   chopped

1 Preheat the oven to 325°F.

2 Sprinkle the lamb with the salt and pepper. Heat a Dutch oven over medium-high heat. Add the oil and tilt the pot to coat the bottom evenly. Add the lamb and cook, turning often, until well browned on all sides, about 10 minutes. Transfer to a plate.

3 Add the carrots, celery, and onion to the Dutch oven and cook, stirring often, until the vegetables soften and begin to brown, 8 minutes. Add the garlic and cook, stirring constantly, until fragrant, 30 seconds. Add the wine and bring to a boil. Cook until most of the liquid evaporates, 2 minutes. Stir in the stock, tomatoes, and chiles. Return the lamb to the Dutch oven. Cover and bring to a boil. Bake until the lamb is very tender, about 2 hours.

4 Transfer the lamb to a platter and cover with foil to keep warm. Using a potato masher, mash the vegetables in the Dutch oven 4 to 5 times, until slightly mashed, but still chunky. Place the Dutch oven over medium-high heat and bring to a boil. Cook, stirring often, until the sauce is slightly thickened, about 5 minutes. Divide the lamb shanks evenly among 6 plates. Spoon the sauce evenly over the lamb and serve at once.

Each serving: 10 g carb, 287 cal, 8 g fat, 3 g sat fat, 110 mg chol, 2 g fib, 36 g pro, 401 mg sod • Carb Choices: ½; Exchanges: 2 veg, 5 lean protein

Braised Lamb with Parsnips and Dried Plums HIGH FIBER

makes 8 servings

This deeply flavored stew is a delicious blend of contrasting tastes: sweet dried plums, slightly bitter parsnips, and a spiced tomato sauce. Serve it over whole wheat couscous or whole wheat orzo with steamed green beans.

1 teaspoon coriander seeds
2 pounds boneless lamb shoulder, trimmed of all visible fat and cut into 1-inch cubes

¾ **teaspoon ground cinnamon**
½ **teaspoon kosher salt**
¼ **teaspoon freshly ground pepper**
4 **teaspoons extra virgin olive oil, divided**
1 **large onion, chopped**
2 **garlic cloves, minced**
1 **tablespoon minced fresh ginger**
4 **cups Beef Stock (page 151) or low-sodium beef broth**
¼ **cup no-salt-added tomato paste**
3 **medium carrots, peeled and chopped**
3 **medium parsnips, peeled and chopped**
1 **cup pitted dried plums, halved**

1 Preheat the oven to 325°F.

2 Place the coriander seeds in a small dry skillet over medium heat and toast, shaking the pan often, until fragrant, about 3 minutes. Transfer to a small dish and allow to cool. Place the seeds in a mortar and crush with a pestle. Alternatively, place the seeds in a small resealable plastic bag. Seal the bag, place on a cutting board, and crush using a meat mallet or the back of a large spoon. Combine the lamb, crushed coriander, cinnamon, salt, and pepper in a large bowl and toss to coat.

3 Heat a Dutch oven over medium-high heat. Add 2 teaspoons of the oil and tilt the pot to coat the bottom evenly. Add half of the lamb and cook, turning occasionally, until browned on all sides, about 6 minutes. Transfer the lamb to a plate. Repeat with the remaining lamb.

4 Add the remaining 2 teaspoons oil to the Dutch oven and tilt the pot to coat the bottom evenly. Add the onion and cook, stirring often, until lightly browned, 8 to 10 minutes. Stir in the garlic and ginger and cook, stirring constantly, until fragrant, 30 seconds. Return the lamb to the Dutch oven. Add the stock and tomato paste. Cover and bake 2 hours. Stir in the carrots, parsnips, and dried plums, cover, and bake

continues on next page

until the lamb is very tender, 1 hour longer. Spoon the stew evenly into 8 shallow bowls and serve at once. The stew can be frozen for up to 3 months.

Each serving: 30 g carb, 319 cal, 10 g fat, 3 g sat fat, 79 mg chol, 5 g fib, 28 g pro, 382 mg sod • Carb Choices: 2; Exchanges: ½ starch, 1 fruit, 1 veg, 3 lean protein, ½ fat

Irish Lamb Stew

makes 8 servings

Giving the lamb a head start on cooking, then adding the vegetables during the last half hour of cooking, ensures that the lamb is fork-tender and the vegetables are not overcooked. For a variation, use beef chuck shoulder roast or bottom round roast instead of the lamb. A slice of Caraway Beer Bread (page 525) is the perfect accompaniment.

2 pounds boneless lamb shoulder, trimmed of all visible fat and cut into 1-inch cubes

¼ cup unbleached all-purpose flour

1½ teaspoons kosher salt, divided

¼ teaspoon plus ⅛ teaspoon freshly ground pepper, divided

6 teaspoons extra virgin olive oil, divided

1 large onion, halved and sliced

4 cups Chicken Stock (page 149) or low-sodium chicken broth

1½ pounds red-skinned potatoes, well scrubbed and cut into 1-inch pieces

2 carrots, peeled and cut into 1-inch pieces

2 stalks celery, cut into 1-inch pieces

¼ cup chopped fresh Italian parsley

1 Place the lamb in a large bowl. Sprinkle with the flour, 1 teaspoon of the salt, and ¼ teaspoon of the pepper and toss to coat.

2 Heat a Dutch oven over medium-high heat. Add 2 teaspoons of the oil and tilt the pot to coat the bottom evenly. Add half of the lamb and cook, turning occasionally, until well browned, about 6 minutes. Transfer the lamb to a plate. Repeat with 2 teaspoons of the remaining oil and the remaining lamb.

3 Add the remaining 2 teaspoons oil to the Dutch oven and tilt the pot to coat evenly. Add the onion and cook, stirring often, until the onion is lightly browned, 5 minutes. Add the stock to the Dutch oven and bring to a boil, stirring to scrape up the browned bits on the bottom of the pan. Return the lamb to the Dutch oven, reduce the heat to low, cover, and simmer until very tender, about 1½ hours. Add the potatoes, carrots, celery, water, if necessary, to cover the vegetables, the remaining ½ teaspoon salt, and remaining ⅛ teaspoon pepper. Cover and simmer until the vegetables are tender, 30 minutes longer. Stir in the parsley. Spoon the stew evenly into 8 shallow bowls and serve at once.

Each serving: 21 g carb, 303 cal, 11 g fat, 4 g sat fat, 82 mg chol, 3 g fib, 29 g pro, 366 mg sod • Carb Choices: 1½; Exchanges: 1 starch, 1 veg, 3 lean protein, ½ fat

Fish and Shellfish Main Dishes

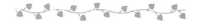

Thin White-Fleshed Fish Fillets

Sautéed Fish Fillets with Lemon Sauce

Fish Fillets with Quick Tomato-Dill Sauce

Cornmeal-Crusted Fish Fillets

Panko-Crusted Fish Fillets

Fish and Chips

Broiled Fish Fillets with Lemon Butter

Broiled Fish Fillets with Chipotle and Lime

Fish Fillets, Potatoes, and Green Beans en Papillote

Fish Tacos

Thick White-Fleshed Fish Fillets

Grilled Fish Fillets with Citrus-Herb Gremolata

Grilled Fish Fillets with Dill Pesto Sauce

Basil-Crusted Fish Fillets with Roasted Cherry Tomatoes

Pan-Seared Fish Fillets with Tomato-Orange Salsa

Fish Fillets with Avocado-Lemon Sauce

Fish Fillets with Tomato, Bell Pepper, and Basil

Potato-Dill-Crusted Fish Fillets

Caper-Crusted Baked Fish

Fish Fillets with Warm Tomato-Lemon Sauce

Mint-Crusted Fish Fillets with Sweet Pea Sauce

Steamed Fish Fillets in Herb Broth

Fish Fillets with Zucchini and Mint en Papillote

Fish Fillets with Roasted Mushrooms

Moroccan-Spiced Fish and Vegetable Kebabs

Salmon and Tuna

Baked Salmon with Cucumber-Grape Tomato Salsa

Baked Salmon with Balsamic Butter Sauce

Pan-Seared Salmon with Chunky Lemon Sauce

Cumin-Crusted Salmon with Cilantro-Chipotle Sauce

Brown Sugar–Spice-Baked Salmon

Salmon Baked in Tomato-Fennel Sauce

Broiled Salmon with Strawberry-Avocado Salsa

Miso-Orange Glazed Salmon

Grilled Salmon with Yogurt Sauce

Salmon with Warm Lentils

Salmon Cakes with Cucumber-Yogurt Sauce

Fresh Salmon Burgers

Asian Salmon Cakes with Cucumber-Sesame Salsa

Tuna with Roasted Lemons

Tuna with Chili-Garlic Roasted Onions

Grilled Tuna with Wasabi Vinaigrette

Grilled Tuna with Anchovy-Caper Sauce

Tuna with Cilantro-Citrus Sauce

Grilled Tuna with Spicy Tomato-Olive Relish

Grilled Chile-Rubbed Tuna with Avocado-Tomato Salsa

Shellfish

BBQ Baked Shrimp

Garlicky Broiled Shrimp

Shrimp in Creole Tomato Sauce

Shrimp in Coconut-Ginger Sauce

Shrimp and Vegetable Stir-Fry

Lemon-Basil Shrimp with Linguini

Mediterranean Shrimp and Pasta

Grilled Shrimp with Spicy Ginger BBQ Sauce

Grilled Shrimp with Thai Slaw

Grilled Shrimp Kebabs with Summer Herb Sauce

Shrimp and Leek Risotto

Shrimp, Asparagus, and Goat Cheese Risotto

Greek Shrimp Risotto

Coconut Shrimp

Pan-Seared Scallops with Pineapple-Mango Salsa

Scallops with Brown Butter–Caper Sauce

Scallops in Cucumber-Dill Broth

Baked Scallops au Gratin

Grilled Scallops with Ponzu Sauce

Steamed Clams or Mussels with Wine and Garlic

Clams or Mussels in Fresh Tomato Broth

Clams or Mussels with Chorizo

Clams or Mussels with Peppers and Feta

Chesapeake Crab Cakes

Easy Seafood Paella

Whole Fish

Whole Roasted Fish with Chermoula Sauce

Salt-Crusted Baked Whole Fish

Whole Grilled Trout with Tarragon and Lemon

Seafood is the ultimate fast food. And, as long as it's prepared using a modest amount of oil, seafood is one of the healthiest foods you can eat. It's lean and packed with nutrients, so you'll do yourself a favor if you enjoy seafood a couple of times a week.

Fatty fish, such as salmon, arctic char, sardines, and lake trout are excellent sources of omega-3 fatty acids, which are thought to lower blood pressure, decrease triglycerides, enhance immune function, and decrease the risk of heart disease. If you are concerned about mercury and other environmental contaminants in seafood, avoid larger predatory fish such as swordfish and albacore tuna (also considered not sustainable; see Choosing Sustainable Seafood, page 330), which contain more mercury than smaller fish. Bigger fish have more mercury because they eat more of the smaller fish (which also contain mercury) and the mercury accumulates over time. The best choice for canned tuna is "light" tuna. "Light" tuna is a smaller species of tuna called skipjack that is caught by the ecologically friendly pole-and-line method of fishing.

When buying fresh seafood, either from a local seafood market or a chain grocery store, shop at a busy store. Lots of business means quick turnover of the stock. When possible, ask the person at the market what the freshest fish is that day and let the answer guide your purchase.

Fish fillets should look solid, with no separation of the flesh. The fillets should look moist all over, with no dry spots. The color should be even throughout with no brown or yellow edges. The best test of fresh seafood is the smell; fish and shellfish should have a clean fragrance with no trace of an unpleasant aroma.

Buy fresh fish no more than a day ahead of when you will cook and serve it. When you bring it home, if you aren't preparing it immediately, remove it from the packaging and place it on a plate. Cover the fish with a piece of parchment paper or a paper towel. Keep the fish in the back of the refrigerator (the coldest part) until ready to cook.

If you buy frozen fish fillets, remove them from the packaging to thaw. Place the fillets on a plate lined with several thicknesses of paper towels, cover, and refrigerate until thawed. Most small fillets will thaw in 8 hours or less in the refrigerator. If you take them out of the freezer in the morning, they'll be ready to cook when you get home from work.

To store live clams or mussels at home, place them in a shallow container and cover them with a damp towel. Do not store them in a plastic bag or a covered container, since they are alive and need to breathe. Use them within 2 days of purchase.

Fish is so flavorful on its own that you don't have to do much to it to make a great meal. Most recipes in this chapter take less than 30 minutes to prepare. You'll find recipes here that are as simple as sprinkling the fish with salt and pepper and serving it with a fresh salsa (Pan-Seared Salmon with Chunky Lemon Sauce, page 342) and recipes for simply grilling it and stirring together an accompanying sauce (try Grilled Scallops with Ponzu Sauce, page 361). There are only two rules to preparing perfect seafood: Buy it fresh and don't overcook it. With the simple and flavorful dishes in this chapter, it will be a pleasure to prepare and serve seafood a couple of times a week.

Thin White-Fleshed Fish Fillets

Sautéed Fish Fillets with Lemon Sauce QUICK

makes 4 servings

Simple, lemony, and fresh, this is an easy dish to make for a weeknight dinner. Spinach with Whole Grain Mustard (page 469) makes a flavorful accompaniment.

¼ cup unbleached all-purpose flour
4 (5-ounce) thin white-fleshed fish fillets
¼ teaspoon plus pinch of kosher salt, divided
⅛ teaspoon plus pinch of freshly ground pepper, divided
2 teaspoons extra virgin olive oil
¾ cup Chicken Stock (page 149) or low-sodium chicken broth
¼ cup lemon juice
1 tablespoon unsalted butter
1 tablespoon chopped fresh Italian parsley

1 Place the flour on a plate. Sprinkle the fish fillets with ¼ teaspoon of the salt and ⅛ teaspoon of the pepper, then dip each one in the flour.

2 Heat a large nonstick skillet over medium heat. Add the oil and tilt the pan to coat the bottom evenly. Add the fish and cook, turning once, until the fish flakes when tested with a fork, about 3 minutes on each side. Transfer to a plate and cover loosely with foil to keep warm.

3 Add the stock and lemon juice to the skillet and bring to a boil, stirring to scrape up the browned bits from the skillet. Cook until the sauce is reduced to about ⅓ cup, about 5 minutes. Remove from the heat and stir in the remaining pinch of salt, pinch of pepper, the butter, and the parsley. Divide the fish among 4 plates, drizzle evenly with the sauce, and serve at once.

Each serving: 6 g carb, 191 cal, 7 g fat, 3 g sat fat, 75 mg chol, 0 g fib, 25 g pro, 218 mg sod • Carb Choices: ½; Exchanges: ½ carb, 3 lean protein, 1 fat

FISH FILLETS WITH WHITE WINE AND HERB SAUCE QUICK: Follow the Sautéed Fish Fillets with Lemon Sauce recipe, at left, through step 2. In step 3, omit the lemon juice, reduce the stock to ½ cup, add ½ cup dry white wine, and proceed with the recipe. You may use Italian parsley or substitute dill, chives, or tarragon.

Each serving: 5 g carb, 210 cal, 7 g fat, 3 g sat fat, 75 mg chol, 0 g fib, 25 g pro, 209 mg sod • Carb Choices: ½; Exchanges: ½ carb, 3 lean protein, 1 fat

Fish Market Options

The recipes here call for either thick or thin white-fleshed fish fillets. Depending on where you live and the availability in your local market, you may not be able to find a specific type of fish. The list below will give you many options when you go shopping, and though the fish in each grouping are not exactly the same in texture and flavor, they can be substituted for each other with great success.

Thin white-fleshed fish fillets are good for sautéing, baking, and broiling. Look for catfish, tilapia, flounder, sole, hake (whiting), striped bass, or rainbow trout.

Thick white-fleshed fish fillets and fish steaks are good for grilling, baking, broiling, and pan-searing. Look for Pacific cod, scrod, pollock, halibut, or turbot.

Fish Fillets with Quick Tomato-Dill Sauce QUICK

makes 4 servings

When friends tell me they don't have time to cook a healthy dinner, I give them this recipe. It's fresh, flavorful, and very low in carbs, calories, and fat. Served with whole wheat couscous and any steamed vegetable, it's a balanced nutritious meal.

¼ cup unbleached all-purpose flour
4 (5-ounce) thin white-fleshed fish fillets
¼ teaspoon plus pinch of kosher salt, divided
⅛ teaspoon plus pinch of freshly ground pepper, divided
4 teaspoons extra virgin olive oil, divided
¼ cup diced onion
1 large tomato, chopped
1 tablespoon chopped fresh dill
1 teaspoon grated lemon zest

1 Place the flour on a plate. Sprinkle the fish fillets with ¼ teaspoon of the salt and ⅛ teaspoon of the pepper, then dip each one in the flour.

2 Heat a large nonstick skillet over medium heat. Add 2 teaspoons of the oil and tilt the pan to coat the bottom evenly. Add the fish and cook, turning once, until the fish flakes when tested with a fork, about 3 minutes on each side. Transfer to a plate and cover loosely with foil to keep warm.

3 Add the remaining 2 teaspoons oil and tilt the pan to coat the bottom evenly. Add the onion, and cook, stirring often, just until softened, about 3 minutes. Add the tomato and cook, stirring often, until heated through, about 2 minutes. Remove from the heat and stir in the dill, lemon zest, and the remaining pinch of salt and pinch of pepper. Divide the fish among 4 plates, spoon the sauce evenly over the fish, and serve at once.

Each serving: 7 g carb, 191 cal, 6 g fat, 1 g sat fat, 67 mg chol, 1 g fib, 25 g pro, 193 mg sod • Carb Choices: ½; Exchanges: ½ carb, 3 lean protein, 1 fat

Cornmeal-Crusted Fish Fillets QUICK

makes 4 servings

Use catfish fillets in this dish for a low-fat version of a Southern-fried favorite. Serve it with Yogurt Tartar Sauce (page 594) and Creamy Coleslaw (page 90) for a home-style, yet healthy meal.

¼ cup yellow cornmeal
4 (5-ounce) thin white-fleshed fish fillets
¼ teaspoon kosher salt
⅛ teaspoon freshly ground pepper
2 teaspoons extra virgin olive oil
Lemon wedges

1 Place the cornmeal on a plate. Sprinkle the fish fillets with the salt and pepper, then dip each one in the cornmeal.

2 Heat a large nonstick skillet over medium heat. Add the oil and tilt the pan to coat the bottom evenly. Add the fish and cook, turning once, until the fish flakes when tested with a fork, about 3 minutes on each side. Divide the fish among 4 plates and serve at once with the lemon wedges.

Each serving: 7 g carb, 166 cal, 4 g fat, 1 g sat fat, 67 mg chol, 1 g fib, 24 g pro, 173 mg sod • Carb Choices: ½; Exchanges: 3 lean protein, ½ fat

SPICED CORNMEAL–CRUSTED FISH FILLETS QUICK : Follow the Cornmeal-Crusted Fish Fillets recipe, above, but in step 1, reduce the cornmeal to 3 tablespoons and omit the pepper. Stir the salt, 1 tablespoon chili powder, 1 teaspoon ground cumin, and ⅛ teaspoon ground cayenne into the cornmeal. Dip the fish fillets into the cornmeal mixture and proceed with the recipe.

Each serving: 7 g carb, 169 cal, 4 g fat, 1 g sat fat, 67 mg chol, 1 g fib, 25 g pro, 218 mg sod • Carb Choices: ½; Exchanges: 3 lean protein, ½ fat

Choosing Sustainable Seafood

Because of overfishing, habitat damage, and poor fisheries management, many kinds of wild fish such as Chilean sea bass, orange roughy, and grouper are in decline and should be avoided so that their species can recover. Other fish, such as monkfish, mahi mahi, and swordfish are caught in ways that damage the environment and result in a large by-catch, the accidental catch and death of sea life.

Eating farm-raised fish may seem like the obvious answer, but it depends on where the farm is located, the species being farmed, and the farming practices used. When carnivorous fish, such as salmon, are farmed, they are often fed wild fish in the form of the fish themselves or meal made from the fish. It can take more than three pounds of wild fish to produce one pound of farmed salmon. This practice is not sustainable and needlessly depletes wild fish stocks.

When buying salmon, the best choice is to look for wild-caught Alaska salmon, or U.S. farmed salmon. U.S. salmon farmers use more ecologically friendly practices than foreign farmers. A good alternative to salmon is Arctic char. It is farmed in a sustainable manner, mostly in the United States, Canada, and Norway and it has a similar pink flesh and rich flavor are similar to salmon's.

Non-fish-eating fish, such as tilapia and catfish, are raised on food that does not contain fish meal and are a more sustainable choice. However, tilapia and catfish farmed in the U.S. are preferable to those famed in other countries. Most fish in the United States are farmed in closed inland systems that prevent the fish from escaping into the wild and the farms have better pollution control standards than Asian or Central American farms. As with farmed tilapia and catfish, look for farmed shrimp that are raised in the United States because of more strict environmental standards than other countries.

Farm-raised mussels, oysters, and clams are a good choice whatever their country of origin, since they collect their own food by filtering the water and they are farmed in an environmentally responsible way.

How do you know where the fish in your supermarket came from? In many stores, it is difficult if not impossible to know. If you have a local seafood market, do your shopping there, since the proprietor will be more likely to know where the fish came from.

More and more retailers are teaming up with the Marine Stewardship Council (MSC), an international organization that works with seafood farmers and fishermen, retailers, and consumers to promote sustainable fishing practices. To buy MSC-certified sustainable seafood, look for the MSC logo on the label of fresh, frozen, and canned seafood. For more information and pocket guides to sustainable seafood for each region of the country, visit the Monterey Bay Aquarium website at seafoodwatch.org.

Panko-Crusted Fish Fillets QUICK

makes 4 servings

This is one of the most crowd-pleasing ways that I know to make fish fillets. Pretoasting the panko crumbs before coating the fillets is what makes the fish extra-crispy.

1 cup panko crumbs

2 teaspoons plus ½ teaspoon extra virgin olive oil, divided

2 tablespoons unbleached all-purpose flour

1 large egg white

1 tablespoon water

2 teaspoons grated lemon zest

½ teaspoon kosher salt

⅛ teaspoon freshly ground pepper

Lemon wedges

1 Preheat the oven to 350°F. Combine the panko crumbs and 2 teaspoons of the oil in a small bowl. Using your fingers, blend the oil evenly into the crumbs. Place the crumbs in a baking pan and bake, stirring once, until toasted, 10 to 12 minutes. Transfer to a dish to cool.

2 Increase the oven temperature to 425°F. Brush a medium rimmed baking sheet with the remaining ½ teaspoon of the oil.

3 Place the flour in a shallow dish. Place the egg white and water in another shallow dish and beat lightly with a fork. Sprinkle the fish evenly with the lemon zest, salt, and pepper. Dip the fillets, one at a time, into the flour, then into the egg white mixture, then into the toasted crumbs, pressing to adhere the crumbs.

4 Arrange the fillets in a single layer in the prepared pan. Bake until the fish flakes easily with a fork, 6 to 8 minutes (do not turn). Divide the fish among 4 plates and serve with the lemon wedges.

Each serving: 15 g carb, 213 cal, 4 g fat, 1 g sat fat, 67 mg chol, 0 g fib, 27 g pro, 291 mg sod • Carb Choices: 1; Exchanges: 1 starch, 3 lean protein, ½ fat

Fish and Chips

makes 4 servings

Fish and chips are not off-limits just because you're watching your carbs and fats. These crispy fish fillets are baked with cornflake crumbs for extra crunch and the "chips" are tossed with olive oil and turned during baking, so they get browned on both sides. If you get the potatoes in the oven by the time you prepare and bake the fish, they'll both be done at the same time.

POTATOES

2 medium baking potatoes (about 1 pound), well scrubbed

2 teaspoons extra virgin olive oil

¼ teaspoon kosher salt

Pinch of freshly ground pepper

FISH

1 teaspoon canola oil

⅓ cup unbleached all-purpose flour

1 large egg white

1 tablespoon water

¾ cup cornflake crumbs

4 (5-ounce) thin white-fleshed fish fillets

½ teaspoon paprika

¼ teaspoon kosher salt

⅛ teaspoon freshly ground pepper

Lemon wedges

1 Preheat the oven to 425°F.

2 To make the potatoes, cut each potato into 8 wedges and place on a medium rimmed baking sheet. Drizzle with the oil, sprinkle with the salt and pepper, and toss to coat. Arrange the potatoes in a single layer.

3 Bake 25 minutes. Turn the wedges and bake until the potatoes are tender and well browned, 8 to 10 minutes longer.

4 Meanwhile, to make the fish, brush a medium rimmed baking sheet with the oil.

continues on next page

5 Place the flour in a shallow dish. Place the egg white and water in another shallow dish and beat lightly with a fork. Place the cornflake crumbs in a third shallow dish. Sprinkle the fish with the paprika, salt, and pepper. Dip the fillets, one at a time, into the flour, then into the egg white mixture, then into the cornflake crumbs, pressing to adhere. Place the fillets on the prepared baking sheet. Bake, without turning, until the crust is golden 12 to 15 minutes. Divide the fish and potatoes among 4 plates and serve at once with the lemon wedges.

Each serving: 24 g carb, 259 cal, 5 g fat, 1 g sat fat, 67 mg chol, 2 g fib, 27 g pro, 450 mg sod • Carb Choices: 1½; Exchanges: 1½ starch, 3 lean protein, ½ fat

Broiled Fish Fillets with Lemon Butter QUICK

makes 4 servings

Make the brightly flavored butter while the fish cooks. Serve the fish with steamed green beans and whole wheat couscous for a satisfying meal in less than 30 minutes.

½ teaspoon canola oil
4 (5-ounce) thin white-fleshed fish fillets
¼ teaspoon plus pinch of kosher salt, divided
⅛ teaspoon freshly ground pepper
2 tablespoons unsalted butter, softened
1 teaspoon grated lemon zest
½ teaspoon lemon juice
Lemon wedges

1 Preheat the broiler. Brush a medium rimmed baking sheet with the oil.

2 Sprinkle the fish with ¼ teaspoon of the salt and the pepper and arrange in a single layer on the prepared baking sheet. Broil, without turning, until the fish flakes easily with a fork, about 8 minutes.

3 Meanwhile, stir together the butter, lemon zest, lemon juice, and remaining pinch of salt in a small bowl. Transfer the fish to 4 plates using a wide spatula, top with the butter mixture, and serve at once with the lemon wedges.

Each serving: 0 g carb, 170 cal, 8 g fat, 4 g sat fat, 82 mg chol, 0 g fib, 24 g pro, 191 mg sod • Carb Choices: 0; Exchanges: 3 lean protein, 1 fat

Broiled Fish Fillets with Chipotle and Lime QUICK

makes 4 servings

Bright and spicy seasonings make this a flavorful dish that is excellent when you use tilapia or catfish. Because the spices in this dish are so pronounced, I wouldn't use a more delicately flavored fish like sole or flounder.

½ teaspoon canola oil
4 (5-ounce) thin white-fleshed fish fillets
1 teaspoon grated lime zest
½ teaspoon chipotle chile powder
¼ teaspoon kosher salt
Lime wedges

1 Preheat the broiler. Brush a medium rimmed baking sheet with the oil.

2 Sprinkle the fish with the lime zest, chile powder, and salt and arrange in a single layer on the prepared baking sheet. Broil, without turning, until the fish flakes easily with a fork, about 8 minutes. Transfer the fish to 4 plates using a wide spatula and serve at once with the lime wedges.

Each serving: 0 g carb, 120 cal, 2 g fat, 0 g sat fat, 67 mg chol, 0 g fib, 24 g pro, 173 mg sod • Carb Choices: 0; Exchanges: 3 lean protein

Fish Fillets, Potatoes, and Green Beans en Papillote

QUICK | HIGH FIBER

makes 4 servings

This is my friend Judy Feagin's go-to recipe for making a healthful—and impressive—dinner with very little effort. If you don't have dried

Italian seasoning, substitute ½ teaspoon each of dried basil and dried oregano—or use fresh herbs if you have them on hand. You really can't go wrong with this simple fresh meal.

8 ounces small red-skinned potatoes, well scrubbed and thinly sliced
8 ounces green beans, trimmed
1 teaspoon Italian seasoning, divided
¾ teaspoon kosher salt, divided
½ teaspoon freshly ground pepper, divided
4 (5-ounce) thin white-fleshed fish fillets
1 cup cherry tomatoes, halved
4 scallions, thinly sliced
2 tablespoons extra virgin olive oil
Lemon wedges

1 Preheat the oven to 450°F.

2 Bring a large saucepan of water to a boil over high heat. Add the potatoes and cook 4 minutes. Add the green beans and cook until the potatoes and beans are just tender, 3 to 4 minutes longer. Drain in a colander and set aside.

3 Tear off four 24 x 12-inch pieces of parchment paper. Fold each piece in half crosswise and cut each one to make a rounded heart shape. Open a parchment "heart" and arrange one-quarter of the potato mixture in the middle of one side. Sprinkle the vegetables with ½ teaspoon of the Italian seasoning, ½ teaspoon of the salt, and ¼ teaspoon of the pepper. Top each portion of vegetables with a fish fillet.

4 Arrange the tomatoes and scallions evenly over the fish. Sprinkle evenly with the remaining ½ teaspoon Italian seasoning, remaining ¼ teaspoon salt, and ¼ teaspoon pepper. Drizzle with the oil.

5 Beginning at the bottom end of each "heart," fold the edges of the parchment in overlapping 1-inch segments, crimping as you go, to form a tight seal. (You can also use aluminum foil to make the packets.)

6 Place the packages on a large rimmed baking sheet and bake until the fish flakes easily with a fork, 10 to 12 minutes. Place the packets on 4 plates and serve at once with the lemon wedges. Use caution when opening the packets, avoiding the steam that escapes.

Each serving: 15 g carb, 247 cal, 9 g fat, 1 g sat fat, 67 mg chol, 4 g fib, 26 g pro, 269 mg sod • Carb Choices: 1; Exchanges: ½ starch, 1 veg, 3 lean protein, 1 fat

Fish Tacos QUICK | HIGH FIBER

makes 4 servings

You can make the tacos with 1 pound of medium peeled and deveined shrimp instead of the fish. The broiling time will be about the same, but turn the shrimp halfway through the cooking time. If you use sturdy fish, such as catfish or tilapia, you can grill the fish instead of broiling. The fish is not seasoned with salt because commercially produced tortillas contain so much sodium. If you make your own tortillas, or have a locally produced brand that is not high in sodium, season the fish with ¼ teaspoon kosher salt.

½ teaspoon canola oil
1 teaspoon grated lime zest
1 tablespoon lime juice
1 garlic clove, minced
2 teaspoons chili powder
½ teaspoon ground cumin
⅛ teaspoon ground cayenne
1¼ pounds thin white-fleshed fish fillets
8 (6-inch) whole wheat flour tortillas, warmed
1 cup thinly sliced cabbage
1 cup Fresh Tomato Salsa (page 41) or Creamy Avocado Sauce (page 596)
Lime wedges

1 Preheat the broiler. Brush a medium rimmed baking sheet with the oil.

2 Combine the lime zest, lime juice, garlic, chili powder, cumin, and cayenne in a medium bowl

continues on next page

and stir to mix well. Add the fish and turn to coat evenly. Arrange the fish in a single layer on the prepared pan. Broil, without turning, until the fish flakes easily with a fork, about 8 minutes.

3 Cut the fish into strips and divide evenly among the tortillas. Top the fish evenly with the cabbage and salsa and serve at once with the lime wedges.

Each serving: 30 g carb, 327 cal, 8 g fat, 1 g sat fat, 67 mg chol, 17 g fib, 30 g pro, 852 mg sod • Carb Choices: 1½; Exchanges: 1½ starch, 1 veg, 3 lean protein, ½ fat

Thick White-Fleshed Fish Fillets

Grilled Fish Fillets with Citrus-Herb Gremolata

makes 4 servings

Make use of this brightly flavored marinade to liven up shrimp, scallops, or any kind of fish. Sprinkle the gremolata over any grilled or baked seafood or chicken to add a dazzle of flavor.

FISH

4 (5-ounce) thick white-fleshed fish fillets
½ cup orange juice
2 tablespoons lemon juice
1 tablespoon chopped fresh tarragon
2½ teaspoons extra virgin olive oil, divided
1 garlic clove, minced
¼ teaspoon kosher salt
⅛ teaspoon freshly ground pepper

GREMOLATA

1 tablespoon chopped fresh Italian parsley
1 tablespoon chopped fresh tarragon
1 teaspoon grated fresh lemon zest
1 teaspoon grated fresh orange zest
½ teaspoon finely minced garlic
Lemon wedges

1 Preheat the grill to medium heat.

2 To make the fish, combine the fish, orange juice, lemon juice, tarragon, 2 teaspoons of the olive oil, and the garlic in a large resealable plastic bag. Seal the bag and refrigerate 30 minutes.

3 To make the gremolata, combine all the ingredients in a small bowl and stir to mix well.

4 Remove the fish from the bag and discard the marinade. Pat the fish dry with paper towels and sprinkle with the salt and pepper.

5 Brush the grill rack with the remaining ½ teaspoon oil. Place the fish on the grill and grill, turning once, until the fish flakes easily with a fork, 3 to 4 minutes on each side. Divide the fish among 4 plates, sprinkle evenly with the parsley mixture, and serve at once with the lemon wedges.

Each serving: 3 g carb, 129 cal, 3 g fat, 0 g sat fat, 54 mg chol, 0 g fib, 23 g pro, 147 mg sod • Carb Choices: 0; Exchanges: 3 lean protein, ½ fat

Grilled Fish Fillets with Dill Pesto Sauce

makes 6 servings

Fresh dill is the perfect partner for any kind of fish, and you can certainly serve this pesto with any grilled or broiled fish or shrimp. In this recipe, the fish is also coated in fresh dill and marinated briefly for a double dose of dill.

FISH

6 (5-ounce) thick white-fleshed fish fillets
2½ teaspoons extra virgin olive oil, divided
1 tablespoon chopped fresh dill
2 garlic cloves, minced
1 teaspoon grated lemon zest
⅛ teaspoon freshly ground pepper
¼ teaspoon kosher salt

SAUCE

1 cup loosely packed fresh dill sprigs

½ cup loosely packed fresh Italian parsley leaves

3 tablespoons extra virgin olive oil

2 tablespoons pine nuts, toasted (page 4)

2 tablespoons freshly grated Parmesan

½ teaspoon grated lemon zest

1 tablespoon lemon juice

1 garlic clove, chopped

¼ teaspoon kosher salt

Lemon wedges

1 Preheat the grill to medium heat.

2 Place the fish in a large shallow dish. Coat with 2 teaspoons of the oil, then with the dill, garlic, lemon zest, and pepper. Cover and refrigerate 30 minutes.

3 Meanwhile, to make the sauce, combine all the ingredients in a food processor and process until the mixture is finely chopped. Transfer to a small bowl. Place a piece of plastic wrap on the surface and refrigerate until ready to serve.

4 Sprinkle the fish with the salt. Brush the grill rack with the remaining ½ teaspoon oil. Place the fish on the grill and grill, turning once, until the fish flakes easily with a fork, 3 to 4 minutes on each side. Divide the fish among 6 plates and serve at once with the sauce and the lemon wedges.

Each serving: 2 g carb, 215 cal, 12 g fat, 2 g sat fat, 55 mg chol, 0 g fib, 24 g pro, 199 mg sod • Carb Choices: 0; Exchanges: 3 lean protein, 2½ fat

Basil-Crusted Fish Fillets with Roasted Cherry Tomatoes QUICK

makes 4 servings

A sprinkling of fresh basil gives this fish terrific flavor. You can use other herbs, too. Try chives, tarragon, or cilantro. The only trick to cooking

this dish is to cook the fish over medium heat so that you don't burn the herbs. The roasted tomatoes pair nicely with the fish, but if you are short on time, you can serve the fish on its own.

TOMATOES

2 cups grape tomatoes

2 teaspoons extra virgin olive oil

1 tablespoon sherry vinegar or white wine vinegar

1 tablespoon capers, rinsed and drained

⅛ teaspoon kosher salt

⅛ teaspoon freshly ground pepper

2 tablespoons chopped fresh basil

FISH

4 (5-ounce) thick white-fleshed fish fillets

¼ teaspoon kosher salt

⅛ teaspoon freshly ground pepper

2 tablespoons chopped fresh basil

2 teaspoons extra virgin olive oil

1 To make the tomatoes, preheat the oven to 400°F.

2 Combine the tomatoes and oil in a medium baking dish and stir to coat. Bake until some of the tomatoes begin to burst, 18 to 20 minutes.

3 Transfer the tomatoes and any pan juices to a medium bowl. Stir in the vinegar, capers, salt, and pepper. Stir in the basil just before serving. Serve warm or at room temperature.

4 Meanwhile, to make the fish, sprinkle the fillets with the salt and pepper, then with the basil, pressing to adhere.

5 Heat a large nonstick skillet over medium heat. Add the oil and tilt the pan to coat the bottom evenly. Add the fillets and cook, turning once, until the fish flakes easily with a fork, about 4 minutes on each side. Divide the fish and tomatoes among 4 plates and serve at once.

Each serving: 3 g carb, 160 cal, 6 g fat, 1 g sat fat, 54 mg chol, 1 g fib, 23 g pro, 249 mg sod • Carb Choices: 0; Exchanges: 1 veg, 3 lean protein, 1 fat

Pan-Seared Fish Fillets with Tomato-Orange Salsa

makes 4 servings

This salsa is a fresh and easy accompaniment for any seafood or chicken. Seafood only needs a short time to pick up the flavors of a marinade, so you can make the salsa while the fish marinates.

FISH

4 (5-ounce) thick fish fillets
½ cup orange juice
¼ cup thinly sliced red onion
2 garlic cloves, minced
4 teaspoons extra virgin olive oil, divided
¼ teaspoon kosher salt
⅛ teaspoon freshly ground pepper

SALSA

3 cups cherry tomatoes, halved
2 tablespoons diced red onion
2 tablespoons chopped fresh cilantro
2 tablespoons white wine vinegar
2 teaspoons freshly grated orange zest
1 garlic clove, minced
¼ teaspoon kosher salt
⅛ teaspoon freshly ground pepper

1 To make the fish, combine the fillets, orange juice, onion, garlic, and 2 teaspoons of the oil in a large resealable plastic bag. Seal the bag and refrigerate 30 minutes.

2 Meanwhile, to make the salsa, combine all the salsa ingredients in a medium bowl and stir to mix well.

3 Remove the fish from the marinade and discard the marinade. Pat the fish dry with paper towels and sprinkle with the salt and pepper.

4 Heat a large nonstick skillet over medium-high heat. Add the remaining 2 teaspoons oil and tilt the pan to coat the bottom evenly. Add the fish and cook, turning once, until the fish flakes easily with a fork, about 4 minutes on each side. Divide the fish and salsa evenly among 4 plates and serve at once.

Each serving: 7 g carb, 166 cal, 5 g fat, 1 g sat fat, 54 mg chol, 2 g fib, 24 g pro, 223 mg sod • Carb Choices: ½; Exchanges: 1 veg, 3 lean protein, ½ fat

Fish Fillets with Avocado-Lemon Sauce HIGH FIBER

makes 4 servings

This rich, tangy, bright green sauce is what makes this dish—or anything else you serve it with—so special. Serve the sauce with steak, shrimp, scallops, or instead of salsa on tacos or tostadas.

FISH

4 (5-ounce) thick white-fleshed fish fillets
½ cup dry white wine
1 teaspoon grated lemon zest
2 tablespoons lemon juice
4 teaspoons extra virgin olive oil, divided
¼ teaspoon kosher salt
⅛ teaspoon freshly ground pepper

SAUCE

1 medium avocado, pitted and peeled
1 cup loosely packed fresh cilantro leaves
⅓ cup cold water
3 tablespoons lemon juice
2 tablespoons thinly sliced scallions
¼ teaspoon ground cumin
½ teaspoon kosher salt

1 To make the fish, combine the fillets, wine, lemon zest, lemon juice, and 2 teaspoons of the oil in a large resealable plastic bag. Seal the bag and refrigerate 30 minutes.

2 Meanwhile, to make the sauce, combine all the sauce ingredients in a food processor and process until a chunky puree forms. Cover and refrigerate until ready to serve.

3 Remove the fish from the marinade and discard the marinade. Pat the fish dry with paper towels and sprinkle with the salt and pepper.

4 Heat a large nonstick skillet over medium-high heat. Add the remaining 2 teaspoons oil and tilt the pan to coat the bottom evenly. Add the fish and cook, turning once, until the fish flakes easily with a fork, about 4 minutes on each side. Divide the fish among 4 plates and serve at once with the sauce.

Each serving: 6 g carb, 233 cal, 12 g fat, 2 g sat fat, 54 mg chol, 4 g fib, 24 g pro, 293 mg sod • Carb Choices: ½; Exchanges: 3 lean protein, 2 fat

Fish Fillets with Tomato, Bell Pepper, and Basil QUICK

makes 4 servings

2 teaspoons extra virgin olive oil
1 medium onion, halved lengthwise and thinly sliced
1 small yellow bell pepper, thinly sliced
1 small red bell pepper, thinly sliced
2 garlic cloves, minced
½ cup dry white wine
1 large tomato, chopped
2 tablespoons chopped fresh basil
½ teaspoon kosher salt, divided
¼ teaspoon freshly ground pepper, divided
4 (5-ounce) thick white-fleshed fish fillets
2 tablespoons chopped fresh basil

1 Heat a large nonstick skillet over high heat. Add the oil and tilt the pan to coat the bottom evenly. Add the onion and bell peppers to the skillet and cook, stirring often, until the vegetables are softened, 5 minutes. Stir in the garlic and cook, stirring constantly, until fragrant, 30 seconds.

2 Add the wine and bring to a boil, stirring to scrape up the browned bits from the bottom of the skillet. Cook until almost all the liquid is evaporated, about 5 minutes. Add the tomato, basil, ¼ teaspoon of the salt, and ⅛ teaspoon of the ground pepper and return to a boil.

3 Sprinkle the fish with the remaining ¼ teaspoon salt and remaining ⅛ teaspoon ground pepper. Arrange the fillets in a single layer on top of the vegetables. Cover, reduce the heat, and simmer until the fish flakes easily with a fork, 6 to 8 minutes. Divide the fish evenly among 4 plates. Stir the basil into the vegetables and spoon evenly over the fish. Serve at once.

Each serving: 9 g carb, 185 cal, 3 g fat, 1 g sat fat, 54 mg chol, 2 g fib, 24 g pro, 222 mg sod • Carb Choices: ½; Exchanges: 1 veg, 3 lean protein, ½ fat

Potato-Dill-Crusted Fish Fillets QUICK

makes 4 servings

There's nothing tricky about getting the shredded potato to stick to the fish. The only awkward step is turning the fish over when you transfer it from the skillet to the pan. A wide spatula makes this easy to do. Cod or halibut are especially good choices for this dish.

4½ teaspoons extra virgin olive oil, divided
2 medium Yukon Gold potatoes
2 tablespoons chopped fresh dill
4 (5-ounce) thick white-fleshed fish fillets
2 teaspoons grated lemon zest
½ teaspoon kosher salt
¼ teaspoon freshly ground pepper

1 Preheat the oven to 400°F. Brush a medium rimmed baking sheet with ½ teaspoon of the oil.

2 Peel the potatoes and shred them on the coarse side of a box grater. Measure 1 cup of the shredded potatoes and place them in a small

continues on next page

bowl (discard any remaining potato). Add the dill and stir to mix well.

3 Sprinkle the fish evenly on one side with the lemon zest, salt, and pepper. Pat ¼ cup of the potato mixture in an even layer over the seasonings on each fillet.

4 Heat a large nonstick skillet over medium heat. Add 2 teaspoons of the remaining oil and tilt the pan to coat the bottom evenly. Carefully place two of the fillets, potato side down, in the skillet. Cook until the potato is tender and browned, about 5 minutes, reducing the heat if the potato begins to brown too quickly.

5 Using a wide spatula, carefully remove the fillets from the skillet and place, potato side up, on the prepared baking sheet. Repeat with the remaining 2 teaspoons oil and remaining fish fillets.

6 Bake until the fish flakes easily with a fork, 6 to 8 minutes (carefully lift the edge of the potato on one of the fillets to test for doneness). Divide the fish among 4 plates and serve at once.

Each serving: 10 g carb, 194 cal, 6 g fat, 1 g sat fat, 54 mg chol, 1 g fib, 23 g pro, 220 mg sod • Carb Choices: ½; Exchanges: ½ starch, 3 lean protein, 1 fat

Caper-Crusted Baked Fish

QUICK

makes 4 servings

You can use any fresh herb in the crust—try 2 tablespoons of basil or Italian parsley or 2 teaspoons of thyme or rosemary.

1 teaspoon plus 2 tablespoons extra virgin olive oil, divided
½ cup plain dry breadcrumbs
2 tablespoons capers, rinsed, drained, and minced
2 tablespoons chopped fresh dill
2 teaspoons grated lemon zest
2 garlic cloves, minced
4 (5-ounce) thick white-fleshed fish fillets
¼ teaspoon kosher salt

⅛ teaspoon freshly ground pepper
Lemon wedges

1 Preheat the oven to 400°F. Brush a medium rimmed baking sheet with 1 teaspoon of the oil.

2 Combine the breadcrumbs and the remaining 2 tablespoons oil in a small bowl. Using your fingers, blend the oil evenly into the breadcrumbs. Stir in the capers, dill, lemon zest, and garlic.

3 Place the fish on the prepared baking sheet. Sprinkle evenly with the salt and pepper. Top each fillet with about ¼ cup of the breadcrumb mixture, pressing to adhere. Bake just until the fish flakes easily with a fork, 10 to 12 minutes. Divide the fish among 4 plates and serve at once with the lemon wedges.

Each serving: 1 g carb, 180 cal, 9 g fat, 1 g sat fat, 54 mg chol, 0 g fib, 23 g pro, 274 mg sod • Carb Choices: 0; Exchanges: 3 lean protein, 1½ fat

Fish Fillets with Warm Tomato-Lemon Sauce QUICK

makes 4 servings

This quick and easy dish is perfect for summer suppers when tomatoes are at their peak and you want to be enjoying the outdoors instead of working in the kitchen. I also like to make this with dill instead of the parsley if I have it on hand.

4 (5-ounce) thick white-fleshed fish fillets
½ teaspoon kosher salt, divided
¼ teaspoon freshly ground pepper, divided
4 teaspoons extra virgin olive oil, divided
2 large tomatoes, chopped
2 tablespoons chopped fresh Italian parsley
1 tablespoon grated lemon zest

1 Sprinkle the fish with ¼ teaspoon of the salt and ⅛ teaspoon of the pepper. Heat a large nonstick skillet over high heat. Add 2 teaspoons of the oil and tilt the pan to coat the bottom evenly. Add the fillets and cook, turning once, just until

the fish flakes easily with a fork, about 4 minutes on each side. Transfer to a plate and cover loosely with foil to keep warm.

2 Add the remaining 2 teaspoons oil to the skillet and tilt the pan to coat the bottom evenly. Add the tomatoes and cook, stirring, just until heated through, about 2 minutes. Remove from the heat and stir in the parsley, lemon zest, remaining ¼ teaspoon salt, and remaining ⅛ teaspoon pepper. Spoon the tomato mixture evenly onto 4 plates and top each with a fish fillet. Serve at once.

Each serving: 4 g carb, 163 cal, 6 g fat, 1 g sat fat, 54 mg chol, 1 g fib, 23 g pro, 222 mg sod • Carb Choices: 0; Exchanges: 1 veg, 3 lean protein, 1 fat

Mint-Crusted Fish Fillets with Sweet Pea Sauce QUICK

makes 4 servings

You can add 2 teaspoons of chopped fresh mint to the pea sauce if you really enjoy the flavor of mint. The vivid green sauce gives the fish a restaurant look with less than 5 minutes work.

1 cup frozen baby green peas, thawed
⅓ cup Chicken Stock (page 149) or low-sodium chicken broth
4 teaspoons extra virgin olive oil, divided
⅛ teaspoon plus ½ teaspoon kosher salt, divided
Pinch plus ⅛ teaspoon freshly ground pepper, divided
4 (5-ounce) thick white-fleshed fish fillets
2 tablespoons chopped fresh mint
2 teaspoons lemon juice

1 Combine the peas, stock, 2 teaspoons of the oil, ⅛ teaspoon of the salt, and the pinch of pepper in a food processor and process until smooth. Transfer to a small saucepan.

2 Sprinkle the fish with the remaining ½ teaspoon salt, and remaining ⅛ teaspoon pepper. Sprinkle with the mint, pressing to adhere.

3 Heat a large nonstick skillet over medium heat. Add the remaining 2 teaspoons oil and tilt the pan to coat the bottom evenly. Add the fillets and cook, turning once, just until the fish flakes easily with a fork, about 4 minutes on each side.

4 Meanwhile, set the pea mixture over low heat and cook, stirring often, just until heated through, about 5 minutes. Remove from the heat and stir in the lemon juice.

5 To serve, place the fillets on 4 plates and drizzle the sauce evenly around the fillets. Serve at once.

Each serving: 5 g carb, 174 cal, 6 g fat, 1 g sat fat, 54 mg chol, 2 g fib, 24 g pro, 263 mg sod • Carb Choices: 0; Exchanges: 3 lean protein, 1 fat

Steamed Fish Fillets in Herb Broth QUICK

makes 4 servings

This fish dish has hardly any calories and yet is tremendously flavorful. It's a good recipe to make with salmon fillets, too. Be sure to drizzle some of the delicious broth over any rice, pasta, or vegetables that you are serving with the fish.

¾ cup Chicken Stock (page 149) or low-sodium chicken broth
¾ cup water
4 sprigs fresh cilantro
4 sprigs fresh dill or basil
½ teaspoon kosher salt
⅛ teaspoon whole black peppercorns
2 tablespoons chopped fresh cilantro
2 tablespoons chopped fresh dill or basil
1 teaspoon grated lemon zest
4 (5-ounce) thick white-fleshed fish fillets

1 Combine the stock, water, cilantro sprigs, dill sprigs, salt, and peppercorns in a large skillet. Bring to a boil. Cover, reduce the heat to low, and simmer 10 minutes.

2 Meanwhile, stir together the chopped cilantro, chopped dill, and lemon zest in a small bowl.

continues on next page

3 Carefully arrange the fish fillets in a single layer in the skillet with the broth mixture. Cover and steam just until the fish flakes easily with a fork, 2 to 3 minutes. Transfer the fish to 4 shallow bowls.

4 Place a wire strainer over a bowl and pour in the stock mixture. Discard the solids. Ladle the broth evenly over the fish fillets. Sprinkle the fish evenly with the cilantro mixture and serve at once.

Each serving: 0 g carb, 108 cal, 1 g fat, 0 g sat fat, 55 mg chol, 0 g fib, 23 g pro, 244 mg sod • Carb Choices: 0; Exchanges: 3 lean protein

Fish Fillets with Zucchini and Mint en Papillote QUICK

makes 4 servings

When you have no time to cook—or to clean up—making dinner in parchment packages is a great idea.

2 medium zucchini, cut in half lengthwise and sliced
⅓ cup thinly sliced red onion
¼ cup thinly sliced fresh basil leaves
1 garlic clove, minced
4 teaspoons extra virgin olive oil
½ teaspoon kosher salt, divided
¼ teaspoon freshly ground pepper, divided
4 (5-ounce) thick white-fleshed fish fillets
1 large lemon, cut into 8 slices

1 Preheat the oven to 450°F.

2 Place the zucchini, onion, basil, garlic, oil, ¼ teaspoon of the salt, and ⅛ teaspoon of the pepper in a large bowl and toss to combine. Sprinkle the fish with the remaining ¼ teaspoon salt and remaining ⅛ teaspoon pepper.

3 Tear off four 24 x 12-inch pieces of parchment paper. Fold each piece in half crosswise and cut each one to make a rounded heart shape. Open a parchment "heart" and arrange one-quarter of the vegetable mixture in the middle of one side. Top each portion of vegetables with a fish fillet. Place 2 lemon slices on top of each fillet.

4 Beginning at the bottom end of each "heart" fold the edges of the parchment in overlapping 1-inch segments, crimping as you go, to form a tight seal. (You can use foil to make the packets.)

5 Place the packages on a large rimmed baking sheet and bake until the fish flakes easily with a fork, 8 to 10 minutes. Place the packets on 4 plates and serve at once. Use caution when opening the packets, avoiding the steam that escapes.

Each serving: 5 g carb, 168 cal, 6 g fat, 1 g sat fat, 54 mg chol, 1 g fib, 24 g pro, 227 mg sod • Carb Choices: 0; Exchanges: 1 veg, 3 lean protein, 1 fat

Fish Fillets with Roasted Mushrooms QUICK

makes 4 servings

You don't often see mushrooms paired with fish, but it's a winning combination. I especially like to make this dish with halibut, so the meaty texture of the fish holds up to the mushrooms. Use any kind of mushrooms, or even a mixture of several types, depending on what's available at your supermarket.

3 teaspoons extra virgin olive oil, divided
1 pound fresh shiitake mushrooms, stemmed and sliced
3 teaspoons chopped fresh rosemary, divided
¾ teaspoon kosher salt, divided
¼ teaspoon freshly ground pepper, divided
4 (5-ounce) thick white-fleshed fish fillets
1 teaspoon grated lemon zest
2 teaspoons lemon juice

1 Preheat the oven to 400°F. Brush a large roasting pan with 1 teaspoon of the oil.

2 Place the mushrooms in the roasting pan. Drizzle with the remaining 2 teaspoons oil. Sprinkle with 2 teaspoons of the rosemary, ¼ teaspoon of the salt, and ⅛ teaspoon of the pepper and toss to coat. Bake 15 minutes.

3 Meanwhile, sprinkle the fish with the remaining 1 teaspoon rosemary, remaining ½ teaspoon salt, and remaining ⅛ teaspoon pepper.

4 Remove the roasting pan from the oven and stir in the mushrooms. Place the fish in a single layer on top of the mushrooms and bake until the fish flakes easily with a fork, 12 minutes.

5 To serve, divide the fish fillets evenly among 4 plates. Stir the lemon zest and lemon juice into the mushrooms and divide the mushrooms evenly among the plates. Serve at once.

Each serving: 5 g carb, 165 cal, 4 g fat, 1 g sat fat, 54 mg chol, 1 g fib, 25 g pro, 293 mg sod • Carb Choices: 0; Exchanges: 1 veg, 3 lean protein, ½ fat

Moroccan-Spiced Fish and Vegetable Kebabs QUICK

makes 4 servings

Choose one of the sturdy fish options for these kebabs. More delicate fish will fall off the skewers as they cook. Serve the kebabs on a bed of Orange-Ginger Couscous (page 420) for a stunning presentation.

2 garlic cloves, minced
1 tablespoon plus ½ teaspoons extra virgin olive oil, divided
1 teaspoon ground cumin
1 teaspoon paprika
1 teaspoon ground coriander
½ teaspoon ground ginger
½ teaspoon kosher salt
1¼ pounds halibut, catfish, tilapia, salmon, or tuna fillets, cut into 1-inch pieces
8 cherry tomatoes
8 whole cremini mushrooms, halved if large
4 scallions, cut into 1-inch pieces
1 small red bell pepper, cut into 1-inch pieces
Lemon wedges

1 Prepare the grill or heat a large grill pan over medium-high heat.

2 Combine the garlic, 1 tablespoon of the oil, the cumin, paprika, coriander, ginger, and salt in a large bowl and stir to mix well. Add the fish, tomatoes, mushrooms, scallions, and bell pepper and toss to coat. Thread the fish and vegetables onto eight 8- to 10-inch metal skewers.

3 Brush the grill rack or grill pan with the remaining ½ teaspoon oil. Place the kebabs on the grill rack or in the grill pan and grill, turning occasionally, until the fish flakes easily with a fork, 6 to 8 minutes. Divide the kebabs evenly among 4 plates and serve at once with the lemon wedges.

Each serving: 7 g carb, 172 cal, 5 g fat, 1 g sat fat, 54 mg chol, 2 g fib, 24 g pro, 224 mg sod • Carb Choices: ½; Exchanges: 1 veg, 3 lean protein, ½ fat

Salmon and Tuna

Baked Salmon with Cucumber-Grape Tomato Salsa QUICK

makes 4 servings

Nothing could be easier than this recipe for baked salmon with a fresh vegetable salsa. Season the fish and put it in the oven. While it bakes, prepare the salsa and some whole wheat couscous and you've got a delicious healthy meal in less than 30 minutes.

2½ teaspoons extra virgin olive oil, divided
4 (4-ounce) salmon fillets
½ teaspoon kosher salt, divided
⅛ teaspoon freshly ground pepper
½ hothouse (English) cucumber, peeled and chopped
1½ cups grape tomatoes, halved
1 jalapeño, seeded and minced
2 tablespoons minced red onion

continues on next page

2 tablespoons lime juice

2 tablespoons chopped fresh cilantro, basil, mint, or Italian parsley

1 Preheat the oven to 400°F. Brush a medium baking dish with ½ teaspoon of the oil.

2 Sprinkle the salmon with ¼ teaspoon of the salt and the pepper. Place in the prepared baking dish and bake until the fish is opaque in the center, 10 to 12 minutes.

3 Meanwhile, combine the cucumber, tomatoes, jalapeño, onion, lime juice, cilantro, remaining 2 teaspoons oil, and remaining ¼ teaspoon salt in a medium bowl and stir to mix well. Divide the salmon and salsa evenly among 4 plates and serve at once.

Each serving: 4 g carb, 229 cal, 11 g fat, 2 g sat fat, 72 mg chol, 1 g fib, 27 g pro, 200 mg sod • Carb Choices: 0; Exchanges: 4 lean protein, ½ fat

Baked Salmon with Balsamic Butter Sauce QUICK

makes 4 servings

Make the addictively delicious sauce just before you are ready to serve it because it thickens as it stands. It's also perfect on grilled steaks or pork chops.

½ teaspoon canola oil

1 cup balsamic vinegar

1 tablespoon unsalted butter

Pinch plus ⅛ teaspoon freshly ground pepper, divided

4 (4-ounce) salmon fillets

½ teaspoon kosher salt

1 Preheat the oven to 400°F. Brush a medium baking dish with the oil.

2 Place the vinegar in a small saucepan. Bring to a boil over medium-high heat and cook until reduced to about ¼ cup, about 15 minutes.

Remove from the heat and whisk in the butter and the pinch of pepper.

3 Meanwhile, sprinkle the salmon with the salt and remaining ⅛ teaspoon pepper. Place in the prepared baking dish and bake until opaque in the center, 10 to 12 minutes.

4 Place the salmon on 4 plates and drizzle evenly with the sauce. Serve at once.

Each serving: 11 g carb, 206 cal, 12 g fat, 3 g sat fat, 79 mg chol, 0 g fib, 26 g pro, 212 mg sod • Carb Choices: ½; Exchanges: ½ carb, 4 lean protein, ½ fat

Pan-Seared Salmon with Chunky Lemon Sauce QUICK

makes 4 servings

Lemon segments may sound too tart to eat, but when sweetened with a little sugar and paired with rich-tasting salmon, they are the perfect counterpoint. I like to have this dish with fresh spinach linguine, which also tastes great with the lemon sauce.

2 large lemons

1 tablespoon water

1 tablespoon sugar

1 tablespoon plus 2 teaspoons extra virgin olive oil, divided

⅛ teaspoon plus ¼ teaspoon kosher salt, divided

¼ teaspoon freshly ground pepper, divided

4 (4-ounce) salmon fillets

1 tablespoon chopped fresh basil, dill, or Italian parsley

1 Cut a thin slice from the top and bottom of the lemons, exposing the flesh. Stand each lemon upright, and using a sharp knife, thickly cut off the peel, following the contour of the fruit and removing all the white pith and membrane. Holding the lemons over a bowl, carefully cut along both sides of each section to free it from the membrane. Discard any seeds and let the sections fall into the bowl. Break the sections into small bits using two forks. Stir in the water,

sugar, 1 tablespoon of the oil, ⅛ teaspoon of the salt, and ⅛ teaspoon of the pepper.

2 Sprinkle the salmon with the remaining ¼ teaspoon salt and the remaining ⅛ teaspoon pepper. Heat a large nonstick skillet over medium-high heat. Add remaining 2 teaspoons oil and tilt the pan to coat the bottom evenly. Add the fish and cook, turning once, until the fish is opaque in the center, about 4 minutes on each side. Place the salmon on 4 plates. Stir the basil into the sauce and drizzle evenly over the salmon. Serve at once.

Each serving: 7 g carb, 261 cal, 14 g fat, 2 g sat fat, 72 mg chol, 1 g fib, 26 g pro, 162 mg sod • Carb Choices: ½; Exchanges: ½ carb, 4 lean protein, 1 fat

Cumin-Crusted Salmon with Cilantro-Chipotle Sauce QUICK

makes 4 servings

A tiny amount of honey rounds out the flavor of this spicy sauce. It's also great on grilled shrimp and chicken. The sauce makes about ¼ cup; if you're serving it to a crowd to accompany other grilled foods, double the recipe.

SAUCE

½ cup tightly packed fresh cilantro leaves
3 tablespoons lime juice
1 tablespoon extra virgin olive oil
1 tablespoon cold water
1 teaspoon honey
½ teaspoon minced chipotle in adobo sauce
1 garlic clove, minced
¼ teaspoon kosher salt
⅛ teaspoon ground cumin

FISH

4 (4-ounce) salmon fillets
¼ teaspoon ground cumin
¼ teaspoon kosher salt
⅛ teaspoon freshly ground pepper
2 teaspoons extra virgin olive oil

1 To make the sauce, combine all the ingredients in a food processor and process until smooth.

2 To make the fish, sprinkle the fillets with the cumin, salt, and pepper. Heat a large nonstick skillet over medium-high heat. Add the oil and tilt the pan to coat the bottom evenly. Add the fish and cook, turning once, until the fish is opaque in the center, about 4 minutes on each side. Place the salmon on 4 plates. Drizzle the sauce evenly over the salmon and serve at once.

Each serving: 3 g carb, 253 cal, 14 g fat, 2 g sat fat, 72 mg chol, 1 g fib, 26 g pro, 238 mg sod • Carb Choices: 0; Exchanges: 4 lean protein, 1 fat

Brown Sugar–Spice-Baked Salmon QUICK

makes 4 servings

If you find that you like the flavor of this rub, make a batch of it to keep on hand in your pantry. It's good on shrimp and steaks, too. Adjust the cayenne depending on your taste. I like a generous pinch because I am especially fond of any dish that is both sweet and spicy.

½ teaspoon canola oil
2 teaspoons light brown sugar
1 teaspoon ground cumin
½ teaspoon kosher salt
½ teaspoon ground coriander
¼ teaspoon freshly ground pepper
Pinch of ground cayenne
4 (4-ounce) salmon fillets
Lime wedges

1 Preheat the oven to 400°F. Brush a medium baking dish with the oil.

2 Stir together the sugar, cumin, salt, coriander, pepper, and cayenne in a shallow dish. Dip the top of each salmon fillet into the sugar mixture and place, sugar side up, in the prepared baking dish.

continues on next page

3 Bake until opaque in the center, 10 to 12 minutes. Place the salmon on 4 plates and serve at once with the lime wedges.

Each serving: 3 g carb, 202 cal, 9 g fat, 1 g sat fat, 72 mg chol, 0 g fib, 26 g pro, 199 mg sod • Carb Choices: 0; Exchanges: 3 lean protein

Wild Salmon and Arctic Char

Consider using wild salmon or Arctic char instead of farmed Atlantic salmon in these and any recipes that call for salmon. Any salmon labeled "Atlantic salmon" is farmed, since there are no longer enough of the fish remaining in the wild to make them commercially viable for fishing.

Most farmed salmon is raised in open cages and waste from the farms is released directly into the ocean. Farmed salmon can escape from the cages and harm wild populations. Parasites and diseases that the salmon carry can spread to wild fish populations. And, farmed salmon are fed wild fish, or feed made from wild fish; it takes up to three pounds of the wild fish to produce one pound of salmon. For these reasons, farmed salmon is not a sustainable seafood choice.

Arctic char is also farm raised, but it is raised in sealed inland waters which prevents release of the fish into the wild, and the farms treat the wastewater to avert pollution. Wild Pacific salmon from Alaska comes from pristine waters and is caught in the best-managed fishery in the world. Either of these fish is a more ocean-friendly choice than farmed Atlantic salmon.

Salmon Baked in Tomato-Fennel Sauce QUICK

makes 4 servings

Fresh fennel gives this ordinary tomato sauce sophisticated flavor. Instead of the salmon, you can make this dish with a pound of medium peeled and deveined shrimp. The dish will cook in about the same time. I like to serve this with fresh whole wheat linguini.

2 teaspoons extra virgin olive oil
1 small onion, halved lengthwise and thinly sliced
1 small bulb fennel, tough outer leaves removed, cored and thinly sliced
1 garlic clove, minced
½ cup dry white wine
½ cup Chicken Stock (page 149) or low-sodium chicken broth
1 large tomato, chopped
¼ teaspoon kosher salt, divided
¼ teaspoon freshly ground pepper, divided
4 (4-ounce) salmon fillets
1 teaspoon grated lemon zest
2 tablespoons chopped fresh Italian parsley

1 Preheat the oven to 350°F.

2 Heat a large ovenproof skillet over medium-high heat. Add the oil and tilt the pan to coat the bottom evenly. Add the onion and fennel and cook, stirring often, until the vegetables are softened, 5 minutes. Add the garlic and cook, stirring constantly, until fragrant, 30 seconds. Add the wine and stock and bring to a boil. Stir in the tomato, ⅛ teaspoon of the salt, and ⅛ teaspoon of the pepper.

3 Sprinkle the salmon with the remaining ⅛ teaspoon salt, the remaining ⅛ teaspoon pepper, and the lemon zest. Place the salmon in a single layer on top of the vegetables. Cover with foil and bake until the fish is opaque in the center, 12 to 15 minutes.

4 Place the salmon in 4 shallow bowls. Stir the parsley into the vegetables remaining in the skillet and spoon evenly around the salmon. Serve at once.

Each serving: 9 g carb, 268 cal, 11 g fat, 2 g sat fat, 72 mg chol, 3 g fib, 28 g pro, 179 mg sod • Carb Choices: ½; Exchanges: 1 veg, 4 lean protein, ½ fat

Broiled Salmon with Strawberry-Avocado Salsa

QUICK

makes 4 servings

Welcome spring with this stunning dish that's perfect for entertaining. If you want to make the salsa a few hours ahead, don't add the avocado until just before serving to keep it from browning. Serve this with steamed asparagus.

½ teaspoon canola oil
2 cups fresh strawberries, quartered or chopped, if large
½ avocado, pitted, peeled, and chopped
1 jalapeño, seeded and minced
2 tablespoons minced red onion
2 tablespoons chopped fresh cilantro
1 tablespoon lime juice
¾ teaspoon ground cumin, divided
4 (4-ounce) salmon fillets
½ teaspoon kosher salt
⅛ teaspoon freshly ground pepper

1 Preheat the broiler. Brush a medium rimmed baking sheet with the oil.

2 Gently toss together the strawberries, avocado, jalapeño, onion, cilantro, lime juice, and ¼ teaspoon of the cumin.

3 Sprinkle the salmon with the remaining ½ teaspoon cumin, the salt, and pepper and place on the prepared baking sheet. Broil until the salmon is opaque in the center, about 5 minutes. Place

the salmon on 4 plates. Spoon the salsa evenly over the salmon and serve at once.

Each serving: 9 g carb, 256 cal, 13 g fat, 2 g sat fat, 72 mg chol, 3 g fib, 27 g pro, 199 mg sod • Carb Choices: ½; Exchanges: ½ fruit, 4 lean protein, 1 fat

Miso-Orange Glazed Salmon QUICK

makes 4 servings

If you keep miso on hand for making miso soup, this is another delicious use for it. The salty miso and sweet orange juice make a perfectly balanced glaze for rich salmon fillets.

½ teaspoon canola oil
4 (4-ounce) salmon fillets
3 tablespoons white miso paste
2 tablespoons orange juice
1 teaspoon reduced-sodium soy sauce
1 teaspoon sugar

1 Preheat the broiler. Brush a medium rimmed baking sheet with the oil.

2 Place the salmon, skin side down, on the prepared baking sheet. Whisk together the miso, orange juice, soy sauce, and sugar in a small bowl. Brush the miso mixture over the salmon.

3 Broil until the salmon is opaque in the center, about 5 minutes. Place the salmon on 4 plates and serve at once.

Each serving: 6 g carb, 222 cal, 9 g fat, 1 g sat fat, 72 mg chol, 0 g fib, 27 g pro, 459 mg sod • Carb Choices: ½; Exchanges: ½ carb, 4 lean protein

Grilled Salmon with Yogurt Sauce QUICK

makes 4 servings

Use this basic grilled salmon recipe, which seasons the fish with only salt, pepper, and bit of cumin, with this tart and creamy yogurt sauce or serve it with any type of salsa, relish, or chutney.

continues on next page

½ cup plain low-fat yogurt

2 tablespoons thinly sliced scallions, green tops only

2 teaspoons lemon juice

½ teaspoon ground cumin, divided

Pinch plus ½ teaspoon kosher salt

Pinch of ground cayenne

4 (4-ounce) salmon fillets

⅛ teaspoon freshly ground pepper

½ teaspoon canola oil

1 Preheat the grill to medium-high heat.

2 Stir together the yogurt, scallions, lemon juice, ¼ teaspoon of the cumin, the pinch of salt, and the cayenne in a small bowl. Cover and refrigerate until ready to serve.

3 Sprinkle the salmon with the remaining ½ teaspoon salt, the remaining ¼ teaspoon cumin, and the pepper. Brush the grill rack with the oil. Place the salmon on the grill and grill until the fish is opaque in the center, about 3 minutes on each side. Place the salmon on 4 plates. Spoon the sauce evenly over the salmon and serve at once.

Each serving: 3 g carb, 211 cal, 9 g fat, 2 g sat fat, 73 mg chol, 0 g fib, 27 g pro, 237 mg sod • Carb Choices: 0; Exchanges: 4 lean protein

Salmon with Warm Lentils

HIGH FIBER

makes 4 servings

Simple pan-seared salmon with French green lentils is a classic restaurant dish that's easy to recreate at home. Watch the lentils carefully as they cook; you want them to be tender, but remain whole. The salad is a delicious one to make for serving on its own for lunch or with grilled chicken instead of the salmon.

2 cups Chicken Stock (page 149) or low-sodium chicken broth

1 cup dried French green lentils, picked over and rinsed

2 plum tomatoes, chopped

2 tablespoons diced red onion

1 tablespoon plus 2 teaspoons extra virgin olive oil, divided

1 tablespoon white wine vinegar

½ teaspoon kosher salt, divided

¼ teaspoon freshly ground pepper, divided

4 (4-ounce) salmon fillets

¼ cup chopped fresh Italian parsley

1 Combine the stock and lentils in a medium saucepan. Bring to a boil over high heat. Cover, reduce the heat to low, and simmer until the lentils are tender but still retain their shape, 15 to 20 minutes. Drain and transfer to a medium bowl. Stir in the tomatoes, onion, 1 tablespoon of the oil, the vinegar, ¼ teaspoon of the salt, and ⅛ teaspoon of the pepper. Let stand at room temperature while preparing the salmon.

2 Sprinkle the salmon with the remaining ¼ teaspoon salt and remaining ⅛ teaspoon pepper. Heat a large nonstick skillet over medium-high heat. Add the remaining 2 teaspoons oil and tilt the pan to coat the bottom evenly. Add the salmon and cook, turning once, until the fish is opaque in the center, about 4 minutes on each side.

3 Stir the parsley into the lentil mixture. Spoon the lentils evenly onto 4 plates and top with the salmon. Serve at once.

Each serving: 29 g carb, 406 cal, 15 g fat, 2 g sat fat, 74 mg chol, 8 g fib, 38 g pro, 267 mg sod • Carb Choices: 1½; Exchanges: 1½ starch, 4 lean protein, 1 plant-based protein, 1 fat

Salmon Cakes with Cucumber-Yogurt Sauce

QUICK

makes 4 servings

Canned salmon is often overlooked, but its ease of preparation, great taste, and superior nutritional profile make it a wonderful choice for healthy meals. Instead of serving these as cakes, put them in buns, add leaf lettuce and tomato slices, and drizzle with the yogurt sauce for a weeknight salmon burger.

1 (14¾-ounce) can wild pink Alaska salmon, drained
¼ cup plain dry breadcrumbs
¼ cup chopped scallions
3 tablespoons chopped fresh Italian parsley, divided
2 teaspoons Dijon mustard
1 large egg
1 teaspoon grated lemon zest
⅛ teaspoon freshly ground pepper
2 teaspoons canola oil
½ cup plain low-fat yogurt
½ hothouse (English) cucumber, peeled, seeded, and shredded
⅛ teaspoon kosher salt
Lemon wedges

1 Place the salmon in a medium bowl and remove and discard the skin and bones. Gently break the salmon into chunks. Add the breadcrumbs, scallions, 2 tablespoons of the parsley, the mustard, egg, lemon zest, and pepper and stir gently to combine. Shape into 4 patties.

2 Heat a large nonstick skillet over medium heat. Add the oil and tilt the pan to coat the bottom evenly. Add the patties and cook, turning once, until well browned and heated through, about 3 minutes on each side.

3 Stir together the yogurt, cucumber, the remaining 1 tablespoon parsley, and the salt. Divide the salmon cakes and the sauce evenly among 4 plates and serve at once with the lemon wedges.

Each serving: 9 g carb, 269 cal, 12 g fat, 3 g sat fat, 101 mg chol, 1 g fib, 29 g pro, 566 mg sod • Carb Choices: ½; Exchanges: ½ carb, 4 lean protein, ½ fat

Fresh Salmon Burgers QUICK

makes 4 servings

Toasted whole wheat English muffins make a delicious base for these sandwiches. Instead of cucumber and cabbage, top them with salad greens or chopped tomatoes, scallions, radishes, or bell pepper.

1 pound skinless salmon fillets, cut into 1-inch pieces
¼ cup plain dry breadcrumbs
1 large egg white
2 tablespoons chopped fresh Italian parsley
2 tablespoons chopped scallion
2 tablespoons lemon juice
¼ teaspoon kosher salt
¼ teaspoon freshly ground pepper
2 teaspoons canola oil
2 whole wheat English muffins, split and toasted
Cucumber slices
Thinly sliced green or napa cabbage

1 Place the salmon in a food processor and pulse until coarsely chopped. Add the breadcrumbs, egg white, parsley, scallion, lemon juice, salt, and pepper and pulse until well blended. Shape into 4 patties.

2 Heat a large nonstick skillet over medium heat. Add the oil and tilt the pan to coat the bottom evenly. Add the burgers and cook, turning once, until well browned and opaque in the centers, 3 to 4 minutes on each side.

3 To serve, place each burger on half an English muffin and top with the cucumber and cabbage.

Each serving: 21 g carb, 314 cal, 12 g fat, 2 g sat fat, 72 mg chol, 3 g fib, 31 g pro, 353 mg sod • Carb Choices: 1½; Exchanges: 1½ starch, 4 lean protein, ½ fat

Asian Salmon Cakes with Cucumber-Sesame Salsa

QUICK

makes 4 servings

If fresh crab cakes are rarely in your budget, these salmon cakes are an inexpensive—though just as delicious and impressive—option. Serve

continues on next page

them with Toasted Coconut–Ginger Rice (page 431) and steamed green beans or asparagus.

SALSA

1 hothouse (English) cucumber, seeded and chopped
2 tablespoons chopped fresh cilantro
1 jalapeño, seeded and minced
1 scallion, thinly sliced
1 tablespoon lime juice
2 teaspoons sesame seeds
¼ teaspoon kosher salt

SALMON CAKES

1 pound skinless salmon fillets, cut into 1-inch pieces
¼ cup plain breadcrumbs
1 large egg white
2 tablespoons chopped fresh cilantro
2 tablespoons chopped red onion
2 tablespoons lime juice
½ teaspoon kosher salt
Pinch of ground cayenne
2 teaspoons canola oil

1 To make the salsa, combine all the ingredients in a medium bowl and stir to combine. Cover and refrigerate until ready to serve.

2 To make the salmon cakes, place the salmon in a food processor and pulse until coarsely chopped. Add the breadcrumbs, egg white, cilantro, onion, lime juice, salt, and cayenne and pulse until well blended. Shape into 4 patties.

3 Heat a large nonstick skillet over medium heat. Add the oil and tilt the pan to coat the bottom evenly. Add the cakes and cook, turning once, until well browned and opaque in the centers, 3 to 4 minutes on each side. Divide the salmon cakes and the salsa evenly among 4 plates and serve at once.

Each serving: 9 g carb, 260 cal, 12 g fat, 2 g sat fat, 72 mg chol, 2 g fib, 29 g pro, 335 mg sod • Carb Choices: ½; Exchanges: ½ starch, 3 lean protein, ½ fat

Tuna with Roasted Lemons

makes 4 servings

This is an exceptionally easy and impressive dish. The roasted lemons are an unexpected and tasty accompaniment for the tuna and they make a good-looking presentation. When you roast the lemons, roast an extra one. Chop a slice or two to add a bright lift to a vinaigrette, a yogurt dip, or a potato or pasta salad.

2 medium lemons, cut into ¼-inch slices
4 teaspoons extra virgin olive oil, divided
4 (5-ounce) tuna steaks
½ teaspoon kosher salt
⅛ teaspoon freshly ground pepper

1 Preheat the oven to 325°F. Line a large rimmed baking sheet with parchment paper. Brush the lemon slices with 2 teaspoons of the oil and arrange in a single layer in the baking pan. Bake until lightly browned, 25 to 30 minutes.

2 Sprinkle the tuna with the salt and pepper. Heat a large skillet over medium-high heat. Add the remaining 2 teaspoons oil and tilt the pan to coat the bottom evenly. Add the tuna and cook, turning once, 2 minutes on each side for medium rare, or to the desired degree of doneness. Place the tuna on 4 plates. Divide the roasted lemons evenly among the plates and serve at once.

Each serving: 3 g carb, 197 cal, 6 g fat, 1 g sat fat, 62 mg chol, 1 g fib, 32 g pro, 193 mg sod • Carb Choices: 0; Exchanges: 4 lean protein, 1 fat

Tuna with Chili-Garlic Roasted Onions

makes 4 servings

These sweet and spicy onions are a delicious accompaniment for steaks or pork chops, too. Make a double batch and store refrigerated, covered, for up to 3 days. Gently reheat them in a small nonstick skillet before serving.

4 teaspoons canola oil, divided
1 tablespoon lime juice
2 teaspoons chili-garlic paste, divided
1 (1¼-pound) tuna steak, about 1-inch thick
2 large sweet onions, halved lengthwise and thinly sliced
½ teaspoon kosher salt, divided
1 tablespoon light brown sugar

1 Preheat the oven to 400°F.

2 Stir together 1 teaspoon of the oil, the lime juice, and 1 teaspoon of the chili-garlic paste in a shallow dish. Add the tuna and turn to coat. Cover and refrigerate 30 minutes.

3 Meanwhile, place the onions on a large rimmed baking sheet. Drizzle with 2 teaspoons of the remaining oil and sprinkle with ¼ teaspoon of the salt. Toss to coat. Arrange the onions in a single layer. Bake, stirring once, until tender and lightly browned, about 30 minutes. Maintain the oven temperature.

4 Transfer the onions to a small bowl. Add the sugar and remaining 1 teaspoon chili-garlic paste and stir to combine.

5 Remove the tuna from the marinade and discard the marinade. Sprinkle the tuna with the remaining ¼ teaspoon salt. Heat a medium ovenproof skillet over medium-high heat. Add the remaining 1 teaspoon oil and tilt the pan to coat the bottom evenly. Place the tuna in the skillet and cook, turning once, 1 minute on each side, or until well browned. Transfer the skillet to the oven and bake 3 minutes for medium rare, or to the desired degree of doneness.

6 Transfer the tuna to a cutting board and cut into thin slices. Divide the tuna and onions evenly among 4 plates and serve at once.

Each serving: 16 g carb, 257 cal, 6 g fat, 1 g sat fat, 62 mg chol, 2 g fib, 33 g pro, 218 mg sod • Carb Choices: 1; Exchanges: 2 veg, 4 lean protein, 1 fat

Grilled Tuna with Wasabi Vinaigrette QUICK

makes 4 servings

The modest amount of wasabi in this vinaigrette allows you to taste the wasabi, but it doesn't overpower the fish. Look for wasabi paste in the supermarket in small jars or tubes in the Asian foods section.

3 tablespoons reduced-sodium soy sauce
2 tablespoons rice vinegar
1 tablespoon plus ½ teaspoon canola oil, divided
2 teaspoons prepared wasabi paste
4 (5-ounce) tuna steaks

1 Whisk together the soy sauce, vinegar, 1 tablespoon of the oil, and the wasabi paste in a medium bowl. Place the tuna in a medium shallow dish and drizzle with 1 tablespoon of the soy sauce mixture. Turn the tuna to coat. Cover and refrigerate 30 minutes.

2 Preheat the grill to medium-high heat.

3 Brush the grill rack with the remaining ½ teaspoon oil. Remove the tuna from the marinade and discard the marinade. Place the tuna on the grill and grill, turning once, 2 minutes on each side for medium rare, or to the desired degree of doneness. Place the tuna on 4 plates, drizzle evenly with the remaining soy sauce mixture, and serve at once.

Each serving: 1 g carb, 191 cal, 5 g fat, 1 g sat fat, 62 mg chol, 0 g fib, 33 g pro, 560 mg sod • Carb Choices: 0; Exchanges: 4 lean protein, 1 fat

Grilled Tuna with Anchovy-Caper Sauce QUICK

makes 4 servings

Anchovy-caper sauce is a traditional Italian accompaniment to grilled steaks and tuna. I made this version one summer when I had an abundance of basil, but you can use Italian parsley instead, or a combination of the two herbs.

2 cups loosely packed whole fresh basil leaves
2 tablespoons plus ½ teaspoon extra virgin olive oil, divided
2 tablespoons cold water
2 tablespoons thinly sliced scallions, green tops only
1 tablespoon white wine vinegar
1 tablespoon capers, rinsed and drained
1 garlic clove, chopped
1 canned anchovy fillet, chopped
4 (5-ounce) tuna steaks
¼ teaspoon kosher salt
⅛ teaspoon freshly ground pepper

1 Prepare the grill or heat a large grill pan over medium-high heat.

2 Combine the basil, 2 tablespoons of the oil, the water, scallion, vinegar, capers, garlic, and anchovy in a food processor and process until smooth.

3 Sprinkle the tuna with the salt and pepper. Brush the grill rack or grill pan with the remaining ½ teaspoon oil. Place the tuna on the grill and grill 2 minutes on each side for medium-rare, or to the desired degree of doneness. Place the tuna on 4 plates, drizzle evenly with the sauce, and serve at once.

Each serving: 1 g carb, 225 cal, 9 g fat, 1 g sat fat, 62 mg chol, 1 g fib, 33 g pro, 223 mg sod • Carb Choices: 0; Exchanges: 4 lean protein, 1½ fat

Tuna with Cilantro-Citrus Sauce QUICK

makes 4 servings

Cilantro lovers will revel in this dish. The sharp citrus tang of the sauce complements the tuna flawlessly, but you can also pair it with shrimp or scallops.

SAUCE

1 cup tightly packed fresh cilantro leaves
¼ cup orange juice
2 tablespoons extra virgin olive oil
1 tablespoon lime juice
¼ teaspoon ground cumin
⅛ teaspoon kosher salt
Pinch of ground cayenne

FISH

4 (5-ounce) tuna steaks
½ teaspoon ground cumin
¼ teaspoon kosher salt
Pinch of ground cayenne
2 teaspoons extra virgin olive oil

1 To make the sauce, combine all the ingredients in a food processor and process until smooth.

2 To make the fish, sprinkle the tuna with the cumin, salt, and cayenne. Heat a large skillet over medium-high heat. Add the oil and tilt the pan to coat the bottom evenly. Add the tuna and cook, turning once, 2 minutes on each side for medium rare, or to the desired degree of doneness. Place the tuna on 4 plates, drizzle evenly with the sauce, and serve at once.

Each serving: 2 g carb, 242 cal, 10 g fat, 1 g sat fat, 62 mg chol, 0 g fib, 32 g pro, 158 mg sod • Carb Choices: 0; Exchanges: 4 lean protein, 1 fat

Grilled Tuna with Spicy Tomato-Olive Relish QUICK

makes 4 servings

This relish is based on the ingredients of the classic Italian puttanesca sauce. It is usually a cooked sauce and served on pasta, but this fresh version with its salty spicy flavors pairs well with grilled tuna.

2 teaspoons grated lemon zest
2 tablespoons lemon juice
1½ teaspoons minced garlic, divided
2 teaspoons chopped fresh oregano or
   ½ teaspoon dried oregano
4 (5-ounce) tuna steaks
2 large tomatoes, chopped
¼ cup Kalamata olives, pitted and sliced
¼ cup chopped fresh Italian parsley
1 tablespoon capers, rinsed and drained
Pinch of crushed red pepper
¼ teaspoon kosher salt
⅛ teaspoon freshly ground pepper
½ teaspoon canola oil

1 Combine the lemon zest, lemon juice, 1 teaspoon of the garlic, and the oregano in a large resealable plastic bag. Add the tuna, turn to coat, and refrigerate 30 minutes.

2 Preheat the grill to medium-high heat.

3 Combine the tomatoes, olives, parsley, capers, remaining ½ teaspoon garlic, and the crushed red pepper in a medium bowl and stir to mix well.

4 Remove the tuna from the marinade and discard the marinade. Sprinkle the tuna with the salt and ground pepper. Brush the grill rack with the oil. Place the tuna on the grill and grill 2 minutes on each side for medium-rare, or to the desired degree of doneness. Divide the tuna and relish evenly among 4 plates and serve at once.

Each serving: 7 g carb, 200 cal, 4 g fat, 1 g sat fat, 62 mg chol, 1 g fib, 33 g pro, 306 mg sod • Carb Choices: ½; Exchanges: 1 veg, 4 lean protein, ½ fat

Grilled Chile-Rubbed Tuna with Avocado-Tomato Salsa QUICK | HIGH FIBER

makes 4 servings

FISH

2 teaspoons grated lime zest
1 tablespoon lime juice
1½ teaspoons ancho chile powder
2½ teaspoons extra virgin olive oil, divided
4 (5-ounce) tuna steaks
¼ teaspoon kosher salt

SALSA

1 avocado, pitted, peeled, and chopped
1 large tomato, chopped
2 tablespoons minced red onion
1 jalapeño, seeded and minced
¼ cup chopped fresh cilantro
2 tablespoons lime juice
¼ teaspoon kosher salt
Lime wedges

1 Preheat the grill to medium-high heat.

2 To make the fish, stir together the lime zest, lime juice, chile powder, and 2 teaspoons of the oil in a shallow dish. Add the tuna and turn to coat. Cover and refrigerate 30 minutes.

3 To make the salsa, combine all the ingredients except the lime wedges in a small bowl.

4 Remove the tuna from the marinade and discard the marinade. Sprinkle the tuna with the salt. Brush the grill rack with the remaining ½ teaspoon oil. Place the tuna on the grill, and grill 2 minutes on each side for medium-rare, or to the desired degree of doneness. Divide the tuna and salsa evenly among 4 plates and serve at once with the lime wedges.

Each serving: 8 g carb, 269 cal, 12 g fat, 2 g sat fat, 62 mg chol, 4 g fib, 33 g pro, 197 mg sod • Carb Choices: ½; Exchanges: 1 veg, 4 lean protein, 2 fat

Shellfish

BBQ Baked Shrimp QUICK

makes 4 servings

The mixture of seasonings in this dish tastes like a light barbecue sauce and it turns ordinary shrimp into an out of the ordinary weeknight meal. Serve it with hot crusty bread to soak up all the delicious cooking juices.

1 tablespoon extra virgin olive oil
1 tablespoon Worcestershire sauce
1 tablespoon lemon juice
1 teaspoon sugar
½ teaspoon paprika
½ teaspoon kosher salt
⅛ teaspoon ground cayenne
1 garlic clove, crushed through a press
1 pound medium peeled deveined shrimp
Lemon wedges

1 Preheat the oven to 400°F.

2 Stir together the oil, Worcestershire sauce, lemon juice, sugar, paprika, salt, cayenne, and garlic in a 13 x 9-inch glass baking dish. Add the shrimp and toss to coat.

3 Bake, stirring once, just until the shrimp are opaque, 12 to 15 minutes. Divide the shrimp among 4 shallow bowls and drizzle evenly with the cooking juices. Serve at once with the lemon wedges.

Each serving: 3 g carb, 127 cal, 4 g fat, 1 g sat fat, 168 mg chol, 0 g fib, 18 g pro, 235 mg sod • Carb Choices: 0; Exchanges: 3 lean protein, ½ fat

Garlicky Broiled Shrimp QUICK

makes 4 servings

This 15-minute dinner is delicious enough for a special occasion. Serve it over fresh whole wheat pasta with steamed green beans or summer squash and you've got a wonderful meal that tastes like it took hours to make.

2 tablespoons extra virgin olive oil
3 garlic cloves, minced
2 teaspoons grated lemon zest
2 tablespoons lemon juice
1 pound medium peeled deveined shrimp
½ teaspoon kosher salt
⅛ teaspoon freshly ground pepper

1 Combine the oil and garlic in a small saucepan and cook over medium-low heat, stirring often, until fragrant, about 2 minutes (do not let the garlic brown). Stir in the lemon zest and lemon juice.

2 Preheat the broiler.

3 Place the shrimp on a medium rimmed baking sheet. Sprinkle with the salt and pepper and toss to coat. Drizzle the shrimp with the oil mixture and toss to coat.

4 Broil, turning once, just until the shrimp turn pink, 6 to 8 minutes. Divide the shrimp among 4 shallow bowls and drizzle evenly with the cooking juices.

Each serving: 2 g carb, 154 cal, 8 g fat, 1 g sat fat, 168 mg chol, 0 g fib, 18 g pro, 334 mg sod • Carb Choices: 0; Exchanges: 3 lean protein, 1½ fat

Shrimp in Creole Tomato Sauce QUICK

makes 4 servings

This dish is traditionally served with rice, but it's good with pasta, too.

2 teaspoons extra virgin olive oil
1 medium onion, chopped
1 green bell pepper, chopped
1 stalk celery, chopped
4 garlic cloves, minced
2 teaspoons Creole seasoning, divided
1 (28-ounce) can no-salt-added whole tomatoes, undrained and chopped
1 cup Chicken Stock (page 149) or low-sodium chicken broth
1 pound medium peeled deveined shrimp
2 tablespoons chopped fresh Italian parsley

1 Heat a large skillet over medium heat. Add the oil and tilt the pan to coat the bottom evenly. Add the onion, bell pepper, and celery and cook, stirring often, until softened, 5 minutes. Add the garlic and 1 teaspoon of the Creole seasoning and cook, stirring constantly, until fragrant, 30 seconds.

2 Add the tomatoes with their juices and the stock and bring to a boil. Reduce the heat to low and simmer, uncovered, stirring occasionally, until the vegetables are tender and the sauce is thickened, about 10 minutes.

3 Meanwhile, place the shrimp in a medium bowl, sprinkle with the remaining 1 teaspoon Creole seasoning, and toss to coat. Add the shrimp to the sauce, cover, and simmer just until the shrimp turn pink, about 2 minutes. Stir in the parsley. Divide the shrimp and sauce evenly among 4 shallow bowls and serve at once.

Each serving: 14 g carb, 170 cal, 4 g fat, 1 g sat fat, 169 mg chol, 3 g fib, 21 g pro, 565 mg sod • Carb Choices: 1; Exchanges: 2 veg, 3 lean protein, ½ fat

Shrimp in Coconut-Ginger Sauce QUICK

makes 4 servings

Made with ordinary pantry ingredients, this creamy shrimp dish tastes like something that takes much more effort than it actually does. Serve it with brown rice and steamed snow peas or broccoli.

2 teaspoons canola oil
2 scallions, thinly sliced
2 garlic cloves, minced
1 jalapeño, seeded and minced
1 tablespoon minced fresh ginger
1 cup reduced-fat coconut milk
½ teaspoon kosher salt
Pinch of ground cayenne
1 pound medium peeled deveined shrimp
2 tablespoons lime juice
2 tablespoons chopped fresh basil or cilantro

Peel Your Own

You can save money by buying shrimp with the shells on and then quickly removing them yourself. The easiest way to peel and devein shrimp in one step is by using scissors. Starting at the head, cut down the center of the back of the shell, cutting through the shell and the flesh to expose the vein. Depending on the dish you're making, you may want to leave the tail on for a pretty presentation or pinch it off to make the shrimp easier to eat. Peel away the shell and open up the cut flesh under cold running water to rinse away the vein.

When buying shell-on shrimp, you will need about 1¼ pounds to yield 1 pound of peeled and deveined shrimp. This will yield about 12 ounces of cooked shrimp.

Always save the shells when you peel your own shrimp and use them to make Shrimp Stock (page 152). You can freeze the flavorful stock for up to 3 months to use in soups or stews.

1 Heat a large nonstick skillet over medium-high heat. Add the oil and tilt the pan to coat the bottom evenly. Add the scallions, garlic, jalapeño, and ginger and cook, stirring constantly, until fragrant, 30 seconds. Add the coconut milk, salt, and cayenne and bring to a boil.

2 Add the shrimp, and cook, stirring often, just until the shrimp turn pink, about 2 minutes. Remove from the heat and stir in the lime juice and basil. Divide the shrimp and sauce evenly among 4 shallow bowls and serve at once.

Each serving: 4 g carb, 150 cal, 6 g fat, 3 g sat fat, 168 mg chol, 0 g fib, 18 g pro, 360 mg sod • Carb Choices: 0; Exchanges: 2 lean protein, 1 fat

continues on next page

THAI GREEN CURRY SHRIMP: Follow the Shrimp in Coconut-Ginger Sauce recipe, on page 353, adding 1 teaspoon green curry paste with the coconut milk in step 1, and proceed as directed.

Each serving: 4 g carb, 150 cal, 6 g fat, 3 g sat fat,168 mg chol, 0 g fib, 18 g pro, 383 mg sod • Carb Choices: 0; Exchanges: 3 lean protein, 1 fat

Shrimp and Vegetable Stir-Fry QUICK

makes 4 servings

⅓ cup Chicken Stock (page 149) or low-sodium chicken broth
2 tablespoons reduced-sodium soy sauce
1 teaspoon Asian sesame oil
½ teaspoon chili-garlic paste
2 teaspoons cornstarch
4 teaspoons canola oil, divided
2 tablespoons minced fresh ginger
2 garlic cloves, minced
1 pound medium peeled deveined shrimp
4 scallions, cut into 2-inch pieces
2 cups snow peas, trimmed
1 red bell pepper, thinly sliced
½ cup chopped fresh cilantro

1 Combine the stock, soy sauce, sesame oil, chili-garlic paste, and cornstarch in a small bowl and stir until the cornstarch dissolves.

2 Heat a large wok or nonstick skillet over medium-high heat. Add 2 teaspoons of the canola oil and tilt the pan to coat the bottom evenly. Add the ginger and garlic and cook, stirring constantly, until fragrant, 30 seconds. Add the shrimp and cook, stirring constantly, until the shrimp just turn pink, about 2 minutes. Transfer the shrimp to a plate and cover with foil to keep warm.

3 Add the remaining 2 teaspoons canola oil to the wok. Add the scallions, snow peas, and bell pepper and cook, stirring constantly, until crisp-tender, 3 minutes. Stir in the stock mixture and add

the shrimp and cook, stirring constantly, until the sauce is thickened, 30 seconds. Remove from the heat and stir in the cilantro. Divide among 4 plates and serve at once.

Each serving: 9 g carb, 156 cal, 2 g fat, 1 g sat fat, 169 mg chol, 2 g fib, 21 g pro, 550 mg sod • Carb Choices: ½; Exchanges: ½ carb, 3 lean protein, 1 fat

Lemon-Basil Shrimp with Linguini QUICK | HIGH FIBER

makes 4 servings

Refrigerated whole wheat pastas are worth seeking out for their fresh flavor and quick cooking time. If you don't like the heaviness of dried whole wheat pasta, give the fresh versions a try—they're just as healthy, but with a lighter wheat flavor.

1 (9-ounce) package fresh whole wheat linguini
2 teaspoons extra virgin olive oil
1 small onion, halved lengthwise and thinly sliced
2 garlic cloves, minced
½ cup dry white wine
¼ teaspoon kosher salt
⅛ teaspoon freshly ground pepper
1 pound medium peeled deveined shrimp
2 teaspoons grated lemon zest
2 tablespoons lemon juice
2 tablespoons chopped fresh basil

1 Cook the linguini according to the package directions.

2 Meanwhile, heat a large nonstick skillet over medium-high heat. Add the oil and tilt the pan to coat the bottom evenly. Add the onion and cook, stirring often, until softened, 5 minutes. Add the garlic and cook, stirring constantly, until fragrant, 30 seconds. Add the wine, salt, and pepper and bring to a boil. Cook until the wine is reduced by half, about 2 minutes.

3 Add the shrimp and cook, stirring constantly, just until the shrimp turn pink, about 2 minutes.

Remove from the heat and stir in the lemon zest, lemon juice, and basil.

4 Divide the linguini among 4 plates and top evenly with the shrimp.

Each serving: 34 g carb, 322 cal, 6 g fat, 1 g sat fat, 206 mg chol, 5 g fib, 28 g pro, 452 mg sod • Carb Choices: 2; Exchanges: 2 starch, 3 lean protein, ½ fat

Mediterranean Shrimp and Pasta QUICK | HIGH FIBER

makes 4 servings

If you have a can of artichokes on hand, they make a nice addition to this dish. Rinse and drain them well, then cut into quarters and add to the tomato mixture in step 2.

6 ounces whole wheat fettuccini
2 large tomatoes, chopped
¼ cup Kalamata olives, pitted and quartered
2 teaspoons grated lemon zest
3 tablespoons lemon juice
1 tablespoon capers, rinsed and drained
¼ teaspoon freshly ground pepper, divided
1 pound medium peeled deveined shrimp
⅛ teaspoon kosher salt
2 teaspoons extra virgin olive oil
2 garlic cloves, minced
¼ cup chopped fresh Italian parsley

1 Cook the fettuccini according to the package directions.

2 Meanwhile, combine the tomatoes, olives, lemon zest, lemon juice, capers, and ⅛ teaspoon of the pepper in a large bowl. Set aside.

3 Sprinkle the shrimp with the salt and remaining ⅛ teaspoon pepper. Heat a large nonstick skillet over medium-high heat. Add the oil and tilt the pan to coat the bottom evenly. Add the garlic and cook, stirring constantly, until fragrant, 30 seconds. Add the shrimp and cook, stirring constantly, just until the shrimp turn pink, about 2 minutes.

4 Add the shrimp, fettuccini, and parsley to the tomato mixture and toss to combine. Divide evenly among 4 shallow bowls and serve at once.

Each serving: 37 g carb, 297 cal, 6 g fat, 1 g sat fat, 168 mg chol, 7 g fib, 25 g pro, 417 mg sod • Carb Choices: 2½; Exchanges: 2 starch, 1 veg, 3 lean protein, 1 fat

Grilled Shrimp with Spicy Ginger BBQ Sauce QUICK

makes 4 servings

This is an amazingly flavorful sauce that puts most American-style barbecue sauces to shame. If you want a mild version, omit the chili-garlic paste. You can use the sauce for making barbecued boneless skinless chicken breasts, too.

2½ teaspoons canola oil, divided
½ cup chopped red onion
2 tablespoons minced fresh ginger
2 garlic cloves, minced
1 jalapeño, seeded and minced
⅓ cup reduced-sodium soy sauce
¼ cup packed light brown sugar
2 tablespoons no-salt-added tomato paste
1 tablespoon lime juice
1 teaspoon Asian sesame oil
1 teaspoon chili-garlic paste
1 pound large peeled deveined shrimp
Lime wedges

1 Heat a medium saucepan over medium heat. Add 2 teaspoons of the canola oil and tilt the pan to coat the bottom evenly. Add the onion, ginger, garlic, and jalapeño and cook, stirring often, until softened, 5 minutes. Add the soy sauce and sugar and bring to a boil. Cover, reduce the heat to low, and simmer until the onion is tender, about 5 minutes.

2 Transfer the onion mixture to a food processor. Add the tomato paste, lime juice, sesame oil, and chili-garlic paste and process until a thick puree forms.

continues on next page

3 Transfer ¼ cup of the sauce to a shallow dish. Add the shrimp and toss to coat. Cover and refrigerate 30 minutes. Reserve the remaining sauce for serving.

4 Preheat the grill to medium-high heat.

5 Brush the grill rack with the remaining ½ teaspoon canola oil. Remove the shrimp from the marinade and discard the marinade. Place the shrimp on the grill and grill, turning once, just until the shrimp turn pink, about 4 minutes. Divide the shrimp among 4 plates and serve with the reserved sauce and the lime wedges.

Each serving: 10 g carb, 149 cal, 3 g fat, 0 g sat fat, 168 mg chol, 0 g fib, 19 g pro, 626 mg sod • Carb Choices: ½; Exchanges: ½ carb, 3 lean protein

Grilled Shrimp with Thai Slaw

makes 4 servings

The slaw looks and tastes best if it's tossed together just before serving. You can prepare the vegetables up to a day ahead and store them in an airtight container in the refrigerator. Then toss with the dressing just before serving. The Asian fish sauce is what gives this dish its distinctive flavor, but it's also very high in sodium. Limit your sodium intake in other foods on a day when you enjoy this dish.

⅓ cup lime juice

¼ cup Asian fish sauce

2 tablespoons cold water

1 tablespoon plus ½ teaspoon canola oil, divided

1 teaspoon chili-garlic paste

1 tablespoon sugar

1 pound large peeled and deveined shrimp

3 cups thinly sliced savoy or napa cabbage

2 scallions, thinly sliced

1 small zucchini, cut into thin strips (about 1 cup)

1 small red bell pepper, cut into thin strips (about 1 cup)

1 small carrot, peeled and coarsely shredded

1 jalapeño, seeded and minced

½ hothouse (English) cucumber, seeded and cut into thin strips (about ½ cup)

¼ cup chopped fresh cilantro

¼ cup chopped fresh mint

1 Combine the lime juice, fish sauce, water, 1 tablespoon of the oil, the chili-garlic paste, and sugar in a large bowl and stir until the sugar dissolves. Transfer ⅓ cup of the lime juice mixture to a shallow dish. Add the shrimp and toss to coat. Cover and refrigerate 30 minutes.

2 Meanwhile, combine the cabbage, scallions, zucchini, bell pepper, carrot, jalapeño, cucumber, cilantro, and mint in a large bowl. Cover and refrigerate until ready to serve. Just before serving, drizzle the vegetables with the remaining lime juice mixture and toss to coat.

3 Preheat the grill to medium-high heat.

4 Brush the grill rack with the remaining ½ teaspoon oil. Remove the shrimp from the marinade and discard the marinade. Place the shrimp on the grill and grill, turning once, just until the shrimp turn pink, about 4 minutes. Divide the shrimp and slaw among 4 plates and serve at once.

Each serving: 12 g carb, 153 cal, 3 g fat, 0 g sat fat, 168 mg chol, 3 g fib, 20 g pro, 940 mg sod • Carb Choices: 1; Exchanges: 2 veg, 3 lean protein

Grilled Shrimp Kebabs with Summer Herb Sauce

makes 4 servings

Once you taste the lively fresh flavor of this herb sauce, you'll make it part of your summer grilling recipe rotation. Serve it with grilled fish, scallops, or chicken breasts.

¾ cup loosely packed fresh basil leaves

½ cup loosely packed fresh mint leaves

¼ cup thinly sliced scallions, green tops only

1 garlic clove, chopped

2 tablespoons plus ½ teaspoon extra virgin olive oil, divided

2 tablespoons cold water

1 tablespoon lemon Juice

¼ teaspoon kosher salt, divided

1 pound large peeled deveined shrimp

⅛ teaspoon freshly ground pepper

Lemon wedges

1 Combine the basil, mint, scallions, garlic, 2 tablespoons of the oil, the water, lemon juice, and ⅛ teaspoon of the salt in a food processor and process until smooth.

2 Place the shrimp in a medium shallow dish and drizzle with 1 tablespoon of the sauce. Toss the shrimp to coat. Cover and refrigerate 30 minutes. Transfer the remaining sauce to a bowl.

3 Preheat the grill to medium-high heat.

4 Thread the shrimp onto four 12-inch metal skewers. Brush the grill rack with the remaining ½ teaspoon oil. Sprinkle the shrimp with the remaining ⅛ teaspoon salt and the pepper. Place the kebabs on the grill and grill, turning once, just until the shrimp turn pink, about 3 minutes on each side.

5 Divide the kebabs among 4 plates. Drizzle evenly with the reserved sauce and serve with the lemon wedges.

Each serving: 2 g carb, 162 cal, 9 g fat, 1 g sat fat, 168 mg chol, 1 g fib, 19 g pro, 334 mg sod • Carb Choices: 0; Exchanges: 3 lean protein, 1½ fat

Shrimp and Leek Risotto

makes 6 servings

3 medium leeks, halved lengthwise, and thinly sliced

4 cups Chicken Stock (page 149) or low-sodium chicken broth

2 teaspoons extra virgin olive oil

1 cup Arborio rice

2 garlic cloves, minced

½ cup dry white wine

¼ teaspoon kosher salt

⅛ teaspoon freshly ground pepper

1 pound medium peeled deveined shrimp

2 tablespoons chopped fresh Italian parsley

2 teaspoons grated lemon zest

1 tablespoon lemon juice

1 Submerge the sliced leeks in a large bowl of water, lift them out and drain in a colander. Repeat, using fresh water, until no grit remains in the bottom of the bowl. Drain the leeks well.

2 Pour the stock into a medium saucepan and bring to a simmer over medium-high heat. Reduce the heat to low and keep the stock warm.

3 Heat a large saucepan over medium heat. Add the oil and tilt the pan to coat the bottom evenly. Add the leeks and cook, stirring often, until softened, 5 minutes. Add the rice and garlic and cook, stirring constantly, 2 minutes. Add the wine, salt, and pepper and cook, stirring often, until the wine is absorbed.

4 Add the stock, ½ cup at a time, stirring frequently, until the liquid is absorbed after each addition before adding more stock. When all the liquid is absorbed and the rice is tender, yet firm to the bite (about 20 minutes), add the shrimp and cook, stirring constantly, just until the shrimp turn pink, about 4 minutes.

5 Remove from the heat and stir in the parsley, lemon zest, and lemon juice. Spoon the risotto evenly into 6 shallow bowls and serve at once.

Each serving: 33 g carb, 247 cal, 3 g fat, 1 g sat fat, 115 mg chol, 2 g fib, 18 g pro, 279 mg sod • Carb Choices: 2; Exchanges: 2 starch, 3 lean protein, 0 fat

Shrimp, Asparagus, and Goat Cheese Risotto

makes 6 servings

4 cups Chicken Stock (page 149) or low-sodium chicken broth

2 teaspoons extra virgin olive oil

1 large onion, chopped

1 cup Arborio rice

continues on next page

2 garlic cloves, minced

¼ teaspoon kosher salt

⅛ teaspoon freshly ground pepper

1 pound medium peeled deveined shrimp

8 ounces asparagus, tough ends trimmed and spears cut into 1½-inch pieces

3 ounces crumbled goat cheese (about ¾ cup), at room temperature

2 teaspoons grated lemon zest

2 tablespoons lemon juice

2 tablespoons fresh chopped dill

1 Pour the stock into a medium saucepan and bring to a simmer over medium-high heat. Reduce the heat to low and keep the stock warm.

2 Heat a large saucepan over medium heat. Add the oil and tilt the pan to coat the bottom. Add the onion and cook, stirring often, 5 minutes. Add the rice and garlic and cook, stirring constantly, 2 minutes. Stir in the salt and pepper.

3 Add the stock, ½ cup at a time, stirring frequently, until the liquid is absorbed after each addition before adding more stock. When all the liquid is absorbed and the rice is tender, yet firm to the bite (about 20 minutes), add the shrimp and asparagus and cook, stirring constantly, just until the shrimp turn pink, 4 minutes.

4 Remove from the heat and stir in the goat cheese, lemon zest, lemon juice, and dill. Spoon the risotto evenly into 6 shallow bowls and serve at once.

Each serving: 31 g carb, 259 cal, 33 g fat, 3 g sat fat, 122 mg chol, 2 g fib, 21 g pro, 333 mg sod • Carb Choices: 2; Exchanges: 2 starch, 3 lean protein, 1 fat

Greek Shrimp Risotto

makes 6 servings

Zucchini, feta, and mint make a winning combination in this one-dish meal. Bring the feta to room temperature before adding it to the risotto so that it will melt into the dish easily.

4 cups Chicken Stock (page 149) or low-sodium chicken broth

2 teaspoons extra virgin olive oil

1 large sweet onion, chopped

1 cup Arborio rice

2 garlic cloves, minced

¼ teaspoon kosher salt

⅛ teaspoon freshly ground pepper

1 pound medium peeled deveined shrimp

1 medium zucchini, halved lengthwise and thinly sliced

2 ounces crumbled feta cheese (about ½ cup), at room temperature

2 teaspoons grated lemon zest

2 tablespoons lemon juice

1 tablespoon chopped fresh mint

1 tablespoon chopped fresh Italian parsley

1 Pour the stock into a medium saucepan and bring to a simmer over medium-high heat. Reduce the heat to low and keep the stock warm.

2 Heat a large saucepan over medium heat. Add the oil and tilt the pan to coat the bottom evenly. Add the onion and cook, stirring often, until softened, 5 minutes. Add the rice and garlic and cook, stirring constantly, 2 minutes. Stir in the salt and pepper.

3 Add the stock, ½ cup at a time, stirring frequently, until the liquid is absorbed after each addition before adding more stock. When all the liquid is absorbed and the rice is tender, yet firm to the bite (about 20 minutes), add the shrimp and zucchini and cook, stirring constantly, just until the shrimp turn pink and the squash is crisp-tender, about 4 minutes.

4 Remove from the heat and stir in the feta, lemon zest, lemon juice, mint, and parsley. Spoon the risotto evenly into 6 shallow bowls and serve at once.

Each serving: 32 g carb, 251 cal, 5 g fat, 2 g sat fat, 124 mg chol, 2 g fib, 20 g pro, 382 mg sod • Carb Choices: 2; Exchanges: 2 starch, 3 lean protein, 1 fat

Coconut Shrimp QUICK

makes 4 servings

This version of typically deep-fried shrimp cooks the shrimp in a small amount of canola oil in a nonstick skillet and gets high marks for flavor and healthfulness. The crust is sweet and crispy and the dish is still low in fat.

3 tablespoons cornstarch
¾ teaspoon kosher salt
⅛ teaspoon ground cayenne
2 large egg whites
2 tablespoons water
¾ cup panko crumbs
½ cup flaked sweetened coconut
1 pound large peeled deveined shrimp
6 teaspoons canola oil, divided

1 Preheat the oven to 200°F.

2 Combine the cornstarch, salt, and cayenne in a large resealable plastic bag. Place the egg whites and water in a shallow dish and beat lightly with a fork. Combine the panko crumbs and coconut in another shallow dish.

3 Place the shrimp in the plastic bag, seal the bag, and shake to coat evenly. Working with a few shrimp at a time, dip the shrimp into the egg white mixture, then into the crumb mixture, pressing to adhere.

4 Heat a large nonstick skillet over medium heat. Add 2 teaspoons of the oil and tilt the pan to coat the bottom evenly. Add about one-third of the shrimp and cook, turning once, until lightly browned, 2 to 3 minutes on each side. Watch the shrimp carefully and adjust the heat if they begin to brown too quickly. Transfer the shrimp to a small baking dish and place in the oven to keep warm. Repeat with the remaining oil and remaining shrimp in two more batches. Divide the shrimp evenly among 4 plates and serve at once.

Each serving: 19 g carb, 261 cal, 11 g fat, 3 g sat fat, 168 mg chol, 1 g fib, 22 g pro, 483 mg sod • Carb Choices: 1; Exchanges: 1 starch, 3 lean protein, 2 fat

Pan-Seared Scallops with Pineapple-Mango Salsa

QUICK

makes 4 servings

This tart fruit salsa makes a delicious paring for rich-tasting scallops. It's especially nice since mango and pineapple are flavorful even in the winter.

1 cup diced pineapple
1 medium mango, peeled, pitted, and diced
2 tablespoons minced red onion
1 tablespoon lime juice
1 tablespoon chopped fresh mint
4 teaspoons canola oil, divided
⅛ teaspoon plus ¼ teaspoon ground cumin, divided
⅛ teaspoon plus ¼ teaspoon ground coriander, divided
Pinch plus ½ teaspoon kosher salt
1 pound sea scallops
Lime wedges

1 Combine the pineapple, mango, onion, lime juice, mint, 2 teaspoons of the oil, ⅛ teaspoon of the cumin, ⅛ teaspoon of the coriander, and the pinch of salt in a large bowl and stir to mix well.

2 Pat the scallops dry and sprinkle with the remaining ½ teaspoon salt, remaining ¼ teaspoon cumin, and remaining ¼ teaspoon coriander. Heat a large skillet over medium-high heat. Add the remaining 2 teaspoons oil and tilt the pan to coat the bottom evenly. Add the scallops and cook, turning once, until just opaque in the centers, about 1½ minutes on each side. Divide

continues on next page

the scallops and salsa among 4 plates and serve at once with the lime wedges.

Each serving: 17 g carb, 196 cal, 6 g fat, 0 g sat fat, 37 mg chol, 1 g fib, 20 g pro, 342 mg sod • Carb Choices: 1; Exchanges: 1 fruit, 3 lean protein, 1 fat

Scallops with Brown Butter–Caper Sauce QUICK

makes 4 servings

Nothing could be simpler than this recipe. The only possible place for error is overbrowning the butter—you want it to be just lightly golden brown and starting to smell nutty before adding the capers and lemon juice.

1 pound sea scallops
½ teaspoon kosher salt
⅛ teaspoon plus pinch of freshly ground pepper, divided
2 teaspoons canola oil
2 tablespoons unsalted butter
1 tablespoon capers, rinsed and drained
1 tablespoon lemon juice

1 Pat the scallops dry and sprinkle with the salt and ⅛ teaspoon of the pepper. Heat a large skillet over medium-high heat. Add the oil and tilt the pan to coat the bottom evenly. Add the scallops and cook, turning once, until just opaque in the centers, about 1½ minutes on each side. Transfer the scallops to a plate and cover loosely with foil to keep warm.

2 Reduce the heat to medium and add the butter to the skillet. Cook, stirring constantly, until the butter is fragrant and lightly browned, about 3 minutes. Stir in the capers, lemon juice, and remaining pinch of pepper. Add any accumulated juices from the scallops to the skillet. Divide the scallops evenly among 4 plates, drizzle evenly with the sauce, and serve at once.

Each serving: 3 g carb, 172 cal, 9 g fat, 4 g sat fat, 52 mg chol, 0 g fib, 19 g pro, 387 mg sod • Carb Choices: 0; Exchanges: 3 lean protein, 1½ fat

Scallops in Cucumber-Dill Broth QUICK

makes 4 servings

This sophisticated dish of warm scallops and crunchy cucumbers in a cool cucumber broth looks like it took hours to make, but it's ready in less than 30 minutes. It's perfect for summer entertaining.

2 large hothouse (English) cucumbers
2 tablespoons lemon juice
1 tablespoon chopped fresh dill
2 teaspoons sugar
Pinch plus ½ teaspoon kosher salt, divided
1 pound sea scallops
¾ teaspoon ground coriander
⅛ teaspoon freshly ground pepper
2 teaspoons canola oil

1 Peel the cucumbers. Using a vegetable peeler, cut the flesh of one of the cucumbers into thin ribbons. Set the ribbons aside. Place the seeds from the cucumber in a food processor. Thickly slice the remaining cucumber and add to the food processor. Process until smooth.

2 Place a fine wire mesh strainer over a bowl and pour in the cucumber mixture. Press the mixture through the strainer, discarding the solids. Add the lemon juice, dill, sugar, and the pinch of salt to the cucumber broth and stir until the sugar dissolves.

3 Divide the cucumber ribbons evenly among 4 shallow bowls. Pour the cucumber broth evenly over the cucumbers.

4 Pat the scallops dry and sprinkle with the coriander, the remaining ½ teaspoon salt, and the pepper. Heat a large skillet over medium-high heat. Add the oil and tilt the pan to coat the bottom evenly. Add the scallops and cook, turning once, until just opaque in the centers, about

1½ minutes on each side. Divide the scallops evenly among 4 bowls and serve at once.

Each serving: 8 g carb, 123 cal, 3 g fat, 0 g sat fat, 28 mg chol, 1 g fib, 15 g pro, 298 mg sod • Carb Choices: ½; Exchanges: ½ carb, 3 lean protein, ½ fat

Baked Scallops au Gratin

QUICK

makes 4 servings

This recipe is from Julia Rutland, the food editor at *Coastal Living* magazine. In her job, Julia tries lots of great seafood recipes and this is one she turns to when she needs something that's really delicious, but super-easy to make. The crumb mixture seems wet when you stir it together, but it crisps when it bakes and is full of vibrant lemon-butter flavor. Try this recipe with large peeled and deveined shrimp, too.

½ teaspoon canola oil
1 pound sea scallops
⅔ cup panko crumbs
2 tablespoons unsalted butter, melted
2 tablespoons lemon juice
1 garlic clove, minced
½ teaspoon kosher salt
¼ teaspoon freshly ground pepper

1 Preheat the oven to 425°F. Brush a 13 x 9-inch baking dish with the oil.

2 Pat the scallops dry and place in the prepared baking dish.

3 Combine the panko crumbs, butter, lemon juice, garlic, salt, and pepper in a small bowl and stir until the crumbs are moistened. Sprinkle the crumb mixture over the scallops.

4 Bake until the scallops are opaque in the center and the crumbs are lightly browned, 15 to 18 minutes. Divide the scallops evenly among 4 plates, top evenly with any crumbs remaining in the dish, and serve at once.

Each serving: 11 g carb, 194 cal, 7 g fat, 4 g sat fat, 52 mg chol, 0 g fib, 21 g pro, 346 mg sod • Carb Choices: ½; Exchanges: ½ starch, 3 lean protein, 1 fat

Grilled Scallops with Ponzu Sauce QUICK

makes 4 servings

Ponzu sauce is a traditional Japanese sauce that is served with grilled meats, poultry, and seafood. This version is simple to make from supermarket ingredients. If you don't have mirin, the sweet Japanese rice wine, you can substitute white wine in this recipe.

2 tablespoons lime juice
2 tablespoons lemon juice
2 tablespoons reduced-sodium soy sauce
1 tablespoon mirin
1 tablespoon sugar
¼ teaspoon Asian fish sauce
1 pound sea scallops
½ teaspoon canola oil
Thinly sliced scallions
Chopped fresh cilantro

1 Preheat the grill to medium-high heat.

2 Whisk together the lime juice, lemon juice, soy sauce, mirin, sugar, and fish sauce in a small bowl.

3 Place the scallops in a medium shallow dish. Add 1 tablespoon of the sauce and toss to coat. Cover and refrigerate 15 minutes.

4 Brush the grill rack with the oil. Remove the scallops from the marinade and discard the marinade. Pat the scallops dry and place on the grill. Grill, turning once, just until the scallops are opaque in the center, 2 to 3 minutes.

5 Divide the scallops among 4 plates and drizzle with the remaining sauce. Sprinkle with the scallions and cilantro and serve at once.

Each serving: 9 g carb, 134 cal, 1 g fat, 0 g sat fat, 37 mg chol, 0 g fib, 20 g pro, 514 mg sod • Carb Choices: ½; Exchanges: ½ carb, 3 lean protein

Steamed Clams or Mussels with Wine and Garlic QUICK

makes 4 servings

If you like to order steamed clams or mussels in a restaurant but have never made them at home, you'll be surprised at how easy it is. You can serve these on their own or over whole wheat linguini or fettuccini.

1 tablespoon extra virgin olive oil
4 garlic cloves, minced
1 cup dry white wine
1 tablespoon lemon juice
½ teaspoon salt
2 pounds small clams or mussels, scrubbed
2 tablespoons chopped fresh Italian parsley

1 Heat a large deep skillet over medium heat. Add the oil and tilt the pan to coat the bottom evenly. Add the garlic and cook, stirring constantly, until fragrant, 30 seconds.

2 Add the wine, lemon juice, and salt and bring to a boil. Add the clams or mussels, cover, and cook until the shells open, 2 to 3 minutes. Discard any clams or mussels that do not open.

3 Remove from the heat and stir in the parsley. Divide the clams or mussels evenly among 4 shallow bowls, spoon the broth evenly over them, and serve at once.

Each serving: 4 g carb, 136 cal, 4 g fat, 1 g sat fat, 23 mg chol, 0 g fib, 9 g pro, 180 mg sod • Carb Choices: 0; Exchanges: 1 lean protein, ½ fat

Clams or Mussels in Fresh Tomato Broth QUICK

makes 4 servings

Don't overlook clams and mussels as a weeknight dish. Though they have a reputation for being hard to cook, few foods are simpler or quicker to cook. Serve the shellfish and broth over pasta or with a slice of crusty bread.

2 teaspoons extra virgin olive oil
1 small onion, chopped
4 garlic cloves, minced
½ cup dry white wine
½ cup clam juice
1 tablespoon no-salt-added tomato paste
¼ teaspoon kosher salt
2 large tomatoes, coarsely chopped
⅛ teaspoon crushed red pepper
2 pounds small clams or mussels, scrubbed
¼ cup chopped fresh Italian parsley

1 Heat a large deep skillet over medium heat. Add the oil and tilt the pan to coat the bottom evenly. Add the onion and cook, stirring often, until softened, 5 minutes. Add the garlic and cook, stirring constantly, until fragrant, 30 seconds.

2 Add the wine, clam juice, tomato paste, and salt and stir until smooth. Stir in the tomatoes and crushed red pepper. Increase the heat to medium-high and bring to a boil. Add the clams or mussels, cover, and cook until the shells open, 2 to 3 minutes. Discard any clams or mussels that do not open.

3 Remove from the heat and stir in the parsley. Divide the clams or mussels evenly among 4 shallow bowls, spoon the tomato mixture evenly over them, and serve at once.

Each serving: 10 g carb, 129 cal, 3 g fat, 0 g sat fat, 24 mg chol, 2 g fib, 10 g pro, 184 mg sod • Carb Choices: ½; Exchanges: 1 veg, 1 lean protein, ½ fat

Clams or Mussels with Chorizo QUICK

makes 4 servings

A tiny bit of chorizo sausage infuses the broth with smoky flavor. If you can't easily find chorizo, use any type of cured sausage you have.

2 teaspoons extra virgin olive oil
1 cured chorizo sausage (about 3 ounces), casing removed, chopped

1 small red onion, halved lengthwise and thinly
   sliced
1 small red bell pepper, chopped
2 garlic cloves, minced
1 teaspoon smoked or regular paprika
¾ cup dry white wine
¾ cup Chicken Stock (page 149) or low-sodium
   chicken broth
¼ teaspoon kosher salt
2 pounds small clams or mussels, scrubbed
2 tablespoons chopped fresh cilantro

1 Heat a large deep skillet over medium heat.
Add the oil and tilt the pan to coat the bottom
evenly. Add the chorizo and cook, stirring often,
until lightly browned, about 3 minutes. Add the
onion and bell pepper and cook, stirring often,
until the vegetables are softened, 5 minutes.
Add the garlic and paprika and cook, stirring
constantly, until fragrant, 30 seconds.

2 Add the wine, stock, and salt. Increase the
heat to medium-high and bring to a boil. Add
the clams or mussels, cover, and cook until the
shells open, 2 to 3 minutes. Discard any clams or
mussels that do not open.

3 Remove from the heat and stir in the cilantro.
Divide the clams or mussels evenly among
4 shallow bowls, spoon the broth and sausage
mixture evenly over them, and serve at once.

Each serving: 6 g carb, 220 cal, 11 g fat, 4 g sat fat, 42 mg chol, 0 g fib,
15 g pro, 398 mg sod • Carb Choices: ½; Exchanges: ½ carb, 1 high-fat
protein, 1 lean protein, ½ fat

Clams or Mussels with Peppers and Feta QUICK

makes 4 servings

Steamed shellfish takes on a Greek flavor with
spicy pepperoncini peppers in the broth and a
sprinkle of feta cheese on top. I like to serve
this as a starter for a dinner party in small bowls
with a slice of crusty bread. As a first course,
this dish will serve six to eight guests.

2 teaspoons extra virgin olive oil
1 small onion, halved lengthwise and thinly sliced
1 small yellow bell pepper, chopped
4 garlic cloves, minced
¾ cup dry white wine
¾ cup Chicken Stock (page 149) or low-sodium
   chicken broth
2 pepperoncini peppers, drained and chopped
2 pounds small clams or mussels, scrubbed
2 tablespoons chopped fresh Italian parsley
2 ounces finely crumbled feta cheese
   (about ½ cup)

1 Heat a large deep skillet over medium heat.
Add the oil and tilt the pan to coat the bottom
evenly. Add the onion and bell pepper and cook,
stirring often, until softened, 5 minutes. Add the
garlic and cook, stirring constantly, until fragrant,
30 seconds.

2 Add the wine, stock, and pepperoncini.
Increase the heat to medium-high and bring to a
boil. Add the clams or mussels, cover, and cook
until the shells open, 2 to 3 minutes. Discard any
clams or mussels that do not open.

3 Remove from the heat and stir in the parsley.
Divide the clams or mussels evenly among
4 shallow bowls. Spoon the broth and vegetables evenly over them, sprinkle evenly with the
feta, and serve at once.

Each serving: 7 g carb, 168 cal, 6 g fat, 3 g sat fat, 36 mg chol, 1 g fib, 12 g
pro, 353 mg sod • Carb Choices: ½; Exchanges: 1 veg, 2 lean protein, 1 fat

Chesapeake Crab Cakes

QUICK

makes 8 servings

Fresh lump crabmeat doesn't need much to
turn it into a delicious crab cake. In this recipe,
a little mayonnaise and just a touch of breadcrumbs hold the crabmeat together. And a dab
of mustard and squeeze of lemon accentuate

continues on next page

rather than detract from the luxurious crab-meat. These sumptuous crab cakes are worthy of any special dinner or celebration.

1 teaspoon canola oil
½ cup mayonnaise
1 large egg
2 teaspoons Dijon mustard
1 teaspoon grated lemon zest
1 tablespoon lemon juice
1 teaspoon Old Bay seasoning
1½ pounds fresh lump crabmeat
¼ cup plain dry breadcrumbs
1 tablespoon chopped fresh Italian parsley
Lemon wedges

1 Preheat the oven to 350°F. Brush a large rimmed baking sheet with the oil.

2 Combine the mayonnaise, egg, mustard, lemon zest, lemon juice, and Old Bay seasoning in a large bowl and whisk until smooth. Add the crabmeat, breadcrumbs, and parsley and stir gently to mix well.

3 Shape into 8 cakes, using a generous ¼ cup of the crab mixture for each cake. Arrange in a single layer on the prepared baking sheet and bake until lightly browned, about 18 minutes. Divide the crab cakes evenly among 8 plates and serve at once with the lemon wedges.

Each serving: 3 g carb, 231 cal, 13 g fat, 2 g sat fat, 128 mg chol, 0 g fib, 22 g pro, 548 mg sod • Carb Choices: 0; Exchanges: 3 lean protein, 2 fat

Easy Seafood Paella

makes 6 servings

You can vary the seafood in this dish depending on what is freshest when you go to the market. You can make it with all clams, all mussels, or instead of the shellfish, use a pound of firm fish such as halibut. If you use fish, follow the instructions here for the shellfish. Cut the fish into cubes and add it with the tomato in step 5—it will cook in about the same amount of time as the clams and shrimp.

½ cup dry white wine
⅛ teaspoon saffron threads, crushed
1 cured chorizo sausage (about 3 ounces), casing removed, thinly sliced
1 small onion, chopped
1 small red bell pepper, chopped
2 garlic cloves, minced
½ teaspoon smoked or hot paprika
1 (8-ounce) bottle clam juice
1 cup Chicken Stock (page 149) or low-sodium chicken broth
1 cup Arborio rice
18 littleneck or cherrystone clams, scrubbed
12 ounces medium peeled deveined shrimp
1 large tomato, chopped

1 Combine the wine and saffron in a small bowl and let stand to soak.

2 Meanwhile, set a large deep skillet over medium heat. Add the chorizo slices and cook, stirring often, until browned, about 5 minutes. Transfer to a plate.

3 Add the onion and bell pepper to the drippings remaining in the skillet and cook, stirring often, until softened, 5 minutes. Add the garlic and paprika and cook, stirring constantly, until fragrant, 30 seconds.

4 Stir in the clam juice, stock, rice, cooked chorizo, and wine mixture and bring to a boil. Cover, reduce the heat to low, and cook until most of the liquid is absorbed, about 15 minutes.

5 Stir in the clams, shrimp, and tomato. Cover and cook until the shrimp turn pink and the clams open, about 4 minutes. Discard any clams that do not open. Divide the paella evenly among 6 plates and serve at once.

Each serving: 30 g carb, 274 cal, 7 g fat, 2 g sat fat, 106 mg chol, 2 g fib, 19 g pro, 396 mg sod • Carb Choices: 2; Exchanges: 2 starch, 2 lean protein, 1 fat

Whole Fish

Whole Roasted Fish with Chermoula Sauce QUICK

makes 4 servings

I understand the trepidation cooks have about cooking a whole fish, and if I didn't do it so often, I would, too. My husband fishes every chance he gets, and if you or someone in your family fishes, you also know the pleasures of cooking fresh whole fish. Nothing could be simpler to make.

2 (2-pound) dressed whole striped bass or
    other small whole fish
2 teaspoons ground cumin, divided
2 teaspoons paprika, divided
1 teaspoon kosher salt, divided
¼ cup loosely packed fresh Italian parsley
¼ cup loosely packed fresh cilantro leaves
3 tablespoons cold water
2 tablespoons extra virgin olive oil
2 tablespoons lemon juice
2 garlic cloves, coarsely chopped
Pinch of ground cayenne pepper

1 Preheat the oven to 400°F.

2 To make the fish, cut 3 diagonal slits in each side of each of the fish. Sprinkle evenly all over with 1 teaspoon of the cumin, 1 teaspoon of the paprika, and ½ teaspoon of the salt. Place the fish in a single layer in a large baking dish. Pour just enough water into the dish to cover the bottom. Bake the fish, uncovered, until the fish flakes easily with a fork, 20 to 25 minutes.

3 Meanwhile, combine the parsley, cilantro, water, oil, lemon juice, garlic, cayenne, remaining 1 teaspoon cumin, remaining 1 teaspoon paprika, and remaining ½ teaspoon salt in a food processor and process until the mixture is finely chopped.

4 Remove the skin from the top side of each of the fish and discard. Run a knife between the flesh and bones of the top half of the fish and lift off the fillet. Turn the fish over and repeat. Divide the fish evenly among 4 plates and drizzle evenly with the sauce.

Each serving: 2 g carb, 214 cal, 10 g fat, 2 g sat fat, 62 mg chol, 0 g fib, 28 g pro, 386 mg sod • Carb Choices: 0; Exchanges: 4 lean protein, 1 fat

Salt-Crusted Baked Whole Fish QUICK

makes 2 servings

A fish prepared in a salt crust will be the most flavorful and moist version you'll ever eat.

4 sprigs fresh rosemary
1 lime, thinly sliced
1 (2-pound) dressed whole striped bass or
    other small whole fish
8 cups kosher salt (about 1½ pounds)
1½ cups cool water
Lime wedges

1 Preheat the oven to 450°F.

2 Place the rosemary sprigs and the lime slices inside the cavity of the fish.

3 Stir together the salt and water in a large bowl. Spread half of the salt into a rectangular shape just larger than the fish onto a large rimmed baking sheet. Place the fish on the salt. Pat the remaining salt mixture over the fish to cover it completely.

4 Bake 30 minutes. Tap around the edge of the salt crust using a meat mallet. Loosen the top of the crust and lift off. Remove the skin from the top side of the fish and discard. Run a knife between the flesh and bones of the top half of the fish and lift off the fillet. Turn the fish over and repeat. Divide the fish evenly among 2 plates and serve at once with the lime wedges.

Each serving: 0 g carb, 144 cal, 3 g fat, 1 g sat fat, 62 mg chol, 0 g fib, 27 g pro, 381 mg sod • Carb Choices: 0; Exchanges: 4 lean protein

Whole Grilled Trout with Tarragon and Lemon QUICK

makes 4 servings

If you have a grill basket, it is convenient to put the fish inside one to make this dish, but it isn't at all necessary. Just be careful when you turn the fish and use a long spatula. You can use any herb you have on hand to stuff the fish—basil, rosemary, thyme, or mint—you can't go wrong with this simple recipe.

½ teaspoon canola oil
4 (7- to 8-ounce) dressed whole trout
¾ teaspoon kosher salt
¼ teaspoon freshly ground pepper
1 large lemon, thinly sliced
4 large sprigs fresh tarragon

1 Preheat the grill to medium-high heat. Brush the grill rack with the oil.

2 Cut 3 diagonal slits in each side of each of the trout. Sprinkle evenly all over with the salt and pepper. Divide the lemon slices evenly among the cavities of the fish and place a tarragon sprig inside each one.

3 Place the fish on the grill rack and grill, turning once, until the fish flakes easily with a fork, 4 to 5 minutes on each side. Place the fish on 4 plates and serve at once.

Each serving: 0 g carb, 169 cal, 7 g fat, 2 g sat fat, 75 mg chol, 0 g fib, 25 g pro, 271 mg sod • Carb Choices: 0; Exchanges: 3 lean protein

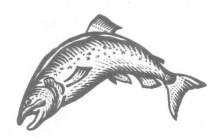

Vegetarian Main Dishes

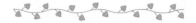

Pasta

Sharp Cheddar Macaroni and Cheese

Macaroni and Cheese Primavera

Tex-Mex Macaroni and Cheese

Pasta Primavera

Pasta with Tomatoes, Baby Spinach, and Feta

Pasta with Artichokes and Tomatoes

Pasta and Zucchini with Creamy Parmesan-Yogurt Sauce

Linguini and Tomatoes with Creamy Ricotta Sauce

Pasta with Squash, Sugar Snaps, and Ricotta Salata

Pasta with Zucchini Ribbons, Tomatoes, and Mint

Pasta with Spinach, Almonds, and Brown Butter

Pasta with Broccoli Rabe and Caramelized Garlic

Pasta with Eggplant and Arugula Sauce

Pasta and Tomatoes with Broccoli Sauce

Pasta with Ricotta and Roasted Tomato Sauce

Pasta, Vegetable, and Goat Cheese Gratin

Lasagna with Greens and Ricotta

Individual Spinach Lasagnas

Manicotti with Ricotta and Kale

Grains

Beet and Barley Chili

Barley Risotto with Asparagus and Peas

Barley Risotto with Summer Squash, Tomatoes, and Pesto

Barley Risotto with Mushrooms and Gorgonzola

Barley and Eggplant–Stuffed Peppers

Portobello Mushrooms Stuffed with Barley and Gruyère

Crisp Polenta Squares with Tomato-Roasted Red Pepper Sauce

Layered Polenta and Vegetable Casserole

Tex-Mex Cheddar, Polenta, and Vegetable Casserole

Polenta-Topped Ratatouille Casserole

Spicy Green Tamale Tart

Farro Risotto with Cherry Tomatoes, Feta, and Herbs

Mushroom and Bulgur–Stuffed Cabbage

Portobello Mushrooms with Couscous, Spinach, and Feta Stuffing

Polenta-Stuffed Portobellos

Quinoa Cakes with Fresh
Tomato–Cilantro Sauce

Basil Quinoa with
Pan-Roasted Tomatoes
and Goat Cheese

Beans

Black and White Bean Chili

Quick Lentil Chili

White Bean, Artichoke, and
Zucchini Stew

Bean and Vegetable Stew
with Crispy Breadcrumbs

Chunky Edamame and
Vegetable Stew

Moroccan Bean Stew

Garbanzo Picadillo

Red Beans and Greens

Lentil and Root
Vegetable Stew

Black Bean Burritos with
Creamy Avocado Sauce

Black Bean and
Poblano Enchiladas

Black Bean and Avocado
Chiles Rellenos

Bean and Spinach Cakes
with Cucumber-Cilantro
Yogurt Sauce

Falafel Burgers

Chipotle Black Bean
Burgers

Tofu

Tofu, Mushroom, and
Broccoli Stir-Fry

Curried Tofu and
Vegetable Stir-Fry

Teriyaki Tofu Stir-Fry

Crispy Tofu with Spicy
Ginger-Lime Soy Sauce

Tofu Baked with Soy,
Ginger, and Garlic

Sesame-Roasted Tofu and
Vegetables with Asian Pesto

Italian Tofu

Eggs and Cheese

Eggplant Rollatini

Mushroom and Fontina
Bread Pudding

Caramelized Onion and Red
Pepper Bread Pudding

Autumn Greens Tart

Leek and Caramelized
Garlic Tart

Crustless Asparagus and
Feta Tart

Most people reading this book aren't vegetarians and probably have no desire to become vegetarian. And that's okay. You don't have to be a full-time vegetarian to reap the benefits of a few meatless meals every week. Don't think of vegetarian meals as lacking in meat, think of them as fiber-rich, nutrient-dense, low-calorie meals that are absolutely delicious!

Replacing some meat-centered meals with lunches and dinners that include foods like dried beans, whole grains, whole wheat pasta, tofu, eggs, and a small amount of cheese will translate into a diet that is higher in fiber, good-for-you carbs, and disease-fighting phytochemicals.

If you are passionate about eating meat, start by having one or two meatless meals a week and try to work your way up slowly to at least three or four a week. If you can't imagine having dinner without meat, then plan a couple of vegetarian lunches into your schedule every week.

If you're worried that you and your family won't get enough protein, you have nothing to be concerned about. Proteins from plants will meet your body's requirements as long as you eat a variety of plant foods. And what about the myth that you have to eat certain complementary foods together to get a "complete protein"? Not true. Even if you are a vegan, meaning that you eat no animal products at all including eggs or cheese, your body will make its own complete protein if you get enough variety in your diet and consume enough calories.

Not only are there health benefits of eating a few meatless meals each week, but you'll be doing your budget and the environment a favor, too. When beans, grains, and pasta are on your shopping list, you'll pay significantly less than when you're shopping for meat, poultry, and seafood. And growing grains and vegetables is more efficient and creates less greenhouse gases than producing meat.

These are all legitimate reasons to eat more vegetables, but the best reason to try the recipes in this chapter is that you'll love how they taste.

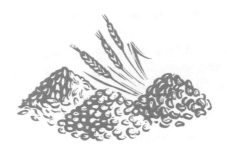

Pasta

Sharp Cheddar Macaroni and Cheese

makes 4 servings

Macaroni and cheese is a staple at my house—at least once a week it finds a place at the table for lunch or dinner. Baking mac and cheese with a crispy crumb crust on top makes it special, but if you are strapped for time, you can skip the crumbs and the baking step.

1 teaspoon canola oil

6 ounces whole wheat macaroni or other short pasta (about 2 cups)

¾ cup 1% low-fat milk

1 tablespoon unbleached all-purpose flour

4 ounces shredded extra-sharp Cheddar cheese (about 1 cup)

2 tablespoons reduced-fat cream cheese (about 1 ounce)

¼ teaspoon kosher salt

¼ teaspoon freshly ground pepper

2 tablespoons plain dry breadcrumbs

1 teaspoon unsalted butter, softened

2 tablespoons freshly grated Parmesan

1 Preheat the oven to 350°F. Brush an 8-inch square baking dish with the oil.

2 Cook the pasta according to the package directions. Transfer to a bowl and keep warm.

3 Meanwhile, combine the milk and flour in a medium saucepan and whisk until smooth. Cook over medium heat, whisking constantly, until the mixture comes to a boil and thickens, about 5 minutes.

4 Remove from the heat. Add the Cheddar, cream cheese, salt, and pepper and whisk until smooth. Add the sauce to the macaroni and stir until well combined.

5 Transfer to the prepared baking dish. Combine the breadcrumbs and butter in a small bowl. Using your fingers, blend the butter evenly into the breadcrumbs. Stir in the Parmesan. Sprinkle the breadcrumb mixture over the pasta and bake until bubbly and heated through, about 25 minutes. Let stand 5 minutes before serving. Divide evenly among 4 plates and serve at once.

Each serving: 38 g carb, 345 cal, 15 g fat, 9 g sat fat, 38 mg chol, 3 g fib, 16 g pro, 365 mg sod • Carb Choices: 2½; Exchanges: 2½ starch, 1 high-fat protein

Macaroni and Cheese Primavera QUICK | HIGH FIBER

makes 4 servings

This veggie-packed mild-flavored mac and cheese is a smart way to get kids to eat their vegetables. For adults or adventurous children, you can make this with a more flavorful cheese such as Gruyère, fontina, or goat cheese.

2 cups loosely packed fresh baby spinach

6 ounces whole wheat macaroni or other short pasta (about 2 cups)

1 cup small broccoli florets

1 cup chopped yellow squash or zucchini

½ cup chopped red bell pepper

¾ cup 1% low-fat milk

1 tablespoon unbleached all-purpose flour

4 ounces shredded mozzarella (about 1 cup)

1 ounce reduced-fat cream cheese (about 2 tablespoons)

¼ teaspoon kosher salt

¼ teaspoon freshly ground pepper

1 Place the spinach in a colander in a sink. Cook the pasta according to the package directions, adding the broccoli, squash, and bell pepper during the last 2 minutes of cooking. Drain the pasta mixture into the colander. Transfer the pasta mixture to a bowl and keep warm.

2 Meanwhile, combine the milk and flour in a medium saucepan and whisk until smooth. Cook over medium heat, whisking constantly, until the mixture comes to a boil and thickens, about 5 minutes.

3 Remove from the heat. Add the mozzarella, cream cheese, salt, and ground pepper and whisk until smooth. Add the sauce to the pasta mixture and stir until well combined. Divide evenly among 4 plates and serve at once.

Each serving: 39 g carb, 328 cal, 12 g fat, 6 g sat fat, 31 mg chol, 5 g fib, 19 g pro, 427 mg sod • Carb Choices: 2½; Exchanges: 2 starch, 1 veg, 1 medium-fat protein

Tex-Mex Macaroni and Cheese HIGH FIBER

makes 4 servings

This is my cheese-loving husband's favorite macaroni and cheese when he's in the mood for something that veers from the classic rendition of the dish. With smoky, spicy chipotles, tomatoes, and cilantro, it is full of flavor. You can double the recipe to make a crowd-pleasing dish for a pot luck.

1 teaspoon canola oil

6 ounces whole wheat macaroni or other short
    pasta (about 2 cups)

¾ cup 1% low-fat milk

1 tablespoon unbleached all-purpose flour

1 teaspoon minced chipotle in adobo sauce

¼ teaspoon ground cumin

¼ teaspoon kosher salt

4 ounces shredded reduced-fat Monterey Jack
    cheese (about 1 cup)

1 ounce reduced-fat cream cheese
    (about 2 tablespoons)

1 (14½-ounce) can no-salt added diced
    tomatoes, drained

¼ cup thinly sliced scallions

2 tablespoons chopped fresh cilantro

2 tablespoons plain dry breadcrumbs

1 teaspoon unsalted butter, softened

2 tablespoons freshly grated Parmesan

1 Preheat the oven to 350°F. Brush an 8-inch square baking dish with the oil.

2 Cook the pasta according to the package directions. Transfer to a bowl and keep warm.

3 Meanwhile, combine the milk, flour, chipotle, cumin, and salt in a medium saucepan and whisk until smooth. Cook over medium heat, whisking constantly, until the mixture comes to a boil and thickens, about 5 minutes.

4 Remove from the heat. Add the Monterey Jack and cream cheese and whisk until smooth. Add the sauce to the pasta and stir until well combined. Stir in the tomatoes, scallions, and cilantro.

5 Transfer to the prepared baking dish. Combine the breadcrumbs and butter in a small bowl. Using your fingers, blend the butter evenly into the breadcrumbs. Stir in the Parmesan. Sprinkle the breadcrumb mixture over the pasta and bake until bubbly and heated through, about 25 minutes. Let stand 5 minutes before serving. Divide evenly among 4 plates and serve at once.

Each serving: 41 g carb, 343 cal, 12 g fat, 6 g sat fat, 31 mg chol, 6 g fib, 18 g pro, 538 mg sod • Carb Choices: 3; Exchanges: 2½ starch, 1 veg, 1 high-fat protein

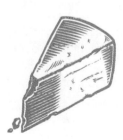

Pasta Primavera $\boxed{\text{QUICK} \mid \text{HIGH FIBER}}$

makes 4 servings

Pasta primavera can be a multistep process hardly worth the effort for the simple dish that it is. In my streamlined version, I cook all the vegetables in the same pot with the pasta, making this a dish that I actually have time to make for dinner. The creamy sauce is made with two cheeses—Parmesan for its sharp flavor and cream cheese for rich creamy texture.

6 ounces whole wheat penne or other short pasta (about 2 cups)

1 pound asparagus, tough ends removed and spears cut into 2-inch pieces

1 red bell pepper, cut into short, thin strips

1 medium yellow squash, halved lengthwise and sliced

½ cup shelled English peas or unthawed frozen petite green peas

½ cup 1% low-fat milk

1 garlic clove, crushed through a press

½ teaspoon kosher salt

¼ teaspoon freshly ground pepper

2 ounces (about ½ cup) plus 2 tablespoons freshly grated Parmesan, divided

¼ cup reduced-fat cream cheese, cut into small pieces

¼ cup chopped fresh basil or Italian parsley

2 teaspoons grated lemon zest

1 Cook the pasta according to the package directions, adding the asparagus, bell pepper, squash, and peas during the last 3 minutes of cooking. Drain and transfer to a large bowl and keep warm.

2 Meanwhile, combine the milk, garlic, salt, and ground pepper in a small saucepan. Set over medium heat until hot (do not boil). Remove from the heat and add ½ cup of the Parmesan and the cream cheese. Whisk until smooth. Add the milk mixture, basil, and lemon zest to the pasta mixture and toss to coat.

3 To serve, divide the pasta mixture evenly among 4 plates. Sprinkle evenly with the remaining 2 tablespoons Parmesan and serve at once.

Each serving: 38 g carb, 293 cal, 8 g fat, 5 g sat fat, 21 mg chol, 8 g fib, 18 g pro, 401 mg sod • Carb Choices: 2; Exchanges: 1½ starch, 1 veg, 1 medium-fat protein

Pasta with Tomatoes, Baby Spinach, and Feta

$\boxed{\text{QUICK} \mid \text{HIGH FIBER}}$

makes 4 servings

When you don't feel like cooking, this is an easy dish to put together. Fresh tomatoes and a sprinkle of feta make it extra flavorful. If you halve the recipe, it makes a light and colorful pasta side dish.

6 ounces whole wheat penne or other short pasta (about 2 cups)

4 cups loosely packed fresh baby spinach

2 teaspoons extra virgin olive oil

2 garlic cloves, minced

2 large tomatoes, chopped

¼ teaspoon kosher salt

⅛ teaspoon freshly ground pepper

2 ounces finely crumbled feta cheese (about ½ cup)

1 Cook the pasta according to the package directions.

2 Place the spinach in a large serving bowl. Drain the pasta and add to the bowl with the spinach. Keep warm.

3 Meanwhile, heat a medium skillet over medium heat. Add the oil and tilt the pan to coat the bottom evenly. Add the garlic and cook, stirring constantly, until fragrant, 30 seconds. Add the tomatoes and cook, stirring often, just until heated through. Stir in the salt and pepper. Add the tomato mixture to the pasta mixture and toss to combine.

4 To serve, divide the pasta mixture evenly among 4 plates. Sprinkle evenly with the feta and serve at once.

Each serving: 31 g carb, 225 cal, 6 g fat, 3 g sat fat, 13 mg chol, 6 g fib, 10 g pro, 259 mg sod • Carb Choices: 2; Exchanges: 1½ starch, 1 veg, 1 medium-fat protein, ½ fat

Pasta with Artichokes and Tomatoes QUICK | HIGH FIBER

makes 4 servings

You've probably got the ingredients to make this dish in your kitchen right now. It's a great weeknight standby that's ready in about 20 minutes. You can speed up the cooking even more if you use fresh whole wheat pasta.

6 ounces whole wheat penne or other short pasta (about 2 cups)

2 teaspoons extra virgin olive oil

1 small red onion, thinly sliced

2 garlic cloves, minced

2 medium tomatoes, chopped

1 (14-ounce) can artichoke hearts, drained and quartered

¼ cup dry white wine

1 tablespoon capers, rinsed and drained

⅛ teaspoon freshly ground pepper

2 tablespoons chopped fresh Italian parsley

1 ounce freshly grated Parmesan (about ¼ cup)

1 Cook the pasta according to the package directions. Transfer to a large bowl and keep warm.

2 Meanwhile, heat a large skillet over medium heat. Add the oil and tilt the pan to coat the bottom evenly. Add the onion and cook, stirring often, until softened, 5 minutes. Add the garlic and cook, stirring constantly, until fragrant, 30 seconds. Add the tomatoes, artichokes, wine, and capers and bring to a boil. Reduce the heat and simmer until the tomatoes are softened,

5 minutes. Remove from the heat and stir in the parsley.

3 Add the sauce to the pasta and toss to combine. Divide the pasta among 4 shallow bowls, sprinkle evenly with the Parmesan and serve at once.

Each serving: 37 g carb, 253 cal, 5 g fat, 2 g sat fat, 4 mg chol, 6 g fib, 12 g pro, 372 mg sod • Carb Choices: 2; Exchanges: 1½ starch, 1 veg, ½ fat

Pasta and Zucchini with Creamy Parmesan-Yogurt Sauce QUICK | HIGH FIBER

makes 4 servings

Thick and creamy Greek yogurt makes an easy no-cook pasta sauce that tastes like it has twice the fat and calories that it actually does. You can add chopped fresh tomatoes or halved cherry tomatoes to this dish if you wish.

6 ounces whole wheat penne or other short pasta (about 2 cups)

2 medium zucchini, cut into short, thin strips

½ cup plain low-fat Greek yogurt or strained yogurt (page 11)

2 ounces freshly grated Parmesan (about ½ cup)

⅛ teaspoon kosher salt

⅛ teaspoon freshly ground pepper

2 tablespoons chopped fresh basil

1 Cook the pasta according to the package directions, adding the zucchini during the last 2 minutes of cooking. Drain.

2 Meanwhile, stir together the yogurt, Parmesan, salt, and pepper in a large bowl. Add the hot pasta mixture and toss to coat. Add the basil and toss to combine. Divide the pasta evenly among 4 shallow bowls and serve at once.

Each serving: 30 g carb, 221 cal, 4 g fat, 3 g sat fat, 11 mg chol, 6 g fib, 14 g pro, 207 mg sod • Carb Choices: 2; Exchanges: 1½ starch, 1 veg

Linguini and Tomatoes with Creamy Ricotta Sauce QUICK | HIGH FIBER

makes 4 servings

If you only use ricotta for making lasagna, this recipe is a fresh new use for the mild-flavored cheese. When hot linguini is tossed with the ricotta, it softens and turns into a creamy sauce that clings to the pasta.

6 ounces whole wheat linguini or other long, thin pasta

⅔ cup part-skim ricotta

1 ounce (about ¼ cup) plus 2 tablespoons freshly grated Parmesan, divided

¼ cup chopped fresh basil

1 garlic clove, crushed through a press

¼ teaspoon kosher salt

⅛ teaspoon freshly ground pepper

2 large tomatoes, chopped

1 Cook the pasta according to the package directions. Drain and keep warm, reserving ⅓ cup of the cooking water.

2 Meanwhile, stir together the ricotta, ¼ cup of the Parmesan, the basil, garlic, salt, and pepper in a large bowl. Add the hot pasta and toss to coat. Add the reserved pasta cooking water 1 tablespoon at a time, as needed, to make a smooth sauce. Add the tomatoes and toss gently to combine.

3 To serve, divide the pasta mixture evenly among 4 plates. Sprinkle evenly with the remaining 2 tablespoons Parmesan and serve at once.

Each serving: 37 g carb, 252 cal, 6 g fat, 3 g sat fat, 19 mg chol, 6 g fib, 15 g pro, 245 mg sod • Carb Choices: 2; Exchanges: 1½ starch, 1 veg, 1 medium-fat protein

Pasta with Squash, Sugar Snaps, and Ricotta Salata QUICK | HIGH FIBER

makes 4 servings

This is a quick summer dish that's ready in the time it takes to cook the pasta. Ricotta salata is a salty Italian sheep's milk cheese. If you can't find it easily, you can substitute crumbled feta cheese.

6 ounces whole wheat penne or other short pasta (about 2 cups)

1 medium yellow squash, halved lengthwise and sliced

12 ounces sugar snap peas, trimmed

2 teaspoons grated lemon zest

3 tablespoons lemon juice

2 tablespoons chopped fresh dill or Italian parsley

¼ teaspoon kosher salt

⅛ teaspoon freshly ground pepper

2 ounces crumbled ricotta salata (about ½ cup)

1 Cook the pasta according to the package directions, adding the squash and peas during the last 4 minutes of cooking. Drain and transfer to a large bowl.

2 Add the lemon zest, lemon juice, dill, salt, and pepper and toss to combine.

3 To serve, divide the pasta mixture evenly among 4 plates. Sprinkle evenly with the ricotta salata and serve at once.

Each serving: 36 g carb, 239 cal, 5 g fat, 3 g sat fat, 15 mg chol, 7 g fib, 12 g pro, 322 mg sod • Carb Choices: 2; Exchanges: 2 starch, 1 fat

Pasta with Zucchini Ribbons, Tomatoes, and Mint QUICK | HIGH FIBER

makes 4 servings

This fresh summery recipe is a delicious way to use up a bounty of zucchini. If you have children old enough to use a vegetable peeler (safely), they'll think it's fun to make the zucchini ribbons. Instead of mint, you can use basil, dill, parsley, or cilantro. And try crumbled goat cheese instead of the feta.

2 medium zucchini
6 ounces whole wheat linguini or other long thin pasta
1 large tomato, chopped
1 teaspoon grated lemon zest
1 tablespoon lemon juice
½ teaspoon kosher salt
2 tablespoons chopped fresh mint
2 ounces finely crumbled feta cheese (about ½ cup)

1 Using a vegetable peeler, cut the zucchini into long, thin ribbons. Set aside.

2 Cook the pasta according to the package directions, adding the zucchini during the last 2 minutes of cooking. Drain and keep warm.

3 Meanwhile, stir together the tomato, lemon zest, lemon juice, and salt in a large bowl. Add the hot pasta mixture and toss to coat. Add the mint and toss to combine.

4 To serve, divide the pasta mixture evenly among 4 plates. Sprinkle evenly with the feta and serve at once.

Each serving: 37 g carb, 219 cal, 5 g fat, 3 g sat fat, 17 mg chol, 7 g fib, 10 g pro, 357 mg sod • Carb Choices: 2; Exchanges: 1½ starch, 1 veg, 1 fat

Pasta with Spinach, Almonds, and Brown Butter QUICK | HIGH FIBER

makes 4 servings

Almonds browned in a small amount of butter add rich flavor and nutty crunch to this simple pasta recipe. It's super-easy to make, but watch the almonds carefully as they cook and reduce the heat if they begin to brown too quickly.

6 ounces whole wheat penne or other short pasta (about 2 cups)
2 tablespoons unsalted butter
2 tablespoons slivered almonds
2 garlic cloves, minced
8 ounces fresh spinach, trimmed and chopped
½ teaspoon kosher salt
¼ teaspoon freshly ground pepper
2 tablespoons freshly grated Parmesan

1 Cook the pasta according to the package directions. Keep warm.

2 Melt the butter in a large nonstick skillet over medium heat. Add the almonds and cook, stirring constantly, until the almonds are lightly browned, 3 minutes. Using a slotted spoon, transfer the almonds to a small dish.

3 Add the garlic to the skillet and cook, stirring constantly, until fragrant, 30 seconds. Add the pasta, spinach, salt, and pepper and cook, stirring constantly, just until the spinach is wilted, about 1 minute.

4 To serve, divide the pasta mixture evenly among 4 plates. Sprinkle evenly with the toasted almonds and the Parmesan.

Each serving: 28 g carb, 235 cal, 9 g fat, 5 g sat fat, 17 mg chol, 6 g fib, 10 g pro, 219 mg sod • Carb Choices: 1½; Exchanges: 1½ starch, 1½ fat

Pasta with Broccoli Rabe and Caramelized Garlic

QUICK | HIGH FIBER

makes 4 servings

Broccoli rabe has a slightly bitter flavor that diminishes significantly if it is cooked until very tender. The greens will lose their vibrant green color, but the flavor is fantastic. Make this dish part of your regular fall and winter weeknight dinner rotation when broccoli rabe is at its peak. Make the grape tomato version of this dish with the last of the tomatoes from your fall garden—or, in winter, use a can of drained diced tomatoes instead of the cherry tomatoes.

6 ounces whole wheat penne or other short pasta (about 2 cups)

1 pound broccoli rabe, tough stems removed, leaves and florets chopped

2 teaspoons extra virgin olive oil

3 garlic cloves, thinly sliced

½ teaspoon kosher salt

⅛ teaspoon crushed red pepper

2 tablespoons freshly grated Parmesan

1 Cook the pasta according to the package directions. Drain, reserving ¼ cup of the cooking water. Transfer the pasta to a large bowl and keep warm.

2 Meanwhile, bring a large pot of water to a boil over high heat. Add the broccoli rabe and cook until barely tender, 5 minutes. Drain in a colander.

3 Heat a large nonstick skillet over medium heat. Add the oil and tilt the pan to coat the bottom evenly. Add the garlic and cook, stirring often, until lightly browned, 3 minutes. Add the broccoli rabe, the reserved pasta cooking water, salt, and crushed red pepper. Cook, stirring constantly until the broccoli rabe is very tender and the liquid evaporates, about 3 minutes.

4 To serve, add the broccoli rabe mixture to the pasta and toss to combine. Divide the pasta among 4 shallow bowls, sprinkle evenly with the Parmesan, and serve at once.

Each serving: 32 g carb, 211 cal, 4 g fat, 2 g sat fat, 2 mg chol, 5 g fib, 12 g pro, 219 mg sod • Carb Choices: 2; Exchanges: 1½ starch, 1 veg, ½ fat

PASTA WITH BROCCOLI RABE AND GRAPE TOMATOES: Follow the Pasta with Broccoli Rabe and Caramelized Garlic recipe, at left, but add 1 cup grape tomatoes, halved, with the broccoli rabe in step 3. Proceed as directed.

Each serving: 33 g carb, 218 cal, 4 g fat, 2 g sat fat, 2 mg chol, 5 g fib, 12 g pro, 221 mg sod • Carb Choices: 2; Exchanges: 1½ starch, 1 veg, ½ fat

Pasta with Eggplant and Arugula Sauce HIGH FIBER

makes 4 servings

In this recipe, eggplant is baked, then simmered to create a silky smooth pasta sauce. Arugula and Kalamata olives add a sharp flavor counterpoint to the sweet eggplant.

1 medium eggplant (about 1¼ pounds)

6 ounces whole wheat penne or other short pasta (about 2 cups)

2 teaspoons extra virgin olive oil

1 small onion, finely chopped

2 garlic cloves, minced

1 cup Vegetable Stock (page 149) or low-sodium vegetable broth

½ teaspoon kosher salt

⅛ teaspoon freshly ground pepper

2 cups chopped arugula

¼ cup Kalamata olives, pitted and coarsely chopped

1 ounce finely shredded Asiago cheese (about ¼ cup)

1 Preheat the oven to 350°F.

2 Using a sharp-pointed knife, prick several holes in the eggplant to prevent bursting. Place the eggplant in a medium baking dish and bake until easily pierced with a knife, about 1 hour. Let stand until cool enough to handle. Cut the eggplant in half and scoop out the flesh. Discard the skin.

3 Cook the pasta according to the package directions. Transfer to a large bowl and keep warm.

4 Meanwhile, heat a large nonstick skillet over medium heat. Add the oil and tilt the pan to coat the bottom evenly. Add the onion and cook, stirring often, until softened, 5 minutes. Add the garlic and cook, stirring constantly, until fragrant, 30 seconds. Add the eggplant pulp, stock, salt, and pepper and bring to a boil. Cover, reduce the heat to low, and simmer 10 minutes. Uncover and simmer until the sauce is thickened, 3 to 4 minutes longer. Add the arugula and olives and cook, stirring constantly, just until the arugula wilts, about 1 minute.

5 To serve, add the eggplant mixture to the pasta and toss to combine. Divide the pasta evenly among 4 shallow bowls, sprinkle evenly with the Asiago, and serve at once.

Each serving: 37 g carb, 257 cal, 8 g fat, 3 g sat fat, 6 mg chol, 9 g fib, 10 g pro, 386 mg sod • Carb Choices: 2; Exchanges: 1½ starch, 1 veg, 1½ fat

Pasta and Tomatoes with Broccoli Sauce QUICK | HIGH FIBER

makes 4 servings

Can't get your kids to eat their broccoli? Try this vibrantly colored broccoli sauce and just call it "green sauce." Instead of the plum tomatoes, you can use 1½ cups cherry tomatoes, halved.

6 ounces whole wheat penne or other short pasta (about 2 cups)

2 large plum tomatoes, chopped

2 teaspoons extra virgin olive oil

1 garlic clove, minced

4 cups broccoli florets (about 8 ounces), cut into 1-inch pieces

About 1 cup Vegetable Stock (page 149) or low-sodium vegetable broth, divided

1 ounce freshly grated Parmesan (about ¼ cup)

1 tablespoon lemon juice

¾ teaspoon kosher salt

⅛ teaspoon freshly ground pepper

2 tablespoons pine nuts, toasted (page 4)

1 Cook the pasta according to the package directions. Place the tomatoes in a large bowl. Add the pasta to the tomatoes and keep warm.

2 Meanwhile, heat a large nonstick skillet over medium-high heat. Add the oil and tilt the pan to coat the bottom evenly. Add the garlic and cook, stirring constantly, until fragrant, 30 seconds. Add the broccoli and ½ cup of the stock. Cover, reduce the heat to low, and simmer until the broccoli is very tender but still bright green, about 5 minutes.

3 Transfer the broccoli mixture to a food processor. Add ¼ cup of the remaining stock, the Parmesan, lemon juice, salt, and pepper and process until smooth, adding the additional ¼ cup stock 1 tablespoon at a time, as needed, to reach a sauce consistency.

4 To serve, add the broccoli mixture to the pasta and toss to combine. Divide the pasta evenly among 4 shallow bowls, sprinkle evenly with the pine nuts, and serve at once.

Each serving: 33 g carb, 247 cal, 8 g fat, 2 g sat fat, 4 mg chol, 7 g fib, 12 g pro, 351 mg sod • Carb Choices: 2; Exchanges: 1½ starch, 1 veg, 1 fat

Pasta with Ricotta and Roasted Tomato Sauce HIGH FIBER

makes 4 servings.

Roasting tomatoes is an easy way to give them great depth of flavor. This method makes a delicious sauce, even if you are using winter tomatoes. When you roast the tomatoes, make a double batch and add the leftovers to salads, soups, or pasta dishes later in the week.

4 large tomatoes, quartered

2 teaspoons extra virgin olive oil

2 garlic cloves, minced

2 teaspoons chopped fresh rosemary or ½ teaspoon crumbled dried rosemary

6 ounces whole wheat penne or other short pasta (about 2 cups)

½ teaspoon kosher salt

⅛ teaspoon freshly ground pepper

8 tablespoons part-skim ricotta, at room temperature

1 Preheat the oven to 400°F.

2 Place the tomatoes on a large rimmed baking sheet. Drizzle with the oil, sprinkle with the garlic and rosemary, and toss to coat. Arrange the tomatoes in a single layer. Bake, turning once, until the tomatoes are soft and well browned, 35 to 40 minutes.

3 Meanwhile, cook the pasta according to the package directions. Transfer to a large bowl and keep warm.

4 Transfer the roasted tomatoes and any cooking juices to a food processor. Add the salt and pepper and pulse until the tomatoes are chunky, but not pureed, 4 to 5 times. Add the tomato mixture to the pasta and toss to combine.

5 To serve, divide the pasta evenly among 4 plates, top each serving with 2 tablespoons of the ricotta, and serve at once.

Each serving: 35 g carb, 242 cal, 6 g fat, 3 g sat fat, 10 mg chol, 7 g fib, 12 g pro, 196 mg sod • Carb Choices: 2; Exchanges: 1½ starch, 1 veg, 1 fat

Pasta, Vegetable, and Goat Cheese Gratin HIGH FIBER

makes 6 servings

This is a comforting dish to make in late summer or early fall when the last of the tomatoes, squash, and eggplant are in the markets and the evenings are just chilly enough that you're craving something from the oven.

3 teaspoons extra virgin olive oil, divided

8 ounces whole wheat penne or other short pasta (about 2⅔ cups)

1 medium eggplant, peeled and cut into ½-inch cubes

1 medium zucchini, quartered lengthwise and sliced

1 medium onion, halved lengthwise and thinly sliced

2 garlic cloves, minced

1 large tomato, chopped

¼ cup Kalamata olives, pitted and quartered

½ teaspoon dried thyme

½ teaspoon kosher salt

⅛ teaspoon freshly ground pepper

4 ounces crumbled goat cheese (about 1 cup)

2 tablespoons freshly grated Parmesan

1 Preheat the oven to 350°F. Brush a 13 x 9-inch baking dish with 1 teaspoon of the oil.

2 Cook the pasta according to the package directions. Transfer to a large bowl.

3 Meanwhile, heat a large nonstick skillet over medium-high heat. Add the remaining 2 teaspoons oil and tilt the pan to coat the bottom

evenly. Add the eggplant, zucchini, and onion and cook, stirring often, until the vegetables are crisp-tender, 8 minutes. Add the garlic and cook, stirring constantly, until fragrant, 30 seconds.

4 Add the vegetable mixture, tomato, olives, thyme, salt, and pepper to the pasta and toss to combine. Add the goat cheese and toss to combine.

5 Transfer to the prepared baking dish. Sprinkle with the Parmesan and bake until the cheese melts and the top is lightly browned, 20 to 25 minutes. Spoon the gratin evenly onto 6 plates and serve at once.

Each serving: 32 g carb, 273 cal, 11 g fat, 5 g sat fat, 16 mg chol, 7 g fib, 12 g pro, 304 mg sod • Carb Choices: 2; Exchanges: 1½ starch, 1 veg, 1 medium-fat protein, ½ fat

Lasagna with Greens and Ricotta HIGH FIBER

makes 6 servings

If you enjoy all the greens in the market in the spring and fall as much as I do, you'll appreciate this recipe for using them. You can make the lasagna with kale, beet greens, or mustard greens, though those may need to cook a few minutes longer than the Swiss chard. Be sure to squeeze the greens dry before assembling the lasagna or they will add too much moisture to the dish.

2 cups Marinara Sauce (page 593)

9 whole wheat lasagna noodles

1 pound Swiss chard, tough stems removed
     and leaves chopped

½ cup water

2 teaspoons canola oil, divided

4 ounces shredded part-skim mozzarella
     (about 1 cup)

1 cup part-skim ricotta

1 ounce (about ¼ cup) plus 2 tablespoons
     freshly grated Parmesan, divided

⅛ teaspoon freshly ground pepper

1 Heat the sauce in a saucepan over medium heat until hot, if necessary.

2 Cook the lasagna noodles according to the package directions. Drain in a colander and rinse with cold water.

3 Meanwhile, combine the chard and water in a large saucepan and bring to a boil over high heat. Cover, reduce the heat to low, and simmer until the chard is tender, about 5 minutes. Drain and let cool. Squeeze the chard dry and transfer to a medium bowl.

4 Preheat the oven to 375°F. Brush an 8-inch square baking dish with 1 teaspoon of the oil.

5 Add the mozzarella, ricotta, ¼ cup of the Parmesan, and the pepper to the chard and stir until well mixed.

6 Spread ½ cup of the sauce in the bottom of the baking dish. Place 3 noodles over the sauce, trimming them as needed to fit the dish. Top the noodles with 1½ cups of the chard mixture and ¾ cup of the remaining sauce. Repeat the layering, ending with the noodles.

7 Brush one side of a sheet of foil with the remaining 1 teaspoon oil. Cover the lasagna with the foil, oiled side down, and place the dish on a large rimmed baking sheet. Bake until the noodles are tender, 30 minutes. Uncover, sprinkle the lasagna with the remaining 2 tablespoons Parmesan, and bake until the Parmesan melts, 5 minutes. Let stand 10 minutes. Cut the lasagna into 6 pieces and serve.

Each serving: 32 g carb, 320 cal, 12 g fat, 6 g sat fat, 27 mg chol, 7 g fib, 20 g pro, 423 mg sod • Carb Choices: 2; Exchanges: 1½ starch, 1 veg, 2 medium-fat protein

Individual Spinach Lasagnas HIGH FIBER

makes 4 servings

I love this lasagna. It's light, fresh—and best of all—easy to make. Don't be daunted by what seems a labor-intensive process; it's all simple. Basically, you boil the noodles, cut them in half, and layer them with quickly sautéed spinach, fresh tomatoes, and ricotta.

6 whole wheat lasagna noodles
1 pound fresh spinach
4 teaspoons extra virgin olive oil, divided
2 garlic cloves, minced
½ teaspoon kosher salt, divided
⅛ teaspoon freshly ground pepper
4 large plum tomatoes, diced (about 2 cups)
¼ cup chopped fresh basil
1 cup part-skim ricotta
1 ounce freshly grated Parmesan (about ¼ cup)
2 ounces shredded part-skim mozzarella
    (about ½ cup)

1 Cook the lasagna noodles according to the package directions. Drain in a colander and rinse with cold water. Cut each noodle crosswise in half and arrange in a single layer on a sheet of wax paper. Cover with plastic wrap.

2 Meanwhile, pinch the tough stems from the spinach. Submerge the spinach in a large bowl of cold water, lift it out and drain in a colander. Repeat, using fresh water, until no grit remains in the bottom of the bowl.

3 Preheat the oven to 375°F. Brush 4 individual gratin or casserole dishes with 2 teaspoons of the oil.

4 Heat a large skillet over medium heat. Add the remaining 2 teaspoons oil and tilt the pan to coat the bottom evenly. Add the garlic and cook, stirring constantly, until fragrant, 30 seconds. Add the spinach in batches and cook, turning with tongs, until the spinach is wilted and most of the liquid evaporates, about 3 minutes. Stir in ¼ teaspoon of the salt and the pepper.

5 Stir together the tomatoes, basil, and remaining ¼ teaspoon salt in a medium bowl. Stir together the ricotta and Parmesan in another medium bowl.

6 Place 1 noodle half in each gratin dish. Spread each of the noodles with 2 tablespoons of the ricotta mixture, then top with ¼ cup of the spinach mixture, then with ¼ cup of the tomato mixture. Top the tomato mixture with 1 noodle half. Spread the noodles with 2 tablespoons of the ricotta mixture, then with ¼ cup of the spinach mixture, then with ¼ cup of the tomato mixture. Top with another noodle half. Sprinkle the lasagnas evenly with the mozzarella. Bake until the lasagnas are heated through and the cheese melts, 12 to 15 minutes. Serve at once.

Each serving: 35 g carb, 360 cal, 15 g fat, 6 g sat fat, 31 mg chol, 8 g fib, 22 g pro, 441 mg sod • Carb Choices: 2; Exchanges: 1½ starch, 1 veg, 2 medium-fat protein, 1 fat

Manicotti with Ricotta and Kale HIGH FIBER

makes 4 servings

You can make this dish a day ahead: you can assemble it, then cover and refrigerate. Let it stand at room temperature about 15 minutes, then bake as directed, adding about 5 minutes to the baking time. You can use Swiss chard instead of kale in this recipe. Be careful not to overcook the manicotti, as they will tear easily if they are too tender.

1¾ cups Marinara Sauce (page 593)
3 teaspoons extra virgin olive oil, divided
8 manicotti shells
1 medium onion, chopped
8 ounces kale, tough stems removed and
    leaves chopped
2 garlic cloves, minced
½ cup Vegetable Stock (page 149) or
    low-sodium vegetable broth
1 cup part-skim ricotta
1 large egg
1 ounce freshly grated Parmesan
    (about ¼ cup)
¼ teaspoon kosher salt
⅛ teaspoon freshly ground pepper
2 ounces shredded part-skim mozzarella
    (about ½ cup)

1 Heat the sauce in a saucepan over medium heat until hot, if necessary. Brush a 13 x 9-inch baking dish with 1 teaspoon of the oil.

2 Cook the manicotti according to the package directions.

3 Preheat the oven to 375°F.

4 Heat a large nonstick skillet over medium heat. Add the remaining 2 teaspoons oil and tilt the pan to coat the bottom evenly. Add the onion and cook, stirring often, until tender, 5 minutes. Stir in the kale and garlic, then add the stock. Cook, stirring often, until the kale is tender and the liquid has evaporated, 5 minutes. Transfer the kale mixture to a large bowl to cool slightly.

5 Add the ricotta, egg, Parmesan, salt, and pepper to the kale mixture and stir until well combined.

6 Spread 1 cup of the sauce in the prepared baking dish. Stuff each manicotti shell with about ¼ cup of the filling. Arrange the manicotti shells on top of the sauce. Spoon the remaining sauce over the shells. Sprinkle with the mozzarella. Bake until the sauce is bubbly and the filling is heated through, 25 to 30 minutes. Divide the manicotti among 4 plates and serve at once.

Each serving: 41 g carb, 389 cal, 17 g fat, 7 g sat fat, 84 mg chol, 4 g fib, 22 g pro, 399 mg sod • Carb Choices: 3; Exchanges: 1½ starch, 2 veg, 2 medium-fat protein, 1 fat

Grains

Beet and Barley Chili HIGH FIBER

makes 6 servings

I got the idea of adding beets to chili from a recipe in the *Hay Day Country Market Cookbook*. It makes the flavor richer and adds nutrients, so it's a great technique to try. Don't be concerned about the large amount of broth in this chili— the barley really soaks it up. If you like chili with smoky heat, stir in ½ teaspoon minced chipotle chile when you add the broth.

2 teaspoons canola oil
1 medium onion, chopped
1 medium green bell pepper, chopped
1 jalapeño, seeded and minced
3 garlic cloves, minced
½ cup pearl barley
2 tablespoons chili powder
2 teaspoons ground cumin
1 teaspoon kosher salt
5 cups Vegetable Stock (page 149) or low-sodium vegetable broth
1 pound beets, peeled and chopped
1 (14½-ounce) can no-salt-added diced tomatoes
1 (15-ounce) can no-salt-added cannellini beans, rinsed and drained
2 teaspoons fine-grind cornmeal
1 tablespoon lime juice
Chopped fresh cilantro

1 Heat a large pot over medium-high heat. Add the oil and tilt the pot to coat the bottom evenly.

2 Add the onion, bell pepper, jalapeño, and garlic and cook, stirring often, until softened, 5 minutes. Stir in the barley, chili powder, cumin, and salt. Add the stock, beets, tomatoes, and beans. Bring to a boil.

3 Cover, reduce the heat to low, and simmer until the beets and barley are tender, about 45 minutes. Sprinkle the cornmeal on top of the chili and stir to combine. Simmer, uncovered, until the chili is slightly thickened, about 3 minutes. Remove from the heat and stir in the lime juice.

4 Ladle evenly into 6 bowls, sprinkle with the cilantro, and serve at once. The chili can be refrigerated, covered, for up to 4 days or frozen for up to 3 months.

Each serving: 38 g carb, 206 cal, 3 g fat, 0 g sat fat, 0 mg chol, 9 g fib, 7 g pro, 454 mg sod • Carb Choices: 2; Exchanges: 1½ starch, 1 veg

Barley Risotto with Asparagus and Peas HIGH FIBER

makes 4 servings

Barley is more forgiving than the typical Arborio rice used to make risotto. You don't have to stir barley as often as you do rice and barley still retains its texture if you overcook it a bit. Serve this dish for a healthful and satisfying springtime entrée or serve it as a side dish to accompany salmon or roast chicken.

4½ cups Vegetable Stock (page 149) or low-sodium vegetable broth
2 teaspoons extra virgin olive oil
1 medium onion, diced
2 garlic cloves, minced
¾ cup pearl barley
½ cup dry white wine
½ teaspoon kosher salt
8 ounces asparagus, tough ends removed and spears cut into 1½-inch pieces
½ cup shelled fresh English peas or frozen green peas, thawed
2 ounces freshly grated Parmesan (about ½ cup)
⅛ teaspoon freshly ground pepper

1 Pour the stock into a medium saucepan and bring to a simmer over medium-high heat. Reduce the heat to low and keep the stock warm.

2 Heat a large saucepan over medium heat. Add the oil and tilt the pan to coat the bottom evenly. Add the onion and cook, stirring often, until softened, 5 minutes. Add the garlic and cook, stirring constantly, until fragrant, 30 seconds.

3 Add the barley and cook, stirring constantly, 2 minutes. Add the wine and salt and cook, stirring frequently, until the liquid is absorbed. Add the stock, ½ cup at a time, stirring frequently, until the liquid is absorbed after each addition before adding more stock.

4 After 30 minutes, stir in the asparagus and peas and continue adding broth and stirring until the barley is tender, about 5 minutes longer. Remove the saucepan from the heat and stir in the Parmesan and pepper. Spoon the risotto evenly into 4 shallow bowls and serve at once.

Each serving: 40 g carb, 278 cal, 6 g fat, 2 g sat fat, 9 mg chol, 8 g fib, 10 g pro, 457 mg sod • Carb Choices: 2½; Exchanges: 2 starch, 1 veg, 1 fat

Barley Risotto with Summer Squash, Tomatoes, and Pesto HIGH FIBER

makes 4 servings

The first time I made barley risotto, I expected a finished dish that would be brown and unappetizing. I could not have been more wrong. Barley risotto is very light in color and has a delicate flavor and texture—the perfect pairing for fresh tomatoes and pesto. To make this dish even more colorful, use a mixture of zucchini and yellow squash.

5 cups Vegetable Stock (page 149) or low-sodium vegetable broth
2 teaspoons extra virgin olive oil
1 medium onion, diced
2 garlic cloves, minced
¾ cup pearl barley
½ teaspoon kosher salt
2 cups diced zucchini or yellow squash
2 tablespoons Basil Pesto (page 597), or purchased pesto
2 ounces freshly grated Parmesan (about ½ cup)
⅛ teaspoon freshly ground pepper
1 medium tomato, chopped

1 Pour the stock into a medium saucepan and bring to a simmer over medium-high heat. Reduce the heat to low and keep the stock warm.

2 Heat a large saucepan over medium heat. Add the oil and tilt the pan to coat the bottom evenly. Add the onion and cook, stirring often, until softened, 5 minutes. Add the garlic and cook, stirring constantly, until fragrant, 30 seconds.

3 Add the barley and cook, stirring constantly, 2 minutes. Add ½ cup of the stock and the salt and cook, stirring frequently, until the liquid is absorbed. Add the remaining stock, ½ cup at a time, stirring frequently, until the liquid is absorbed after each addition before adding more stock.

4 After 30 minutes, stir in the zucchini and continue adding broth and stirring until the barley is tender, about 5 minutes longer. Remove the saucepan from the heat and stir in the pesto, Parmesan, and pepper. Gently stir in the tomato. Spoon the risotto evenly into 4 shallow bowls and serve at once.

Each serving: 37 g carb, 294 cal, 10 g fat, 3 g sat fat, 11 mg chol, 8 g fib, 10 g pro, 548 mg sod • Carb Choices: 2½; Exchanges: 2 starch, 1 veg, 2 fat

Barley Risotto with Mushrooms and Gorgonzola HIGH FIBER

makes 4 servings

This is a hearty and filling vegetarian main dish. The pungent blue cheese and earthy mushrooms also make this dish delicious alongside Grilled T-Bone with Green Peppercorn–Garlic Crust (page 266) or Filets Mignons with Cabernet-Butter Sauce (page 269).

4½ cups Vegetable Stock (page 149) or low-sodium vegetable broth

2 teaspoons extra virgin olive oil

8 ounces cremini mushrooms, thinly sliced

1 medium onion, diced

2 garlic cloves, minced

¾ cup pearl barley

½ cup dry white wine

½ teaspoon kosher salt

3 tablespoons crumbled Gorgonzola or other blue cheese

1 teaspoon fresh minced thyme or ¼ teaspoon dried thyme

⅛ teaspoon freshly ground pepper

1 Pour the stock into a medium saucepan and bring to a simmer over medium-high heat. Reduce the heat to low and keep the stock warm.

2 Heat a large saucepan over medium heat. Add the oil and tilt the pan to coat the bottom evenly. Add the mushrooms and onion and cook, stirring often, until the mushrooms are tender and most of the liquid has evaporated, about 8 minutes. Add the garlic and cook, stirring constantly, until fragrant, 30 seconds.

3 Add the barley and cook, stirring constantly, 2 minutes. Add the wine and salt and cook, stirring frequently, until the liquid is absorbed. Add the stock, ½ cup at a time, stirring frequently,

until the liquid is absorbed after each addition before adding more stock.

4 When all the liquid is absorbed and the barley is tender (about 35 minutes), remove the saucepan from the heat and stir in the Gorgonzola, thyme, and pepper. Spoon the risotto evenly into 4 shallow bowls and serve at once.

Each serving: 39 g carb, 247 cal, 4 g fat, 2 g sat fat, 5 mg chol, 7 g fib, 6 g pro, 377 mg sod • Carb Choices: 2; Exchanges: 2 starch, 1 veg, 1 fat

Barley and Eggplant–Stuffed Peppers HIGH FIBER

makes 4 servings

No one will miss the meat in these homey vegetable-and-grain filled peppers. Make this dish in late summer when you can find all the vegetables at your local farmers' market.

4 medium green, red, or yellow bell peppers

4 teaspoons extra virgin olive oil, divided

1 small eggplant, peeled and chopped (about 4 cups)

1 small onion, diced

2 garlic cloves, chopped

1 cup cooked pearl barley (page 108)

1 large tomato, chopped

½ cup low-sodium tomato juice

¼ cup chopped fresh basil

½ teaspoon kosher salt

⅛ teaspoon freshly ground pepper

2 ounces freshly grated Parmesan (about ½ cup)

1 Preheat the broiler. Line a large rimmed baking sheet with foil.

2 Cut the bell peppers in half lengthwise and remove the ribs and seeds. Place the peppers, skin side up, on the foil. Broil until the skins are charred, about 15 minutes. Cover the pan with foil and let the peppers stand until cool enough to handle. Peel away the skins.

3 Preheat the oven to 400°F. Brush a 13 x 9-inch baking dish with 2 teaspoons of the oil.

4 Heat a large nonstick skillet over medium high heat. Add the remaining 2 teaspoons oil and tilt the pan to coat the bottom evenly. Add the eggplant and onion, and cook, stirring frequently, until softened, 5 minutes. Add the garlic and cook, stirring constantly, until fragrant, 30 seconds. Add the barley, tomato, and tomato juice and cook, stirring often, until heated through, about 3 minutes. Stir in the basil, salt, and ground pepper.

5 Spoon about ½ cup of the eggplant mixture into each bell pepper half. Arrange the peppers in the baking dish. Sprinkle with the Parmesan and bake until the peppers are hot, 20 to 25 minutes. Divide the peppers evenly among 4 plates and serve at once.

Each serving: 24 g carb, 204 cal, 8 g fat, 3 g sat fat, 9 mg chol, 8 g fib, 8 g pro, 320 mg sod • Carb Choices: 1½; Exchanges: 1 starch, 2 veg, 1 fat

Portobello Mushrooms Stuffed with Barley and Gruyère HIGH FIBER

makes 4 servings

Stuffed portobello mushrooms, with their meaty texture and rich flavor, make a satisfying vegetarian entrée. These are topped with nutty tasting Gruyère cheese, but you can use whatever you have on hand—sharp white Cheddar, fontina, or feta would all be delicious options. Add a leafy green salad as an accompaniment.

4 large portobello mushrooms (about 4½-inch diameter)

4 teaspoons extra virgin olive oil, divided

1 medium bulb fennel

1 medium onion, diced

1 small red bell pepper, diced

2 garlic cloves, minced

1 cup cooked pearl barley (page 108)

¼ cup Vegetable Stock (page 149) or low-sodium vegetable broth

½ teaspoon kosher salt

¼ teaspoon freshly ground pepper

2 tablespoons chopped fresh basil or parsley

2 ounces shredded Gruyère (about ½ cup)

1 Cut away and discard the tough stems of the mushrooms. Using a spoon, gently scrape away and discard the dark gills on the underside of each mushroom.

2 Heat a large nonstick skillet over medium-high heat. Add 2 teaspoons of the oil and tilt the pan to coat the bottom evenly. Add the mushrooms, cover, and cook, turning once, until tender, 6 to 8 minutes. Transfer the mushrooms, stem side up, to a medium rimmed baking sheet. Cover with foil to keep warm.

3 Meanwhile, trim the tough outer stalks from the fennel. Cut the fennel bulb in half vertically and cut away and discard the core. Chop the fennel.

4 Add the remaining 2 teaspoons oil to the skillet. Add the fennel, onion, and bell pepper and cook, stirring often, until the vegetables are softened, 8 minutes. Add the garlic and cook, stirring constantly, until fragrant, 30 seconds.

5 Add the barley, stock, salt, and ground pepper and cook, stirring often, until the vegetables are tender and the barley is heated through, about 3 minutes. Remove from the heat and stir in the basil.

6 Preheat the broiler.

7 Spoon about 1 cup of the vegetable mixture into each of the mushroom caps. Sprinkle evenly with the cheese. Broil until the cheese melts, about 2 minutes. Divide the mushrooms evenly among 4 plates and serve at once.

Each serving: 25 g carb, 217 cal, 10 g fat, 3 g sat fat, 16 mg chol, 6 g fib, 9 g pro, 236 mg sod • Carb Choices: 1½; Exchanges: 1 starch, 1 veg, 1 medium-fat protein, 1 fat

Crisp Polenta Squares with Tomato–Roasted Red Pepper Sauce HIGH FIBER

makes 4 servings

Cut into squares and cooked until crisp and golden, this polenta elevates cornmeal to a gourmet meal. For a vegetarian entrée, you can top the polenta with almost any kind of sauce or vegetables. Try simple Marinara Sauce (page 593), Roasted Broccoli Rabe with Lemon and Olives (page 452), or Sautéed Mixed Mushrooms with Rosemary (page 473).

5 teaspoons extra virgin olive oil, divided

1 recipe Parmesan Polenta (page 422)

1 small onion, chopped

2 garlic cloves, minced

1 (14½-ounce) can no-salt-added diced tomatoes

¾ cup red Roasted Bell Peppers (page 21) or roasted red peppers from a jar, cut into short, thin strips

¼ teaspoon kosher salt

⅛ teaspoon freshly ground pepper

1 tablespoon chopped fresh basil

½ teaspoon sherry vinegar or white wine vinegar

2 tablespoons freshly grated Parmesan

1 Line an 8-inch square metal baking dish with foil, allowing the foil to extend over the rim of the pan by 2 inches. Brush the foil with 1 teaspoon of the oil. Prepare the polenta as directed and pour into the prepared pan. Let cool to room temperature. Cover and refrigerate at least 4 hours or up to 3 days.

2 Meanwhile, heat a medium skillet over medium heat. Add 2 teaspoons of the remaining oil and tilt the pan to coat the bottom evenly. Add the onion and cook, stirring often, until softened, 5 minutes. Add the garlic and cook, stirring constantly, until fragrant, 30 seconds. Add the tomatoes, bell peppers, salt, and ground pepper and bring to a boil. Cover, reduce the heat to low and simmer 10 minutes. Uncover and simmer until the sauce is thickened, 3 to 4 minutes longer. Remove from the heat and stir in the basil and vinegar.

3 Lift the polenta from the pan using the foil overhang as handles. Cut into 4 squares. Cut each square into 2 triangles. Heat a large nonstick skillet over medium-high heat. Add the remaining 2 teaspoons oil and tilt the pan to coat the bottom evenly. Add the polenta triangles in two batches, and cook, turning once, until the polenta is lightly browned, about 4 minutes.

4 To serve, place 2 polenta triangles on each of 4 plates. Spoon the sauce evenly over the polenta. Sprinkle evenly with the Parmesan and serve at once.

Each serving: 24 g carb, 190 cal, 8 g fat, 2 g sat fat, 7 mg chol, 4 g fib, 5 g pro, 437 mg sod • Carb Choices: 1½; Exchanges: 1 starch, 1 veg, 1½ fat

Quick- vs. Long-Cooking Polenta

The polenta recipes in this section all use quick-cooking fine-grind cornmeal, which is also called instant polenta. The difference in fine-grind and medium- or coarse-grind polenta is the size of the particles that the corn is ground into. The finer the grind, the quicker the polenta cooks. If you'd like to try making a side dish of long-cooking medium or coarse-grind polenta, I've given an easy no-stir method in the Oven-Baked Polenta (page 424).

Layered Polenta and Vegetable Casserole HIGH FIBER

makes 8 servings

Perfect for a potluck or any casual get-together, this casserole is an easy-to-make crowd-pleaser. You can assemble it a day ahead and cover and refrigerate. If you make it ahead, let it stand at room temperature for about 15 minutes before baking and add 10 to 15 minutes to the baking time.

5 teaspoons extra virgin olive oil, divided
1 large onion, chopped
1 red bell pepper, chopped
1 medium zucchini, chopped
1 medium yellow squash, chopped
2 garlic cloves, minced
1 (14½-ounce) can no-salt added diced tomatoes
½ cup chopped fresh basil
¾ teaspoon kosher salt, divided
¼ teaspoon freshly ground pepper, divided
8 cups Vegetable Stock (page 149) or low-sodium vegetable broth
2 cups fine-grind yellow cornmeal
2 ounces freshly grated Parmesan (about ½ cup)
8 ounces shredded part-skim mozzarella, divided (about 2 cups)

1 Preheat the oven to 375°F. Brush a 13 x 9-inch baking dish with 2 teaspoons of the oil.

2 Heat a large nonstick skillet over medium-high heat. Add 2 teaspoons of the remaining oil and tilt the pan to coat the bottom evenly. Add the onion, bell pepper, zucchini, and yellow squash and cook, stirring occasionally, until the vegetables are crisp-tender, 3 minutes. Add the garlic, and cook, stirring constantly, until fragrant, 30 seconds. Add the tomatoes and bring to a boil. Reduce the heat to low and simmer until most of the liquid has evaporated, 8 minutes. Remove from the heat and stir in the basil, ¼ teaspoon of the salt, and ⅛ teaspoon of the ground pepper.

3 Combine the stock, remaining ½ teaspoon salt, and remaining ⅛ teaspoon ground pepper in a large saucepan and bring to a boil over high heat. Slowly sprinkle the cornmeal into the stock, whisking constantly. Reduce the heat to low and cook, stirring constantly, until the polenta is thickened, about 3 minutes. Remove from the heat and stir in the Parmesan.

4 Spread half of the polenta in the prepared baking dish. Top with the vegetable mixture. Sprinkle the vegetables with 1½ cups of the mozzarella. Spread the remaining polenta evenly over the vegetables. Brush one side of a sheet of foil with the remaining 1 teaspoon oil. Cover the casserole with the foil, oiled side down, and bake 30 minutes. Uncover, sprinkle with the remaining ½ cup of the mozzarella, and bake until the cheese melts, 5 minutes. Let stand 10 minutes before serving. Spoon the casserole evenly onto 8 plates and serve at once.

Each serving: 39 g carb, 305 cal, 11 g fat, 5 g sat fat, 20 mg chol, 5 g fib, 13 g pro, 568 mg sod • Carb Choices: 2½; Exchanges: 2 starch, 1 veg, 1 medium fat protein, 1 fat

Tex-Mex Cheddar, Polenta, and Vegetable Casserole

makes 6 servings

This spicy casserole is reminiscent of creamy Southern spoon bread, but it's loaded with healthful vegetables and flavored with just a smidgen of cheese. It makes a great side dish, too.

3 teaspoons canola oil, divided
1 medium onion, diced
1 medium red bell pepper, diced
1 medium zucchini, diced
1 jalapeño, seeded and minced
2 cloves garlic, minced
2 teaspoons chili powder
1 teaspoon ground cumin
2 cups Vegetable Stock (page 149) or
     low-sodium vegetable broth
½ teaspoon kosher salt
½ cup fine-grind yellow cornmeal
3 large egg whites
4 ounces shredded reduced-fat sharp Cheddar
     cheese (about 1 cup)
2 large eggs
¼ cup chopped fresh cilantro

1 Preheat the oven to 375°F. Brush an 11 x 7-inch baking dish with 1 teaspoon of the oil.

2 Heat a large nonstick skillet over medium-high heat. Add the remaining 2 teaspoons oil and tilt the pan to coat. Add the onion, bell pepper, zucchini, and jalapeño and cook, stirring occasionally, until the vegetables are tender, 8 to 10 minutes. Add the garlic, chili powder, and cumin and cook, stirring constantly, until fragrant, 1 minute longer. Transfer the vegetable mixture to a bowl. Do not wash the skillet.

3 Add the broth and salt to the skillet and bring to a boil. Slowly whisk in the cornmeal and cook, whisking constantly, until the polenta is thickened, 2 to 3 minutes. Transfer the polenta to a large bowl and let stand to cool slightly.

4 Place the egg whites in a large bowl and beat at high speed with an electric mixer until stiff peaks form. Stir the vegetable mixture, Cheddar, eggs, and cilantro into the polenta. Fold the egg whites into the polenta mixture in 3 additions, stirring until no white streaks appear.

5 Spoon into the prepared baking dish and bake for 30 minutes or until the center is set and the edges are lightly browned. Let stand 5 minutes before serving. Spoon the casserole evenly onto 6 plates and serve at once.

Each serving: 16 g carb, 181 cal, 8 g fat, 3 g sat fat, 84 mg chol, 2 g fib, 10 g pro, 357 mg sod • Carb Choices: 1; Exchanges: ½ starch, 1 veg, 1 high-fat protein, ½ fat

Polenta-Topped Ratatouille Casserole HIGH FIBER

makes 4 servings

This dish is like a ratatouille topped with polenta and baked. Instead of the fontina cheese, you can use Gruyère or for a milder flavor, part-skim mozzarella.

3 teaspoons extra virgin olive oil, divided
1 medium onion, chopped
1 large yellow or red bell pepper, chopped
1 medium eggplant (about 1¼ pounds), cut
     into ½-inch pieces
2 garlic cloves, minced
1 (14½-ounce) can no-salt-added diced tomatoes
¾ teaspoon kosher salt, divided
¼ teaspoon freshly ground pepper, divided
2 tablespoons chopped fresh basil or
     1 teaspoon dried basil
2 cups Vegetable Stock (page 149) or
     low-sodium vegetable broth
½ cup fine-grind yellow cornmeal
½ cup (2 ounces) plus 2 tablespoons shredded
     fontina, divided

1 Preheat the oven to 375°F. Brush an 8-inch square baking dish with 1 teaspoon of the oil.

2 Heat a large nonstick skillet over medium heat. Add the remaining 2 teaspoons oil and tilt the pan to coat. Add the onion, bell pepper, eggplant, and garlic and cook, covered, stirring occasionally, until the vegetables are softened, 6 to 8 minutes. Add the tomatoes, ¼ teaspoon of the salt, and ⅛ teaspoon of the ground pepper and cook, covered, stirring occasionally, until the vegetables are tender, about 5 minutes. Stir in the basil and spoon the mixture into the prepared baking dish.

3 Combine the stock, remaining ½ teaspoon salt, and remaining ⅛ teaspoon ground pepper in a medium saucepan and bring to a boil over medium-high heat.

4 Slowly sprinkle the cornmeal into the stock, whisking constantly. Reduce the heat and cook, stirring constantly, until the polenta is thickened, about 3 minutes. Remove from the heat and stir in ½ cup of the fontina.

5 Spoon the polenta over the vegetables in the baking dish. Sprinkle the polenta with the remaining 2 tablespoons fontina. Bake until the casserole is hot and the cheese melts, about 15 minutes. Let stand 5 minutes before serving. Spoon the casserole evenly onto 4 plates and serve at once.

Each serving: 32 g carb, 239 cal, 10 g fat, 4 g sat fat, 20 mg chol, 8 g fib, 9 g pro, 466 mg sod • Carb Choices: 2; Exchanges: 1 starch, 3 veg, 1 high-fat protein, ½ fat

Spicy Green Tamale Tart

makes 6 servings

Accompany this tart with a green salad tossed with Cilantro-Lime Vinaigrette (page 139) for a south of the border lunch menu. You can also cut the tart into very thin wedges and serve it as an hors d'oeuvre.

1 teaspoon canola oil

3 cups Vegetable Stock (page 149) or low-sodium vegetable broth

½ teaspoon minced chipotle in adobo sauce

1 teaspoon kosher salt, divided

1 cup fine-grind yellow cornmeal

4 poblano chiles, roasted (page 21) and finely chopped

4 ounces shredded reduced-fat Monterey Jack cheese (about 1 cup)

¼ cup thinly sliced scallions

¼ cup chopped fresh cilantro

1 Brush a 9-inch tart pan with removable bottom with the oil.

2 Combine the stock, chipotle, and ¾ teaspoon of the salt in a medium saucepan and bring to a boil over medium-high heat. Slowly sprinkle the cornmeal into the stock, whisking constantly. Reduce the heat to low and cook, stirring constantly, until the polenta is thickened, about 3 minutes. Spoon into the prepared tart pan and spread evenly in the bottom and up the side of the pan. Let cool 15 minutes.

3 Preheat the oven to 375°F.

4 Combine the chiles, Monterey Jack, scallions, cilantro, and remaining ¼ teaspoon salt in a large bowl. Toss to combine. Spread the chile mixture evenly in the polenta crust (the pan will be very full). Place the tart pan on a rimmed baking sheet and bake until the tart is heated through and the cheese melts, about 15 minutes. Let stand 5 minutes before slicing. Cut the tart into 6 wedges and serve at once.

Each serving: 22 g carb, 158 cal, 6 g fat, 2 g sat fat, 14 mg chol, 2 g fib, 7 g pro, 447 mg sod • Carb Choices: 1½; Exchanges: 1½ starch, 1 fat

Farro Risotto with Cherry Tomatoes, Feta, and Herbs HIGH FIBER

makes 6 servings

Farro is a grain similar to wheat that is often used in Italian cooking. It lends a nutty flavor to risotto. You can serve this risotto in smaller portions as a side dish.

2 medium leeks, halved lengthwise and thinly sliced

4 cups Vegetable Stock (page 149) or low-sodium vegetable broth

2 teaspoons extra virgin olive oil

1 cup farro

½ cup dry white wine

½ teaspoon kosher salt

3 cups cherry tomatoes, halved

2 ounces finely crumbled feta cheese (about ½ cup)

2 tablespoons any combination of chopped fresh basil, dill, mint, or Italian parsley

1 tablespoon lemon juice

1 Submerge the sliced leeks in a large bowl of water, lift them out, and drain in a colander. Repeat, using fresh water, until no grit remains in the bottom of the bowl. Drain the leeks well.

2 Pour the stock into a medium saucepan and bring to a simmer over medium-high heat. Reduce the heat to low and keep the stock warm.

3 Heat a large saucepan over medium heat. Add the oil and tilt the pan to coat the bottom evenly. Add the leeks and cook, stirring often, until softened, 5 minutes.

4 Add the farro and cook, stirring constantly, 2 minutes. Add the wine and salt and cook, stirring frequently, until the liquid is absorbed. Add the stock, ½ cup at a time, and cook, stirring frequently, until the liquid is absorbed after each addition before adding more stock. When all the liquid is absorbed and the farro is tender, stir in the tomatoes, feta, and herbs and cook until the tomatoes are heated through, 2 minutes. Stir in the lemon juice. Divide among 6 bowls and serve at once.

Each serving: 32 g carb, 214 cal, 4 g fat, 2 g sat fat, 8 mg chol, 5 g fib, 7 g pro, 302 mg sod • Carb Choices: 2; Exchanges: 1½ starch, 1 veg, 1 fat

Mushroom and Bulgur– Stuffed Cabbage HIGH FIBER

makes 4 servings

1 large head savoy cabbage

4 teaspoons extra virgin olive oil, divided

1 small onion, chopped

8 ounces cremini or white mushrooms, chopped

1 garlic clove, minced

¾ teaspoon ground cinnamon

1½ cups Vegetable Stock (page 149) or low-sodium vegetable broth

⅓ cup medium- or coarse-grind bulgur

¼ cup golden raisins

½ teaspoon kosher salt

⅛ teaspoon freshly ground pepper

¼ cup pine nuts, toasted (page 4)

2 tablespoons lemon juice

1 (15-ounce) can no-salt-added crushed tomatoes

1 tablespoon white wine vinegar

1 tablespoon honey

1 Remove 8 large outer leaves from the cabbage and set aside. From the remaining cabbage, chop 4 cups of cabbage. Reserve the remaining cabbage for another use.

2 Bring a large pot of water to a boil over high heat. Add the large outer cabbage leaves and cook until soft and pliable, about 3 minutes.

Drain the cabbage leaves in a colander and rinse under cold running water until cool. Dry the cabbage leaves with paper towels.

3 Heat a large nonstick skillet over medium-high heat. Add 2 teaspoons of the oil and the onion, mushrooms, and chopped cabbage and cook, stirring often, until most of the liquid has evaporated, 8 minutes. Add the garlic and cinnamon and cook, stirring constantly, 30 seconds. Stir in the stock, bulgur, raisins, salt, and pepper and bring to a boil. Cover, reduce the heat, and simmer until the bulgur is tender, 15 minutes. Stir in the pine nuts and lemon juice.

4 Preheat the oven to 350°F. Brush a large casserole dish with the remaining 2 teaspoons oil.

5 Place ½ cup of the bulgur mixture in the center of each cabbage leaf. Fold in the sides of the leaf and roll up. Place the rolls, seam side down, in the prepared dish.

6 Stir together the tomatoes, vinegar, and honey in a bowl. Pour the tomato mixture over the cabbage rolls. Cover and bake 45 minutes.

7 Divide the cabbage rolls and sauce evenly among 4 plates.

Each serving: 40 g carb, 285 cal, 11 g fat, 1 g sat fat, 0 mg chol, 8 g fib, 8 g pro, 361 mg sod • Carb Choices: 2½; Exchanges: ½ starch, 1 carb, 3 veg, 2 fat

Portobello Mushrooms with Couscous, Spinach, and Feta Stuffing HIGH FIBER

makes 4 servings

4 large portobello mushrooms (about 4-inch diameter)

½ cup Vegetable Stock (page 149) or low-sodium vegetable broth

½ cup whole wheat couscous

1 tablespoon capers, rinsed and drained

2 teaspoons grated lemon zest

¼ teaspoon freshly ground pepper, divided

2 teaspoons extra virgin olive oil

¼ cup diced onion

2 garlic cloves, minced

1 pound fresh prewashed spinach

1 tablespoon lemon juice

¼ teaspoon kosher salt

2 ounces crumbled feta cheese (about ½ cup)

1 Cut away and discard the tough stems of the mushrooms. Using a spoon, scrape away and discard the gills on the underside of each mushroom.

2 Place the stock in a small saucepan and bring to a boil. Remove from the heat and stir in the couscous, capers, lemon zest, and ⅛ teaspoon of the pepper. Cover and let stand 5 minutes.

3 Meanwhile, heat a large nonstick skillet over medium-high heat. Add the oil and the mushrooms, cover, and cook, turning once, until tender, 8 minutes. Transfer the mushrooms, stem side up, to a rimmed baking sheet.

4 Reduce the heat to medium. Add the onion and garlic to the mushroom liquid remaining in the pan and cook, until softened, 3 minutes. Add the spinach in batches and cook, turning with tongs, until most of the liquid evaporates, 3 minutes. Stir in the lemon juice, salt, and remaining ⅛ teaspoon pepper.

5 Preheat the broiler.

6 Spoon about ⅓ cup of the couscous into each of the mushroom caps, pressing the mixture to pack it into each cap. Mound about ½ cup of the spinach mixture on top of the couscous. Top the spinach evenly with the feta. Broil until the feta melts, about 3 minutes. Divide the mushrooms evenly among 4 plates and serve at once.

Each serving: 22 g carb, 180 cal, 7 g fat, 3 g sat fat, 17 mg chol, 5 g fib, 9 g pro, 431 mg sod • Carb Choices: 1½; Exchanges: 1 starch, 2 veg, 1½ fat

Polenta-Stuffed Portobellos [HIGH FIBER]

makes 4 servings

Creamy polenta and rich meaty mushrooms give this dish contrasting textures and flavors. Serve two mushrooms as a main dish, or one mushroom as an appetizer. Served with a salad of baby lettuces alongside, these tomato-topped mushrooms make a striking presentation.

8 large portobello mushrooms (about 4½-inch diameter)

6 teaspoons extra virgin olive oil, divided

1 small onion, chopped

1 garlic clove, minced

2 cups Vegetable Stock (page 149) or low-sodium vegetable broth

½ teaspoon kosher salt

⅛ teaspoon freshly ground pepper

½ cup fine-grind yellow cornmeal

2 ounces shredded fontina or Gruyère (about ½ cup)

2 tablespoons chopped fresh basil

4 small plum tomatoes, thinly sliced

1 ounce freshly grated Parmesan (about ¼ cup)

1 Cut away and discard the tough stems of the mushrooms. Using a spoon, gently scrape away and discard the dark gills on the underside of each mushroom.

2 Heat a large nonstick skillet over medium-high heat. Add 2 teaspoons of the oil and tilt the pan to coat the bottom evenly. Add 4 of the mushrooms, cover, and cook, turning once, until tender, 6 to 8 minutes. Transfer the mushrooms, stem side up, to a large rimmed baking sheet. Cover to keep warm. Repeat with 2 teaspoons of the remaining oil and the remaining 4 mushrooms.

3 Meanwhile, heat a medium saucepan over medium-high heat. Add the remaining 2 teaspoons oil and tilt the pan to coat the bottom evenly. Add the onion and cook, stirring often, until softened, 5 minutes. Add the garlic and cook, stirring constantly, until fragrant, 30 seconds. Add the stock, salt, and pepper and bring to a boil.

4 Slowly sprinkle the cornmeal into the stock, whisking constantly. Reduce the heat to low and cook, stirring constantly, until the polenta is thickened, about 3 minutes. Remove from the heat and stir in the fontina and basil.

5 Preheat the broiler.

6 Spoon about ¼ cup of the polenta into each of the mushroom caps. Top with the tomatoes and sprinkle evenly with the Parmesan. Broil until the cheese melts, about 2 minutes. Divide the mushrooms among 4 plates and serve at once.

Each serving: 29 g carb, 283 cal, 14 g fat, 5 g sat fat, 21 mg chol, 5 g fib, 12 g pro, 415 mg sod • Carb Choices: 2; Exchanges: 1 starch, 2 veg, 2 fat

Quinoa Cakes with Fresh Tomato–Cilantro Sauce

makes 4 servings

This recipe puts a Southwestern spin on quinoa. The cheese in the quinoa cakes melts and browns as the cakes cook, creating a crispy crust. You can serve this dish to 8 people as an out-of-the-ordinary starter to a Tex-Mex meal.

1½ cups Vegetable Stock (page 149) or low-sodium vegetable broth

1 cup quinoa, rinsed

¼ teaspoon plus pinch of kosher salt, divided

4 ounces shredded reduced-fat Monterey Jack cheese (about 1 cup)

2 large egg whites

¼ cup plain dry breadcrumbs

Pinch of ground cayenne

2¼ teaspoons canola oil, divided

1 large tomato, chopped

2 tablespoons chopped fresh cilantro

2 tablespoons thinly sliced scallions

2 teaspoons lime juice

1 Combine the stock, quinoa, and ¼ teaspoon of the salt in a medium saucepan and bring to a boil over high heat. Reduce the heat to low, cover, and simmer until the quinoa is tender, 12 to 15 minutes. Transfer to a medium bowl to cool.

2 Add the Monterey Jack, egg whites, breadcrumbs, and cayenne to the quinoa and stir to mix well.

3 Brush a ¼-cup measuring cup with ¼ teaspoon of the oil. Spoon the quinoa mixture into the cup, pressing until it is lightly packed. Invert the quinoa cakes onto a large plate. Cover and refrigerate 30 minutes.

4 Meanwhile, place the tomato, cilantro, scallions, lime juice, and the remaining pinch of salt in a food processor. Pulse until coarsely chopped, but not pureed, 4 to 5 times. Set the sauce aside.

5 Heat a large nonstick skillet over medium heat. Add the remaining 2 teaspoons oil and tilt the pan to coat the bottom evenly. Add the quinoa cakes and cook, turning once, until well browned, 3 to 4 minutes on each side. Spoon the sauce evenly onto 4 plates, top evenly with the quinoa cakes, and serve at once.

Each serving: 39 g carb, 317 cal, 12 g fat, 4 g sat fat, 20 mg chol, 3 g fib, 16 g pro, 475 mg sod • Carb Choices: 2½; Exchanges: 2½ starch, 1 high-fat protein, ½ fat

Basil Quinoa with Pan-Roasted Tomatoes and Goat Cheese HIGH FIBER

makes 4 servings

Browning tomatoes in a skillet is a quick way to caramelize them and add robust flavor. This dish is fantastic with summer tomatoes, but even with winter tomatoes, it's an enjoyable no-brainer dinner. Instead of the quinoa, you can serve the tomatoes with any kind of grain or pasta—try whole wheat couscous, orzo, or barley.

1¾ cups Vegetable Stock (page 149) or low-sodium vegetable broth, divided
1 cup quinoa, rinsed
½ teaspoon plus ⅛ teaspoon kosher salt, divided
4 teaspoons extra virgin olive oil, divided
4 large plum tomatoes, halved lengthwise
2 scallions, thinly sliced
1 garlic clove, minced
½ cup dry white wine
Pinch of freshly ground pepper
2 tablespoons chopped fresh basil
4 ounces crumbled goat cheese (about 1 cup), at room temperature

1 Combine 1½ cups of the stock, the quinoa, and ¼ teaspoon of the salt in a medium saucepan and bring to a boil. Reduce the heat, cover, and simmer until tender, 12 to 15 minutes.

2 Meanwhile, heat a large nonstick skillet over medium-high heat. Add 2 teaspoons of the oil and tilt the pan to coat the bottom. Add the tomatoes, cut side down, and cook until browned, 3 minutes. Turn and cook 1 minute longer. Sprinkle the tomatoes with ¼ teaspoon of the remaining salt. Transfer the tomatoes to 4 plates and keep warm.

3 Wipe out the skillet with several thicknesses of paper towels and heat over medium-high heat. Add the remaining 2 teaspoons oil to the skillet and tilt the pan to coat the bottom evenly. Add the scallions and garlic to the skillet and cook, stirring constantly, until softened, about 1 minute. Add the wine, the remaining ¼ cup stock, remaining ⅛ teaspoon salt and the pepper and bring to a boil. Cook until reduced to about ¼ cup, about 4 minutes.

4 Stir the basil into the quinoa. Divide the quinoa among the plates. Drizzle the tomatoes and quinoa with the wine mixture. Sprinkle with the goat cheese and serve at once.

Each serving: 35 g carb, 352 cal, 16 g fat, 7 g sat fat, 22 mg chol, 4 g fib, 12 g pro, 396 mg sod • Carb Choices: 2; Exchanges: 2 starch, 1 high-fat protein, 1 fat

Beans

Black and White Bean Chili QUICK | HIGH FIBER

makes 6 servings

Beer and chili are perfect partners—especially if you put the beer in the chili. The dark beer gives this quick-cooking chili a rich, deep flavor that makes this dish taste like it simmered for hours.

2 teaspoons canola oil
1 large onion, chopped
1 red bell pepper, chopped
1 green bell pepper, chopped
1 jalapeño, seeded and minced
2 garlic cloves, minced
2 tablespoons chili powder
2 tablespoons ground cumin
½ teaspoon kosher salt
⅛ teaspoon freshly ground pepper
2 cans (14½-ounces) no-salt-added diced tomatoes
2 (15-ounce) cans no-salt-added cannellini beans, rinsed and drained
2 (15-ounce) cans no-salt-added black beans, rinsed and drained
1 (12-ounce) bottle dark beer
Thinly sliced scallions

1 Heat a large pot over medium-high heat. Add the oil and tilt the pot to coat the bottom evenly.

2 Add the onion, bell peppers, jalapeño, and garlic and cook, stirring often, until softened, 5 minutes. Add the chili powder, cumin, salt, and ground pepper and cook, stirring constantly, until fragrant, 30 seconds. Add the tomatoes, cannellini beans, black beans, and beer and bring to a boil over high heat. Cover, reduce the heat to low, and simmer until the vegetables are very tender and the chili is thickened, about 20 minutes.

3 Ladle the chili evenly into 6 bowls, sprinkle with the scallions, and serve at once. The chili can be refrigerated, covered, for up to 4 days or frozen for up to 3 months.

Each serving: 54 g carb, 327 cal, 4 g fat, 0 g sat fat, 0 mg chol, 17 g fib, 17 g pro, 274 mg sod • Carb Choices: 3; Exchanges: 2½ starch, 1 veg, 2 plant-based protein

Quick Lentil Chili QUICK | HIGH FIBER

makes 6 servings

Lentils are so quick cooking, they can easily be part of a weeknight meal. This fast and filling chili will certainly become a family favorite. You can dress it up with a sprinkle of chopped fresh cilantro or thinly sliced scallions, or a spoonful of plain low-fat yogurt.

2 teaspoons canola oil
1 medium onion, chopped
1 small green bell pepper, chopped
2 garlic cloves, minced
2 tablespoons chili powder
1 tablespoon ground cumin
½ teaspoon dried oregano
½ teaspoon kosher salt
5 cups Vegetable Stock (page 149) or low-sodium vegetable broth
2 (15-ounce) cans no-salt-added crushed tomatoes
1 cup dried brown lentils, picked over and rinsed
1 tablespoon lime juice
2 ounces shredded reduced-fat extra-sharp Cheddar cheese (about ¼ cup)

1 Heat a large pot over medium-high heat. Add the oil and tilt the pot to coat the bottom evenly.

2 Add the onion and bell pepper and cook, stirring often, until softened, 5 minutes. Add the garlic, chili powder, cumin, oregano, and salt and

cook, stirring constantly, until fragrant, 30 seconds. Add the stock, tomatoes, and lentils and bring to a boil over high heat. Cover, reduce the heat to low, and simmer until the lentils are tender and the chili is thickened, 20 to 25 minutes. Remove from the heat and stir in the lime juice.

3 Ladle the chili into 6 bowls, sprinkle evenly with the Cheddar, and serve at once. The chili can be refrigerated, covered, for up to 4 days or frozen for up to 3 months.

Each serving: 34 g carb, 255 cal, 6 g fat, 2 g sat fat, 9 mg chol, 11 g fib, 13 g pro, 462 mg sod • Carb Choices: 2; Exchanges: 1 starch, 2 veg, 1 plant-based protein, 1 fat

White Bean, Artichoke, and Zucchini Stew QUICK | HIGH FIBER

makes 6 servings

Artichoke hearts offer an unusual addition to this Mediterranean-inspired bean stew. Fresh rosemary adds a piney flavor and a touch of balsamic vinegar adds a little sparkle.

2 teaspoons extra virgin olive oil

1 medium onion, chopped

1 medium red bell pepper, chopped

2 garlic cloves, chopped

3 cups Vegetable Stock (page 149) or low-sodium vegetable broth

2 (15-ounce) cans no-salt-added cannellini beans, rinsed and drained

1 (14½-ounce) can no-salt-added diced tomatoes, drained

¼ cup no-salt-added tomato paste

2 teaspoons chopped fresh rosemary

1 (14-ounce) can artichoke hearts

1 medium zucchini, quartered lengthwise and sliced

2 cups chopped fresh spinach

1½ teaspoons balsamic vinegar

Pinch of crushed red pepper

1 Heat a large pot over medium heat. Add the oil and tilt the pan to coat the bottom evenly. Add the onion and bell pepper and cook, stirring often, until the vegetables are softened, 5 minutes. Add the garlic and cook, stirring constantly, until fragrant, 30 seconds. Add the stock, beans, tomatoes, tomato paste, and rosemary and bring to a boil over high heat. Cover, reduce the heat, and simmer until the vegetables are tender, 15 minutes.

2 Meanwhile, drain and rinse the artichoke hearts and cut into quarters. Place the artichokes on several thicknesses of paper towels and gently blot dry.

3 Add the artichoke hearts and zucchini to the pot and return to a simmer. Cook until the zucchini is crisp-tender, about 3 minutes. Stir in the spinach and cook just until the spinach wilts, about 1 minute. Stir in the vinegar and crushed red pepper. Ladle the stew evenly into 6 bowls and serve at once.

Each serving: 34 g carb, 201 cal, 3 g fat, 0 g sat fat, 0 mg chol, 8 g fib, 10 g pro, 311 mg sod • Carb Choices: 2; Exchanges: 1 starch, 3 veg, 1 plant-based protein

Bean and Vegetable Stew with Crispy Breadcrumbs

QUICK | HIGH FIBER

makes 4 servings

The crispy baked breadcrumbs turn an already delicious soup into a distinctive lunch or dinner. Don't add them until you're ready to serve the soup so they will stay crisp. The crumbs are a delicious topping for almost any kind of soup or pasta dish.

4 teaspoons extra virgin olive oil, divided

1 large onion, chopped

2 garlic cloves, minced

2 carrots, peeled and chopped

1 stalk celery, chopped

1 medium turnip, peeled and chopped

2 (15-ounce) cans no-salt-added navy beans, rinsed and drained

1½ cups Vegetable Stock (page 149) or low-sodium vegetable broth

2 tablespoons no-salt-added tomato paste

½ teaspoon kosher salt

¼ teaspoon freshly ground pepper

¾ cup fresh whole wheat breadcrumbs

1 garlic clove, crushed through a press

4 plum tomatoes, chopped

2 tablespoons chopped fresh basil

1 Heat a large pot over medium-high heat. Add 2 teaspoons of the oil and tilt the pot to coat the bottom evenly. Add the onion and cook, stirring often, until the onion is softened, 5 minutes. Stir in the garlic and cook, stirring constantly, until fragrant, 30 seconds.

2 Add the carrots, celery, turnip, beans, stock, tomato paste, salt, and pepper and bring to a boil over high heat. Cover, reduce the heat to low, and simmer until the vegetables are very tender, about 15 minutes.

3 Preheat the oven to 350°F.

4 Stir together the breadcrumbs, garlic, and the remaining 2 teaspoons oil in a small bowl until the crumbs are moist. Place the crumbs in a small rimmed baking sheet and bake, stirring once, until crisp, 8 to 10 minutes.

5 Add the tomatoes to the stew and cook just until heated through, about 2 minutes. Remove the stew from the heat and stir in the basil. Ladle the stew into 4 bowls, sprinkle evenly with the crumbs, and serve at once. The stew can be refrigerated, covered, for up to 4 days.

Each serving: 32 g carb, 228 cal, 6 g fat, 1 g sat fat, 0 mg chol, 10 g fib, 9 g pro, 303 mg sod • Carb Choices: 2; Exchanges: 1½ starch, 1 veg, 1 plant-based protein, 1 fat

Chunky Edamame and Vegetable Stew

QUICK | HIGH FIBER

makes 4 servings

Edamame is given a decidedly American treatment in this summer stew. If you prefer, you can use baby lima beans for this recipe, but take into account the extra carbs. One ½ cup of edamame has just 7 grams of carbs and the same amount of baby limas has 21 grams.

8 dry-packed sun-dried tomatoes, finely chopped

½ cup water

2 teaspoons extra virgin olive oil

1 small onion, chopped

2 garlic cloves, minced

3 cups Vegetable Stock (page 149) or low-sodium vegetable broth

½ teaspoon kosher salt

¼ teaspoon freshly ground pepper

2 cups frozen shelled edamame

1 medium yellow squash, quartered lengthwise and sliced

1 medium zucchini, quartered lengthwise and sliced

½ small eggplant, peeled and cut into ½-inch pieces (about 2 cups)

1 large tomato, chopped

2 tablespoons finely shredded Parmesan

2 tablespoons chopped fresh basil or Italian parsley

1 Combine the sun-dried tomatoes and water in a small saucepan. Set over medium heat and bring to a boil. Remove from the heat, cover, and let stand 15 minutes.

2 Meanwhile, heat a large pot over medium heat. Add the oil and tilt the pan to coat the bottom evenly. Add the onion and cook, stirring often, until softened, 5 minutes. Add the garlic and cook, stirring constantly, until fragrant, 30 seconds. Add the stock, sun-dried tomato mixture, salt, and pepper and bring to a boil over high heat.

3 Add the edamame, yellow squash, zucchini, and eggplant and bring to a boil. Cook until the vegetables are crisp-tender, about 5 minutes. Stir in the tomato and cook just until heated through, about 1 minute.

4 To serve, ladle the soup into 4 bowls, sprinkle evenly with the Parmesan and basil, and serve at once. The stew is best on the day it is made.

Each serving: 20 g carb, 172 cal, 7 g fat, 1 g sat fat, 3 mg chol, 7 g fib, 10 g pro, 396 mg sod • Carb Choices: 1; Exchanges: ½ starch, 1 veg, 1 plant-based protein, 1 fat

Moroccan Bean Stew

HIGH FIBER

makes 4 servings

Navy beans are commonly used to make baked beans, but you can use them in any soup, stew, or chili that calls for cannellini beans. Navy beans are smaller than cannellini beans—they're about the size of a large pea. In this recipe, they lend their creamy texture to a vibrantly spiced bean and vegetable stew.

2 teaspoons extra virgin olive oil

2 stalks celery, chopped

1 large carrot, peeled and chopped

1 medium onion, chopped

2 garlic cloves, minced

2 teaspoons ground cumin

1 teaspoon paprika

1 teaspoon ground ginger

¼ teaspoon ground turmeric

¼ teaspoon freshly ground pepper

¼ teaspoon kosher salt

⅛ teaspoon ground cinnamon

2 (15-ounce) cans no-salt-added navy beans, rinsed and drained

1½ cups Vegetable Stock (page 149) or low-sodium vegetable broth

1 (14½-ounce) can no-salt-added diced tomatoes

2 tablespoons no-salt-added tomato paste

1 tablespoon lime juice

2 teaspoons honey

Chopped fresh cilantro

1 Heat a large saucepan over medium heat. Add the oil and tilt the pan to coat the bottom evenly. Add the celery, carrot, and onion and cook, stirring often, until softened, 5 minutes. Add the garlic, cumin, paprika, ginger, turmeric, pepper, salt, and cinnamon and cook, stirring constantly, until fragrant, 30 seconds. Add the beans, stock, tomatoes, and tomato paste and bring to a boil over high heat.

2 Cover, reduce the heat to low, and simmer until the vegetables are tender and the stew is thickened, 20 to 25 minutes. Remove from the heat and stir in the lime juice and honey.

3 Ladle the stew evenly into 4 bowls, sprinkle with the cilantro, and serve at once. The stew can be refrigerated, covered, for up to 4 days or frozen for up to 3 months.

Each serving: 47 g carb, 265 cal, 4 g fat, 0 g sat fat, 0 mg chol, 15 g fib, 13 g pro, 225 mg sod • Carb Choices: 2½; Exchanges: 2 starch, 2 veg, 2 plant-based protein, ½ fat

Garbanzo Picadillo

QUICK | HIGH FIBER

makes 6 servings

Picadillo is a spicy Cuban dish usually made with ground beef and used as a filling for tacos or served over rice. This stew is a take on the sweet and spicy flavors of picadillo and uses healthful fiber-rich beans instead of ground beef.

2 teaspoons extra virgin olive oil

1 medium onion, chopped

2 garlic cloves, minced

2 teaspoons ground cumin

1 teaspoon ground coriander

½ teaspoon kosher salt

¼ teaspoon freshly ground pepper

¼ teaspoon ground cinnamon

Pinch of ground cayenne

2 cups Vegetable Stock (page 149) or low-sodium vegetable broth

2 (14½-ounce) cans no-salt-added diced tomatoes

2 (15-ounce) cans no-salt-added garbanzo beans, rinsed and drained

¼ cup golden raisins

2 tablespoons capers, rinsed and drained

2 tablespoons no-salt-added tomato paste

2 medium zucchini, chopped

1 tablespoon honey

1 tablespoon sherry vinegar or white wine vinegar

Chopped fresh cilantro

1 Heat a large saucepan over medium heat. Add the oil and tilt the pan to coat the bottom evenly. Add the onion and cook, stirring often, until softened, 5 minutes. Add the garlic, cumin, coriander, salt, pepper, cinnamon, and cayenne and cook, stirring constantly, until fragrant, 30 seconds. Add the stock, tomatoes, beans, raisins, capers, and tomato paste and bring to a boil over high heat.

2 Cover, reduce the heat to low, and simmer until the stew is slightly thickened, about 20 minutes. Add the zucchini and cook until just crisp-tender, about 3 minutes longer. Remove from the heat and stir in the honey and vinegar.

3 Ladle the stew evenly into 6 bowls, sprinkle with the cilantro, and serve at once. The stew can be refrigerated, covered, for up to 4 days or frozen for up to 3 months.

Each serving: 42 g carb, 252 cal, 3 g fat, 0 g sat fat, 0 mg chol, 9 g fib, 11 g pro, 324 mg sod • Carb Choices: 3; Exchanges: 2 starch, 2 veg, 1 plant-based protein

Red Beans and Greens HIGH FIBER

makes 6 servings

Red kidney beans are one of the best sources of fiber you can eat—a ½-cup serving has a whopping 8 grams of fiber. Their meaty texture and earthy flavor is a perfect match to the spicy Cajun-inspired flavors of this stew.

2 teaspoons extra virgin olive oil

1 large onion, chopped

1 red or yellow bell pepper, chopped

1 stalk celery, chopped

2 garlic cloves, minced

2 (15-ounce) cans no-salt-added red kidney beans, rinsed and drained

3 cups Vegetable Stock (page 149) or low-sodium vegetable broth

2 (14½-ounce) cans no-salt-added diced tomatoes

2 tablespoons no-salt-added tomato paste

1½ teaspoons dried oregano

1 teaspoon kosher salt

1 teaspoon dried thyme

2 teaspoons paprika

⅛ teaspoon ground cayenne

1 pound kale, tough stems removed and leaves chopped

½ teaspoon hot sauce

1 Heat a large pot over medium heat. Add the oil and tilt the pan to coat the bottom evenly. Add the onion, bell pepper, and celery and cook, stirring often, until softened, 5 minutes. Add the garlic and cook, stirring constantly, until fragrant, 30 seconds.

2 Meanwhile, place ¼ cup of the beans in a small bowl and mash with a fork. Add the mashed beans, whole beans, stock, tomatoes, tomato paste, oregano, salt, thyme, paprika, and cayenne to the pot and bring to a boil over high heat. Add the kale in batches and return to a boil. Cover, reduce the heat to low, and simmer until the kale is very tender, about 30 minutes. Remove from the heat and stir in the hot sauce. Ladle the stew evenly into 6 bowls and serve at once. The stew can be refrigerated, covered, for up to 4 days.

Each serving: 41 g carb, 222 cal, 3 g fat, 0 g sat fat, 0 mg chol, 12 g fib, 13 g pro, 287 mg sod • Carb Choices: 2; Exchanges: 1½ starch, 2 veg, 1 plant-based protein, ½ fat

Lentil and Root Vegetable Stew HIGH FIBER

makes 6 servings

This stew has a long ingredient list, but many of the ingredients are spices, so the dish comes together quickly. Warm spices, sweet currants, and earthy lentils make it perfect for a chilly fall or winter evening.

2 teaspoons extra virgin olive oil
1 medium onion, chopped
1 yellow bell pepper, chopped
2 garlic cloves, minced
1 tablespoon minced fresh ginger
1 teaspoon kosher salt
½ teaspoon ground cumin
½ teaspoon ground coriander
½ teaspoon ground cinnamon
½ teaspoon paprika
¼ teaspoon freshly ground pepper
⅛ teaspoon ground allspice
Pinch of ground cayenne
5 cups Vegetable Stock (page 149) or low-sodium vegetable broth
1 (14½-ounce) can no-salt-added diced tomatoes
¾ cup dried brown lentils, picked over and rinsed
1 medium turnip, peeled and chopped
1 medium sweet potato, peeled and chopped
¼ cup dried currants
¼ cup no-salt-added tomato paste
2 tablespoons lemon juice
Chopped fresh cilantro

1 Heat a large pot over medium heat. Add the oil and tilt the pan to coat the bottom evenly. Add the onion and bell pepper and cook, stirring often, until softened, 5 minutes. Add the garlic, ginger, salt, cumin, coriander, cinnamon, paprika, ground pepper, allspice, and cayenne and cook, stirring constantly, until fragrant, 30 seconds.

2 Add the stock, tomatoes, lentils, turnip, sweet potato, currants, and tomato paste and bring to a boil over high heat. Cover, reduce the heat to low, and simmer until the lentils are tender, about 30 minutes.

3 Remove from the heat and stir in the lemon juice. Ladle the stew evenly into 6 bowls, sprinkle with the cilantro, and serve at once. The stew can be refrigerated, covered, for up to 4 days.

Each serving: 31 g carb, 168 cal, 2 g fat, 0 g sat fat, 0 mg chol, 8 g fib, 8 g pro, 223 mg sod • Carb Choices: 2; Exchanges: 1 starch, 2 veg, 1 plant-based protein

Black Bean Burritos with Creamy Avocado Sauce

QUICK | HIGH FIBER

makes 4 servings

Made with canned beans and loads of quick-cooking vegetables, these burritos are a fast and convenient dinner to make when you've got other activities planned for the evening. If your kids say no to avocados, serve the burritos with Fresh Tomato Salsa (page 41) or to save time, serve them with purchased salsa.

2 teaspoons canola oil

1 red bell pepper, thinly sliced

1 medium red onion, thinly sliced

1 jalapeño, seeded and minced

2 garlic cloves, minced

2 teaspoons chili powder

1 teaspoon ground cumin

1 (15-ounce) can no-salt-added black beans, rinsed and drained

½ cup Vegetable Stock (page 149) or low-sodium vegetable broth

2 plum tomatoes, chopped

8 (6-inch) whole wheat flour tortillas, warmed

1 recipe Creamy Avocado Sauce (page 596)

1 Heat a large nonstick skillet over medium-high heat. Add the oil and tilt the pan to coat the bottom evenly. Add the bell pepper, onion, and jalapeño and cook, stirring often, until softened, 5 minutes. Add the garlic, chili powder, and cumin and cook, stirring constantly, until fragrant, 30 seconds.

2 Add the beans and stock and bring to a boil over high heat. Reduce the heat to low and simmer until the vegetables are tender and most of the liquid has absorbed, about 5 minutes. Add the tomatoes and cook, stirring often, just until heated through, about 3 minutes.

3 Spoon the bean mixture evenly down the center of each tortilla. Roll up and place 2 burritos seam side down on each of 4 plates. Drizzle with the sauce and serve at once.

Each serving: 39 g carb, 364 cal, 11 g fat, 1 g sat fat, 2 mg chol, 25 g fib, 15 g pro, 644 mg sod • Carb Choices: 2½; Exchanges: 2 starch, 1 veg, 1 plant-based protein, ½ fat

Black Bean and Poblano Enchiladas HIGH FIBER

makes 4 servings

Enchiladas are typically made with corn tortillas, but you can use whole wheat flour tortillas for these instead. To save time, you can use a purchased tomatillo sauce or an enchilada sauce instead of the fresh Tomatillo Sauce.

4 teaspoons canola oil, divided

1 large poblano chile, cut into short, thin strips

1 small red onion, halved lengthwise and thinly sliced

2 garlic cloves, minced

1 (14½-ounce) can no-salt-added diced tomatoes

1 cup canned no-salt-added black beans, drained and rinsed

½ teaspoon minced chipotle in adobo sauce

¼ teaspoon kosher salt

¼ cup chopped fresh cilantro

1 cup Tomatillo Sauce (page 596)

8 (6-inch) corn tortillas, warmed

2 ounces shredded reduced-fat Monterey Jack cheese (about ½ cup)

1 Preheat the oven to 375°F. Brush a 13 x 9-inch baking dish with 2 teaspoons of the oil.

2 Heat a large nonstick skillet over medium heat, add the remaining 2 teaspoons oil, and tilt the pan to coat the bottom evenly. Add the poblano and onion and cook, stirring often, until softened, 5 minutes. Add the garlic and cook,

stirring constantly, until fragrant, 30 seconds. Add the tomatoes, beans, chipotles, and salt and cook, stirring often, until heated through, about 3 minutes. Remove from the heat and stir in the cilantro.

3 Spoon ½ cup of the sauce in the bottom of the prepared baking dish. Spoon about ⅓ cup of the vegetable mixture down the center of each tortilla. Roll up and place seam side down in the baking dish. Spoon the remaining ½ cup of the sauce over the enchiladas and bake until heated through, 20 minutes. Sprinkle with the Monterey Jack and bake until the cheese melts, 5 minutes longer. Divide the enchiladas evenly among 4 plates and serve at once.

Each serving: 52 g carb, 351 cal, 12 g fat, 2 g sat fat, 10 mg chol, 9 g fib, 11 g pro, 519 mg sod • Carb Choices: 3; Exchanges: 2½ starch, 2 veg, 1 plant-based protein, 2 fat

Black Bean and Avocado Chiles Rellenos HIGH FIBER

makes 4 servings

These chiles rellenos are the antithesis of the typical heavy batter-fried version. Filled with fiber-rich beans, fresh tomatoes, and avocado and baked instead of fried, these are just as delicious as they are healthful.

8 large poblano chiles
1 teaspoon canola oil
1 cup canned no-salt-added black beans, rinsed and drained
3 ounces shredded reduced-fat extra-sharp Cheddar cheese (about ¾ cup)
1 large tomato, diced
½ avocado, peeled, pitted, and diced
½ cup chopped fresh cilantro
1 tablespoon lime juice
1 cup Tomatillo Sauce (page 596)
1 ounce shredded reduced-fat Monterey Jack cheese (about ¼ cup)

1 Roast the poblanos according to the procedure for Roasted Bell Peppers (page 21). When peeling the peppers, leave them whole and cut a slit lengthwise in each pepper to remove the seeds.

2 Preheat the oven to 350°F. Brush a 13 x 9-inch baking dish with the oil.

3 Stir together the beans, Cheddar, tomato, avocado, cilantro, and lime juice in a medium bowl.

4 Spread ½ cup of the sauce in the bottom of the prepared dish. Fill the cavity of each pepper with about ½ cup of the bean mixture. Place the peppers, slit side up, in a single layer in the prepared baking dish. Drizzle the peppers with the remaining ½ cup sauce.

5 Cover with foil and bake until the stuffing is heated through and the sauce is bubbly, about 20 minutes. Uncover, sprinkle with the Monterey Jack, and bake until the cheese melts, about 5 minutes longer. Divide the chiles evenly among 4 plates and serve at once.

Each serving: 27 g carb, 268 cal, 13 g fat, 5 g sat fat, 20 mg chol, 9 g fib, 14 g pro, 425 mg sod • Carb Choices: 1½; Exchanges: ½ starch, 3 veg, 1 high-fat protein, 1 plant-based protein, 1 fat

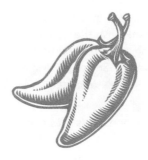

Bean and Spinach Cakes with Cucumber-Cilantro Yogurt Sauce HIGH FIBER

makes 4 servings

You can shape these into four "cakes" instead of eight to turn them into burgers. Serve them in buns with lettuce, tomatoes, and the yogurt sauce. The frozen spinach and canned beans make these a speedy weeknight supper.

1 (15-ounce) can no-salt-added garbanzo beans, rinsed and drained
1 (10-ounce) package frozen chopped spinach, thawed and squeezed dry
1 large egg
¼ cup plain dry breadcrumbs
1 small garlic clove, crushed through a press
½ teaspoon ground cumin
½ teaspoon kosher salt
Pinch of ground cayenne
2 teaspoons extra virgin olive oil
½ cup low-fat plain yogurt
¼ cup peeled seeded shredded cucumber
2 tablespoons chopped fresh cilantro
2 teaspoons lime juice
Lime wedges

1 Place the beans in a medium bowl. Using a potato masher, mash the beans until chunky. Stir in the spinach, egg, breadcrumbs, garlic, cumin, salt, and cayenne. Shape into eight 2-inch cakes. Place on a large plate, cover, and refrigerate for 30 minutes.

2 Heat a large nonstick skillet over medium heat. Add the oil and tilt the pan to coat the bottom evenly. Add the cakes and cook, turning once, until well browned, 2 to 3 minutes on each side.

3 Meanwhile, to make the sauce, stir together the yogurt, cucumber, cilantro, and lime juice in a small bowl. Divide the cakes and sauce among 4 plates and serve at once with the lime wedges.

Each serving: 23 g carb, 201 cal, 6 g fat, 1 g sat fat, 55 mg chol, 5 g fib, 11 g pro, 480 mg sod • Carb Choices: 1½; Exchanges: 1 starch, 1 plant-based protein, ½ fat

Falafel Burgers QUICK | HIGH FIBER

makes 4 servings

Falafel is one of my favorite vegetarian dishes and this version, which turns falafel into a burger, is a dinner that I make often. Cooked in just a tiny amount of oil, these are lower in calories and fat than deep-fried restaurant versions. Serve them with Greek Salad (page 84).

1 (15-ounce) can no-salt-added garbanzo beans, rinsed and drained
2 tablespoons diced red onion
1 garlic clove, minced
1 large egg
3 tablespoons fresh Italian parsley leaves
¼ cup plain dry breadcrumbs
2 teaspoons lemon juice
1 teaspoon ground cumin
¼ teaspoon kosher salt
Pinch of ground cayenne
2 teaspoons canola oil
4 whole wheat kaiser rolls, split and toasted
Lettuce leaves
Cucumber slices

1 Place the beans in a large bowl and mash with a potato masher until chunky. Stir in the onion, garlic, egg, parsley, breadcrumbs, lemon juice, cumin, salt, and cayenne. Shape into 4 patties.

2 Heat a large nonstick skillet over medium-high heat. Add the oil and tilt the pan to coat the bottom evenly. Add the burgers and cook, turning once, until lightly browned, 2 to 3 minutes on each side. Serve the burgers in the rolls, topped with the lettuce and cucumber.

Each serving: 43 g carb, 257 cal, 5 g fat, 1 g sat fat, 53 mg chol, 8 g fib, 12 g pro, 463 mg sod • Carb Choices: 2½; Exchanges: 2½ starch, 1 plant-based protein

Chipotle Black Bean Burgers QUICK | HIGH FIBER

makes 4 servings

You can serve these delicious vegetarian burgers to any meat lover. Chipotle, cumin, and cilantro add lots of flavor and an egg makes them super-moist. Turn them into cheeseburgers by topping them with a little shredded Monterey Jack or sharp Cheddar cheese during the last 2 minutes of cooking.

1 (15-ounce) can no-salt-added black beans, rinsed and drained
⅓ cup plain dry breadcrumbs
2 tablespoons chopped fresh cilantro
3 tablespoons chopped scallions
1 garlic clove, minced
1 large egg
½ teaspoon ground cumin
¼ to ½ teaspoon minced chipotle in adobo sauce
¼ teaspoon kosher salt
2 teaspoons canola oil
4 whole wheat kaiser rolls, split and toasted
1 cup Winter Tomato Salsa (page 41) or purchased salsa
Lettuce leaves

1 Place the beans in a large bowl and mash with a potato masher until chunky. Stir in the breadcrumbs, cilantro, scallion, garlic, egg, cumin, chipotle, and salt. Shape into 4 patties.

2 Heat a large nonstick skillet over medium-high heat. Add the oil and tilt the pan to coat the bottom evenly. Add the burgers and cook, turning once, until lightly browned, 2 to 3 minutes on each side. Serve the burgers in the rolls, topped with the salsa and lettuce.

Each serving: 46 g carb, 289 cal, 6 g fat, 1 g sat fat, 53 mg chol, 10 g fib, 13 g pro, 401 mg sod • Carb Choices: 3; Exchanges: 3 starch, 1 plant-based protein

Tofu

Tofu, Mushroom, and Broccoli Stir-Fry

QUICK | HIGH FIBER

makes 4 servings

If you love Thai-inspired coconut soup, here's a new way to enjoy those same flavors in a stir-fry. Serve it over brown jasmine rice or soba noodles. If you're not a vegetarian, you can substitute Asian fish sauce for the soy sauce.

1 cup reduced-fat coconut milk
2 tablespoons reduced-sodium soy sauce
2 teaspoons grated lime zest
1 tablespoon lime juice
½ teaspoon chili-garlic paste
1 (1-pound) package firm reduced-fat tofu, cut into 1-inch cubes
6 teaspoons canola oil, divided
3 tablespoons minced fresh ginger
8 ounces fresh shiitake mushrooms, stemmed and sliced
4 cups broccoli florets
4 scallions, cut into 2-inch pieces
¼ cup chopped fresh cilantro

1 Stir together the coconut milk, soy sauce, lime zest, lime juice, and chili-garlic paste in a small bowl. Set aside.

2 Pat the tofu dry with paper towels. Heat a large wok or nonstick skillet over medium-high heat. Add 2 teaspoons of the oil and tilt the pan to coat the bottom evenly. Add half of the tofu and cook, stirring often, until lightly browned, about 5 minutes. Transfer the tofu to a plate. Repeat with 2 teaspoons of the remaining oil and the remaining tofu.

continues on next page

3 Add the remaining 2 teaspoons oil to the wok. Add the ginger and cook, stirring constantly, until fragrant, 30 seconds. Add the mushrooms and cook, stirring frequently, until the mushrooms are softened and the liquid has evaporated, about 3 minutes. Add the broccoli and scallions and cook, stirring constantly, until crisp-tender, 5 minutes. Stir in the tofu and the coconut milk mixture and cook, stirring constantly, until the mixture comes to a boil. Remove from the heat and stir in the cilantro. Divide evenly among 4 plates and serve at once.

Each serving: 16 g carb, 257 cal, 16 g fat, 4 g sat fat, 0 mg chol, 6 g fib, 17 g pro, 386 mg sod • Carb Choices: 1; Exchanges: ½ starch, 1 veg, 2 plant-based protein, 2 fat

Curried Tofu and Vegetable Stir-Fry

QUICK | HIGH FIBER

makes 4 servings

Green curry paste gives this dish fantastic flavor in an instant. You can make it with red curry paste, too, but use only 1 teaspoon of red curry paste, unless you love spicy food.

⅔ cup reduced-fat coconut milk

1 tablespoon lime juice

2 teaspoons green curry paste

1 (1-pound) package extra-firm reduced-fat tofu, cut into 1-inch cubes

6 teaspoons canola oil, divided

2 garlic cloves, minced

2 cups small broccoli florets

1 small red onion, halved lengthwise and thinly sliced

1 red bell pepper, cut into short, thin strips

1 small yellow squash, halved lengthwise and sliced

½ teaspoon kosher salt

¼ cup chopped fresh basil

1 Stir together the coconut milk, lime juice, and curry paste in a small bowl. Set aside. Pat the tofu dry with paper towels.

2 Heat a large wok or nonstick skillet over medium-high heat. Add 2 teaspoons of the oil and tilt the pan to coat the bottom evenly. Add half of the tofu and cook, stirring often, until lightly browned, about 5 minutes. Transfer the tofu to a plate. Repeat with 2 teaspoons of the remaining oil and the remaining tofu.

3 Add the remaining 2 teaspoons oil to the wok. Add the garlic and cook, stirring constantly, until fragrant, 30 seconds. Add the broccoli, onion, bell pepper, and squash and cook, stirring often, until crisp-tender, 5 minutes. Stir in the tofu, the coconut milk mixture, and the salt and cook, stirring constantly, until the mixture comes to a boil. Remove from the heat and stir in the basil. Divide evenly among 4 plates and serve at once.

Each serving: 14 g carb, 232 cal, 14 g fat, 3 g sat fat, 0 mg chol, 5 g fib, 15 g pro, 220 mg sod • Carb Choices: 1; Exchanges: ½ starch, 1 veg, 2 fat

Teriyaki Tofu Stir-Fry QUICK

makes 4 servings

Soy sauce, fresh ginger, and a touch of sugar give this stir-fry the flavor of a typical teriyaki but with a lot less sodium and sugar than bottled teriyaki sauce. Serve this with steamed broccoli and brown rice.

2 tablespoons reduced-sodium soy sauce

1 tablespoon water

1 tablespoon rice vinegar

1 tablespoon sugar

½ teaspoon Asian sesame oil

1 (1-pound) package extra-firm reduced-fat tofu, cut into 1-inch cubes

6 teaspoons canola oil, divided

1 garlic clove, minced

1 tablespoon minced fresh ginger

2 scallions, thinly sliced

1 tablespoon sesame seeds, toasted (page 4)

1 Combine the soy sauce, water, vinegar, sugar, and sesame oil in a small bowl and stir until the sugar dissolves. Set aside.

2 Pat the tofu dry with paper towels. Heat a large wok or nonstick skillet over medium-high heat. Add 2 teaspoons of the canola oil and tilt the pan to coat the bottom evenly. Add half of the tofu and cook, stirring often, until lightly browned, about 5 minutes. Transfer to a serving platter. Repeat with 2 teaspoons of the remaining canola oil and the remaining tofu.

3 Add the remaining 2 teaspoons canola oil to the wok and tilt the pan to coat the bottom evenly. Add the garlic and ginger and cook, stirring constantly, until fragrant, 30 seconds. Add the soy sauce mixture and bring to a boil. Pour the sauce over the tofu. Sprinkle with the scallions and sesame seeds. Divide the tofu and sauce evenly among 4 plates and serve at once.

Each serving: 10 g carb, 214 cal, 14 g fat, 1 g sat fat, 0 mg chol, 3 g fib, 14 g pro, 311 mg sod • Carb Choices: ½; Exchanges: ½ carb, 2 plant-based protein, 1½ fat

Crispy Tofu with Spicy Ginger-Lime Soy Sauce

QUICK

makes 4 servings

In about 20 minutes from start to finish, you can make this incredibly flavored Asian dish. The texture of plain tofu is off-putting to some (including me), but browning it to create a crispy crust, as in this recipe, makes it really satisfying. Serve this dish with brown rice and sautéed spinach, bok choy, or Chinese broccoli to make it a meal.

2 tablespoons reduced-sodium soy sauce
2 tablespoons lime juice
2 tablespoons water
2 teaspoons light brown sugar
1 teaspoon grated fresh ginger
1 teaspoon cornstarch
¼ teaspoon chili-garlic paste
1 (1-pound) package extra-firm reduced-fat tofu
2 teaspoons canola oil
2 tablespoons chopped fresh cilantro
2 tablespoons thinly sliced scallion

1 Combine the soy sauce, lime juice, water, sugar, ginger, cornstarch, and chili-garlic paste in a small saucepan and stir until the sugar dissolves. Set aside.

2 Cut the tofu in half lengthwise, then cut each piece in half crosswise. Pat dry with paper towels.

3 Heat a large wok or nonstick skillet over medium-high heat. Add the oil and tilt the pan to coat the bottom evenly. Add the tofu and cook, turning once, until well browned, 3 to 4 minutes on each side.

4 Meanwhile, set the soy sauce mixture over medium-high heat and cook, whisking often, until the mixture comes to a boil and thickens, about 3 minutes.

5 Place the tofu on a serving platter, drizzle with the sauce, and sprinkle with the cilantro and scallion. Divide the tofu and sauce evenly among 4 plates and serve at once.

Each serving: 9 g carb, 153 cal, 7 g fat, 0 g sat fat, 0 mg chol, 3 g fib, 13 g pro, 311 mg sod • Carb Choices: ½; Exchanges: ½ carb, 2 plant-based protein, ½ fat

Tofu Baked with Soy, Ginger, and Garlic

makes 4 servings

This tofu soaks up the flavors of the cooking liquid as it bakes, making this a delicious discovery for those who think tofu has to taste bland. Serve it with any kind of steamed or sautéed greens and brown basmati rice.

1 (1-pound) package firm reduced-fat tofu
1 teaspoon canola oil
2 tablespoons reduced-sodium soy sauce
2 tablespoons orange juice
1 tablespoon rice vinegar
1 teaspoon grated fresh ginger
1 garlic clove, crushed through a press

1 Cut the tofu in half lengthwise, then cut each piece in half crosswise.

2 Brush an 8-inch square baking dish with the oil. Place the tofu in the prepared baking dish. Stir together the soy sauce, orange juice, vinegar, ginger, and garlic in a small bowl. Pour over the tofu and turn to coat. Let stand at room temperature, turning occasionally, 30 minutes.

3 Preheat the oven to 375°F.

4 Bake, turning the tofu once, until most of the sauce is absorbed and the tofu is lightly browned, about 40 minutes. Transfer the tofu to 4 plates and drizzle evenly with the sauce remaining in the baking dish. Serve at once.

Each serving: 7 g carb, 134 cal, 6 g fat, 0 g sat fat, 0 mg chol, 3 g fib, 13 g pro, 309 mg sod • Carb Choices: ½; Exchanges: ½ starch, 2 plant-based protein

Sesame-Roasted Tofu and Vegetables with Asian Pesto HIGH FIBER

makes 4 servings

Roasting tofu with sesame oil gives it a hearty, chewy texture and great sesame flavor. If you don't have time to make the pesto with this recipe (it's definitely worth the effort if you do have time), drizzle the tofu and vegetables with reduced-sodium soy sauce just before serving.

2 teaspoons canola oil
1 (1-pound) package firm reduced-fat tofu
3 teaspoons Asian sesame oil, divided
6 thin scallions, white and light green parts cut into 2-inch pieces
1 large red bell pepper, thinly sliced
½ teaspoon kosher salt
4 tablespoons Asian Pesto (page 598)

1 Preheat the oven to 425°F. Brush a large rimmed baking sheet with the canola oil.

2 Cut the tofu in half lengthwise, then cut each piece in half crosswise. Pat the tofu dry with paper towels.

3 Brush the tofu with 1 teaspoon of the sesame oil and arrange in a single layer on one end of the prepared baking sheet. Place the scallions and bell pepper on the other end of the baking sheet. Drizzle with the remaining 2 teaspoons sesame oil, sprinkle with the salt, and toss to coat. Arrange the vegetables in a single layer. Bake, stirring the vegetables and turning the tofu once, until tender and lightly browned, 30 to 35 minutes.

4 To serve, divide the tofu and vegetables evenly among 4 plates. Top each serving of tofu with 1 tablespoon of the pesto.

Each serving: 10 g carb, 228 cal, 15 g fat, 2 g sat fat, 2 mg chol, 4 g fib, 15 g pro, 301 mg sod • Carb Choices: ½; Exchanges: ½ starch, 1 veg, 2 plant-based protein, 2 fat

Italian Tofu [HIGH FIBER]

makes 4 servings

If you think you'll never get your family to eat tofu, try this recipe. It tastes just like chicken Parmesan. Well, almost. The Italian-seasoned panko crumbs make the tofu crisp and flavorful and the marinara sauce and grated Parmesan topping take it as far away from Asian flavors as tofu can go. Serve it with whole wheat pasta, of course.

2 cups Marinara Sauce (page 593)
1 large egg white
2 tablespoons water
⅔ cup panko crumbs
¼ cup plus 2 tablespoons freshly grated
    Parmesan, divided
¼ teaspoon dried oregano
¼ teaspoon dried basil
⅛ teaspoon freshly ground pepper
1 (1-pound) package firm reduced-fat tofu, cut
    crosswise into 8 slices
4 teaspoons extra virgin olive oil, divided

1 Heat the sauce in a saucepan over medium heat until hot, if necessary.

2 Place the egg white and water in a shallow dish and beat lightly with a fork. Stir together the panko crumbs, ¼ cup of the Parmesan, the oregano, basil, and pepper in another shallow dish. Dip the tofu, 1 slice at a time, into the egg white mixture, then into the crumb mixture, pressing to adhere the crumbs.

3 Heat a large nonstick skillet over medium heat. Add 2 teaspoons of the oil and tilt the pan to coat the bottom evenly. Add 4 slices of the tofu and cook, turning once, until the crumbs are lightly browned, 6 to 8 minutes. Transfer to a plate keep warm. Repeat with the remaining oil and tofu.

4 Divide the tofu among 4 plates, top with the sauce and the remaining 2 tablespoons Parmesan. Serve at once.

Each serving: 20 g carb, 269 cal, 14 g fat, 2 g sat fat, 7 mg chol, 4 g fib, 19 g pro, 222 mg sod • Carb Choices: 1; Exchanges: ½ starch, 1 veg, 2 plant-based protein, 1 fat

Eggs and Cheese

Eggplant Rollatini [HIGH FIBER]

makes 6 servings

Let's face it, eggplant rollatini is just an excuse to eat a little eggplant and a lot of cheese. This recipe uses low-fat cheeses and very little oil to make the healthiest possible version that's delicious enough to serve to your Italian grandmother.

3 teaspoons plus 1 tablespoon extra virgin
    olive oil, divided
2 medium eggplants
2 cups Marinara Sauce (page 593)
1¼ cups part-skim ricotta
1 ounce freshly grated Parmesan (about ¼ cup)
3 tablespoons chopped fresh basil
1 garlic clove, crushed through a press
¼ teaspoon kosher salt
⅛ teaspoon freshly ground pepper
2 ounces shredded part-skim mozzarella
    (about ½ cup)

1 Preheat the oven to 400°F. Brush each of 2 large rimmed baking sheets with 1 teaspoon of the oil.

2 Cut each eggplant lengthwise into six ¼-inch slices, discarding the end slices, which have too much skin. Brush the eggplant slices with 1 tablespoon of the remaining oil. Arrange the eggplant in a single layer on the prepared baking sheets and bake until they begin to brown, 15 to 20 minutes. Using a long metal spatula, carefully turn the eggplant slices and bake until tender and well browned, 8 to 10 minutes longer. Reduce the oven temperature to 350°F. Let the eggplant stand at room temperature until cool enough to handle.

3 Heat the sauce in a saucepan over medium heat until hot, if necessary.

continues on next page

4 Brush a 13 x 9-inch baking dish with the remaining 1 teaspoon oil.

5 Stir together the ricotta, Parmesan, basil, garlic, salt, and pepper in a medium bowl. Spoon 1 cup of the sauce into the prepared baking dish. Spoon about 2 tablespoons of the ricotta mixture onto one end of each eggplant slice. Roll up the slices and place seam side down in the baking dish. Spoon the remaining 1 cup sauce over the eggplant. Sprinkle evenly with the mozzarella.

6 Bake, uncovered, until the eggplant is heated through and the sauce is bubbly, 20 to 25 minutes. Divide the rollatini and sauce evenly among 6 plates and serve at once.

Each serving: 15 g carb, 216 cal, 13 g fat, 5 g sat fat, 26 mg chol, 6 g fib, 12 g pro, 282 mg sod • Carb Choices: 1; Exchanges: 2 veg, 2 medium-fat protein, 1 fat

Mushroom and Fontina Bread Pudding

makes 6 servings

This hearty pudding makes a comforting dinner, but it's just as well suited to serving for brunch. Serve it with Bibb and Whole Herb Salad (page 88) at either meal.

3 teaspoons extra virgin olive oil, divided

1 cup 1% low-fat milk

2 large eggs

2 large egg whites

¾ teaspoon kosher salt, divided

¼ teaspoon freshly ground pepper

5 slices day-old whole wheat bread, cut into ½-inch cubes (about 4 cups)

1½ pounds mixed mushrooms, sliced (such as shiitake, cremini, or oyster)

1 small onion, chopped

2 garlic cloves, minced

2 teaspoons chopped fresh thyme or ½ teaspoon dried thyme

3 ounces shredded fontina (about ¾ cup), divided

2 tablespoons chopped fresh Italian parsley

1 Preheat the oven to 350°F. Brush an 11 x 7-inch baking dish with 1 teaspoon of the oil.

2 Whisk together the milk, eggs, egg whites, ¼ teaspoon of the salt, and the pepper in a large bowl. Add the bread cubes and toss to combine. Let stand while you prepare the mushrooms, stirring occasionally.

3 Heat a large nonstick skillet over medium heat. Add the remaining 2 teaspoons oil and tilt the pan to coat the bottom evenly. Add the mushrooms, onion, garlic, thyme, and remaining ½ teaspoon salt and cook, stirring often, until the mushrooms are tender and the liquid has evaporated, about 8 minutes. Spoon the mushroom mixture into a bowl and let cool slightly.

4 Stir the mushroom mixture, ½ cup of the fontina, and the parsley into the bread mixture. Spoon into the prepared baking dish. Sprinkle the top of the pudding with the remaining ¼ cup fontina. Bake, uncovered, until the pudding is bubbly and the top is lightly browned, 30 to 35 minutes. Let stand 5 minutes before serving. Divide the bread pudding among 6 plates and serve at once.

Each serving: 23 g carb, 233 cal, 10 g fat, 4 g sat fat, 89 mg chol, 3 g fib, 15 g pro, 489 mg sod • Carb Choices: 1½; Exchanges: 1 starch, 1 veg, 1 high-fat protein, ½ fat

Caramelized Onion and Red Pepper Bread Pudding

makes 6 servings

To make this bread pudding the centerpiece of a weekend brunch or lunch, make the caramelized onions the day before and cover and refrigerate them. The next day, the bread pudding can be assembled with just a few minutes prep. Serve it with Orchard Fruit Salad (page 30) and mimosas.

3 teaspoons extra virgin olive oil, divided

2 large onions, halved and thinly sliced

¾ teaspoon kosher salt, divided

1 cup 1% low-fat milk

2 large eggs

2 large egg whites

¾ teaspoon kosher salt, divided

¼ teaspoon freshly ground pepper

5 slices day-old 100% whole wheat bread, cut into ½-inch cubes (about 4 cups)

1 cup red Roasted Bell Peppers (page 21) or roasted red peppers from a jar, sliced

3 ounces shredded part-skim mozzarella (about ¾ cup), divided

¼ cup chopped fresh basil

1 Heat a large nonstick skillet over medium heat. Add 2 teaspoons of the oil and tilt the pan to coat the bottom evenly. Add the onions and ½ teaspoon of the salt and cook, stirring often, until the onions are very tender and lightly browned, about 30 minutes. Spoon the onion mixture into a bowl and let cool slightly.

2 Preheat the oven to 350°F. Brush an 11 x 7-inch baking dish with the remaining 1 teaspoon oil.

3 Whisk together the milk, eggs, egg whites, remaining ¼ teaspoon salt, and the ground pepper in a large bowl. Add the bread cubes and toss to combine. Let stand until most of the liquid is absorbed, stirring occasionally, about 10 minutes.

4 Stir the onions, roasted peppers, ½ cup of the mozzarella, and the basil into the bread mixture. Spoon into the prepared baking dish. Sprinkle the top of the pudding with the remaining ¼ cup of mozzarella. Bake, uncovered, until the pudding is bubbly and the top is lightly browned, 30 to 35 minutes. Let stand 5 minutes before serving. Divide the bread pudding among 6 plates and serve at once.

Each serving: 24 g carb, 213 cal, 8 g fat, 3 g sat fat, 80 mg chol, 3 g fib, 12 g pro, 399 mg sod • Carb Choices: 1½; Exchanges: 1 starch, 1 veg, 1 medium-fat protein, ½ fat

Autumn Greens Tart

HIGH FIBER

makes 6 servings

My husband, Nick, who usually covers his eyes at the sight of a green vegetable, wanted a second slice of this tart. It's delicious for brunch, lunch, or a light supper. You can even cut it into very thin slices and serve it at room temperature with wine or cocktails.

1 Pastry Crust (page 546), prepared without sugar

2 teaspoons extra virgin olive oil

1 small onion, chopped

2 garlic cloves, minced

½ cup water

8 ounces kale, tough stems removed and leaves chopped

8 ounces Swiss chard, tough stems removed and leaves chopped

1 cup low-fat cottage cheese

⅓ cup freshly grated Parmesan

2 large egg whites

1 large egg

½ teaspoon kosher salt

⅛ teaspoon crushed red pepper

1 Preheat the oven to 400°F.

2 Place the pastry dough between two sheets of wax paper. Roll the dough into a 12-inch circle. Remove the top layer of wax paper and place the dough, with the remaining sheet of wax paper facing up, into a 9-inch tart pan with a removable bottom. Trim the edge of the crust to fit the pan. Prick the bottom of the crust all over with a fork. Line the crust with parchment paper and fill with pie weights or dried beans. Place the tart pan on a rimmed baking sheet and bake 20 minutes. Remove the parchment and weights and bake until the crust is lightly browned, 5 to 8 minutes. Maintain the oven temperature.

continues on next page

3 Meanwhile, heat a large nonstick skillet over medium heat. Add the oil and tilt the pan to coat the bottom evenly. Add the onion and cook, stirring often, until softened, 5 minutes. Add the garlic and cook, stirring constantly, until fragrant, 30 seconds.

4 Add the water, then add the kale and chard in batches and cook, stirring constantly, until wilted. Cover and cook, stirring frequently, until the greens are tender, 6 to 8 minutes. Transfer to a colander and let stand until cool enough to handle. Squeeze the greens mixture dry.

5 Combine the greens mixture, cottage cheese, Parmesan, egg whites, egg, salt, and crushed red pepper in a large bowl and add to the stir to mix well.

6 Spoon the greens mixture into the prepared crust, spreading evenly. Place the tart pan on a large rimmed baking sheet and bake until the tart is set, 25 to 28 minutes. Let stand 5 minutes before slicing. Cut into 6 wedges and serve hot, warm, or at room temperature.

Each serving: 25 g carb, 259 cal, 12 g fat, 6 g sat fat, 61 mg chol, 4 g fib, 13 g pro, 527 mg sod • Carb Choices: 1½; Exchanges: 1½ starch, 1 veg, 2 fat

Leek and Caramelized Garlic Tart HIGH FIBER

makes 6 servings

In this version of the classic quiche Lorraine, crispy caramelized garlic stands in for the bacon. You can cut the tart into 16 slices to serve as an hors d'oeuvre—it tastes just as good at room temperature as it does when hot.

1 Pastry Crust (page 546), prepared without sugar

3 medium leeks, halved lengthwise and thinly sliced (about 3 cups)

1 tablespoon extra virgin olive oil

3 garlic cloves, thinly sliced

3 large eggs

3 large egg whites

⅔ cup 1% low-fat milk

2 ounces freshly grated Parmesan (about ½ cup)

½ teaspoon kosher salt

⅛ teaspoon freshly ground pepper

1 Preheat the oven to 400°F.

2 Place the pastry dough between two sheets of wax paper. Roll the dough into a 12-inch-diameter circle. Remove the top layer of wax paper and place the dough, with the remaining sheet of wax paper facing up, into a 9-inch tart pan with a removable bottom. Trim the edge of the crust to fit the pan. Prick the bottom of the crust all over with a fork. Line the crust with parchment paper and fill with pie weights or dried beans. Place the tart pan on a rimmed baking sheet and bake 20 minutes. Remove the parchment and weights and bake until the crust is lightly browned, 5 to 8 minutes. Remove the crust and maintain the oven temperature.

3 Meanwhile, submerge the sliced leeks in a large bowl of water, lift them out, and drain in a colander. Repeat, using fresh water, until no grit remains in the bottom of the bowl. Drain the leeks well.

4 Heat a medium nonstick skillet over medium heat. Add the oil and tilt the pan to coat the bottom evenly. Add the garlic and cook, stirring often, until lightly browned, about 3 minutes. Using a slotted spoon, transfer the garlic to a small dish.

5 Add the leeks to the skillet and cook, covered, over medium heat, stirring often, until very tender, 15 to 20 minutes. Transfer to the plate with the garlic to cool slightly.

6 Whisk together the eggs, egg whites, milk, Parmesan, salt, and pepper in a large bowl. Stir in the cooked leeks and garlic.

7 Pour the egg mixture into the crust. Place the tart pan on a large rimmed baking sheet and bake until the tart is set, about 25 minutes. Let stand 5 minutes before slicing. Cut into 6 wedges and serve hot, warm, or at room temperature.

Each serving: 28 g carb, 294 cal, 15 g fat, 7 g sat fat, 133 mg chol, 4 g fib, 12 g pro, 381 mg sod • Carb Choices: 2; Exchanges: 1½ starch, 1 veg, 1 medium-fat protein, 2 fat

Crustless Asparagus and Feta Tart

makes 6 servings

You can use 3 cups of small broccoli florets in this recipe instead of the asparagus, following the same procedure for cooking the asparagus. A couple tablespoons of fresh chopped dill or basil make a nice addition if you have them on hand.

½ teaspoon canola oil

1½ pounds asparagus, tough ends removed and spears cut into ¾-inch pieces (about 3 cups)

4 large eggs

4 large egg whites

¾ cup 1% low-fat milk

2 tablespoons unbleached all-purpose flour

1 garlic clove, crushed through a press

½ teaspoon kosher salt

¼ teaspoon freshly ground pepper

4 ounces finely crumbled feta cheese (about 1 cup)

1 Preheat the oven to 350°F. Brush a 9- or 10-inch ceramic quiche pan or a 10-inch glass or ceramic pie plate with the oil.

2 Bring a large saucepan of water to a boil over high heat. Add the asparagus and cook until crisp-tender, 3 to 4 minutes. Drain in a colander and rinse with cold running water until cool. Pat the asparagus dry with paper towels.

3 Combine the eggs, egg whites, milk, flour, garlic, salt, and pepper in a large bowl and whisk until smooth. Add the asparagus and the feta and stir to combine. Pour into the prepared pan and arrange the asparagus evenly.

4 Place the quiche pan on a large rimmed baking sheet. Bake until the top is golden and the center is set, 30 to 35 minutes. Let stand 5 minutes. Cut the tart into 6 wedges using a serrated knife. Serve hot, warm, or at room temperature.

Each serving: 7 g carb, 153 cal, 8 g fat, 4 g sat fat, 159 mg chol, 1 g fib, 12 g pro, 407 mg sod • Carb Choices: ½; Exchanges: 1 veg, 1 medium-fat protein, 1 fat

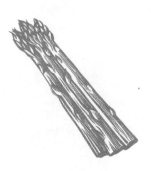

Grain Sides

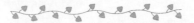

Barley

Barley with Asparagus and Almonds

Tomato-Basil Barley

Barley with Cherry Tomatoes, Rosemary, and Feta

Barley with Roasted Red Peppers and Red Onion

Barley with Pear, Dried Cranberries, and Toasted Walnuts

Barley Risotto with Spinach and Feta

Bulgur

Bulgur Pilaf with Spinach

Lemony Bulgur Pilaf with Kalamata Olives

Bulgur Pilaf with Fresh Tomatoes and Goat Cheese

Spiced Bulgur Pilaf with Almonds

Couscous

Kalamata Olive Couscous

Pistachio-Herb Couscous

Orange-Ginger Couscous

Couscous with Jalapeño and Cilantro

Chutney Couscous

Couscous with Currants and Almonds

Polenta

Basic Polenta

Creamy Polenta with Goat Cheese and Tomatoes

Polenta with Cheddar and Roasted Poblano

Oven-Baked Polenta

Fresh Corn Spoon Bread

Quinoa

Quinoa with Toasted Almonds and Lemon

Quinoa with Spinach and Pine Nuts

Spicy Quinoa with Zucchini and Bell Pepper

Quinoa with Tomato and Dill

Rice

Rice with Corn and Zucchini

Rice with Shiitakes and Spinach

Rice with Mushrooms and Roasted Peppers

Rice with Tomato and Saffron

Rice with Apple, Pecans, and Rosemary

Raisin-Spice Rice

Rice with Roasted Grapes
and Coriander

Toasted Coconut–Ginger
Rice

Oven-Baked Rice with
Tomatoes and Rosemary

Southwestern Oven-
Baked Rice

Baked Butternut Squash
Risotto

Wheat Berries

Wheat Berry, Green Bean,
and Lemon Sauté

Wheat Berries with Fennel
and Apple

Wheat Berries with Broccoli
Rabe and Currants

Wheat Berries and
Vegetables with Moroccan
Spices

Farro and Vegetable Risotto

Wild Rice

Wild Rice with Caramelized
Fennel and Onions

Wild Rice with Apricots and
Almonds

Wild Rice with Butternut
Squash and Sage

Wild Rice with Mushrooms
and Thyme

Whole grains are "good carbs." Making the switch from eating processed grains to whole and less refined grains will increase your intake of fiber, phytochemicals, B vitamins, and minerals. By choosing brown rice, barley, wheat berries, and bulgur over white rice or white pasta, you'll be doing your blood sugar and your waistline a favor, too. The fiber in whole grains can help lower blood glucose levels since high-fiber foods take longer to digest. And fiber gives a feeling of fullness, which helps you eat less and control your weight.

If those are not reasons enough to eat more whole grains, they taste great, too. Whole grains have not had their bran, germ, and endosperm stripped away, so their natural texture, flavor, and unique character are still intact. As you'll see when you try the dishes in this chapter, whole grain does not equate with "no flavor." I've used the grains in this chapter as a canvas on which to paint a world of exciting flavors. Once you try a few of these recipes, you'll see that you can add almost any flavorful vegetable, herb, spice, or citrus to a cooked whole grain to create a delicious side dish.

Because many grains take a long time to cook, in most recipes, I cook the grain first, and then add it to whatever seasonings I'm using to flavor the dish. This method keeps the vegetables and herbs fresh, flavorful, and attractive. Another great advantage to this method is that you can cook a large batch of one or two grains on the weekend and use them throughout the week to make super-quick side dishes. When you're in a hurry, try the recipes for quinoa, instant polenta, or whole wheat couscous for a side dish that's ready in less than 15 minutes. If you have leftovers, most of these dishes will reheat beautifully in the microwave for lunch the next day.

Don't just think of these dishes as sides, either. You can add cooked chopped leftover chicken, pork loin, or lean beef or rinsed and drained canned dried beans to many of these recipes to turn them into main dishes.

A note on the "whole grains" in this chapter: whole wheat couscous and polenta included here are not whole grains and bulgur is also not strictly a whole grain, since a small amount of its bran is removed during processing. But these foods are rich enough in nutrients, convenient to cook, and low in calories that it would be a mistake not to include them. You'll find a side dish here to pair healthfully with whatever you're serving for dinner tonight.

Also, note that there are grain dishes in other chapters such as Vegetarian Main Dishes (page 367) that you could be serve as sides in smaller servings, but the recipes here are intentionally simpler and servings and nutrition information are calculated for smaller portions.

Barley

Barley with Asparagus and Almonds

makes 6 servings

Pearl barley refers to barley that has had the hull removed and the outside of the grains polished or "pearled." This processing makes barley relatively quick-cooking (less than 30 minutes), yet it is still a good source of fiber and B vitamins. In this recipe, fresh asparagus and a smattering of almonds turn barley into a warm weather side dish for salmon or grilled shrimp.

2 teaspoons extra virgin olive oil
½ cup diced onion
1 garlic clove, minced
1 pound asparagus, tough stems removed and cut into 1-inch pieces
¼ cup Vegetable Stock (page 149) or low-sodium vegetable broth
½ teaspoon kosher salt
⅛ teaspoon freshly ground pepper
2 cups cooked pearl barley (page 108)
2 tablespoons sliced almonds, toasted (page 4)
2 teaspoons lemon juice

1 Heat a medium nonstick skillet over medium heat. Add the oil and tilt the pan to coat the bottom evenly. Add the onion and cook, stirring often, until softened, 5 minutes. Add the garlic and cook, stirring constantly, until fragrant, 30 seconds.

2 Add the asparagus, stock, salt, and pepper and cook, stirring often, until the asparagus is crisp-tender, about 3 minutes.

3 Add the barley and cook, stirring often, until heated through. Remove from the heat and stir in the almonds and lemon juice. Spoon the barley into a serving dish and serve at once.

Each serving: 19 g carb, 109 cal, 3 g fat, 0 g sat fat, 0 mg chol, 3 g fib, 3 g pro, 102 mg sod • Carb Choices: 1; Exchanges: 1 starch, ½ fat

Tomato-Basil Barley

makes 6 servings

In the heat of summer, I love to put tomatoes and basil into almost any dish that I cook, so I don't miss an opportunity to savor the short season for real tomatoes. This simple recipe makes a wonderful side dish to serve with grilled chicken or fish. But I also sometimes turn it into a vegetarian main dish by adding some canned cannellini beans when I add the tomato, and then I top it with a sprinkle of crumbled goat cheese.

2 teaspoons extra virgin olive oil
½ cup diced onion
1 garlic clove, minced
2 cups cooked pearl barley (page 108)
1 large tomato, chopped
½ teaspoon kosher salt
⅛ teaspoon freshly ground pepper
2 tablespoons pine nuts, toasted (page 4)
2 tablespoons chopped fresh basil
2 teaspoons lemon juice

1 Heat a medium nonstick skillet over medium heat. Add the oil and tilt the pan to coat the bottom evenly. Add the onion and cook, stirring often, until softened, 5 minutes. Add the garlic and cook, stirring constantly, until fragrant, 30 seconds.

2 Add the barley, tomato, salt, and pepper and cook, stirring often, until heated through. Remove from the heat and stir in the pine nuts, basil, and lemon juice. Spoon the barley into a serving dish and serve at once.

Each serving: 18 g carb, 111 cal, 4 g fat, 0 g sat fat, 0 mg chol, 3 g fib, 2 g pro, 97 mg sod • Carb Choices: 1; Exchanges: 1 starch, ½ fat

Barley with Cherry Tomatoes, Rosemary, and Feta

makes 6 servings

If you're tired of serving lamb or chicken kebabs on a bed of boring rice, try this colorful dish to accompany them next time. Lemon and rosemary accentuate the flavors of almost anything grilled, so try this with grilled salmon or pork tenderloin, too.

2 teaspoons extra virgin olive oil
½ cup diced onion
1 garlic clove, minced
2 cups cooked pearl barley (page 108)
2 cups cherry tomatoes, halved
½ teaspoon kosher salt
⅛ teaspoon freshly ground pepper
2 teaspoons lemon juice
1 teaspoon chopped fresh rosemary
3 tablespoons finely crumbled feta cheese

1 Heat a medium nonstick skillet over medium heat. Add the oil and tilt the pan to coat the bottom evenly. Add the onion and cook, stirring often, until softened, 5 minutes. Add the garlic and cook, stirring constantly, until fragrant, 30 seconds.

2 Add the barley, tomatoes, salt, and pepper and cook, stirring often, until heated through. Remove from the heat and stir in the lemon juice and rosemary. Spoon the barley into a serving dish and sprinkle with the feta. Serve at once.

Each serving: 19 g carb, 108 cal, 3 g fat, 1 g sat fat, 4 mg chol, 3 g fib, 3 g pro, 151 mg sod • Carb Choices: 1; Exchanges: 1 starch, ½ fat

Barley with Roasted Red Peppers and Red Onion

makes 6 servings

This flavorful and pretty side dish is perfect for almost any occasion. Serve it with Herb-Crusted Sautéed Chicken (page 207) for a quick weeknight family dinner or with Spinach and Feta–Stuffed Chicken (page 234) when company comes.

2 teaspoons extra virgin olive oil
½ cup diced red onion
1 garlic clove, minced
2 cups cooked pearl barley (page 108)
1 cup chopped red Roasted Bell Peppers (page 21) or roasted red peppers from a jar
½ teaspoon kosher salt
⅛ teaspoon freshly ground pepper
2 tablespoons chopped fresh Italian parsley
2 teaspoons lemon juice
3 tablespoons freshly grated Parmesan

1 Heat a medium nonstick skillet over medium heat. Add the oil and tilt the pan to coat the bottom evenly. Add the onion and cook, stirring often, until softened, 5 minutes. Add the garlic and cook, stirring constantly, until fragrant, 30 seconds.

2 Add the barley, roasted peppers, salt, and ground pepper and cook, stirring often, until heated through, 2 minutes. Remove from the heat and stir in the parsley and lemon juice. Spoon the barley into a shallow serving bowl and sprinkle with the Parmesan. Serve at once.

Each serving: 18 g carb, 103 cal, 3 g fat, 1 g sat fat, 2 mg chol, 3 g fib, 3 g pro, 135 mg sod • Carb Choices: 1; Exchanges: 1 starch, ½ fat

Barley with Pear, Dried Cranberries, and Toasted Walnuts HIGH FIBER

makes 6 servings

Pair this colorful side dish with a holiday turkey or pork roast, or for a more casual meal, it's perfect with a weeknight roast chicken. The cranberries add a pleasant tartness and the toasted walnuts lend crunch and substance.

2 teaspoons extra virgin olive oil
½ cup diced onion
1 garlic clove, minced
1 large ripe pear, peeled and chopped
2 tablespoons dried cranberries
¼ cup Vegetable Stock (page 149) or low-sodium vegetable broth
1 teaspoon minced fresh sage
½ teaspoon kosher salt
⅛ teaspoon freshly ground pepper
2 cups cooked pearl barley (page 108)
2 tablespoons walnuts, toasted and chopped (page 4)
2 teaspoons lemon juice

1 Heat a medium nonstick skillet over medium heat. Add the oil and tilt the pan to coat the bottom evenly. Add the onion and cook, stirring often, until softened, 5 minutes. Add the garlic and cook, stirring constantly, until fragrant, 30 seconds.

2 Add the pear, cranberries, stock, sage, salt, and pepper and cook, stirring often, until the pear is tender, about 5 minutes.

3 Add the barley and cook, stirring often, until heated through, about 2 minutes. Remove from the heat and stir in the walnuts and lemon juice. Spoon the barley into a serving dish and serve at once.

Each serving: 24 g carb, 130 cal, 3 g fat, 0 g sat fat, 0 mg chol, 4 g fib, 2 g pro, 102 mg sod • Carb Choices: 1½; Exchanges: 1 starch, ½ fruit, ½ fat

Barley Risotto with Spinach and Feta HIGH FIBER

makes 6 servings

Barley risotto is lighter in texture and flavor than you would imagine. Serve this to accompany a simple grilled steak or salmon fillet.

4½ cups Vegetable Stock (page 149) or low-sodium vegetable broth
2 teaspoons extra virgin olive oil
½ cup minced shallots
¾ cup pearl barley
½ cup dry white wine
½ teaspoon kosher salt
2 cups chopped fresh spinach
1 large tomato, chopped
2 tablespoons crumbled feta cheese
2 teaspoons grated lemon zest
⅛ teaspoon freshly ground pepper

1 Pour the stock into a medium saucepan and bring to a simmer over medium-high heat. Reduce the heat to low and keep the stock warm.

2 Heat a large saucepan over medium heat. Add the oil and tilt the pan to coat the bottom evenly. Add the shallots and cook, stirring often, until softened, 5 minutes.

3 Add the barley and cook, stirring constantly, 2 minutes. Add the wine and salt and cook, stirring frequently until absorbed. Add the stock, ½ cup at a time, stirring frequently, until the liquid is absorbed after each addition before adding more. When all the liquid is absorbed and the barley is tender, yet firm to the bite (about 35 minutes), add the spinach, tomato, and feta and cook, stirring constantly, until the spinach is wilted and the tomato is heated through, about 2 minutes. Remove from the heat and stir in the lemon zest and pepper. Spoon the risotto into a serving dish and serve at once.

Each serving: 26 g carb, 159 cal, 3 g fat, 1 g sat fat, 3 mg chol, 5 g fib, 4 g pro, 247 mg sod • Carb Choices: 2; Exchanges: 2 starch, ½ fat

Bulgur

Bulgur Pilaf with Spinach

QUICK | HIGH FIBER

makes 6 servings

Bulgur is made by steaming grains of wheat, then drying and crushing them into small bits. Because bulgur has been steamed—basically precooked—all you have to do is rehydrate it by soaking it or cooking it quickly in a flavorful both. Fine-grind bulgur is usually used in recipes for Tabbouleh (page 107), where the grain is soaked, and medium- and coarse-grind bulgur is used in pilafs, where the grain is cooked.

2 teaspoons extra virgin olive oil
½ cup diced onion
1 garlic clove, minced
2 cups Vegetable Stock (page 149) or
    low-sodium vegetable broth
¾ cup medium- or coarse-grind bulgur
½ teaspoon kosher salt
Pinch of freshly ground pepper
2 cups chopped fresh spinach
1 tablespoon lemon juice

1 Heat a medium nonstick skillet over medium heat. Add the oil and tilt the pan to coat the bottom evenly. Add the onion and cook, stirring often, until softened, 5 minutes. Add the garlic and cook, stirring constantly, until fragrant, 30 seconds.

2 Stir in the stock, bulgur, salt, and pepper and bring to a boil over high heat. Cover, reduce the heat to low, and simmer until the liquid has absorbed and the bulgur is tender, 15 to 18 minutes.

3 Add the spinach, stirring just until wilted, about 1 minute. Remove from the heat and stir in the lemon juice. Spoon the bulgur into a serving dish and serve at once.

Each serving: 16 g carb, 90 cal, 2 g fat, 0 g sat fat, 0 mg chol, 4 g fib, 3 g pro, 152 mg sod • Carb Choices: 1; Exchanges: 1 starch

Lemony Bulgur Pilaf with Kalamata Olives

QUICK | HIGH FIBER

makes 6 servings

The tart lemon zest and juice along with the salty olives make this dish a good pairing for any kind of seafood or lamb chops. If you have an orange on hand when you make this, you can use a teaspoon of lemon zest and a teaspoon of orange zest for more complex citrus flavor.

2 teaspoons extra virgin olive oil
½ cup diced onion
1 garlic clove, minced
2 cups Vegetable Stock (page 149) or
    low-sodium vegetable broth
¾ cup medium- or coarse-grind bulgur
¼ teaspoon kosher salt
Pinch of freshly ground pepper
3 tablespoons Kalamata olives, pitted and
    sliced
2 tablespoons chopped fresh Italian parsley
2 teaspoons grated lemon zest
1 tablespoon lemon juice

1 Heat a medium nonstick skillet over medium heat. Add the oil and tilt the pan to coat the bottom evenly. Add the onion and cook, stirring often, until softened, 5 minutes. Add the garlic and cook, stirring constantly, until fragrant, 30 seconds.

2 Stir in the stock, bulgur, salt, and pepper and bring to a boil over high heat. Cover, reduce the heat to low, and simmer until the liquid has absorbed and bulgur is tender, 15 to 18 minutes.

3 Remove from the heat and stir in the olives, parsley, lemon zest, and lemon juice. Spoon the pilaf into a serving dish and serve at once.

Each serving: 17 g carb, 103 cal, 3 g fat, 0 g sat fat, 0 mg chol, 4 g fib, 2 g pro, 174 mg sod • Carb Choices: 1; Exchanges: 1 starch, ½ fat

Bulgur Pilaf with Fresh Tomatoes and Goat Cheese QUICK | HIGH FIBER

makes 6 servings

This is a mind-changing dish for people who think they don't like the flavor of whole grains. Bulgur is very mild tasting and paired with juicy tomatoes, fresh basil, and goat cheese, it makes a delectable side dish for summer grilling.

2 teaspoons extra virgin olive oil
1 garlic clove, minced
2 cups Vegetable Stock (page 149) or low-sodium vegetable broth
¾ cup medium- or coarse-grind bulgur
½ teaspoon kosher salt
Pinch of freshly ground pepper
1 large tomato, chopped
1 scallion, thinly sliced
2 tablespoons chopped fresh basil
1 tablespoon lemon juice
3 tablespoons finely crumbled goat cheese

1 Heat a medium nonstick skillet over medium heat. Add the oil and tilt the pan to coat the bottom evenly. Add the garlic and cook, stirring constantly, until fragrant, 30 seconds.

2 Stir in the stock, bulgur, salt, and pepper and bring to a boil over high heat. Cover, reduce the heat to low, and simmer until the liquid has absorbed and the bulgur is tender, 15 to 18 minutes.

3 Add the tomato and scallion and cook, stirring often, until heated through. Remove from the heat and stir in the basil and lemon juice. Spoon the pilaf into a serving dish, sprinkle with the goat cheese, and serve at once.

Each serving: 16 g carb, 98 cal, 3 g fat, 1 g sat fat, 2 mg chol, 4 g fib, 3 g pro, 159 mg sod • Carb Choices: 1; Exchanges: 1 starch, ½ fat

Spiced Bulgur Pilaf with Almonds QUICK | HIGH FIBER

makes 6 servings

Exotic allspice, sweet raisins, crunchy toasted almonds, and fresh cilantro come together to make a versatile pilaf that goes well with grilled meat kebabs, tagines, or vegetable stews.

2 teaspoons extra virgin olive oil
½ cup diced onion
1 garlic clove, minced
¼ teaspoon ground allspice
Pinch of ground cayenne
2 cups Vegetable Stock (page 149) or low-sodium vegetable broth
¾ cup medium- or coarse-grain bulgur
¼ cup golden raisins
½ teaspoon kosher salt
2 tablespoons sliced almonds, toasted (page 4)
2 tablespoons chopped fresh cilantro
2 teaspoons lime juice

1 Heat a medium nonstick skillet over medium heat. Add the oil and tilt the pan to coat the bottom evenly. Add the onion and cook, stirring often, until softened, 5 minutes. Add the garlic, allspice, and cayenne and cook, stirring constantly, until fragrant, 30 seconds.

2 Stir in the stock, bulgur, raisins, and salt and bring to a boil over high heat. Cover, reduce the heat, and simmer until the liquid has absorbed and the bulgur is tender, 15 to 18 minutes.

3 Remove from the heat and stir in the almonds, cilantro, and lime juice. Spoon the pilaf into a serving dish and serve at once.

Each serving: 21 g carb, 117 cal, 3 g fat, 0 g sat fat, 0 mg chol, 4 g fib, 3 g pro, 145 mg sod • Carb Choices: 1½; Exchanges: 1 starch, ½ fruit, ½ fat

Couscous

Kalamata Olive Couscous

QUICK

makes 6 servings

Great for serving with anything Greek, this simple couscous is packed with flavor. It's good with green olives, too—try manzanillas or picholines.

1¼ cups Vegetable Stock (page 149) or
    low-sodium vegetable broth
¼ teaspoon kosher salt
1 cup whole wheat couscous
6 Kalamata olives, pitted and coarsely chopped
1 teaspoon grated lemon zest
Pinch of freshly ground pepper
2 tablespoons chopped fresh Italian parsley
2 tablespoons lemon juice
1 teaspoon extra virgin olive oil

1 Combine the stock and salt in a medium saucepan and bring to a boil over high heat. Remove from the heat and stir in the couscous, olives, lemon zest, and pepper. Cover and let stand 5 minutes.

2 Fluff the couscous with a fork and stir in the parsley, lemon juice, and oil. Spoon the couscous into a serving dish and serve at once.

Each serving: 17 g carb, 98 cal, 2 g fat, 0 g sat fat, 0 mg chol, 2 g fib, 3 g pro, 153 mg sod • Carb Choices: 1; Exchanges: 1 starch, ½ fat

Pistachio-Herb Couscous

QUICK

makes 6 servings

Pistachios and fresh herbs give this dish a fresh green color and terrific flavor. If you don't have pistachios on hand, use slivered almonds instead. Use this as a bed for serving grilled or broiled salmon or pork tenderloin.

2 teaspoons extra virgin olive oil
⅓ cup minced shallots
1¼ cups Vegetable Stock (page 149) or
    low-sodium vegetable broth
1 cup whole wheat couscous
2 teaspoons grated lemon zest
½ teaspoon kosher salt
Pinch of freshly ground pepper
3 tablespoons shelled pistachios, toasted and
    chopped (page 4)
2 tablespoons lemon juice
1 tablespoon chopped fresh basil
1 tablespoon chopped fresh dill
1 tablespoon chopped fresh Italian parsley

1 Heat a medium nonstick skillet over medium heat. Add the oil and tilt the pan to coat the bottom evenly. Add the shallots and cook, stirring often, until softened, 5 minutes.

2 Add the stock and bring to a boil over high heat. Remove from the heat and stir in the couscous, lemon zest, salt, and pepper. Cover and let stand 5 minutes.

3 Fluff the couscous with a fork and stir in the pistachios, lemon juice, basil, dill, and parsley. Spoon the couscous into a serving dish and serve at once.

Each serving: 19 g carb, 119 cal, 4 g fat, 0 g sat fat, 0 mg chol, 3 g fib, 4 g pro, 124 mg sod • Carb Choices: 1; Exchanges: 1 starch, 1 fat

Orange-Ginger Couscous

QUICK

makes 6 servings

When you need a quick, flavorful side dish for ordinary weeknight chicken breasts or pork chops, make this your go-to recipe. Simmering the orange juice concentrates the citrus flavor, so you really do taste the fresh orange juice.

¾ cup orange juice

1 cup Vegetable Stock (page 149) or low-sodium vegetable broth

½ teaspoon kosher salt

2 teaspoons grated fresh ginger

½ teaspoon grated orange zest

½ teaspoon ground cumin

1 cup whole wheat couscous

2 tablespoons chopped fresh cilantro

1 teaspoon extra virgin olive oil

1 Pour the orange juice into a medium saucepan and bring to a boil over high heat. Cook, uncovered, until reduced to ¼ cup, about 6 minutes. Add the stock and salt and return to a boil. Remove from the heat and stir in the ginger, orange zest, and cumin, then stir in the couscous. Cover and let stand 5 minutes.

2 Fluff the couscous with a fork and stir in the cilantro and oil. Spoon the couscous into a serving dish and serve at once.

Each serving: 19 g carb, 96 cal, 1 g fat, 0 g sat fat, 0 mg chol, 3 g fib, 3 g pro, 118 mg sod • Carb Choices: 1; Exchanges: 1 starch

Couscous with Jalapeño and Cilantro QUICK

makes 6 servings

The jalapeño makes this dish quite spicy. If you don't like so much spice, use only half of a jalapeño or leave it out. Serve this as a side dish with Cumin-and Lime Grilled Chicken (page 238).

1¼ cups Vegetable Stock (page 149) or low-sodium vegetable broth

1 jalapeño, seeded and minced

1 garlic clove, crushed through a press

½ teaspoon ground cumin

½ teaspoon kosher salt

1 cup whole wheat couscous

2 tablespoons thinly sliced scallion tops

2 tablespoons chopped fresh cilantro

2 tablespoons lime juice

1 Combine the stock, jalapeño, garlic, cumin, and salt in a medium saucepan and bring to a boil over high heat. Remove from the heat and stir in the couscous. Cover and let stand 5 minutes.

2 Fluff the couscous with a fork and stir in the scallions, cilantro, and lime juice. Spoon the couscous into a serving dish and serve at once.

Each serving: 16 g carb, 78 cal, 0 g fat, 0 g sat fat, 0 mg chol, 3 g fib, 3 g pro, 123 mg sod • Carb Choices: 1; Exchanges: 1 starch

Chutney Couscous QUICK

makes 6 servings

Major Grey's chutney is an Indian chutney made from mangoes, sugar, vinegar, and lots of spices. It adds an instant burst of Indian flavor to this quick couscous dish. If your chutney has large pieces of mangoes, finely chop the chutney before adding it to the couscous.

1¼ cups Vegetable Stock (page 149) or low-sodium vegetable broth

½ teaspoon kosher salt

⅓ cup Major Grey's chutney

⅛ teaspoon ground cayenne

1 cup whole wheat couscous

2 tablespoons chopped fresh cilantro

2 tablespoons sliced almonds, toasted (page 4)

1 tablespoon lime juice

1 Combine the stock and salt in a medium saucepan and bring to a boil over high heat. Remove from the heat and stir in the chutney and cayenne, then stir in the couscous. Cover and let stand 5 minutes.

2 Fluff the couscous with a fork and stir in the cilantro, almonds, and lime juice. Spoon the couscous into a serving dish and serve at once.

Each serving: 26 g carb, 122 cal, 1 g fat, 0 g sat fat, 0 mg chol, 3 g fib, 3 g pro, 158 mg sod • Carb Choices: 2; Exchanges: 1 starch, 1 carb

Couscous with Currants and Almonds QUICK

makes 6 servings

Sweet and spicy flavors and crunchy almonds make this couscous a complementary side dish to serve with Indian dishes or with roast chicken or pork. Whole wheat couscous tends to stick together as it absorbs the cooking liquid, so always fluff it with a fork to separate the grains and give it a light texture.

1¼ cups Vegetable Stock (page 149) or
    low-sodium vegetable broth

3 tablespoons currants

½ teaspoon kosher salt

¼ teaspoon ground cumin

⅛ teaspoon ground cinnamon

1 cup whole wheat couscous

2 tablespoons chopped fresh Italian parsley

2 tablespoons slivered almonds, toasted
    (page 4)

1 Combine the stock, currants, salt, cumin, and cinnamon in a medium saucepan and bring to a boil over high heat. Remove from the heat and stir in the couscous. Cover and let stand 5 minutes.

2 Fluff the couscous with a fork and stir in the parsley and almonds. Spoon the couscous into a serving dish and serve at once.

Each serving: 19 g carb, 100 cal, 1 g fat, 0 g sat fat, 0 mg chol, 3 g fib, 3 g pro, 123 mg sod • Carb Choices: 1; Exchanges: 1 starch

Polenta

Basic Polenta QUICK

makes 4 servings

These recipes use fine-grind yellow cornmeal or instant polenta (both the same thing), making it possible to have a satisfying side dish in less than 10 minutes. Fine-grind cornmeal is not a whole grain, since the skin of the corn kernel and the germ are removed. Using fine cornmeal still results in a healthful, low-calorie side dish.

2 cups Vegetable Stock (page 149) or
    low-sodium vegetable broth

¾ teaspoon kosher salt

Pinch of freshly ground pepper

½ cup fine-grind yellow cornmeal

1 Combine the stock, salt, and pepper in a medium saucepan and bring to a boil over medium-high heat.

2 Slowly sprinkle the cornmeal into the stock, whisking constantly. Reduce the heat to low and cook, stirring constantly, until the polenta is thickened, about 3 minutes. Spoon the polenta into a serving dish and serve at once.

Each serving: 16 g carb, 70 cal, 0 g fat, 0 g sat fat, 0 mg chol, 1 g fib, 1 g pro, 280 mg sod • Carb Choices: 1; Exchanges: 1 starch

PARMESAN POLENTA: Follow the Basic Polenta recipe, above, decreasing the salt to ½ teaspoon. When the polenta is thickened, remove it from the heat and stir in ¼ cup freshly grated Parmesan.

Each serving: 16 g carb, 92 cal, 2 g fat, 1 g sat fat, 4 mg chol, 1 g fib, 3 g pro, 286 mg sod • Carb Choices: 1; Exchanges: 1 starch

POLENTA WITH FRESH CORN AND THYME: Follow the Basic Polenta recipe, above, adding the corn kernels from 1 medium ear corn and ½ teaspoon chopped fresh thyme to the stock in step 1. Proceed with the recipe.

Each serving: 20 g carb, 93 cal, 1 g fat, 0 g sat fat, 0 mg chol, 2 g fib, 2 g pro, 280 mg sod • Carb Choices: 1; Exchanges: 1 starch

Creamy Polenta with Goat Cheese and Tomatoes

QUICK

makes 4 servings

Using milk and stock in this recipe as well as adding some creamy goat cheese results in an especially rich and velvety dish. It elevates any ordinary entrée to a special meal.

1 cup Vegetable Stock (page 149) or low-sodium vegetable broth
1 cup 1% low-fat milk
¾ teaspoon kosher salt
Pinch of freshly ground pepper
½ cup fine-grind yellow cornmeal
2 tablespoons crumbled goat cheese
1 small plum tomato, chopped
1 tablespoon chopped fresh basil

1 Combine the stock, milk, salt, and pepper in a medium saucepan and bring to a boil over medium-high heat.

2 Slowly sprinkle the cornmeal into the stock mixture, whisking constantly. Reduce the heat to low and cook, stirring constantly, until the polenta is thickened, about 3 minutes. Remove from the heat and stir in the goat cheese. Gently stir in the tomato and basil. Spoon the polenta into a serving dish and serve at once.

Each serving: 19 g carb, 110 cal, 2 g fat, 1 g sat fat, 5 mg chol, 2 g fib, 5 g pro, 300 mg sod • Carb Choices: 1; Exchanges: 1 starch

Polenta with Cheddar and Roasted Poblano QUICK

makes 4 servings

Instead of serving rice with Tex-Mex meals, serve this quick and creamy side dish. It tastes like it takes much more effort than it does.

2 cups Vegetable Stock (page 149) or low-sodium vegetable broth
¾ teaspoon kosher salt
½ teaspoon ground cumin
½ cup fine-grind yellow cornmeal
1 poblano chile, roasted (page 21) and chopped
1 ounce shredded reduced-fat extra-sharp Cheddar cheese (about ¼ cup)
1 tablespoon chopped fresh cilantro

1 Combine the stock, salt, and cumin in a medium saucepan and bring to a boil over medium-high heat.

2 Slowly sprinkle the cornmeal into the stock mixture, whisking constantly. Stir in the poblano. Reduce the heat to low and cook, stirring constantly, until the polenta is thickened, about 3 minutes. Remove from the heat and stir in the Cheddar and cilantro. Spoon the polenta into a serving dish and serve at once.

Each serving: 17 g carb, 101 cal, 3 g fat, 2 g sat fat, 8 mg chol, 2 g fib, 3 g pro, 326 mg sod • Carb Choices: 1; Exchanges: 1 starch, ½ fat

Oven-Baked Polenta

makes 8 servings

This recipe uses medium- or coarse-grind cornmeal, which, if cooked on top of the stove, takes constant attention, and almost constant stirring for 30 to 45 minutes. This carefree—and just as creamy—polenta is as good as the stovetop version. Serve it plain or stir in almost any kind of cheese and/or fresh herb just before serving. Coarse-grind cornmeal is not a whole grain—the skin of the corn kernel is left on but the germ has been removed.

1 teaspoon extra virgin olive oil
4 cups Vegetable Stock (page 149) or
    low-sodium vegetable broth
1 cup coarse-grind yellow cornmeal
1½ teaspoons kosher salt

1 Preheat the oven to 350°F. Brush an 8-inch square baking dish with the oil.

2 Add the stock, cornmeal, and salt to the prepared dish and stir until well mixed. Bake, uncovered, for 45 minutes. Stir and bake until the polenta is thickened and creamy, about 15 minutes longer. Serve the polenta at once.

Each serving: 13 g carb, 70 cal, 1 g fat, 0 g sat fat, 0 mg chol, 1 g fib, 1 g pro, 285 mg sod • Carb Choices: 1; Exchanges: 1 starch

Fresh Corn Spoon Bread

makes 6 servings

If you're not familiar with spoon bread, it's like a cornbread soufflé. This one is creamy in the center with a crisp cheesy exterior, perfect for serving alongside any roasted or grilled meats or as the centerpiece of a summer vegetable plate.

1 teaspoon canola oil
1 cup Vegetable Stock (page 149) or
    low-sodium vegetable broth
1 cup 1% low-fat milk
½ cup fine-grind yellow cornmeal
1 medium ear corn, kernels cut from
    the cob
2 tablespoons chopped fresh basil
1 teaspoon baking powder
¾ teaspoon kosher salt
⅛ teaspoon freshly ground pepper
2 large egg whites
1 tablespoon freshly grated Parmesan

1 Preheat the oven to 375°F. Brush a 1½-quart soufflé dish with the oil.

2 Combine the stock and milk in a medium saucepan and bring to a boil over medium-high heat.

3 Slowly sprinkle the cornmeal into the stock, whisking constantly. Reduce the heat to low and cook, stirring constantly, until thickened, about 3 minutes. Tansfer to a large bowl and stir in the corn, basil, baking powder, salt and pepper.

4 Place the egg whites in a medium bowl and beat at high speed with an electric mixer until stiff peaks form. Fold the egg whites into the cornmeal mixture in three additions, stirring until no white streaks appear.

5 Spoon into the prepared soufflé dish, sprinkle with the Parmesan, and bake until puffed and golden, 35 to 40 minutes. Serve the spoon bread at once.

Each serving: 15 g carb, 95 cal, 2 g fat, 1 g sat fat, 2 mg chol, 1 g fib, 5 g pro, 285 mg sod • Carb Choices: 1; Exchanges: 1 starch

Quinoa

Quinoa with Toasted Almonds and Lemon QUICK

makes 6 servings

When you are in a hurry, quinoa is one of the quickest and healthiest grains to make. It cooks in about 15 minutes and its mild flavor pairs well with almost any vegetable or herb. Serve this lively lemony side dish alongside sautéed chicken or baked fish.

1½ cups Vegetable Stock (page 149) or low-sodium vegetable broth
1 cup quinoa, rinsed
½ teaspoon kosher salt
2 teaspoons extra virgin olive oil
1 scallion, thinly sliced
1 teaspoon grated lemon zest
1 tablespoon lemon juice
¼ teaspoon freshly ground pepper
2 tablespoons sliced almonds, toasted (page 4)
1 tablespoon chopped fresh Italian parsley

1 Combine the stock, quinoa, and salt in a medium saucepan and bring to a boil over high heat. Reduce the heat to low, cover, and simmer until the quinoa is tender, 12 to 15 minutes.

2 Heat a medium nonstick skillet over medium heat. Add the oil and tilt the pan to coat the bottom evenly. Add the scallion and cook, stirring often, until softened, 1 minute.

3 Add the quinoa, lemon zest, lemon juice, and pepper and stir to combine. Remove from the heat and stir in the almonds and parsley. Spoon the quinoa into a serving dish and serve at once.

Each serving: 21 g carb, 138 cal, 4 g fat, 0 g sat fat, 0 mg chol, 2 g fib, 4 g pro, 135 mg sod • Carb Choices: 1½; Exchanges: 1½ starch, ½ fat

Quinoa with Spinach and Pine Nuts QUICK

makes 6 servings

1½ cups Vegetable Stock (page 149) or low-sodium vegetable broth
1 cup quinoa, rinsed
½ teaspoon kosher salt
2 teaspoons extra virgin olive oil
¼ cup minced shallots
2 cups chopped fresh spinach
2 tablespoons pine nuts, toasted (page 4)
2 teaspoons lemon juice
⅛ teaspoon freshly ground pepper

1 Combine the stock, quinoa, and salt in a medium saucepan and bring to a boil over high heat. Reduce the heat to low, cover, and simmer until the quinoa is tender, 12 to 15 minutes.

2 Heat a medium nonstick skillet over medium heat. Add the oil and shallots and cook, stirring often, 5 minutes.

3 Add the spinach and cook, until wilted, 1 minute. Stir in the quinoa, pine nuts, lemon juice, and pepper. Spoon into a serving dish and serve at once.

Each serving: 21 g carb, 147 cal, 5 g fat, 1 g sat fat, 0 mg chol, 2 g fib, 4 g pro, 142 mg sod • Carb Choices: 1½; Exchanges: 1½ starch, 1 fat

Removing Bitterness from Quinoa

Quinoa contains a naturally occurring and harmless substance called saponin, which lends a bitter note to its flavor. Rinsing the quinoa thoroughly will eliminate the bitterness. To rinse quinoa, place it in a bowl and cover with cold water. Swirl the quinoa, and pour off the water. Repeat the rinsing until the water is clear. Drain the quinoa in a fine wire mesh strainer before cooking.

Spicy Quinoa with Zucchini and Bell Pepper QUICK

makes 6 servings

When a traditional Mexican rice dish is too heavy, serve this fresh and spicy quinoa with your Tex-Mex menu. It's colorful, nutritious, and very easy to make.

1½ cups Vegetable Stock (page 149) or
    low-sodium vegetable broth
1 cup quinoa, rinsed
½ teaspoon kosher salt
2 teaspoons extra virgin olive oil
½ cup diced red bell pepper
¼ cup diced onion
1 jalapeño, seeded and minced
½ cup diced zucchini
1 garlic clove, minced
½ teaspoon ground cumin
Pinch of ground cayenne
2 tablespoons chopped fresh cilantro
2 teaspoons lime juice

1 Combine the stock, quinoa, and salt in a medium saucepan and bring to a boil over high heat. Reduce the heat to low, cover, and simmer until the quinoa is tender, 12 to 15 minutes.

2 Heat a medium nonstick skillet over medium heat. Add the oil and tilt the pan to coat the bottom evenly. Add the bell pepper, onion, and jalapeño and cook, stirring often, until softened, 5 minutes. Add the zucchini, garlic, cumin, and cayenne and cook, stirring often, until the zucchini is crisp-tender, 2 minutes.

3 Remove from the heat and stir in the quinoa, cilantro, and lime juice. Spoon the quinoa into a serving dish and serve at once.

Each serving: 22 g carb, 135 cal, 3 g fat, 0 g sat fat, 0 mg chol, 2 g fib, 4 g pro, 137 mg sod • Carb Choices: 1½; Exchanges: 1½ starch, ½ fat

Quinoa with Tomato and Dill QUICK

makes 6 servings

Dill and tomatoes is one of my favorite summertime flavor pairings. In winter, make this dish with halved cherry or grape tomatoes, which always seem to have at least some tomato flavor even when there's snow on the ground.

1½ cups Vegetable Stock (page 149) or
    low-sodium vegetable broth
1 cup quinoa, rinsed
½ teaspoon kosher salt
2 teaspoons extra virgin olive oil
¼ cup diced onion
1 garlic clove, minced
1 large tomato, chopped
1 tablespoon chopped fresh dill
1 teaspoon grated lemon zest
2 teaspoons lemon juice

1 Combine the stock, quinoa, and salt in a medium saucepan and bring to a boil over high heat. Reduce the heat to low, cover, and simmer until the quinoa is tender, 12 to 15 minutes.

2 Heat a medium nonstick skillet over medium heat. Add the oil and tilt the pan to coat the bottom evenly. Add the onion and cook, stirring often, until softened, 5 minutes. Add the garlic and cook, stirring often, until fragrant, 30 seconds. Add the tomato and cook, stirring often, just until heated through, 1 minute.

3 Remove from the heat and stir in the quinoa, dill, lemon zest, and lemon juice. Spoon the quinoa into a serving dish and serve at once.

Each serving: 22 g carb, 134 cal, 3 g fat, 0 g sat fat, 0 mg chol, 2 g fib, 4 g pro, 136 mg sod • Carb Choices: 1½; Exchanges: 1½ starch

Rice

Rice with Corn and Zucchini

makes 6 servings

When you run out of ideas for summer's bounty, make a batch of this rice to serve alongside anything grilled. If you've got extra tomatoes, chop one and stir it in when you add the cooked rice.

2 teaspoons extra virgin olive oil

¼ cup minced onion

1 garlic clove, minced

1 teaspoon ground cumin

Pinch of ground cayenne

¼ cup Vegetable Stock (page 149) or low-sodium vegetable broth

1 medium ear corn, kernels cut from the cob

1 small zucchini, diced

1½ cups cooked brown rice (page 108)

1 teaspoon kosher salt

2 tablespoons chopped fresh cilantro

1 tablespoon lime juice

1 Heat a medium nonstick skillet over medium heat. Add the oil and tilt the pan to coat the bottom evenly. Add the onion and cook, stirring often, until softened, 5 minutes. Add the garlic, cumin, and cayenne and cook, stirring constantly, until fragrant, 30 seconds.

2 Add the stock, corn, and zucchini and bring to a boil over high heat. Reduce the heat to low and simmer, uncovered, until the vegetables are tender and most of the liquid has evaporated, about 3 minutes. Add the rice and salt and cook, stirring often, until heated through, 2 minutes. Remove from the heat and stir in the cilantro and lime juice. Spoon the rice into a serving dish and serve at once.

Each serving: 16 g carb, 93 cal, 3 g fat, 0 g sat fat, 0 mg chol, 2 g fib, 2 g pro, 196 mg sod • Carb Choices: 1; Exchanges: 1 starch

Rice with Shiitakes and Spinach

makes 4 servings

Shiitake mushrooms always add elegance to a dish. Here they are paired with vibrant spinach and earthy brown rice for a terrific side dish for simple baked salmon or sautéed chicken.

2 teaspoons extra virgin olive oil

1 cup sliced shiitake mushroom caps

¼ cup minced onion

1 garlic clove, minced

4 cups chopped fresh spinach

2 cups cooked brown rice (page 108)

½ teaspoon kosher salt

2 teaspoons lemon juice

1 Heat a medium nonstick skillet over medium heat. Add the oil and tilt the pan to coat the bottom evenly. Add the mushrooms and onion and cook, stirring often, until softened, 5 minutes. Add the garlic and cook, stirring constantly, until fragrant, 30 seconds.

2 Add the spinach, rice, and salt and cook, stirring constantly, until the spinach is wilted and the rice is heated through, 2 minutes. Remove from the heat and stir in the lemon juice. Spoon the rice into a serving dish and serve at once.

Each serving: 26 g carb, 147 cal, 3 g fat, 1 g sat fat, 0 mg chol, 3 g fib, 4 g pro, 166 mg sod • Carb Choices: 2; Exchanges: 2 starch, ½ fat

MIX AND MATCH FRIED RICE

Heat a large nonstick skillet over medium-high heat. Add 2 teaspoons canola oil and tilt the pan to coat the bottom evenly. Add 2 teaspoons minced fresh ginger and 1 garlic clove, minced, and cook, stirring constantly, until fragrant, 30 seconds. Add a vegetable from each of the Vegetable columns in the chart below and cook, stirring often, until the vegetables are crisp-tender, about 5 minutes. Add 2 cups cooked brown rice and a Flavor Booster from the chart and cook, stirring constantly, until the rice is heated through. Remove from the heat, stir in a Finishing Touch and 1 tablespoon lime juice, and serve at once. The rice dishes make enough to serve 4 as a side dish. Each serving has 2 Carb Choices (about 28 grams of carbs) and about 150 calories.

Vegetable 1 Choose 1	Vegetable 2 Choose 1	Flavor Booster Choose 1	Finishing Touch Choose 1
¾ cup thinly sliced red onion	½ cup ½-inch pieces cooked green beans	2 tablespoons reduced-sodium soy sauce	2 tablespoons chopped fresh cilantro
1 cup thinly sliced red bell pepper	1 cup sliced zucchini squash	1 tablespoon hoisin sauce	2 tablespoons chopped fresh basil
1 cup snow peas, trimmed and cut in half on the diagonal	1 cup small broccoli florets	1 tablespoon black bean sauce	2 tablespoons thinly sliced scallion tops
1 cup sugar snap peas, trimmed	1 cup ½-inch pieces asparagus	2 tablespoons oyster sauce	1 jalapeño, seeded and minced
¾ cup ¼-inch-thick carrot sticks	1 cup sliced white or shiitake mushroom caps	1 tablespoon Asian fish sauce	½ cup bean sprouts

Rice with Mushrooms and Roasted Peppers

makes 4 servings

Use any variety of mushrooms for this recipe. If you use portobello mushrooms, use a spoon to scrape out the gills underneath the caps, then coarsely chop the mushrooms.

2 teaspoons extra virgin olive oil

1 cup sliced cremini or white mushroom caps

¼ cup diced onion

¼ cup Vegetable Stock (page 149) or low-sodium vegetable broth

2 cups cooked brown rice (page 108)

¼ cup diced red Roasted Bell Peppers (page 21) or roasted red peppers from a jar

½ teaspoon kosher salt

Pinch of freshly ground pepper

1 tablespoon chopped fresh Italian parsley

1 Heat a medium nonstick skillet over medium heat. Add the oil and tilt the pan to coat the bottom evenly. Add the mushrooms and onion and cook, stirring often, until softened, 5 minutes.

2 Add the stock and bring to a boil over high heat. Reduce the heat to low and simmer, uncovered, until the vegetables are very tender and most of the liquid has evaporated, about 3 minutes. Add the rice, roasted pepper, salt, and ground pepper and cook, stirring often, until heated through, 2 minutes. Remove from the heat and stir in the parsley. Spoon the rice into a serving dish and serve at once.

Each serving: 26 g carb, 146 cal, 3 g fat, 1 g sat fat, 0 mg chol, 2 g fib, 3 g pro, 153 mg sod • Carb Choices: 2; Exchanges: 2 starch, ½ fat

Rice with Tomato and Saffron

makes 4 servings

A pinch of luxurious saffron elevates this rice to a special dish. If you don't have saffron, leave it out—the sautéed onion, bell pepper, and fresh tomato give it plenty of flavor.

¼ cup Vegetable Stock (page 149) or low-sodium vegetable broth
Pinch of saffron threads
2 teaspoons extra virgin olive oil
¼ cup diced onion
¼ cup diced red bell pepper
1 garlic clove, minced
2 cups cooked brown rice (see page 108)
1 plum tomato, chopped
½ teaspoon kosher salt
Pinch of freshly ground pepper
1 tablespoon chopped fresh Italian parsley

1 Pour the stock into a small bowl and microwave on high until hot, about 30 seconds. Add the saffron and set aside.

2 Heat a medium nonstick skillet over medium heat. Add the oil and tilt the pan to coat the bottom evenly. Add the onion and bell pepper and cook, stirring often, until softened, 5 minutes. Add the garlic and cook, stirring constantly, until fragrant, 30 seconds.

3 Add the stock mixture and bring to a boil over high heat. Reduce the heat to low and simmer, uncovered, until the vegetables are tender and most of the liquid has evaporated, about 3 minutes. Add the rice, tomato, salt, and ground pepper and cook, stirring often, until heated through, 2 minutes. Remove from the heat and stir in the parsley. Spoon the rice into a serving dish and serve at once.

Each serving: 26 g carb, 142 cal, 3 g fat, 1 g sat fat, 0 mg chol, 2 g fib, 3 g pro, 152 mg sod • Carb Choices: 2; Exchanges: 2 starch, ½ fat

Rice with Apple, Pecans, and Rosemary

makes 4 servings

This autumnal side dish makes a colorful accompaniment for pork loin or roast chicken. When you cook the apple, watch it carefully so it doesn't get too tender—you want to see the pieces of apple in the finished dish. Thyme is a nice substitute for the rosemary in this dish.

2 teaspoons extra virgin olive oil
1 small apple, peeled, cored, and chopped
¼ cup diced onion
¼ cup Vegetable Stock (page 149) or low-sodium vegetable broth
2 teaspoons chopped fresh rosemary or ½ teaspoon crumbled dried rosemary
2 cups cooked brown rice (page 108)
½ teaspoon kosher salt
Pinch of freshly ground pepper
2 tablespoons pecans, toasted and chopped (page 4)

1 Heat a medium nonstick skillet over medium heat. Add the oil and tilt the pan to coat the bottom evenly. Add the apple and onion and cook, stirring often, until softened, 5 minutes.

2 Add the stock and rosemary and bring to a boil over high heat. Reduce the heat and simmer, uncovered, until the apple is tender and most of the liquid has evaporated, about 3 minutes. Add the rice, salt, and pepper and cook, stirring often, until heated through, 2 minutes. Stir in the pecans. Spoon the rice into a serving dish and serve at once.

Each serving: 28 g carb, 173 cal, 6 g fat, 1 g sat fat, 0 mg chol, 3 g fib, 3 g pro, 150 mg sod • Carb Choices: 2; Exchanges: 1½ starch, ½ fruit, 1 fat

Beyond Brown Rice

The recipes here all call for ordinary brown rice. It's the most common and the most economical variety of whole grain rice. But wherever you shop, be it at a suburban supermarket or a specialty store, you'll find many types of whole grain rice on the shelves.

Look for brown basmati, brown jasmine, black japonica, Bhutanese red, and Wehani rice. Give them a try as a substitute for the ordinary brown rice in any of the recipes here and as a change of pace from plain brown rice. All of these varieties have about the same carbohydrate content of regular brown rice—about 23 grams of carbs in ½ cup serving.

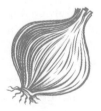

Raisin-Spice Rice

makes 4 servings

This intensely flavored rice is a delicious backdrop for Tandoori-Style Chicken (page 237) or Indian-Spiced Turkey Cutlets with Sautéed Peaches (page 251).

2 teaspoons extra virgin olive oil
¼ cup diced onion
1 garlic clove, minced
⅛ teaspoon ground cardamom
⅛ teaspoon ground cinnamon
⅛ teaspoon ground cloves
½ cup Vegetable Stock (page 149) or
    low-sodium vegetable broth
2 tablespoons golden raisins
2 cups cooked brown rice (page 108)
½ teaspoon kosher salt
2 teaspoons lemon juice
1 tablespoon chopped fresh Italian
    parsley

1 Heat a medium nonstick skillet over medium heat. Add the oil and tilt the pan to coat the bottom evenly. Add the onion and cook, stirring often, until softened, 5 minutes. Add the garlic, cardamom, cinnamon, and cloves and cook, stirring constantly, until fragrant, 30 seconds.

2 Add the stock and raisins and bring to a boil over high heat. Reduce the heat to low and simmer, uncovered, until the raisins are plumped and most of the liquid has evaporated, about 3 minutes. Add the rice and salt and cook, stirring often, until heated through, 2 minutes. Remove from the heat and stir in the lemon juice and parsley. Spoon the rice into a serving dish and serve at once.

Each serving: 29 g carb, 154 cal, 3 g fat, 1 g sat fat, 0 mg chol, 2 g fib, 3 g pro, 160 mg sod • Carb Choices: 2; Exchanges: 2 starch, ½ fat

Rice with Roasted Grapes and Coriander

makes 4 servings

The idea for pairing rice and grapes came from Mangia, one of my favorite spots for lunch in Manhattan. My friend Nancy Jessup is the chef there and she keeps the menu so fresh and ever-changing that you could eat there every day and never have the same dish twice.

1 cup seedless red or green grapes
3 teaspoons extra virgin olive oil, divided
¼ cup minced shallot
1 teaspoon ground coriander
¼ cup Vegetable Stock (page 149) or
    low-sodium vegetable broth
2 cups cooked brown rice (page 108)
½ teaspoon kosher salt
2 tablespoons pine nuts, toasted (page 4)
1 tablespoon chopped fresh Italian parsley

1 Preheat the oven to 400°F.

2 Place the grapes on a small rimmed baking sheet. Drizzle with 1 teaspoon of the oil and stir to coat. Roast until the grapes begin to shrivel and the skins begin to break, 25 minutes.

3 About 10 minutes before the grapes are done, heat a medium nonstick skillet over medium heat. Add the remaining 2 teaspoons oil and the shallot and cook, stirring, until softened, 5 minutes. Stir in the coriander.

4 Add the stock and bring to a boil over high heat. Reduce the heat to low and simmer, uncovered, until most of the liquid has evaporated, about 3 minutes. Add the rice and salt and cook, stirring often, until heated through, 2 minutes. Remove from the heat and stir in the roasted grapes and their pan juices, the pine nuts, and parsley. Spoon the rice into a serving dish and serve at once.

Each serving: 33 g carb, 206 cal, 7 g fat, 1 g sat fat, 0 mg chol, 2 g fib, 3 g pro, 152 mg sod • Carb Choices: 2; Exchanges: 1½ starch, ½ fruit, 1 fat

Toasted Coconut–Ginger Rice

makes 4 servings

Coconut milk gives this dish a rich creamy texture—think of it as an Asian risotto. Serve it with any simple seafood or chicken or with a stir-fry.

2 tablespoons flaked sweetened coconut
2 teaspoons canola oil
1 scallion, thinly sliced
2 teaspoons minced fresh ginger
2 cups cooked brown rice (page 108)
¼ cup reduced-fat coconut milk
1 tablespoon Asian fish sauce
1 tablespoon chopped fresh cilantro
1 tablespoon lime juice

1 Preheat the oven to 350°F. Place the coconut in a small baking pan and bake, stirring once, until lightly toasted, 6 to 8 minutes.

2 Heat a medium nonstick skillet over medium heat. Add the oil and tilt the pan to coat the bottom evenly. Add the scallion and ginger and cook, stirring often, until the scallion is softened, 1 minute.

3 Add the rice, coconut milk, and fish sauce and cook, stirring often, until the rice is heated through, about 2 minutes. Remove from the heat and stir in the toasted coconut, cilantro, and lime juice. Spoon the rice into a serving dish and serve at once.

Each serving: 26 g carb, 158 cal, 5 g fat, 2 g sat fat, 0 mg chol, 2 g fib, 3 g pro, 363 mg sod • Carb Choices: 2; Exchanges: 2 starch, 1 fat

Oven-Baked Rice with Tomatoes and Rosemary

makes 6 servings

When you need a delicious side dish that doesn't take any tending, this one is a satisfying choice. A larger portion, sprinkled with a little feta cheese, makes a tasty vegetarian main dish.

2 teaspoons extra virgin olive oil
½ cup diced onion
2 garlic cloves, minced
1¼ cups Vegetable Stock (page 149) or low-sodium vegetable broth
1 (14½-ounce) can no-salt-added diced tomatoes, drained
2 teaspoons minced fresh rosemary or ½ teaspoon crumbled dried rosemary
½ teaspoon kosher salt
Pinch of freshly ground pepper
¾ cup long-grain brown rice

1 Preheat the oven to 375°F.

2 Heat a medium nonstick skillet over medium heat. Add the oil and tilt the pan to coat the bottom evenly. Add the onion and cook, stirring often, until softened, 5 minutes. Add the garlic and cook, stirring constantly, until fragrant, 30 seconds.

3 Add the stock, tomatoes, rosemary, salt, and pepper and bring to a boil over high heat. Place the rice in a 1½-quart baking dish. Pour the hot stock mixture over the rice and stir to mix well. Cover with foil and bake until the liquid has absorbed and the rice is tender, 1 hour. Fluff with a fork before serving. Serve the rice at once.

Each serving: 23 g carb, 125 cal, 2 g fat, 0 g sat fat, 0 mg chol, 3 g fib, 3 g pro, 154 mg sod • Carb Choices: 1½; Exchanges: 1 starch, 1 veg

Southwestern Oven-Baked Rice

makes 6 servings

Many people, including myself, tend to mess up rice on top of the stove. This baked rice is foolproof—just put it in the oven and set the timer while you make the rest of dinner. This rice reheats beautifully in the microwave, so it's great to have for leftovers.

2 teaspoons extra virgin olive oil
½ cup diced onion
½ cup diced green bell pepper
1 jalapeño, seeded and minced
2 garlic cloves, minced
1 teaspoon ground cumin
1¼ cups Vegetable Stock (page 149) or low-sodium vegetable broth
1 (14½-ounce) can no-salt-added diced tomatoes, drained
½ teaspoon kosher salt
Pinch of ground cayenne
¾ cup long-grain brown rice
¼ cup chopped fresh cilantro
2 teaspoons lime juice

1 Preheat the oven to 375°F.

2 Heat a medium nonstick skillet over medium heat. Add the oil and tilt the pan to coat the bottom evenly. Add the onion, bell pepper, and jalapeño and cook, stirring often, until softened, 5 minutes. Add the garlic and cumin and cook, stirring constantly, until fragrant, 30 seconds.

3 Add the stock, tomatoes, salt, and cayenne and bring to a boil over high heat. Place the rice in a 1½-quart baking dish. Pour the hot stock mixture over the rice and stir to mix well. Cover and bake until the liquid has absorbed and the rice is tender, 1 hour. Fluff with a fork and stir in the cilantro and lime juice. Serve the rice at once.

Each serving: 24 g carb, 128 cal, 2 g fat, 0 g sat fat, 0 mg chol, 3 g fib, 3 g pro, 155 mg sod • Carb Choices: 1½; Exchanges: 1 starch, 1 veg

Baked Butternut Squash Risotto

makes 8 servings

Cut the remaining squash that you'll have from preparing this recipe into chunks, toss with olive oil, and sprinkle with salt. Bake it on a rimmed baking sheet while you bake the risotto and serve it for a side dish later in the week.

2 teaspoons extra virgin olive oil
1 medium onion, diced
2 garlic cloves, minced
1 cup short- or medium-grain brown rice
2 cups cubed butternut squash
1⅔ cups Vegetable Stock (page 149) or low-sodium vegetable broth
1 ounce freshly grated Parmesan (about ¼ cup)
2 teaspoons chopped fresh rosemary
1 teaspoon kosher salt
⅛ teaspoon freshly ground pepper

1 Preheat the oven to 375°F.

2 Heat a Dutch oven over medium-high heat. Add the oil and tilt the pan to coat the bottom evenly. Add the onion and cook, stirring often, until softened, 5 minutes. Add the garlic and cook, stirring constantly, until fragrant, 30 seconds.

3 Add the rice and cook, stirring constantly, 2 minutes. Add the squash and stock and bring to a boil over high heat. Cover, reduce the heat to low, and simmer 5 minutes. Remove the Dutch oven from the heat and stir in the Parmesan, rosemary, salt, and pepper. Cover and bake until the rice is tender and almost all the liquid is absorbed, 1 hour. Fluff with a fork before serving. Serve the risotto at once.

Each serving: 21 g carb, 122 cal, 2 g fat, 1 g sat fat, 2 mg chol, 1 g fib, 3 g pro, 208 mg sod • Carb Choices: 1½; Exchanges: 1½ starch

Wheat Berries

Wheat Berry, Green Bean, and Lemon Sauté HIGH FIBER

makes 6 servings

Wheat berries are chewy and nutty—a real grain lover's treat. Fresh green beans, lemon, and parsley lightens them up in this summery side dish. Serve it with grilled fish or baked chicken.

6 ounces green beans, trimmed and cut into ½-inch pieces
2 teaspoons extra virgin olive oil
⅓ cup minced shallots
2 cups cooked wheat berries (page 108)
2 tablespoons water
1 teaspoon grated lemon zest
1 teaspoon lemon juice
2 tablespoons chopped fresh Italian parsley
½ teaspoon kosher salt
Pinch of freshly ground pepper

1 Fill a medium saucepan half full with water and bring to a boil over high heat. Add the green beans, return to a boil, and cook just until crisp-tender, about 3 minutes. Drain in a colander.

2 Meanwhile, heat a medium nonstick skillet over medium heat. Add the oil and tilt the pan to coat the bottom evenly. Add the shallots and cook, stirring often, until softened, 5 minutes.

3 Add the wheat berries and water. Cook, stirring often, until the wheat berries are heated through, about 2 minutes. Add the green beans, lemon zest, lemon juice, parsley, salt, and pepper and stir to combine. Spoon the wheat berries into a serving dish and serve at once.

Each serving: 21 g carb, 120 cal, 2 g fat, 0 g sat fat, 0 mg chol, 4 g fib, 4 g pro, 97 mg sod • Carb Choices: 1½; Exchanges: 1½ starch

Wheat Berries with Fennel and Apple

makes 6 servings

Sweet apple and savory fennel make this a perfectly balanced side dish. It's a natural with roast pork or pork chops. If you're feeling indulgent, stir in 2 tablespoons toasted chopped walnuts just before serving.

2 teaspoons extra virgin olive oil
½ cup chopped fennel bulb
1 small Granny Smith apple, peeled, cored, and chopped
2 cups cooked wheat berries (page 108)
2 tablespoons water
1 tablespoon chopped fresh Italian parsley
1 teaspoon lemon juice
½ teaspoon kosher salt
Pinch of freshly ground pepper

1 Heat a medium nonstick skillet over medium heat. Add the oil and tilt the pan to coat the bottom evenly. Add the fennel and cook, stirring often, until softened, 5 minutes. Add the apple and cook, stirring often, until the apple just begins to soften, 3 minutes.

2 Add the wheat berries and water. Cook, stirring often until the wheat berries are heated through, about 2 minutes. Remove from the heat and stir in the parsley, lemon juice, salt, and pepper. Spoon the wheat berries into a serving dish and serve at once.

Each serving: 21 g carb, 118 cal, 2 g fat, 0 g sat fat, 0 mg chol, 3 g fib, 4 g pro, 98 mg sod • Carb Choices: 1½; Exchanges: 1½ starch

Wheat Berries with Broccoli Rabe and Currants

makes 6 servings

For anyone who finds broccoli rabe to be bitter, this is a great dish to serve. Combined with nutty wheat berries, sweet currants, and rich Parmesan, broccoli rabe is mellow enough to appeal to any palate.

8 ounces broccoli rabe, tough stems removed, leaves and florets chopped
2 teaspoons extra virgin olive oil
2 garlic cloves, minced
2 tablespoons currants
⅓ cup Vegetable Stock (page 149) or low-sodium vegetable broth
½ teaspoon kosher salt
2 cups cooked wheat berries (page 108)
1 teaspoon lemon juice
2 tablespoons freshly grated Parmesan

1 Bring a medium pot of water to a boil over high heat. Add the broccoli rabe and cook until barely tender, 5 minutes. Drain in a colander.

2 Heat a medium nonstick skillet over medium heat. Add the oil and tilt the pan to coat the bottom evenly. Add the garlic and cook, stirring often, until fragrant and lightly browned, about 1 minute. Add the broccoli rabe, currants, stock, and salt. Cook, stirring occasionally, until the broccoli rabe is very tender and the liquid evaporates, about 2 minutes. Add the wheat berries and cook, stirring often, until heated through, 2 minutes. Remove from the heat and stir in the lemon juice. Spoon onto a serving platter, sprinkle with the Parmesan, and toss to coat. Serve at once.

Each serving: 22 g carb, 134 cal, 3 g fat, 1 g sat fat, 1 mg chol, 3 g fib, 6 g pro, 139 mg sod • Carb Choices: 1½; Exchanges: 1½ starch, ½ fat

Wheat Berries and Vegetables with Moroccan Spices

makes 6 servings

The yellow and green squash add a light summery flavor and vibrant color to wheat berries. Spoon this onto a platter, then top with grilled meat or seafood kebabs for an excellent and easy summer meal.

2 teaspoons extra virgin olive oil
½ cup diced onion
1 garlic clove, minced
¼ teaspoon ground ginger
¼ teaspoon ground cumin
⅛ teaspoon ground cinnamon
⅛ teaspoon ground cayenne
¼ cup Vegetable Stock (page 149) or
    low-sodium vegetable broth
2 cups cooked wheat berries (page 108)
1 small zucchini, cut into ½-inch cubes
1 small yellow squash, cut into ½-inch cubes
½ teaspoon kosher salt
2 tablespoons chopped fresh cilantro
1 teaspoon lime juice

1 Heat a medium nonstick skillet over medium heat. Add the oil and tilt the pan to coat the bottom evenly. Add the onion and cook, stirring often, until softened, 5 minutes. Add the garlic, ginger, cumin, cinnamon, and cayenne and cook, stirring constantly, until fragrant, 30 seconds.

2 Add the stock, then add the wheat berries, zucchini, yellow squash, and salt. Cook, stirring occasionally, until the squash is crisp-tender and the liquid evaporates, about 3 minutes. Remove from the heat and stir in the cilantro and lime juice. Spoon the wheat berries into a serving dish and serve at once.

Each serving: 21 g carb, 119 cal, 2 g fat, 0 g sat fat, 0 mg chol, 3 g fib, 4 g pro, 105 mg sod • Carb Choices: 1½; Exchanges: 1½ starch

Farro and Vegetable Risotto

makes 8 servings

Farro is a type of wheat similar to wheat berries. It has had part of the bran removed, so it cooks faster than wheat berries.

4 cups Vegetable Stock (page 149) or
    low-sodium vegetable broth
2 teaspoons extra virgin olive oil
8 ounces sliced mushrooms, any variety
1 small onion, diced
1 cup farro
½ teaspoon kosher salt
8 ounces asparagus, tough stems removed and
    spears cut into 1½-inch pieces
2 packed cups chopped fresh spinach
2 ounces freshly grated Parmesan
    (about ½ cup)
⅛ teaspoon freshly ground pepper

1 Pour the stock into a medium saucepan and bring to a simmer over medium-high heat. Reduce the heat to low and keep the stock warm.

2 Heat a large saucepan over medium heat. Add the oil, mushrooms, and onion and cook, stirring often, until the vegetables are softened, 8 minutes.

3 Add the farro and salt and cook, stirring constantly, 2 minutes. Add the stock, ½ cup at a time, stirring frequently, until the liquid is absorbed after each addition before adding more broth. After 30 minutes, stir in the asparagus and continue adding broth and stirring until the farro is tender, about 5 minutes longer. Stir in the spinach and cook, stirring constantly, until the spinach is wilted, about 1 minute. Remove the saucepan from the heat and stir in the Parmesan and pepper. Spoon the farro into a serving dish and serve at once.

Each serving: 17 g carb, 125 cal, 3 g fat, 1 g sat fat, 4 mg chol, 3 g fib, 6 g pro, 225 mg sod • Carb Choices: 1; Exchanges: 1 starch, ½ fat

Wild Rice

Wild Rice with Caramelized Fennel and Onions HIGH FIBER

makes 6 servings

Licorice-flavored fennel is caramelized to maximize its sweetness in this dish that's ideal for serving with lamb chops or roast pork.

2 teaspoons extra virgin olive oil
1 bulb fennel, tough outer leaves removed, cored and thinly sliced
1 small onion, halved lengthwise and thinly sliced
½ teaspoon kosher salt, divided
2 tablespoons water
2 cups cooked wild rice (page 108)
Pinch freshly ground pepper
2 tablespoons chopped fresh Italian parsley
1 teaspoon lemon juice

1 Heat a medium nonstick skillet over medium heat. Add the oil and tilt the pan to coat the bottom evenly. Add the fennel, onion, and ¼ teaspoon of the salt and cook, covered, stirring occasionally, until the vegetables are very tender, about 25 minutes.

2 Add the water and bring to a boil, stirring to scrape up the browned bits from the bottom of the skillet. Add the rice, remaining ¼ teaspoon salt, and the pepper and cook, stirring often, until heated through, 2 minutes. Remove from the heat and stir in the parsley and lemon juice. Spoon the rice into a serving dish and serve at once.

Each serving: 24 g carb, 130 cal, 3 g fat, 0 g sat fat, 0 mg chol, 4 g fib, 4 g pro, 175 mg sod • Carb Choices: 1½; Exchanges: 1½ starch, ½ fat

Wild Rice with Apricots and Almonds

makes 4 servings

Dried apricots and just a smidgen of maple syrup lend sweetness to this nutty side dish. Instead of the apricots, you can use ¼ cup of dried cranberries or golden raisins.

1 medium leek, halved lengthwise, and thinly sliced
2 teaspoons extra virgin olive oil
6 dried apricots, chopped
½ cup Vegetable Stock (page 149) or low-sodium vegetable broth
1 teaspoon chopped fresh thyme or ¼ teaspoon dried thyme
2 cups cooked wild rice (page 108)
½ teaspoon kosher salt
Pinch of teaspoon freshly ground pepper
2 tablespoons slivered almonds, toasted (page 4)
2 teaspoons real maple syrup
2 teaspoons lemon juice

1 Submerge the sliced leek in a medium bowl of cold water, lift it out, and drain in a colander. Repeat, using fresh water, until no grit remains in the bottom of the bowl. Drain the leek well.

2 Heat a medium nonstick skillet over medium heat. Add the oil and tilt the pan to coat the bottom evenly. Add the leek and cook, stirring occasionally, until softened, 5 minutes.

3 Add the apricots, stock, and thyme and bring to a boil over high heat. Reduce the heat to low and simmer, uncovered, until the apricots are plumped and most of the liquid has evaporated, about 5 minutes. Add the rice, salt, and pepper and cook, stirring often, until heated through, 2 minutes. Remove from the heat and stir almonds, maple syrup, and lemon juice. Spoon the rice into a serving dish and serve at once.

Each serving: 30 g carb, 177 cal, 4 g fat, 1 g sat fat, 0 mg chol, 3 g fib, 5 g pro, 166 mg sod • Carb Choices: 2; Exchanges: 1½ starch, ½ fruit, 1 fat

Wild Rice with Butternut Squash and Sage

makes 4 servings

Taking the extra step of lightly browning the squash cubes gives this dish added flavor and color. Make a double batch and serve this instead of stuffing alongside a holiday turkey.

1 cup cubed butternut squash
3 teaspoons extra virgin olive oil, divided
½ cup diced onion
1 garlic clove, minced
½ teaspoon ground coriander
¼ cup Vegetable Stock (page 149) or low-sodium vegetable broth
1 teaspoon minced fresh sage
1½ cups cooked wild rice (page 108)
2 tablespoons orange marmalade
½ teaspoon kosher salt

1 Bring a medium saucepan of water to a boil over high heat. Add the squash and cook until just tender, 5 minutes. Drain in a colander.

2 Heat a medium nonstick skillet over medium-high heat. Add 2 teaspoons of the oil and tilt the pan to coat the bottom evenly. Add the squash and cook, stirring occasionally, until browned, 5 minutes. Transfer to a plate.

3 Reduce the heat to medium and add the remaining 1 teaspoon oil to the pan. Add the onion and cook, stirring often, until softened, 5 minutes. Add the garlic and coriander and cook, stirring constantly, until fragrant, 30 seconds.

4 Add the stock and sage and bring to a boil over high heat. Reduce the heat to low and simmer, uncovered, until most of the liquid has evaporated, about 3 minutes. Add the squash, rice, marmalade, and salt and cook, stirring often, until heated through, 2 minutes. Spoon the rice into a serving dish and serve at once.

Each serving: 25 g carb, 141 cal, 4 g fat, 1 g sat fat, 0 mg chol, 2 g fib, 3 g pro, 158 mg sod • Carb Choices: 1½; Exchanges: 1½ starch, ½ carb, ½ fat

Wild Rice with Mushrooms and Thyme

makes 4 servings

Nutty chewy wild rice, earthy mushrooms, and thyme make a delicious side dish for Cornish hens, roast beef tenderloin, or a holiday turkey.

½ cup Vegetable Stock (page 149) or low-sodium vegetable broth
½ ounce dried porcini mushrooms (about ½ cup)
2 teaspoons extra virgin olive oil
4 ounces shiitake mushrooms, stemmed and thinly sliced
2 shallots, minced
½ teaspoon kosher salt, divided
2 cups cooked wild rice (page 108)
1 teaspoon chopped fresh thyme or ¼ teaspoon dried thyme
Pinch of freshly ground pepper

1 Bring the stock to a boil in a small saucepan. Remove from the heat, add the porcini mushrooms, cover, and let stand 30 minutes.

2 Place a coffee filter in a fine wire mesh strainer and place over a bowl. Pour the mushroom mixture through the filter. Finely chop the mushrooms and set aside and reserve the strained mushroom soaking liquid.

3 Heat a medium nonstick skillet over medium heat. Add the oil and the shiitake mushrooms, shallots, and ¼ teaspoon of the salt and cook, stirring often, until the mushrooms are browned 8 minutes.

4 Add the reserved mushroom soaking liquid and cook until most of the liquid has evaporated, about 2 minutes. Add the porcini mushrooms, rice, thyme, remaining ¼ teaspoon salt, and the pepper and cook, stirring often, until heated through, 2 minutes. Spoon the rice into a serving dish and serve at once.

Each serving: 23 g carb, 137 cal, 3 g fat, 0 g sat fat, 0 mg chol, 3 g fib, 5 g pro, 163 mg sod • Carb Choices: 1½; Exchanges: 1½ starch, 1 veg, ½ fat

Vegetable Sides

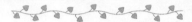

Artichokes

Grilled Artichokes with
Olive Oil and Lemon

Artichoke Hearts with
Garlic, Olive Oil, and
Parsley

Braised Baby Artichokes

Asparagus

Stir-Fried Asparagus with
Sesame and Lime

Grilled Asparagus with
Lemon Vinaigrette

Steamed Asparagus with
Asiago Vinaigrette

Asparagus with Sautéed
Shiitake Mushrooms

Beets

Foil-Roasted Beets

Basic Boiled Beets

Beets with Sautéed Beet
Greens

Pomegranate-Glazed Beets

Roasted Beets with
Apple-Walnut Dressing

Roasted Beets with
Grapefruit and Mint

Broccoli and
Broccoli Rabe

Two-Minute Microwave
Broccoli with Lemon Butter

Roasted Broccoli with
Balsamic-Dijon Vinaigrette

Stir-Fried Broccoli with
Ginger Sauce

Sesame Broccoli

Broccoli and Sweet Onion
Puree

Stewed Broccoli Rabe with
Ancho and Manchego

Broccoli Rabe with Garlic
and Sun-Dried Tomatoes

Roasted Broccoli Rabe with
Lemon and Olives

Brussels Sprouts

Brussels Sprouts with Apple
Cider Glaze

Roasted Brussels Sprouts
with Toasted Walnuts

Shaved Brussels Sprouts
with Garlic and Lemon

Brussels Sprouts with
Caraway

Carrots

Carrot and Orange Puree

Carrot Puree with Maple
and Cardamom

Mango and Ginger–Glazed
Carrots

Roasted Carrots with
Coriander and Cilantro

Carrots with Moroccan
Spices

Cauliflower

Cauliflower Mash

Spicy Roasted Cauliflower with Lime

Baked Cauliflower with Parmesan

Corn

Microwave Corn-on-the-Cob

Corn with Basil and Lemon

Corn with Roasted Jalapeño and Lime

Eggplant

Roasted Eggplant with Tomato Vinaigrette

Eggplant Gratin

Grilled Eggplant Rounds with Basil and Caper Sauce

Baby Eggplants Stuffed with Zucchini and Dried Tomatoes

Spicy Eggplant with Ginger and Sesame

Fennel

Grilled Fennel with Orange-Olive Vinaigrette

Sautéed Fennel with Ginger

Roasted Fennel with Pernod

Fennel Gratin

Green Beans

Steamed Green Beans with Walnuts and Parmesan

Lemon-Dill Green Beans

Green Beans with Caramelized Onions and Cider Vinegar

Green Beans with Grape Tomatoes

Thin-Sliced Green Beans with Pine Nuts and Mint

Green Beans with Feta Vinaigrette

Stir-Fried Green Beans

Roasted Green Beans

Slow-Cooked Italian Pole Beans with Tomatoes and Oregano

Greens

Spinach with Whole Grain Mustard

Spinach with Garlic, Lemon, and Cracked Pepper

Kale with Crispy Crumbs and Pine Nuts

Wilted Escarole with Anchovies

Swiss Chard with Raisins and Pine Nuts

Roasted Radicchio with Balsamic-Garlic Vinaigrette

Sautéed Greens with Vinegar and Garlic

Chinese Broccoli in Oyster Sauce

Steamed Baby Bok Choy with Ginger Sauce

Mushrooms

Sautéed Mixed Mushrooms with Rosemary

Bacon-Basil Mushrooms

Roasted Cremini Mushrooms with Thyme

Roasted Portobello Mushrooms with Balsamic Vinegar

Vegetable-Stuffed Portobello Mushrooms

Grilled Mushrooms with Parmesan

Shiitake Mushrooms with Ginger

Okra

Grilled Okra with Yogurt-Cilantro Sauce

Cajun Roasted Okra with Holy Trinity Salsa

Onions

Crispy Oven-Fried Onion Rings

Balsamic-Baked Sweet Onions

Grilled Sweet Onion Slices with Sherry Vinegar and Thyme

Cipolline Onions with Wine and Rosemary

Leeks Braised in White Wine

Peas

Fresh English Peas

English Pea Puree

Sugar Snap Peas with Ginger and Orange

Potatoes

Buttermilk Mashed Potatoes

Roasted Garlic Mashed Potatoes

Two-Potato Puree

Potato-Cauliflower Mash

Chile-Lime Oven Fries

Roasted Potatoes with Fresh Herbs and Lemon

Rutabagas and Turnips

Roasted Rutabagas with Molasses

Rutabaga-Apple Puree

Roasted Turnips with Honey and Toasted Spices

Summer Squash

Sautéed Zucchini with Cilantro and Lime

Summer Squash with Onion and Dill en Papillote

Roasted Summer Squash Spears with Basil and Mint

Grilled Summer Squash with Corn Vinaigrette

Roasted Zucchini with Toasted Cumin and Basil

Sweet Potatoes

Roasted Sweet Potatoes with Ginger and Lime

Sweet Potato and Pear Puree

Sweet Potato Puree with Cranberries

Tomatoes

Broiled Beefsteak Tomatoes with Basil and Parmesan

Braised Plum Tomatoes

Roasted Plum Tomatoes with Garlic and Capers

Blistered Cherry Tomatoes with Rosemary

Oven-Fried Green Tomatoes

Winter Squash

Roasted Acorn Squash with Ginger Butter

Masala-Roasted Acorn Squash

Butternut Squash and Gruyère Gratin

Roasted Butternut Squash with Goat Cheese

Butternut Squash Hash

Winter Squash Puree with Olive Oil and Rosemary

Roasted Delicata Squash with Sage and Garlic

Mixed Vegetable Dishes

Corn and Bell Peppers with Thyme

Summer Succotash

Carrots and Fennel Braised with White Wine and Garlic

Roasted Root Vegetables with Kale

Fruit and Honey–Roasted Vegetables

Roasted Broccoli and Cauliflower with Indian Spices

Eggplant and Tomatoes with Herb Sauce

Summer Garden Vegetable Gratin

Stewed Okra and Tomatoes

Root Vegetable Hash with Brussels Sprouts

Asian Vegetable Stir-Fry

Eating a generous variety of vegetables is a deliciously rewarding way for people with diabetes to help keep blood sugar and blood lipids under control and to get fiber, vitamins, and other micronutrients they need.

Non-starchy vegetables, such as broccoli, greens, eggplant, and cucumbers, contain very little carbohydrate, and unless eaten in massive amounts, have virtually no effect on blood sugars. Starchy vegetables, such as peas, potatoes, and winter squash, contain important vitamins, minerals, and fiber and should be consumed regularly, but remember to take the carbohydrates into consideration when eating them.

Many people with diabetes are also at risk for or already have heart disease. Studies have shown conclusively that people who eat a low-fat diet with lots of vegetables and fruits reduce their risk for heart attack and stroke.

Vegetables, as well as fruits, whole grains, and beans contain vital phytochemicals found only in plant foods that are believed to reduce the risk of diabetes, heart disease, and certain cancers.

If you need yet another reason to eat more vegetables, they can help you lose weight. You've probably heard the recommendation to fill your plate at least half full with vegetables at lunch and dinner. That's great advice in order to get all the nutrients you need, but it's a great weight-loss tip, too.

The recipes in this chapter are meant to keep your taste buds excited meal after meal with new and appetizing ways to cook vegetables. I believe in big flavors, so I use spice rubs, herbs, sauces, and dressings to give

vegetables great taste. For many of the vegetables in this chapter, you'll find at least one recipe for roasting. It's one of the easiest ways to coax great flavor out of vegetables you thought you didn't even like (think beets, cauliflower, and Brussels sprouts).

Almost all the vegetable recipes here include some oil or butter. Adding a touch of fat to vegetables helps make the fat-soluble nutrients easier for your body to absorb—and it just makes them taste better. Most of these vegetable recipes have about ½ teaspoon of olive or canola oil or butter per serving, which adds about 20 extra calories. For what you lose in the additional calories, you'll enjoy the flavor of the vegetables more and get more nutrients from them.

As with other recipes, I use only extra virgin olive oil for its great flavor and high level of monounsaturated (good for you) fat. For Asian-influenced recipes where olive oil would be overwhelmed by stronger flavors, I use virtually tasteless canola oil (which is also high in monounsaturated fats). And some vegetables—like corn, mashed potatoes, and fresh English peas—just have to have a little butter.

The serving sizes for the recipes in this chapter are side-dish servings (about ½ cup), but you can turn many of them into main courses, too. Because I don't eat a lot of meat, especially in summer and early fall, when vegetables are available in abundance, many of the recipes in this chapter are dishes that I make and serve alongside pasta, rice, wheat berries, quinoa, or polenta as a main dish. I've noted many of those recipes throughout the chapter.

You can think of some of these vegetable recipes as salads, too and serve them warm or at room temperature. I love drizzling vegetables with dressings made with citrus juices and vinegars to bring out their wonderful flavors. You'll find serving directions with each recipe stating whether it should be served at once, or if it can also be served warm or at room temperature.

No matter what the season, whether you're shopping for fresh vegetables at a humdrum neighborhood grocery store, a gourmet produce shop, or a farmers' market, you'll find wholesome, health-giving, and delicious dishes here to create with whatever vegetables you've brought home.

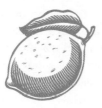

Artichokes

Grilled Artichokes with Olive Oil and Lemon HIGH FIBER

makes 4 servings

Grilling adds a smoky nuance to the nutty flavor of artichokes. You must boil the artichokes before grilling them, since they take so long to cook that they would burn before they got tender on the grill. To save time, boil the artichokes up to 2 days ahead. When you're ready to grill, bring the artichokes to room temperature and proceed with the recipe.

4 medium artichokes
2 teaspoons plus 1 tablespoon extra virgin olive oil, divided
3 tablespoons lemon juice
½ teaspoon kosher salt

1 Place the artichokes in a large pot and add water to cover. Bring to a boil over high heat, reduce the heat, cover, and simmer until just tender when pierced with a knife, 35 to 45 minutes. Drain the artichokes and let stand until cool enough to handle. Cut each one in half lengthwise and remove the fuzzy center choke using a spoon or a melon baller.

2 Prepare the grill or heat a large grill pan over medium-high heat.

3 Brush the artichokes with 2 teaspoons of the oil. Grill, turning occasionally, until the artichokes are well browned and very tender, about 15 minutes. Place the artichokes in a serving dish.

4 Whisk together the remaining 1 tablespoon oil, the lemon juice, and salt in a small bowl. Drizzle the mixture over the artichokes and serve hot or at room temperature.

Each serving: 14 g carb, 115 cal, 6 g fat, 1 g sat fat, 0 mg chol, 7 g fib, 4 g pro, 254 mg sod • Carb Choices: 1; Exchanges: 2 veg, 1 fat

Artichoke Hearts with Garlic, Olive Oil, and Parsley HIGH FIBER

makes 4 servings

This easy method of cooking takes all the work out of eating an artichoke, since you trim away all the inedible parts before cooking. It's perfect as an elegant side dish for fish fillets or roast chicken. Or make this dish an entrée for two served over pasta.

1 small lemon
4 medium artichokes
1 tablespoon extra virgin olive oil
2 garlic cloves, minced
1½ cups dry white wine
½ teaspoon kosher salt
2 tablespoons chopped fresh Italian parsley

1 Squeeze the juice from the lemon into a large bowl and fill the bowl three-quarters full with cold water.

2 Working with one at a time, snap off the outer petals of each artichoke including the light inner leaves. Trim away the brown tip of the stem and peel the stem. Quarter the artichokes and use a spoon or a melon baller to scoop out the fuzzy choke. As you finish, place the artichokes in the lemon water.

3 Heat a large skillet over medium heat. Add the oil and tilt the pan to coat the bottom evenly. Add the garlic and cook, stirring constantly, until fragrant, 30 seconds. Add the wine and salt. Drain the artichokes and add to the skillet. Bring to a boil, cover, reduce the heat to low, and simmer until the artichokes are tender, about 30 minutes. If excess liquid remains in the pan, uncover and cook until most of the liquid evaporates. Spoon the artichokes onto a serving platter and sprinkle with the parsley. Serve at once.

Each serving: 16 g carb, 166 cal, 4 g fat, 1 g sat fat, 0 mg chol, 7 g fib, 4 g pro, 255 mg sod • Carb Choices: 1; Exchanges: 2 veg, ½ fat

Braised Baby Artichokes

HIGH FIBER

makes 4 servings

When you first see baby artichokes in the market in the springtime, make this dish as a celebration of the season.

1 small lemon
12 baby artichokes
1 tablespoon extra virgin olive oil
1 small onion, halved and thinly sliced
2 garlic cloves, minced
½ cup Chicken Stock (page 149) or low-sodium chicken broth
¼ teaspoon kosher salt
1 teaspoon lemon juice
1 tablespoon chopped fresh basil or 1 teaspoon chopped fresh rosemary

1 Squeeze the juice from the lemon into a large bowl and fill the bowl three-quarters full with cold water.

2 Working with one at a time, snap off the outer petals of each artichoke until you reach leaves that are half green and half yellow. Cut away and discard the top third of each artichoke. Trim away the brown tip of the stem and peel the stem. Cut each artichoke in half, and remove any pink- or purple-tinted leaves inside. As you finish, place each artichoke in the lemon water.

3 Heat a large skillet over medium heat. Add the oil and tilt the pan to coat the bottom evenly. Add the onion and cook, stirring occasionally, until softened, 5 minutes. Stir in the garlic and cook until fragrant, 30 seconds. Drain the artichokes and add to the pan. Add the stock and salt and bring to a boil over high heat. Cover, reduce the heat to low, and simmer until the artichokes are tender, 8 to 10 minutes. Stir in the lemon juice and basil. Spoon the artichokes into a serving dish. Serve hot, warm, or at room temperature.

Each serving: 12 g carb, 104 cal, 4 g fat, 1 g sat fat, 1 mg chol, 5 g fib, 5 g pro, 202 mg sod • Carb Choices: 1; Exchanges: 2 veg, 1 fat

Asparagus

Stir-Fried Asparagus with Sesame and Lime QUICK

makes 4 servings

A few drops of toasted sesame oil and fresh lime juice accentuate the earthy flavors of asparagus in this easy side dish. Serve it to accompany any Asian-inspired entrée, or make it an entrée for two served over rice or soba noodles.

2 teaspoons canola oil
1 pound asparagus, tough ends removed, cut into 1-inch pieces
1 garlic clove, minced
2 teaspoons lime juice
¼ teaspoon Asian sesame oil
¼ teaspoon kosher salt

1 Heat a large wok or nonstick skillet over medium-high heat. Add the canola oil and tilt the pan to coat the bottom evenly. Add the asparagus and garlic and cook, stirring constantly, until crisp-tender, 4 minutes.

2 Spoon the asparagus into a serving bowl. Add the lime juice, sesame oil, and salt and toss gently to coat. Serve hot or warm.

Each serving: 3 g carb, 40 cal, 3 g fat, 0 g sat fat, 0 mg chol, 1 g fib, 1 g pro, 71 mg sod • Carb Choices: 0; Exchanges: 1 veg, ½ fat

Grilled Asparagus with Lemon Vinaigrette QUICK

makes 4 servings

The flavors of asparagus and lemon both say springtime to me and this is a delicious combination of two favorites. You can also roast the asparagus: Place the spears in a medium roasting pan, drizzle with 1 teaspoon of olive oil, turn to coat, and bake at 425°F for 15 to 20 minutes, shaking the pan once while baking.

1 pound asparagus, tough ends removed
1 teaspoon plus 1 tablespoon extra virgin olive oil, divided
1 teaspoon grated lemon zest
2 teaspoons lemon juice
½ teaspoon kosher salt
Pinch of freshly ground pepper

1 Prepare the grill or heat a large grill pan over medium-high heat.

2 Place the asparagus in a shallow dish and drizzle with 1 teaspoon of the oil. Turn to coat.

3 Grill, turning often, until the asparagus is crisp-tender, about 6 minutes.

4 Whisk together the lemon zest, lemon juice, salt, and pepper in a small bowl. Slowly whisk in the remaining 1 tablespoon oil.

5 Arrange the asparagus on a serving platter and drizzle with the dressing. Serve hot, warm, or at room temperature.

Each serving: 3 g carb, 58 cal, 5 g fat, 1 g sat fat, 0 mg chol, 1 g fib, 1 g pro, 141 mg sod • Carb Choices: 0; Exchanges: 1 veg, 1 fat

Trimming Asparagus

If you've ever cooked asparagus and found the ends of the spears to be tough and stringy, here's how to get rid of them before they end up on your plate. Bend each spear about three-quarters of the way down from the top of the spear and it will naturally break off where the tough part of the spear starts.

Steamed Asparagus with Asiago Vinaigrette QUICK

makes 4 servings

Adding grated aged sharp cheese to a vinaigrette makes one of my favorite toppings for simply prepared vegetables. Try the vinaigrette over steamed green beans, grilled or roasted eggplant rounds, or grilled or roasted fennel.

1 pound asparagus, tough ends removed

2 teaspoons white wine vinegar

1 garlic clove, crushed through a press

¼ teaspoon kosher salt

Pinch of freshly ground pepper

1 tablespoon extra virgin olive oil

2 tablespoons freshly grated aged Asiago cheese or Parmigiano-Reggiano

2 teaspoons chopped fresh Italian parsley

1 In a saucepan fitted with a steamer basket, bring 1 inch of water to a boil over medium-high heat. Add the asparagus, reduce the heat to low, cover, and steam until tender, 4 to 5 minutes.

2 Meanwhile, whisk together the vinegar, garlic, salt, and pepper in a small bowl. Slowly whisk in the oil. Stir in the Asiago and parsley.

3 Arrange the asparagus on a serving platter and drizzle with the vinaigrette. Serve hot, warm, or at room temperature.

Each serving: 3 g carb, 57 cal, 4 g fat, 1 g sat fat, 2 mg chol, 1 g fib, 2 g pro, 101 mg sod • Carb Choices: 0; Exchanges: 1 veg, 1 fat

Asparagus with Sautéed Shiitake Mushrooms QUICK

makes 4 servings

This is an attractive and easy dish to serve at any springtime celebration. The bright green spears peeking out from under the lightly sautéed mushrooms make an inviting dish that can accompany almost any entrée. And it tastes as good hot as it does at room temperature, making it a perfect side dish for a buffet. The recipe can be easily doubled.

1 pound asparagus, tough ends removed

2 teaspoons extra virgin olive oil

6 ounces shiitake mushrooms, stemmed and thinly sliced

1 small shallot, finely chopped

¼ teaspoon kosher salt

2 teaspoons chopped fresh Italian parsley

1 In a saucepan fitted with a steamer basket, bring 1 inch of water to a boil over medium-high heat. Add the asparagus, reduce the heat to low, cover, and steam until tender, 4 to 5 minutes.

2 Meanwhile, heat a medium nonstick skillet over medium-high heat. Add the oil and tilt the pan to coat the bottom evenly. Add the mushrooms, shallots, and salt. Cook, stirring often, until the mushrooms are barely tender, 3 minutes. Remove from the heat and stir in the parsley.

3 To serve, arrange the asparagus on a serving platter and spoon the mushrooms over them. Serve hot, warm, or at room temperature.

Each serving: 7 g carb, 56 cal, 3 g fat, 0 g sat fat, 0 mg chol, 2 g fib, 2 g pro, 73 mg sod • Carb Choices: ½; Exchanges: 1 veg, ½ fat

Beets

Foil-Roasted Beets

makes 4 servings

Roasted beets have a more concentrated sweet and earthy flavor than boiled beets. Boiled beets are quicker to make and easier to peel, but both are delicious and exceedingly better than anything in a can. Use roasted or boiled beets interchangeably in any recipe calling for cooked beets. When you're baking something else, bake some beets at the same time. Add or subtract 10 to 15 minutes to the baking time, depending on the temperature you are using to bake other foods.

1 pound beets, well scrubbed (about 3 medium)

1 Preheat the oven to 400°F. Wrap the beets in a sheet of aluminum foil, place them in a roasting pan, and bake until tender when pierced with a knife, 1 hour 15 minutes to 1 hour 30 minutes.

2 Let the beets rest until cool enough to handle and peel.

Each serving: 7 g carb, 33 cal, 0 g fat, 0 g sat fat, 0 mg chol, 2 g fib, 1 g pro, 59 mg sod • Carb Choices: ½; Exchanges: 1 vegetable

Basic Boiled Beets

makes 4 servings

As a child, I always thought it was magical the way the skins of boiled beets slid right off using just your hands. I guess that's why I always got that job—there was no danger of sharp knives harming my small hands. (Your kids may like this job, too.) You'll find boiled beets are a little less sweet than roasted beets because the sugars do not concentrate as much as they do when roasted.

1 pound beets, well scrubbed (about 3 medium)

1 Place the beets in a large saucepan and add water to cover. Bring to a boil over high heat.

Reduce the heat to low, cover, and simmer until the beets are tender when pierced with a knife, about 1 hour.

2 Drain the beets in a colander. Cool slightly and use your hands to slip the skins off under cold running water.

Each serving: 7 g carb, 33 cal, 0 g fat, 0 g sat fat, 0 mg chol, 2 g fib, 1 g pro, 59 mg sod • Carb Choices: ½; Exchanges: 1 vegetable

Beets with Sautéed Beet Greens

makes 6 servings

When you find beets in the market with their green tops attached, try this recipe. It's a perfect balance of sweet, bitter, and sour.

1½ pounds beets with green tops attached
2 teaspoons extra virgin olive oil
½ small onion, thinly sliced
1 garlic clove, minced
½ cup Vegetable Stock (page 149) or low-sodium vegetable broth
¼ teaspoon kosher salt
½ teaspoon red wine vinegar

1 Thinly slice the tops of the beets and set aside. Prepare the beets using either the recipe for Foil-Roasted Beets (at left) or Basic Boiled Beets (at left). Cut the beets into bite-size pieces.

2 Heat a large nonstick skillet over medium heat. Add the oil and tilt the pan to coat the bottom evenly. Add the onion and cook, stirring often, until softened, 5 minutes. Add the garlic and cook, stirring constantly, 30 seconds. Add the stock and the beet greens and cook, stirring often, until the greens are tender, 5 minutes.

3 Add the beets and salt and cook, stirring often, until heated through, about 3 minutes. Remove from the heat and stir in the vinegar. Spoon the beets into a serving dish and serve at once.

Each serving: 7 g carb, 47 cal, 2 g fat, 0 g sat fat, 0 mg chol, 2 g fib, 2 g pro, 158 mg sod • Carb Choices: ½; Exchanges: 1 veg, ½ fat

Pomegranate-Glazed Beets

makes 4 servings

A touch of brown sugar rounds out the tart flavor of the pomegranate juice in this recipe. The rich red color of this dish makes a beautiful presentation for a Thanksgiving buffet. You can cook the beets a day ahead and glaze them just before serving. Garnish them with strips of orange zest for a more festive presentation.

1 recipe Foil-Roasted Beets (page 447) or Basic Boiled Beets (page 447)
2 teaspoons extra virgin olive oil
¼ teaspoon kosher salt
1 cup pomegranate juice
6 whole cloves
1 (3-inch) cinnamon stick
1 packed teaspoon light brown sugar

1 Cut the beets into bite-size pieces.

2 Heat a large nonstick skillet over medium-high heat. Add the oil and tilt the pan to coat the bottom evenly. Add the beets and salt and cook, stirring occasionally, until the beets are lightly browned, 6 minutes.

3 Add the pomegranate juice, cloves, cinnamon, and sugar and bring to a boil over high heat. Reduce the heat to medium and cook, uncovered, stirring occasionally, until the liquid is almost evaporated, about 10 minutes. Remove and discard the cloves and cinnamon. Spoon the beets into a serving dish and serve at once.

Each serving: 17 g carb, 93 cal, 3 g fat, 0 g sat fat, 0 mg chol, 2 g fib, 1 g pro, 137 mg sod • Carb Choices: 1; Exchanges: ½ fruit, 1 veg, ½ fat

Roasted Beets with Apple-Walnut Dressing

makes 4 servings

Simmering apple cider concentrates its sweetness and flavor to make this distinctive dressing. You can serve the dressing over room-temperature beets and skip the reheating in step 4 if you wish.

½ cup apple cider
1 teaspoon apple cider vinegar
½ teaspoon kosher salt, divided
Pinch of freshly ground pepper
1 tablespoon walnut oil or extra virgin olive oil
1 recipe Foil-Roasted Beets (page 447) or Basic Boiled Beets (page 447)
2 teaspoons extra virgin olive oil
2 tablespoons walnuts, toasted and chopped (page 4)

1 To make the dressing, place the cider in a small skillet and bring to a boil over high heat. Reduce the heat to low and simmer, uncovered, until the cider is thickened and reduced to about 2 tablespoons, 6 minutes. Transfer to a medium bowl and allow to cool.

2 Whisk in the vinegar, ¼ teaspoon of the salt, and the pepper. Slowly whisk in the walnut oil.

3 Cut the beets into bite-size pieces.

4 Heat a large nonstick skillet over medium-high heat. Add the olive oil and tilt the pan to coat the bottom evenly. Add the beets and remaining ¼ teaspoon salt and cook, stirring occasionally, until the beets are lightly browned, 6 minutes. Add the beets to the dressing and toss gently to coat.

5 To serve, spoon the beets onto a serving platter and sprinkle with the walnuts. Serve hot or warm.

Each serving: 11 g carb, 119 cal, 8 g fat, 1 g sat fat, 0 mg chol, 2 g fib, 2 g pro, 133 mg sod • Carb Choices: 1; Exchanges: ½ carb, 1 veg, 1½ fat

Roasted Beets with Gragefruit and Mint HIGH FIBER

makes 6 servings

Here's another way—and I think the most delicious—to make beets. If you use this method, you either have to wear gloves or not mind having pink hands for a while. The beets are peeled while raw, cut into chunks, and then roasted.

3 pounds beets, peeled and cut into ½-inch pieces
2 teaspoons plus 1 tablespoon extra virgin olive oil, divided
½ teaspoon kosher salt, divided
1 large pink grapefruit
2 teaspoons chopped fresh mint
¼ teaspoon honey
⅛ teaspoon freshly ground pepper

1 Preheat the oven to 425°F.

2 Place the beets in a large roasting pan. Drizzle with 2 teaspoons of the oil, sprinkle with ¼ teaspoon of the salt, toss to coat evenly, and spread in an even layer. Bake, stirring occasionally, until the beets are browned and tender, 1 hour.

3 Meanwhile, cut a thin slice from the top and bottom of the grapefruit, exposing the flesh. Stand the grapefruit upright, and using a sharp knife, thickly cut off the peel, following the contour of the fruit and removing all the white pith and membrane. Holding the grapefruit over a bowl, carefully cut along both sides of each section to free it from the membrane. Discard any seeds and let the sections fall into the bowl. Break the sections into small bits using two forks. Stir in the remaining 1 tablespoon olive oil, remaining ¼ teaspoon salt, the mint, honey, and pepper.

4 Arrange the beets on a serving platter and spoon the grapefruit mixture over them. Serve hot, warm, or at room temperature.

Each serving: 19 g carb, 119 cal, 4 g fat, 1 g sat fat, 0 mg chol, 5 g fib, 3 g pro, 212 mg sod • Carb Choices: 1; Exchanges: 2 veg, 1 fat

Broccoli and Broccoli Rabe

Two-Minute Microwave Broccoli with Lemon Butter QUICK

makes 2 servings

This is my side dish (or sometimes my dinner with leftover pasta or rice) when I'm absolutely too tired to make anything else. With a recipe this easy, there's no reason not to eat your vegetables. Resist the urge to add water to the broccoli when cooking it—it's absolutely not necessary. Two minutes is the time for crisp-tender broccoli; cook yours longer depending on your preference.

2 cups broccoli florets, cut into bite-size pieces
2 teaspoons lemon juice
1 teaspoon unsalted butter
¼ teaspoon kosher salt

1 Place the broccoli in a microwave-safe bowl and cover with plastic wrap. Microwave on high for 2 minutes.

2 Meanwhile, place the lemon juice, butter, and salt in a medium bowl.

3 Carefully uncover the broccoli and drain in a colander. Return to the bowl; add the lemon juice, butter, and salt; and toss gently to coat. Serve at once.

Each serving: 3 g carb, 24 cal, 1 g fat, 1 g sat fat, 3 mg chol, 2 g fib, 2 g pro, 85 mg sod • Carb Choices: 0; Exchanges: 1 vegetable

Roasted Broccoli with Balsamic-Dijon Vinaigrette

QUICK

makes 4 servings

Roasting transforms broccoli, browning the outer buds and caramelizing the natural sugars. You can serve this plain and skip the vinaigrette if you prefer.

5 cups broccoli florets, cut into bite-size pieces
1 teaspoon plus 1 tablespoon extra virgin olive oil, divided
2 teaspoons balsamic vinegar
½ teaspoon Dijon mustard
¼ teaspoon kosher salt
Pinch of freshly ground pepper

1 Preheat the oven to 425°F.

2 Place the broccoli in a medium roasting pan. Drizzle with 1 teaspoon of the oil and toss to coat. Bake, stirring once, until the broccoli is lightly browned and tender, about 15 minutes.

3 Meanwhile, whisk together the vinegar, mustard, salt, and pepper in a medium bowl. Slowly whisk in the remaining 1 tablespoon oil. Add the broccoli to the bowl and toss to coat. Serve at once.

Each serving: 5 g carb, 66 cal, 5 g fat, 1 g sat fat, 0 mg chol, 3 g fib, 3 g pro, 110 mg sod • Carb Choices: 0; Exchanges: 1 veg, 1 fat

Stir-Fried Broccoli with Ginger Sauce QUICK

makes 4 servings

Adding just a touch of cornstarch to the sauce ensures that the delicious gingery flavor clings to each piece of the broccoli. This is another side dish that can easily become dinner for two when paired with cooked rice.

2 tablespoons Chicken Stock (page 149) or low-sodium chicken broth
1 teaspoon reduced-sodium soy sauce

1 teaspoon hoisin sauce
¼ teaspoon cornstarch
2 teaspoons canola oil
2 teaspoons minced fresh ginger
1 garlic clove, minced
3 cups broccoli florets, cut into bite-size pieces

1 Stir together the stock, soy sauce, hoisin sauce, and cornstarch in a small bowl and set aside.

2 Heat a large nonstick skillet over medium-high heat. Add the oil and tilt the pan to coat the bottom evenly. Add the ginger and garlic and cook, stirring constantly, until fragrant, 30 seconds.

3 Add the broccoli and cook, stirring constantly, until the broccoli is crisp-tender, 3 minutes. Stir the stock mixture and add to the skillet. Cook, stirring constantly, until the sauce comes to a boil and thickens slightly, 1 minute. Spoon the broccoli and sauce into a serving dish and serve at once.

Each serving: 4 g carb, 43 cal, 3 g fat, 0 g sat fat, 0 mg chol, 2 g fib, 2 g pro, 91 mg sod • Carb Choices: 0; Exchanges: 1 veg, ½ fat

Sesame Broccoli QUICK

makes 4 servings

Flavorful, pretty, and straightforward—this is a great way to dress up plain broccoli to accompany any Asian-inspired entrée.

2 teaspoons reduced-sodium soy sauce
1 teaspoon fresh lime juice
¼ teaspoon Asian sesame oil
2 teaspoons canola oil
1 garlic clove, minced
1 teaspoon sesame seeds
3 cups broccoli florets, cut into bite-size pieces

1 Combine the soy sauce, lime juice, and sesame oil in a medium serving bowl and set aside.

2 Heat a large nonstick skillet over medium-high heat. Add the canola oil and tilt the pan to coat the bottom evenly. Add the garlic and sesame seeds and cook, stirring constantly, until fragrant, 30 seconds.

3 Add the broccoli and cook, stirring constantly, until the broccoli is crisp-tender, about 3 minutes. Add the broccoli mixture to the soy sauce mixture and toss to coat. Serve at once.

Each serving: 4 g carb, 45 cal, 3 g fat, 0 g sat fat, 0 mg chol, 2 g fib, 2 g pro, 115 mg sod • Carb Choices: 0; Exchanges: 1 veg, ½ fat

Broccoli and Sweet Onion Puree

makes 4 servings

Cooking the vegetables in chicken stock gives this dish an unexpected richness. Serve it with anything you'd serve mashed potatoes with: roast chicken, meatloaf, fish fillets, or steak.

12 ounces broccoli

2 teaspoons extra virgin olive oil

1 cup chopped sweet onion

1 garlic clove, chopped

1 cup Chicken Stock (page 149) or low-sodium chicken broth

1 medium baking potato, peeled and chopped (about 1 cup)

½ teaspoon kosher salt

½ teaspoon lemon juice

Pinch of freshly ground pepper

1 Cut the florets from the broccoli and peel and chop the stems, keeping the florets and stems separate. Set aside.

2 Heat a medium saucepan over medium heat. Add the oil and tilt the pan to coat the bottom evenly. Add the onion and cook, stirring often, until softened, 5 minutes. Stir in the garlic and cook, stirring constantly, until fragrant, 30 seconds.

3 Add the stock, potato, and salt and bring to a boil over high heat. Reduce the heat to low, cover, and simmer 15 minutes. Add the broccoli stems to the potato mixture and cook 5 minutes longer. Add the broccoli florets and cook until the vegetables are tender, 5 minutes. Drain the vegetables, reserving the cooking liquid.

4 Transfer the vegetables to a food processor. Add the lemon juice and pepper and process until smooth, adding the reserved cooking liquid a few teaspoons at a time, if needed, to reach a smooth consistency. Spoon into a serving bowl and serve at once.

Each serving: 15 g carb, 94 cal, 3 g fat, 1 g sat fat, 1 mg chol, 3 g fib, 4 g pro, 198 mg sod • Carb Choices: 1; Exchanges: ½ starch, 1 veg, ½ fat

Stewed Broccoli Rabe with Ancho and Manchego QUICK | HIGH FIBER

makes 2 servings

Ancho chile and grated Manchego cheese elevate lowly broccoli rabe into a stunning side dish. With a kick from the chile and richness from the cheese, it's a complex side to pair with a simple entrée, such as roast pork or chicken.

2 teaspoons extra virgin olive oil

4 garlic cloves, thinly sliced

1 pound broccoli rabe, tough stems removed, leaves and florets chopped

½ cup Chicken Stock (page 149) or low-sodium chicken broth

1 small dried ancho chile, seeded and chopped, or ⅛ teaspoon crushed red pepper

¼ teaspoon kosher salt

2 tablespoons freshly grated aged manchego or Parmesan

1 Heat a large saucepan over medium heat. Add the oil and tilt the pan to coat the bottom evenly. Add the garlic and cook, stirring constantly, until lightly browned, about 3 minutes.

2 Add the broccoli rabe, stock, chile, and salt and bring to a boil. Reduce the heat to low, partially cover, and cook, stirring occasionally, until the broccoli rabe is tender and most of the liquid is evaporated, 10 minutes. Spoon the broccoli rabe into a serving bowl and sprinkle with the manchego. Serve at once.

Each serving: 10 g carb, 129 cal, 8 g fat, 2 g sat fat, 6 mg chol, 5 g fib, 8 g pro, 296 mg sod • Carb Choices: ½; Exchanges: 2 veg, 1½ fat

Broccoli Rabe with Garlic and Sun-Dried Tomatoes

QUICK | HIGH FIBER

makes 2 servings

This is one of my favorite "emergency" dinners and I vary it in numerous ways, depending on my mood and what's on hand. No broth? Use water instead. No sun-dried tomatoes? Use fresh cherry tomatoes or coarsely chopped plum tomatoes. No Parmesan? Use provolone, Asiago, or fontina. It's almost impossible to make this dish less than delicious.

1 pound broccoli rabe, tough stems removed, leaves and florets chopped

2 teaspoons extra virgin olive oil

4 garlic cloves, thinly sliced

¼ cup Chicken Stock (page 149) or low-sodium chicken broth

4 dry-packed sun-dried tomatoes, thinly sliced

½ teaspoon kosher salt

⅛ teaspoon crushed red pepper

2 tablespoons freshly grated Parmesan

1 Bring a large pot of water to a boil over high heat. Add the broccoli rabe and cook until barely tender, 5 minutes. Drain in a colander.

2 Meanwhile, heat a large nonstick skillet over medium heat. Add the oil and tilt the pan to coat the bottom evenly. Add the garlic and cook, stirring often, until lightly browned, 3 minutes. Add the broccoli rabe, stock, tomatoes, salt, and crushed red pepper. Cook, stirring occasionally, until the broccoli rabe is very tender and the liquid evaporates, about 5 minutes. Spoon the broccoli rabe into a serving bowl and sprinkle with the Parmesan.

Each serving: 8 g carb, 113 cal, 7 g fat, 2 g sat fat, 5 mg chol, 4 g fib, 7 g pro, 358 mg sod • Carb Choices: ½; Exchanges: 1 veg, 1½ fat

Roasted Broccoli Rabe with Lemon and Olives QUICK

makes 2 servings

Roasted broccoli rabe loses all its bright green color, but the fabulous flavor more than makes up for its less than stellar looks. This is wonderful as a side dish or with pasta as an entrée for two. You can even turn it into bruschetta: spoon it on top of toasted baguette slices, top with grated Parmesan, and broil until the cheese melts.

1 pound broccoli rabe, tough stems removed

2 teaspoons extra virgin olive oil

4 Kalamata olives, pitted and chopped

½ teaspoon grated lemon zest

½ teaspoon lemon juice

¼ teaspoon kosher salt

⅛ teaspoon crushed red pepper

1 Preheat the oven to 400°F.

2 Place the broccoli rabe in a large roasting pan. Drizzle with the oil and toss to coat. Bake, stirring once, until the broccoli rabe is lightly browned and tender, 18 to 20 minutes. When stirring, move the broccoli rabe to the center of the pan to prevent over-browning of the thin tender leaves.

3 Place the olives, lemon zest, lemon juice, salt, and crushed red pepper in a medium serving bowl. Add the broccoli rabe and toss gently to coat. Serve at once.

Each serving: 4 g carb, 90 cal, 7 g fat, 1 g sat fat, 0 mg chol, 3 g fib, 4 g pro, 302 mg sod • Carb Choices: 0; Exchanges: 1 veg, 1½ fat

Brussels Sprouts

Brussels Sprouts with Apple Cider Glaze QUICK

makes 6 servings

Sweet apple cider is a good partner for Brussels sprouts, taming their bitterness. Don't overcook them—the 3-minute cooking time here leaves them a little crunchy, but don't cook them too much longer or they begin to give off their characteristic cabbagey odor and turn olive green.

1 pound Brussels sprouts, trimmed and halved lengthwise, if large
2 teaspoons extra virgin olive oil
1 small red onion, halved and thinly sliced
1 garlic clove, minced
⅓ cup apple cider
2 teaspoons apple cider vinegar
½ teaspoon kosher salt
Pinch of freshly ground pepper

1 Bring a medium saucepan half full of water to a boil over high heat. Add the Brussels sprouts and cook until crisp-tender, about 3 minutes. Drain in a colander.

2 Meanwhile, heat a large nonstick skillet over medium heat. Add the oil and tilt the pan to coat the bottom evenly. Add the onion, and cook, stirring often, until softened, 5 minutes. Stir in the garlic and cook, stirring constantly, until fragrant, 30 seconds. Add the cider and vinegar. Increase the heat to medium-high and bring to a boil. Cook until the liquid is almost evaporated, 2 to 3 minutes. Add the Brussels sprouts, salt, and pepper and stir to coat. Spoon the Brussels sprouts into a serving bowl and serve at once.

Each serving: 9 g carb, 55 cal, 2 g fat, 2 g sat fat, 0 mg chol, 3 g fib, 2 g pro, 112 mg sod • Carb Choices: ½; Exchanges: 1 vegetable

Roasted Brussels Sprouts with Toasted Walnuts

HIGH FIBER

makes 4 servings

Cutting the sprouts in half allows for more surface area to brown and create the caramelized crust that makes these taste so wonderful.

1 pound Brussels sprouts, trimmed and halved
2 teaspoons extra virgin olive oil
½ teaspoon kosher salt
⅛ teaspoon freshly ground pepper
2 tablespoons walnuts, toasted and chopped (page 4)
½ teaspoon grated lemon zest
2 teaspoons lemon juice

1 Preheat the oven to 425°F.

2 Place the Brussels sprouts in a large roasting pan. Drizzle with the oil and sprinkle with the salt and pepper. Toss to coat. Arrange the Brussels sprouts in a single layer.

3 Roast, stirring once, until the Brussels sprouts are tender and lightly browned, 35 to 40 minutes.

4 Place the Brussels sprouts in a serving bowl. Add the walnuts, lemon zest, and lemon juice and toss to coat. Serve at once.

Each serving: 10 g carb, 86 cal, 5 g fat, 1 g sat fat, 0 mg chol, 4 g fib, 4 g pro, 166 mg sod • Carb Choices: ½; Exchanges: 2 veg, 1 fat

ROASTED BRUSSELS SPROUTS AND SHALLOTS HIGH FIBER: Follow the Roasted Brussels Sprouts with Toasted Walnuts recipe, above, but add 4 large shallots, quartered, to the Brussels sprouts in step 1. Omit the walnuts.

Each serving: 14 g carb, 84 cal, 3 g fat, 0 g sat fat, 0mg chol, 4 g fib, 4 g pro, 166 mg sod • Carb Choices: 1; Exchanges: 2 veg, ½ fat

Shaved Brussels Sprouts with Garlic and Lemon QUICK

makes 6 servings

Make this recipe only if you can slice the Brussels sprouts in a food processor; otherwise, it's too much work. You can shred them on a box grater, but it takes a long time, especially if your sprouts are small.

1 pound Brussels sprouts, trimmed
1 tablespoon extra virgin olive oil
1 garlic clove, minced
¾ teaspoon kosher salt
Pinch of freshly ground pepper
½ teaspoon grated lemon zest
1 teaspoon lemon juice

1 Working with a few at a time, feed the Brussels sprouts through the feed tube of a food processor fitted with a thin slicing disc.

2 Heat a large nonstick skillet over medium heat. Add the oil and tilt the pan to coat the bottom evenly. Add the garlic and cook, stirring constantly, until lightly browned, about 1 minute. Add the Brussels sprouts, salt, and pepper and cook, stirring often, until lightly browned and crisp-tender, 6 to 8 minutes.

3 Spoon the Brussels sprouts into a serving bowl. Sprinkle with the lemon zest and lemon juice and toss to combine. Serve at once.

Each serving: 6 g carb, 51 cal, 3 g fat, 0 g sat fat, 0 mg chol, 3 g fib, 2 g pro, 157 mg sod • Carb Choices: ½; Exchanges: 1 veg, ½ fat

Brussels Sprouts with Caraway QUICK

makes 6 servings

Delicately anise-flavored caraway seeds in these Brussels sprouts will remind you of German or Hungarian dishes. Continue the theme and pair them with grilled chicken sausages or roast pork tenderloin.

1 tablespoon extra virgin olive oil
1 small onion, halved and thinly sliced
½ teaspoon caraway seeds
1 pound Brussels sprouts, trimmed and quartered
½ cup Chicken Stock (page 149) or low-sodium chicken broth
½ teaspoon kosher salt
⅛ teaspoon freshly ground pepper

1 Heat a large nonstick skillet over medium heat. Add the oil and tilt the pan to coat the bottom evenly. Add the onion and caraway seeds and cook, stirring occasionally, until the onion is tender, 5 minutes.

2 Add the Brussels sprouts, stock, salt, and pepper. Cover and cook, stirring often, until the Brussels sprouts are crisp-tender, about 5 minutes. If excess liquid remains in the pan, uncover and cook until most of the liquid evaporates. Spoon the Brussels sprouts into a serving bowl and serve at once.

Each serving: 7 g carb, 50 cal, 2 g fat, 0 g sat fat, 0 mg chol, 3 g fib, 3 g pro, 122 mg sod • Carb Choices: 1; Exchanges: 1 vegetable

Carrots

Carrot and Orange Puree

makes 4 servings

Vibrant and flavorful, this puree is just as good as a kid-pleasing side dish as it is for the fanciest holiday dinner. Add a pinch of cloves, ginger, cinnamon, or nutmeg to the puree if you wish.

1 pound carrots, peeled and sliced
1 cup orange juice
2 garlic cloves, sliced
1 small navel orange
2 teaspoons unsalted butter
Pinch of kosher salt

1 Combine the carrots, orange juice, and garlic in a medium saucepan. Bring to a boil over high heat. Reduce the heat to medium, cover, and cook until the carrots are very tender, 20 to 25 minutes. Drain the carrots in a colander, reserving the cooking liquid.

2 Meanwhile, remove ½ teaspoon of zest from the orange and reserve. Cut a thin slice from the top and bottom of the orange, exposing the flesh. Stand the orange upright, and using a sharp knife, thickly cut off the peel, following the contour of the fruit and removing all the white pith and membrane. Holding the orange over a bowl, carefully cut along both sides of each section to free it from the membrane. Discard any seeds and let the sections fall into the bowl.

3 Place the carrot mixture, the orange segments, orange zest, butter, and salt in a food processor. Process until smooth, adding the reserved cooking liquid a few teaspoons at a time, if needed, to reach a smooth consistency. Spoon the carrots into a serving bowl and serve hot or warm.

Each serving: 19 g carb, 96 cal, 2 g fat, 1 g sat fat, 5 mg chol, 3 g fib, 2 g pro, 88 mg sod • Carb Choices: 1; Exchanges: ½ fruit, 2 veg, ½ fat

Carrot Puree with Maple and Cardamom

makes 4 servings

This dish is a perfect example of where a little bit of sweetener (maple syrup) and a tiny amount of butter goes a long way in taking an ordinary vegetable to a new level of flavor.

2 teaspoons extra virgin olive oil
1 small onion, chopped
2 garlic cloves, chopped
1 pound carrots, peeled and sliced
½ to ⅔ cup orange juice
¼ teaspoon kosher salt
1 tablespoon real maple syrup
2 teaspoons unsalted butter
¼ teaspoon ground cardamom

1 Heat a medium saucepan over medium heat. Add the oil and tilt the pan to coat the bottom evenly. Add the onion and cook, stirring often, until softened, 5 minutes. Add the garlic and cook, stirring constantly, until fragrant, 30 seconds. Add the carrots, ½ cup of the orange juice, and the salt and bring to a boil. Reduce the heat to medium, cover, and cook until the carrots are very tender, 15 to 20 minutes.

2 Place the carrot mixture, the maple syrup, butter, and cardamom in a food processor and process until smooth, adding the remaining orange juice a few teaspoons at a time, if needed, to reach a smooth consistency. Spoon the carrots into a serving bowl and serve hot or warm.

Each serving: 17 g carb, 110 cal, 5 g fat, 2 g sat fat, 5 mg chol, 3 g fib, 1 g pro, 141 mg sod • Carb Choices: 1; Exchanges: ½ carb, 2 veg, 1 fat

Mango and Ginger–Glazed Carrots QUICK

makes 4 servings

You can use orange or apple juice instead of mango nectar, in this kid-friendly dish.

2 teaspoons canola oil
2 teaspoons minced fresh ginger
1 pound baby carrots
½ cup mango nectar
½ teaspoon kosher salt

1 Heat a medium skillet over medium heat. Add the oil and tilt the pan to coat the bottom evenly. Add the ginger and cook, stirring constantly, until fragrant, 30 seconds. Add the carrots, mango nectar, and salt and bring to a boil.

2 Reduce the heat to medium-low, cover, and simmer until the carrots are almost tender, about 8 minutes. Uncover and cook until the carrots are tender and the mango nectar is thickened to a light glaze consistency, 2 minutes. Spoon the carrots into a serving bowl and serve at once.

Each serving: 14 g carb, 77 cal, 3 g fat, 0 g sat fat, 0 mg chol, 3 g fib, 1 g pro, 230 mg sod • Carb Choices: 1; 2 veg, ½ fat

Roasted Carrots with Coriander and Cilantro

makes 4 servings

Coriander seeds produce the cilantro plant and both seed and leaf pair well with sweet roasted carrots. They make a colorful and easy-to-prepare side dish for almost any entrée.

1 pound baby carrots or 1 pound regular carrots, peeled and cut into ½-inch-thick sticks
2 teaspoons extra virgin olive oil
½ teaspoon ground coriander
½ teaspoon kosher salt
2 tablespoons chopped fresh cilantro

1 Preheat the oven to 425°F.

2 Place the carrots in a large roasting pan. Add the oil, coriander, and salt, and toss to coat. Arrange the carrots in a single layer.

3 Roast, stirring once, until the carrots are tender and lightly browned, 30 to 35 minutes.

4 Arrange the carrots on a serving platter and sprinkle with the cilantro. Serve hot or warm.

Each serving: 9 g carb, 61 cal, 3 g fat, 0 g sat fat, 0 mg chol, 3 g fib, 1 g pro, 229 mg sod • Carb Choices: ½; Exchanges: 2 veg, ½ fat

Carrots with Moroccan Spices QUICK

makes 4 servings

1 pound baby carrots or 1 pound regular carrots, peeled and cut into ½-inch-thick sticks
2 teaspoons extra virgin olive oil
1 garlic clove, minced
¼ teaspoon ground cumin
½ teaspoon kosher salt
⅛ teaspoon paprika
⅛ teaspoon ground cinnamon
1 tablespoon chopped fresh Italian parsley

1 Place the carrots in a medium saucepan and add water to cover. Bring to a boil over high heat. Reduce the heat to medium, cover, and cook until the carrots are tender, 10 to 12 minutes. Drain the carrots in a colander.

2 Heat a large nonstick skillet over medium heat. Add the oil and tilt the pan to coat the bottom evenly. Add the garlic, cumin, salt, paprika, and cinnamon and cook, stirring constantly, until the mixture is fragrant, 1 minute.

3 Add the carrots and stir to coat. Spoon the carrots into a serving bowl and sprinkle with the parsley. Serve at once.

Each serving: 10 g carb, 62 cal, 3 g fat, 0 g sat fat, 0 mg chol, 3 g fib, 1 g pro, 229 mg sod • Carb Choices: ½; Exchanges: 2 veg, ½ fat

Cauliflower

Cauliflower Mash QUICK

makes 4 servings

Even if you don't like cauliflower, you'll love this recipe. Keep quiet when you serve this dish, and your family will probably tell you how delicious the mashed potatoes are.

1 pound cauliflower, cut into 1-inch florets (about 4 cups)
1 cup Chicken Stock (page 149) or low-sodium chicken broth
¼ teaspoon kosher salt
3 to 5 tablespoons 1% low-fat milk
Pinch of freshly ground pepper
1 teaspoon unsalted butter

1 Place the cauliflower, stock, and salt in a medium saucepan and add water to cover. Bring to a boil over high heat. Reduce the heat to medium, cover, and cook until the cauliflower is tender, 10 to 12 minutes. Drain the cauliflower in a colander.

2 Place the cauliflower in a food processor. Add 3 tablespoons of the milk and the pepper and process until smooth, adding the remaining 2 tablespoons milk, if needed, to reach a smooth consistency. Transfer to a serving bowl and stir in the butter. Serve at once.

Each serving: 6 g carb, 44 cal, 1 g fat, 1 g sat fat, 4 mg chol, 3 g fib, 3 g pro, 140 mg sod • Carb Choices: ½; Exchanges: 1 vegetable

Spicy Roasted Cauliflower with Lime

makes 4 servings

Cumin, coriander, and lime take cauliflower in an Indian-inspired direction in this dish. You can roast the cauliflower plain, too. Drizzle the florets with oil, sprinkle with salt and pepper, and roast for a simple side dish.

½ teaspoon ground coriander
½ teaspoon ground cumin
⅛ to ¼ teaspoon ground cayenne
½ teaspoon kosher salt
1 pound cauliflower, cut into 2-inch florets
2 teaspoons extra virgin olive oil
2 teaspoons lime juice

1 Preheat the oven to 425°F.

2 Stir together the coriander, cumin, cayenne, and salt in a small dish. Place the cauliflower in a large roasting pan. Drizzle with the oil, sprinkle with the spice mixture, and toss to coat. Arrange the cauliflower in a single layer.

3 Roast, stirring once, until the cauliflower is tender and well browned, 20 to 25 minutes.

4 Spoon the cauliflower into a serving bowl, drizzle with the lime juice, and toss to coat. Serve at once.

Each serving: 6 g carb, 47 cal, 2 g fat, 0 g sat fat, 0 mg chol, 3 g fib, 2 g pro, 170 mg sod • Carb Choices: ½; Exchanges: 1 veg, ½ fat

Baked Cauliflower with Parmesan HIGH FIBER

makes 4 servings

Baking vegetables topped with cheese is one of my favorite—and one of the simplest—ways to make a delicious side dish. Here, the cauliflower gets a salty sprinkle of capers and a fresh finishing touch of Italian parsley.

1 pound cauliflower, cut into 1-inch florets
1 tablespoon capers, rinsed and drained
2 teaspoons extra virgin olive oil
¼ teaspoon kosher salt
⅛ teaspoon freshly ground pepper
1 ounce freshly grated Parmesan (about ¼ cup)
1 tablespoon chopped fresh Italian parsley

1 Preheat the oven to 400°F.

2 In a saucepan fitted with a steamer basket, bring 1 inch of water to a boil over high heat. Add the cauliflower, reduce the heat to low, cover, and steam until tender, 6 to 8 minutes.

3 Place the cauliflower in a shallow 2-quart baking dish. Add the capers, oil, salt, and pepper and toss to coat. Arrange the cauliflower evenly in the dish and sprinkle with the Parmesan.

4 Bake, uncovered, until the cheese is melted, 15 to 20 minutes. Sprinkle with the parsley and serve hot or warm.

Each serving: 6 g carb, 68 cal, 4 g fat, 1 g sat fat, 4 mg chol, 4 g fib, 4 g pro, 240 mg sod • Carb Choices: ½; Exchanges: 1 veg, 1 fat

Corn

Microwave Corn-on-the-Cob QUICK

makes 2 servings

This is a technique I discovered after coming home from the farmers' market with the first corn of the season. I couldn't wait for water to boil to enjoy the first sweet crunchy ears, so I tried the microwave. This works perfectly for 2 ears of corn—add more and the kernels cook unevenly. Removing the husks under cold running water cools the corn enough to handle, but not so much that the butter won't melt—and you can eat it immediately.

2 ears corn with husks
1 teaspoon butter
⅛ teaspoon salt

1 Place the corn with the husks intact in the microwave and cook on high 5 minutes.

2 Carefully remove from the microwave using tongs or an oven mitt, place under cold running water, and remove the husks. The corn will cool, but just enough to be ready to eat immediately.

3 Rub each ear with ½ teaspoon of the butter and sprinkle evenly with the salt. Serve at once.

Each serving: 17 g carb, 94 cal, 3 g fat, 1 g sat fat, 5 mg chol, 2 g fib, 3 g pro, 159 mg sod • Carb Choices: 1; Exchanges: 1 starch, ½ fat

Corn with Basil and Lemon [QUICK]

makes 4 servings

The trio of corn, basil, and lemon makes this dish a perfect partner for fish fillets, shrimp, or scallops.

2 large ears corn, kernels cut from the cob
¼ cup water
1 tablespoon chopped fresh basil
1 teaspoon unsalted butter
1 teaspoon grated lemon zest
1 teaspoon lemon juice
¼ teaspoon kosher salt

1 Combine the corn and water in a medium skillet. Cook over medium-high heat, stirring often, until the corn is crisp-tender and most of the liquid has evaporated, about 5 minutes.

2 Remove from the heat and stir in the basil, butter, lemon zest, lemon juice, and salt. Spoon the corn into a serving bowl and serve at once.

Each serving: 14 g carb, 70 cal, 2 g fat, 1 g sat fat, 3 mg chol, 2 g fib, 2 g pro, 81 mg sod • Carb Choices: 1; Exchanges: 1 starch

Corn with Roasted Jalapeño and Lime

makes 4 servings

You can roast the jalapeño on the stovetop if you have a gas range. Leave the pepper whole and place it directly on the flame. Turn it often, using long-handled tongs, until the skin is blistered.

1 jalapeño, cut in half lengthwise and seeded
2 large ears corn, kernels cut from the cob
¼ cup water
1 teaspoon unsalted butter
½ teaspoon grated lime zest
1 teaspoon lime juice
¼ teaspoon kosher salt

1 Preheat the broiler.

2 Cover a broiler pan with foil and place the jalapeño on the pan. Broil, turning occasionally, until the skin blisters and it is charred all over, about 10 minutes. Put the pepper in a small bowl, cover, and let stand until cool enough to handle. Peel off the skin and mince the pepper.

3 Combine the corn and water in a medium skillet. Cook over medium-high heat, stirring often, until the corn is crisp-tender and most of the liquid has evaporated, about 5 minutes. Remove from the heat and stir in the jalapeño, butter, lime zest, lime juice, and salt. Spoon the corn into a serving bowl and serve at once.

Each serving: 14 g carb, 71 cal, 2 g fat, 1 g sat fat, 3 mg chol, 2 g fib, 2 g pro, 81 mg sod • Carb Choices: 1; Exchanges: 1 starch

Eggplant

Roasted Eggplant with Tomato Vinaigrette

HIGH FIBER

makes 6 servings

This dish is a delicious way to use a bumper crop of eggplant. You can roast the eggplant a day ahead and let it come to room temperature before serving. Instead of the vinaigrette in this recipe, try topping the roasted eggplant with Romesco Sauce (page 593) or Chimichurri Sauce (page 594).

1 teaspoon plus 3 tablespoons extra virgin olive oil, divided

1 large eggplant (about 1¾ pounds), cut into ½-inch rounds

½ teaspoon kosher salt, divided

¼ teaspoon freshly ground pepper, divided

1 tablespoon red wine vinegar

1 garlic clove, crushed through a press

½ teaspoon Dijon mustard

¼ cup peeled diced fresh tomato

2 teaspoons chopped fresh rosemary

1 Preheat the oven to 425°F. Brush a large rimmed baking sheet with 1 teaspoon of the oil.

2 Brush the eggplant slices with 1 tablespoon of the remaining oil. Sprinkle with ¼ teaspoon of the salt and ⅛ teaspoon of the pepper. Arrange in a single layer on the baking sheet. Bake, turning once, until tender and well browned, 35 to 40 minutes.

3 Meanwhile, whisk together the vinegar, garlic, mustard, remaining ¼ teaspoon salt, and remaining ⅛ teaspoon pepper in a medium bowl. Slowly whisk in the remaining 2 tablespoons oil. Stir in the tomato and rosemary.

4 To serve, arrange the eggplant slices on a serving platter. Spoon the vinaigrette evenly over the eggplant. Serve hot, warm, or at room temperature.

Each serving: 8 g carb, 97 cal, 7 g fat, 1 g sat fat, 0 mg chol, 5 g fib, 1 g pro, 108 mg sod • Carb Choices: ½; Exchanges: 1 veg, 1½ fat

Eggplant Gratin

makes 6 servings

Vary this dish according to what you have on hand. Add diced bell pepper, fresh fennel, or zucchini and cook them along with the onion. Instead of basil, use 1 teaspoon chopped fresh thyme or oregano or 2 tablespoons chopped fresh Italian parsley.

4½ teaspoons extra virgin olive oil, divided

1 small onion, diced

2 garlic cloves, minced

¼ teaspoon crushed red pepper

1 medium eggplant (about 1¼ pounds), peeled and cut into ½-inch cubes

1 medium tomato, chopped

2 tablespoons chopped fresh basil

½ teaspoon kosher salt

½ cup fresh whole wheat breadcrumbs

1 ounce freshly grated Parmesan (about ¼ cup)

1 Preheat the oven to 400°F. Brush a shallow 1½- to 2-quart baking dish with ½ teaspoon of the oil.

2 Heat a small nonstick skillet over medium heat. Add 2 teaspoons of the remaining oil and tilt the pan to coat the bottom evenly. Add the onion and cook, stirring often, until softened, 5 minutes. Stir in the garlic and crushed red pepper and cook, stirring constantly, until fragrant, 30 seconds. Transfer to a large bowl.

3 Meanwhile, in a pot fitted with a steamer basket, bring 1 inch of water to a boil over high heat. Add the eggplant cubes, reduce the heat to low, cover, and steam until they are tender but still retain their shape, about 5 minutes. Transfer to a colander to drain. Add to the bowl with the onion mixture. Stir in the tomato, basil, and salt. Spoon into the prepared baking dish.

4 Stir together the breadcrumbs, Parmesan, and remaining 2 teaspoons olive oil in a small bowl and sprinkle evenly over the eggplant mixture. Bake, uncovered, until the crumbs are browned, 20 to 25 minutes. Serve the gratin at once.

Each serving: 9 g carb, 85 cal, 5 g fat, 1 g sat fat, 3 mg chol, 3 g fib, 3 g pro, 173 mg sod • Carb Choices: ½; Exchanges: 1 veg, 1 fat

Grilled Eggplant Rounds with Basil and Caper Sauce

QUICK | HIGH FIBER

makes 6 servings

When fresh tomatoes are at their peak, alternate slices of the grilled eggplant with tomato slices on a platter and drizzle with the sauce to make a beautiful presentation for a summer cookout.

1 large eggplant (about 1¾ pounds), cut into ½-inch rounds

3 tablespoons plus ½ teaspoon extra virgin olive oil, divided

½ teaspoon kosher salt, divided

⅛ teaspoon plus a pinch of freshly ground pepper, divided

1 tablespoon red wine vinegar

1 garlic clove, crushed through a press

2 tablespoons chopped fresh basil

2 teaspoons capers, rinsed and drained

1 Prepare the grill or heat a large grill pan over medium-high heat.

2 Brush the eggplant with 1 tablespoon of the oil. Sprinkle with ¼ teaspoon of the salt and ⅛ teaspoon of the pepper. Brush the grill rack or grill pan with ½ teaspoon of the remaining oil. Place the eggplant on the grill rack or in the grill pan and grill, turning often, until the eggplant is tender and well browned, 8 to 10 minutes.

3 Meanwhile, whisk together the vinegar, garlic, remaining ¼ teaspoon salt, and remaining pinch of pepper in a small bowl. Slowly whisk in the remaining 2 tablespoons oil. Stir in the basil and capers.

4 To serve, arrange the eggplant slices on a serving platter. Spoon the sauce evenly over the eggplant. Serve hot, warm, or at room temperature.

Each serving: 8 g carb, 103 cal, 8 g fat, 1 g sat fat, 0 mg chol, 5 g fib, 1 g pro, 125 mg sod • Carb Choices: ½; Exchanges: 1 veg, 1½ fat

Baby Eggplants Stuffed with Zucchini and Dried Tomatoes

makes 8 servings

These baby eggplants make an impressive presentation, but if you don't want to bother with the extra steps it takes, make this dish using a 1½-pound eggplant, peeled and chopped, and just make the filling. Spoon the vegetable mixture onto a serving platter, sprinkle with the cheese, and you've got a delicious summer vegetable side dish that's ready in about 20 minutes. Or serve it on top of pasta for a dinner for two.

continues on next page

4 small eggplants (6 to 8 ounces each), cut in half lengthwise

3 teaspoons extra virgin olive oil, divided

1 small zucchini, chopped

1 small onion, chopped

1 garlic clove, minced

1 medium tomato, chopped

¼ cup chopped fresh basil

¾ teaspoon kosher salt

Pinch of freshly ground pepper

1 ounce freshly grated Parmesan (about ¼ cup)

1 Preheat the broiler.

2 Scoop out the flesh of the eggplant halves using a small spoon or a melon baller, leaving ½-inch-thick shells. Reserve the flesh. Brush a broiler rack with ½ teaspoon of the oil. Place the eggplant shells on the rack, cut side up, and broil until softened, about 5 minutes.

3 Preheat the oven to 400°F.

4 Meanwhile, chop the flesh of the eggplants. Heat a medium nonstick skillet over medium heat. Add 2 teaspoons of the remaining oil and tilt the pan to coat the bottom evenly. Add the eggplant, zucchini, and onion and cook, stirring often, until softened, 8 minutes. Add the garlic and cook, stirring constantly, until fragrant, 30 seconds. Stir in the tomato, basil, salt, and pepper and cook until heated through, 1 minute.

5 Brush a large shallow baking dish with the remaining ½ teaspoon oil. Spoon about ½ cup of the vegetable mixture into each of the eggplant shells. Sprinkle evenly with the Parmesan. Place in the baking dish in a single layer and bake, uncovered, until the cheese melts, 20 minutes. Serve at once.

Each serving: 7 g carb, 56 cal, 3 g fat, 1 g sat fat, 2 mg chol, 3 g fib, 2 g pro, 148 mg sod • Carb Choices: ½; Exchanges: 1 veg, ½ fat

Spicy Eggplant with Ginger and Sesame QUICK

makes 4 servings

Serve this with any entrée that features Asian flavors or over soba noodles or brown rice as quick and flavorful dinner for two.

1 (1-pound) eggplant, peeled and cut into ½-inch cubes

2 teaspoons reduced-sodium soy sauce

1 teaspoon rice vinegar

½ teaspoon chili-garlic paste

⅛ teaspoon Asian sesame oil

2 teaspoons canola oil

1 tablespoon minced fresh ginger

2 garlic cloves, minced

¼ teaspoon kosher salt

1 small scallion, thinly sliced

1 In a pot fitted with a steamer basket, bring 1 inch of water to a boil over high heat. Add the eggplant cubes, reduce heat to low, cover, and steam until tender but still retain their shape, about 5 minutes. Transfer to a colander and drain.

2 Meanwhile, stir together the soy sauce, vinegar, chili-garlic paste, and sesame oil in a small dish. Set aside.

3 Heat a large nonstick skillet over medium-high heat. Add the canola oil and tilt the pan to coat the bottom evenly. Add the ginger and garlic and cook, stirring constantly, until fragrant, 30 seconds. Add the eggplant, sprinkle with the salt, and stir to coat. Remove from the heat and stir in the soy sauce mixture.

4 Spoon into a serving bowl and sprinkle with the scallion. Serve at once.

Each serving: 6 g carb, 49 cal, 3 g fat, 3 g sat fat, 0 mg chol, 3 g fib, 1 g pro, 200 mg sod • Carb Choices: ½; Exchanges: 1 veg, ½ fat

Fennel

Grilled Fennel with Orange-Olive Vinaigrette

HIGH FIBER

makes 4 servings

Brightly flavored citrus and salty green olives are a good match for sweet grilled fennel. Any kind of green olive you have on hand will give the saltiness this dish needs. The manzanilla, or common Spanish olive, works very well, and milder flavored French picholine olives are excellent. This is a perfect accompaniment to grilled salmon or shrimp.

¾ cup orange juice
¼ teaspoon kosher salt, divided
Pinch of freshly ground pepper
1 tablespoon plus 2½ teaspoons extra virgin olive oil, divided
4 large green olives, pitted and chopped
2 large bulbs fennel

1 Place the orange juice in a small saucepan and boil over medium-high heat until reduced to about ¼ cup, 6 to 8 minutes. Transfer to a small bowl and let stand to cool. Whisk in ⅛ teaspoon of the salt and the pepper. Slowly whisk in 1 tablespoon of the oil. Stir in the olives. Set aside.

2 Prepare the grill or preheat a large grill pan over medium-high heat.

3 Trim the tough outer stalks from the fennel bulbs. Cut each one in half vertically and discard the cores. Cut each half lengthwise into ½-inch slices.

4 Place the fennel in a medium bowl, drizzle with 2 teaspoons of the remaining oil, sprinkle with the remaining ⅛ teaspoon salt, and toss to coat. Place the fennel on a grill rack or grill pan brushed with the ½ teaspoon remaining oil. Grill, turning often, until the fennel is tender and well browned, 12 to 15 minutes.

5 Arrange the fennel on a serving platter and drizzle with the dressing. Serve hot, warm, or at room temperature.

Each serving: 14 g carb, 122 cal, 7 g fat, 1 g sat fat, 0 mg chol, 4 g fib, 2 g pro, 205 mg sod • Carb Choices: 1; Exchanges: 2 veg, 1½ fat

Sautéed Fennel with Ginger QUICK HIGH FIBER

makes 4 servings

Anise and ginger make a surprisingly good pairing in this intensely flavored side dish. For an easy, yet sophisticated entrée, spoon the fennel evenly onto four serving plates and top each one with a simply sautéed chicken breast or fish fillet. If you have fresh fennel fronds, sprinkle them on top for a garnish.

2 large bulbs fennel
1 tablespoon extra virgin olive oil
1 tablespoon minced fresh ginger
½ teaspoon kosher salt
1 teaspoon lemon juice

1 Trim the tough outer stalks from the fennel bulbs. Cut each one in half vertically and discard the cores. Cut each half lengthwise into ½-inch slices.

2 Heat a large nonstick skillet over medium heat. Add the oil and tilt the pan to coat the bottom evenly. Add the ginger and cook, stirring constantly, until fragrant, 30 seconds. Add the fennel and salt and cook, stirring frequently, until tender and lightly browned, 8 to 10 minutes. Stir in the lemon juice. Spoon the fennel into a serving dish and serve at once.

Each serving: 9 g carb, 69cal, 4 g fat, 1 g sat fat, 0 mg chol, 4 g fib, 2 g pro, 201 mg sod • Carb Choices: ½; Exchanges: 2 veg, ½ fat

Roasted Fennel with Pernod HIGH FIBER

makes 4 servings

With a double hit of anise from the fennel and the Pernod liqueur, this is a dish for licorice lovers. It's just right for serving with fish or shellfish.

2 large bulbs fennel
2 teaspoons plus 1 tablespoon extra virgin olive oil, divided
¼ teaspoon plus ⅛ teaspoon kosher salt, divided
Pinch of freshly ground pepper
2 teaspoons Pernod or other anise liqueur
1 teaspoon lemon juice
⅛ teaspoon sugar

1 Preheat the oven to 425°F.

2 Trim the tough outer stalks from the fennel bulbs. Cut each one in half vertically and discard the cores. Cut each half lengthwise into ½-inch slices.

3 Place the fennel in a large roasting pan. Drizzle with 2 teaspoons of the oil and sprinkle with ¼ teaspoon of the salt and the pepper. Toss to coat. Arrange the fennel in a single layer. Roast, stirring once, until the fennel is tender and lightly browned, 25 to 30 minutes.

4 Meanwhile, whisk together the Pernod, lemon juice, sugar, and remaining ⅛ teaspoon salt in a small bowl. Slowly whisk in the remaining 1 tablespoon oil.

5 Arrange the fennel on a serving plate and drizzle with the Pernod mixture. Serve hot or at room temperature.

Each serving: 10 g carb, 97 cal, 6 g fat, 1 g sat fat, 0 mg chol, 4 g fib, 1 g pro, 166 mg sod • Carb Choices: ½; Exchanges: 2 veg, 1 fat

Fennel Gratin HIGH FIBER

makes 4 servings

In this dish, fennel is first steamed, then topped with Parmesan and baked in the oven, giving it a silky melt-in-your-mouth texture.

2 large bulbs fennel
1 teaspoon extra virgin olive oil
½ teaspoon kosher salt
Pinch of freshly ground pepper
1 ounce freshly grated Parmesan (about ¼ cup)

1 Preheat the oven to 400°F.

2 Trim the tough outer stalks from the fennel bulbs. Cut each one in half vertically and discard the cores. Cut each half lengthwise into ½-inch slices.

3 In a saucepan fitted with a steamer basket, bring 1 inch of water to a boil over high heat. Add the fennel, reduce the heat to low, cover, and steam until tender, about 5 minutes.

4 Place the fennel in a shallow 2-quart baking dish. Drizzle with the oil, sprinkle with the salt and pepper, and toss to coat. Arrange the fennel evenly in the dish and sprinkle with the Parmesan.

5 Bake, uncovered, until the cheese is melted, 15 to 20 minutes. Serve hot or warm.

Each serving: 9 g carb, 68 cal, 3 g fat, 1 g sat fat, 4 mg chol, 4 g fib, 3 g pro, 277 mg sod • Carb Choices: ½; Exchanges: 2 veg, ½ fat

Green Beans

Steamed Green Beans with Walnuts and Parmesan `QUICK` `HIGH FIBER`

makes 4 servings

This recipe dresses up green beans just enough so that they taste fantastic—yet there's little effort involved. Toasting walnuts in a skillet is quicker than toasting them in the oven. Watch them carefully, though, as they can burn quickly.

1 pound green beans, trimmed
2 teaspoons extra virgin olive oil
2 tablespoons chopped walnuts
½ teaspoon kosher salt
Pinch of freshly ground pepper
2 tablespoons finely shredded Parmesan

1 In a saucepan fitted with a steamer basket, bring 1 inch of water to a boil over high heat. Add the green beans, reduce the heat to low, cover, and steam until tender, 4 to 5 minutes.

2 Meanwhile, heat a medium nonstick skillet over medium heat. Add the oil and tilt the pan to coat the bottom evenly. Add the walnuts and cook, stirring often, until toasted and fragrant, 2 minutes. Add the green beans, salt, and pepper and stir to coat. Spoon onto a serving platter and sprinkle with the Parmesan. Serve at once.

Each serving: 8 g carb, 87 cal, 6 g fat, 1 g sat fat, 2 mg chol, 4 g fib, 3 g pro, 184 mg sod • Carb Choices: ½; Exchanges: 1 veg, 1 fat

Lemon-Dill Green Beans

`QUICK`

makes 4 servings

These beans are delicious as a cold salad, too. Steam the green beans as directed, drain, and cool them under cold running water. Don't cook the garlic; just mince it and combine it with all the other ingredients in a large bowl. Blot the beans dry and add to the garlic mixture. You can add some penne, rotini, or bow-tie pasta and halved cherry tomatoes to make a summer pasta salad, if you wish.

1 pound green beans, trimmed
2 teaspoons extra virgin olive oil
1 garlic clove, minced
½ teaspoon grated lemon zest
1 tablespoon lemon juice
1 tablespoon chopped fresh dill
½ teaspoon kosher salt
Pinch of freshly ground pepper

1 In a saucepan fitted with a steamer basket, bring 1 inch of water to a boil over high heat. Add the green beans, reduce the heat to low, cover, and steam until tender, 4 to 5 minutes.

2 Meanwhile, heat a medium nonstick skillet over medium heat. Add the oil and tilt the pan to coat the bottom evenly. Add the garlic and cook, stirring constantly, until fragrant, 30 seconds. Add the beans, lemon zest, lemon juice, dill, salt, and pepper and stir to coat. Transfer the beans to a serving dish. Serve hot, warm, or at room temperature.

Each serving: 8 g carb, 54 cal, 3 g fat, 0 g sat fat, 0 mg chol, 3 g fib, 2 g pro, 146 mg sod • Carb Choices: ½; Exchanges: 1 veg, ½ fat

Green Beans with Caramelized Onions and Cider Vinegar HIGH FIBER

makes 4 servings

This is an excellent recipe for making green beans in the fall and winter months. The onions lend sweetness and the vinegar adds a sour note to make a dish of perfectly balanced flavors. Try the same technique with steamed Brussels sprouts.

2 teaspoons extra virgin olive oil
1 medium onion, halved and thinly sliced
1 pound green beans, trimmed
2 teaspoons apple cider vinegar
½ teaspoon kosher salt
Pinch of freshly ground pepper

1 Heat a medium nonstick skillet over medium heat. Add the oil and tilt the pan to coat the bottom evenly. Add the onion and cook, stirring often, until very soft and browned, about 20 minutes.

2 Meanwhile, in a saucepan fitted with a steamer basket, bring 1 inch of water to a boil over high heat. Add the green beans, reduce the heat to low, cover, and steam until tender, 4 to 5 minutes.

3 Add the green beans, vinegar, salt, and pepper to the onion and stir to combine. Spoon the green beans and onion into a serving dish and serve hot or warm.

Each serving: 10 g carb, 63 cal, 3 g fat, 0 g sat fat, 0 mg chol, 4 g fib, 2 g pro, 147 mg sod • Carb Choices: ½; Exchanges: 2 veg, ½ fat

Green Beans with Grape Tomatoes QUICK HIGH FIBER

makes 4 servings

Made from two abundant summer staples, this side dish is as colorful as it is delicious. Pair it with anything you've got going on the outdoor grill.

1 pound green beans, trimmed
2 teaspoons extra virgin olive oil
1 garlic clove, minced
1 cup grape or small cherry tomatoes
½ teaspoon kosher salt
Pinch of freshly ground pepper

1 In a saucepan fitted with a steamer basket, bring 1 inch of water to a boil over high heat. Add the green beans, reduce the heat to low, cover, and steam until tender, 4 to 5 minutes.

2 Meanwhile, heat a large nonstick skillet over medium heat. Add the oil and tilt the pan to coat the bottom evenly. Add the garlic and cook, stirring constantly, 1 minute. Add the tomatoes and cook, stirring occasionally, until the skins just begin to burst, about 3 minutes. Stir in the green beans, salt, and pepper. Spoon the green beans and tomatoes into a serving dish and serve at once.

Each serving: 9 g carb, 60 cal, 3 g fat, 0 g sat fat, 0 mg chol, 4 g fib, 2 g pro, 148 mg sod • Carb Choices: ½; Exchanges: 2 veg, ½ fat

Thin-Sliced Green Beans with Pine Nuts and Mint

QUICK | HIGH FIBER

makes 4 servings

Cutting the green beans into thin slices makes this dish almost like eating a chopped salad—you get the satisfying crunch of the beans, the rich flavor of pine nuts, and the refreshing taste of mint in every bite.

2 teaspoons extra virgin olive oil
1 pound green beans, trimmed and cut on the diagonal into ½-inch slices
½ teaspoon kosher salt
2 tablespoons pine nuts, toasted (page 4)
2 teaspoons chopped fresh mint or 1 tablespoon chopped fresh basil or Italian parsley
Pinch of freshly ground pepper

1 Heat a medium nonstick skillet over medium-high heat. Add the oil and tilt the pan to coat the bottom evenly.

2 Add the green beans and salt and cook, stirring constantly, until the beans are crisp-tender, about 4 minutes. (If you like beans more tender, add 2 tablespoons water, cover, and cook an additional 1 to 2 minutes.) Remove from the heat and stir in the pine nuts, mint, and pepper. Spoon the green beans into a serving dish and serve hot or warm.

Each serving: 8 g carb, 81 cal, 5 g fat, 1 g sat fat, 0 mg chol, 4 g fib, 2 g pro, 146 mg sod • Carb Choices: ½; Exchanges: 1 veg, 1 fat

Green Beans with Feta Vinaigrette QUICK

makes 4 servings

Using a combination of herbs will make the flavor more complex, but if you only have a single herb on hand, the dish will still be delicious.

1 pound green beans, trimmed
1 tablespoon white wine vinegar
¼ teaspoon kosher salt
Pinch of freshly ground pepper
2 tablespoons extra virgin olive oil
2 tablespoons finely crumbled feta cheese
1 tablespoon any combination of chopped fresh basil, dill, mint, or Italian parsley

1 In a saucepan fitted with a steamer basket, bring 1 inch of water to a boil over high heat. Add the green beans, reduce the heat to low, cover, and steam until tender, 4 to 5 minutes.

2 Meanwhile, whisk together the vinegar, salt, and pepper in a small bowl. Slowly whisk in the oil. Stir in the feta and herbs.

3 To serve, arrange the beans on a serving platter and drizzle with the vinaigrette. Serve hot, warm, or at room temperature.

Each serving: 7 g carb, 103 cal, 8 g fat, 2 g sat fat, 3 mg chol, 3 g fib, 2 g pro, 116 mg sod • Carb Choices: ½; Exchanges: 1 veg, 1½ fat

Stir-Fried Green Beans QUICK

makes 4 servings

The secret to the great flavor of these beans is adding them to a hot skillet, so that they brown lightly. Once browned, they finish cooking by steaming in a little ginger, garlic, and water—simple and delicious.

2 teaspoons canola oil
1 pound green beans, trimmed
2 tablespoons water
2 teaspoons minced fresh ginger
1 garlic clove, minced
1 tablespoon reduced-sodium soy sauce
½ teaspoon Asian sesame oil

1 Heat a large wok or nonstick skillet over medium-high heat. Add the canola oil and tilt the pan to coat the bottom evenly. Add the green beans and cook, stirring constantly, until the beans are lightly browned, 2 to 3 minutes.

2 Add the water, ginger, and garlic. Cover and cook, stirring often, until the beans are crisp-tender, 2 to 3 minutes. Remove from the heat and stir in the soy sauce and sesame oil. Spoon the green beans into a serving dish and serve at once.

Each serving: 8 g carb, 61 cal, 3 g fat, 0 g sat fat, 0 mg chol, 3 g fib, 2 g pro, 158 mg sod • Carb Choices: ½; Exchanges: 1 veg, ½ fat

Roasted Green Beans QUICK

makes 4 servings

As with other vegetables, roasting concentrates the flavors and caramelizes the natural sugars of green beans. If you've never roasted them before, you're in for a treat. Enjoy them plain, as in this recipe, or sprinkle them with crumbled feta or finely shredded Parmesan.

1 pound green beans, trimmed
2 teaspoons extra virgin olive oil
½ teaspoon kosher salt
Pinch of freshly ground pepper

1 Preheat the oven to 425°F.

2 Place the beans in a large roasting pan. Drizzle with the oil and sprinkle with the salt and pepper. Toss to coat. Arrange the beans in a single layer.

3 Roast, stirring once, until lightly browned and crisp-tender, 18 to 20 minutes. Spoon the green beans into a serving dish and serve hot or warm.

Each serving: 7 g carb, 52 cal, 3 g fat, 0 g sat fat, 0 mg chol, 3 g fib, 2 g pro, 146 mg sod • Carb Choices: ½; Exchanges: 1 veg, ½ fat

Slow-Cooked Italian Pole Beans with Tomatoes and Oregano HIGH FIBER

makes 4 servings

Pole beans are wide, flat green beans that contain a larger seed than regular green beans. The pods are edible, but they are not as tender as the pod of regular green beans. I like to simmer them until they are quite soft in a flavorful tomato sauce spiked with oregano.

2 teaspoons extra virgin olive oil
1 medium red onion, halved and thinly sliced
1 garlic clove, minced
1 pound flat Italian pole beans, trimmed and broken into 2-inch pieces
1 large tomato, peeled and chopped, or 1 (14½-ounce) can no-salt-added diced tomatoes
½ cup water
1 teaspoon chopped fresh oregano or ¼ teaspoon dried oregano
½ teaspoon kosher salt
Pinch of freshly ground pepper

1 Heat a large saucepan over medium heat. Add the oil and tilt the pan to coat the bottom evenly.

2 Add the onion and cook, stirring often, until softened, 5 minutes. Add the garlic and cook, stirring constantly, until fragrant, 30 seconds.

3 Add the beans, tomato, water, oregano, salt, and pepper and bring to a boil over high heat. Reduce the heat to low, cover, and simmer until the beans are very tender, 25 to 30 minutes. Check the beans often, adding additional water if necessary. Spoon the green beans into a serving dish and serve at once.

Each serving: 12 g carb, 73 cal, 3 g fat, 0 g sat fat, 0 mg chol, 5 g fib, 3 g pro, 150 mg sod • Carb Choices: 1; Exchanges: 2 veg, ½ fat

Greens

Spinach with Whole Grain Mustard QUICK

makes 4 servings

This vibrant spinach dish makes a perfect "bed" on which to serve baked salmon or white fish fillets. The Dijon adds a little tang that pairs nicely with seafood.

1 pound fresh spinach
2 teaspoons extra virgin olive oil
¼ cup diced onion
2 garlic cloves, minced
1 tablespoon whole grain Dijon mustard
½ teaspoon kosher salt
Pinch of freshly ground pepper

1 Pinch the tough stems from the spinach. Submerge the spinach in a large bowl of cold water, lift it out, and drain in a colander. Repeat, using fresh water, until no grit remains in the bottom of the bowl.

2 Heat a large nonstick skillet over medium heat. Add the oil and tilt the pan to coat the bottom evenly. Add the onion and cook, stirring often, until softened, 5 minutes. Stir in the garlic and cook, stirring constantly, until fragrant, 30 seconds.

3 Add the spinach in batches and cook, turning with tongs, until the spinach is wilted and most of the liquid has evaporated, about 2 minutes. Remove from the heat and stir in the mustard, salt, and pepper. Spoon the spinach into a serving dish and serve at once.

Each serving: 6 g carb, 52 cal, 3 g fat, 0 g sat fat, 0 mg chol, 2 g fib, 3 g pro, 295 mg sod • Carb Choices: ½; Exchanges: 1 veg, ½ fat

Spinach with Garlic, Lemon, and Cracked Pepper QUICK

makes 4 servings

Spinach varieties are either flat-leaved or what is called "savoyed," a wrinkle-leaved variety. I prefer the flat-leaved variety because it's easier to wash the grit from the flat leaves. There is no difference in taste between the two varieties, but if you buy the crinkly variety, wash it well.

⅛ teaspoon whole black peppercorns
1 pound fresh spinach
2 teaspoons canola oil
2 garlic cloves, minced
½ teaspoon grated lemon zest
½ teaspoon kosher salt

1 Place the peppercorns in a mortar and crush with a pestle. Alternatively, place the peppercorns in a small resealable plastic bag. Seal the bag, place on a cutting board, and crush using a meat mallet or the back of a large spoon. Set aside.

2 Pinch the tough stems from the spinach. Submerge the spinach in a large bowl of cold water, lift it out, and drain in a colander. Repeat, using fresh water, until no grit remains in the bottom of the bowl.

3 Heat a large nonstick skillet over medium heat. Add the oil and tilt the pan to coat the bottom evenly. Add the garlic and cook, stirring constantly, until fragrant, 30 seconds.

4 Add the spinach in batches and cook, turning with tongs, until the spinach is wilted and most of the liquid has evaporated, about 2 minutes. Remove from the heat and stir in the lemon zest, salt, and peppercorns. Spoon the spinach into a serving dish and serve at once.

Each serving: 4 g carb, 41 cal, 3 g fat, 0 g sat fat, 0 mg chol, 2 g fib, 2 g pro, 205 mg sod • Carb Choices: ½; Exchanges: 1 veg, ½ fat

Kale with Crispy Crumbs and Pine Nuts

makes 4 servings

As part of my community-supported agriculture program, I look forward to fall and the bounty of greens that are in my produce box every week. This dish is a favorite that I serve often. The toasted breadcrumbs and pine nuts add crunch and they make the greens look more interesting when you serve them. You can easily double this recipe—just be sure to cook the greens in your largest skillet.

4 teaspoons extra virgin olive oil, divided
¼ cup fresh whole wheat breadcrumbs
1 tablespoon pine nuts
2 garlic cloves, thinly sliced
¾ cup Vegetable Stock (page 149) or low-
    sodium vegetable broth
½ teaspoon kosher salt
⅛ teaspoon crushed red pepper
1 pound kale, tough stems removed and leaves
    chopped

1 Heat a large nonstick skillet over medium heat. Add 2 teaspoons of the oil and tilt the pan to coat the bottom evenly. Add the breadcrumbs and pine nuts and cook, stirring often, until lightly toasted, 5 minutes. Transfer the bread-crumb mixture to a small bowl.

2 Wipe out the skillet with paper towels and set over medium heat. Add the remaining 2 teaspoons oil and tilt the pan to coat the bottom evenly. Add the garlic and cook, stirring often, until lightly browned, 3 minutes. Using a slotted spoon, transfer the garlic to a small plate.

3 Add the stock, salt, and crushed red pepper to the skillet and bring to a boil over medium-high heat. Add the kale in batches and cook, stirring occasionally, until the kale is tender and most of the liquid has evaporated, 8 to 10 minutes. Stir in the reserved garlic.

4 Transfer the kale to a serving platter, sprinkle with the breadcrumb mixture and serve at once.

Each serving: 10 g carb, 106 cal, 7 g fat, 1 g sat fat, 0 mg chol, 2 g fib, 3 g pro, 213 mg sod • Carb Choices: ½; Exchanges: 1 veg, 1 fat

Wilted Escarole with Anchovies QUICK

makes 4 servings

Add at least one anchovy to this dish, even if you don't like anchovies. The fish dissolves as it cooks with the escarole, leaving behind a complex and indefinable (except to the cook) saltiness. If you want to keep the aromatic fish away from your cutting board, place the anchovies in a small dish and break them into small pieces using two forks.

1 pound escarole, coarsely chopped
2 teaspoons extra virgin olive oil
2 garlic cloves, thinly sliced
1 to 2 canned anchovy fillets, drained and
    minced
½ teaspoon kosher salt
⅛ teaspoon crushed red pepper

1 Submerge the escarole in a large bowl of cold water, lift it out, and drain in a colander. Repeat, using fresh water, until no grit remains in the bottom of the bowl.

2 Heat a large nonstick skillet over medium heat. Add the oil and tilt the pan to coat the bottom evenly. Add the garlic and cook, stirring constantly, until lightly browned, 2 minutes.

3 Add the escarole, anchovy, salt, and crushed red pepper. Cook, stirring often, until the escarole is tender and most of the liquid has evaporated, about 5 minutes. Spoon the escarole into a serving dish and serve at once.

Each serving: 4 g carb, 42 cal, 3 g fat, 0 g sat fat, 0 mg chol, 3 g fib, 2 g pro, 198 mg sod • Carb Choices: 0; Exchanges: 1 veg, ½ fat

Swiss Chard with Raisins and Pine Nuts QUICK

makes 4 servings

Golden raisins add a touch of sweetness to this dish that erases the slight bitterness of the chard. Serve this tossed with penne and sprinkled with some finely shredded Parmesan for a quick vegetarian dinner for two. In a well-stocked produce market you might find red, golden, and white varieties of Swiss chard bundled together in bunches and sold as "rainbow chard."

12 ounces Swiss chard
2 tablespoons pine nuts
2 teaspoons extra virgin olive oil
1 medium red onion, halved and thinly sliced
¼ cup golden raisins
¼ cup Chicken Stock (page 149) or low-sodium chicken broth or water
¼ teaspoon kosher salt
Pinch of freshly ground pepper
½ teaspoon red wine vinegar

1 Cut the stems away from the tender leaves of the chard. Chop the stems and thinly slice the leaves, keeping the stems and leaves separate. Set aside.

2 Place the pine nuts in a large nonstick skillet and toast over medium heat, stirring frequently, until lightly browned and fragrant. Transfer to a plate to cool.

3 Increase the heat under the skillet to medium-high. Add the oil and tilt the pan to coat the bottom evenly. Add the chard stems and onion and cook, stirring often, until softened, 5 minutes. Add the chard leaves, raisins, stock, salt, and pepper. Cover and cook, stirring frequently, until the chard is tender, 6 to 8 minutes. Remove from the heat and stir in the vinegar and pine nuts. Spoon the Swiss chard into a serving dish and serve at once.

Each serving: 14 g carb, 88 cal, 3 g fat, 0 g sat fat, 0 mg chol, 3 g fib, 3 g pro, 303 mg sod • Carb Choices: 1; Exchanges: ½ fruit, 1 veg, ½ fat

Roasted Radicchio with Balsamic-Garlic Vinaigrette

makes 4 servings

Radicchio loses its striking red color in this dish, but the caramelized flavor is fantastic. This is a good companion to roast pork or chicken.

2 heads radicchio, each cut into 4 wedges with core intact
2 garlic cloves, halved
2 teaspoons plus 1 tablespoon extra virgin olive oil, divided
½ teaspoon kosher salt, divided
2 teaspoons balsamic vinegar
Pinch of freshly ground pepper

1 Preheat the oven to 425°F.

2 Place the radicchio and garlic in a large roasting pan. Drizzle with 2 teaspoons of the oil and turn to coat. Sprinkle with ¼ teaspoon of the salt. Arrange the radicchio cut side up and roast, turning once, until the radicchio is lightly browned and tender and the garlic is soft, 20 to 25 minutes.

3 Transfer the garlic to a medium bowl and mash to a paste with a fork. Whisk in the vinegar, remaining ¼ teaspoon salt, and the pepper. Slowly whisk in the remaining 1 tablespoon oil.

4 Arrange the radicchio wedges on a serving platter and drizzle with the vinaigrette. Serve at once.

Each serving: 6 g carb, 80 cal, 6 g fat, 1 g sat fat, 0 mg chol, 1 g fib, 2 g pro, 164 mg sod • Carb Choices: ½; Exchanges: 1 veg, 1 fat

Sautéed Greens with Vinegar and Garlic

makes 4 servings

This is an infinitely versatile dish that you can make with a single type of green or a variety of greens. It's not necessary to remove the stems of the greens for this rustic dish, unless they are particularly thick and tough. This is especially delicious and pretty if made with baby versions of the greens. If you are lucky enough to have those, leave them whole and cook just until they are wilted.

1 pound any combination Swiss chard, collard greens, kale, beet greens, or mustard greens, tough stems removed and leaves coarsely chopped

2 teaspoons extra virgin olive oil

2 garlic cloves, thinly sliced

½ teaspoon kosher salt

⅛ teaspoon crushed red pepper

1 teaspoon red wine vinegar

1 Submerge the greens in a large bowl of cold water, lift them out and drain in a colander. Repeat, using fresh water, until no grit remains in the bottom of the bowl.

2 Heat a large nonstick skillet over medium heat. Add the oil and tilt the pan to coat the bottom evenly. Add the garlic and cook, stirring constantly, until lightly browned, 2 minutes.

3 Add the greens, salt, and crushed red pepper. For young, tender greens, cook, stirring often, until the greens are tender, 3 to 5 minutes. (For mature greens, add about ½ cup water, cover, and simmer until the greens are tender, 15 to 20 minutes.) Remove from the heat and stir in the vinegar. Spoon the greens into a serving dish and serve at once.

Each serving: 4 g carb, 43 cal, 3 g fat, 0 g sat fat, 0 mg chol, 2 g fib, 2 g pro, 363 mg sod • Carb Choices: 0; Exchanges: 1 veg, ½ fat

Chinese Broccoli in Oyster Sauce QUICK

makes 4 servings

Chinese broccoli looks like broccoli rabe, but it is less bitter and has thinner stems and fewer buds. This recipe uses the stems and the leaves in a dish that's salty, sweet, and spicy.

1 pound Chinese broccoli

2 tablespoons Chicken Stock (page 149) or low-sodium chicken broth

2 tablespoons oyster sauce

½ teaspoon chili-garlic paste

½ teaspoon cornstarch

2 teaspoons canola oil

2 teaspoons minced fresh ginger

1 garlic clove, minced

1 Coarsely chop the leaves and tender stems of the Chinese broccoli. Peel and thinly slice the larger stems and keep them separate.

2 In a saucepan fitted with a steamer basket, bring 1 inch of water to a boil. Add the Chinese broccoli stems, reduce the heat to low, cover, and steam 2 minutes. Add the leaves and tender stems, cover, and steam until tender, 3 minutes.

3 Meanwhile, stir together the stock, oyster sauce, chili-garlic paste, and cornstarch in a small bowl and set aside.

4 Heat a large wok or nonstick skillet over medium-high heat. Add the oil and tilt the pan to coat the bottom evenly. Add the ginger and garlic and cook, stirring constantly, until fragrant, 30 seconds.

5 Add the Chinese broccoli. Stir the broth mixture and add to the skillet. Cook, stirring constantly, until the sauce comes to a boil and thickens slightly, 1 minute. Spoon the Chinese broccoli into a serving dish and serve at once.

Each serving: 10 g carb, 73 cal, 3 g fat, 0 g sat fat, 0 mg chol, 3 g fib, 3 g pro, 166 mg sod • Carb Choices: ½; Exchanges: 2 veg, ½ fat

Steamed Baby Bok Choy with Ginger Sauce QUICK

makes 4 servings

This simple and flavorful sauce accentuates almost any vegetable. Try it with steamed broccoli, green beans, or summer squash. You can also make it ahead, let it cool, and serve as a dipping sauce with fresh cut-up vegetables.

1 pound baby bok choy, quartered with core intact
¼ cup water
2 tablespoons reduced-sodium soy sauce
2 teaspoons grated fresh ginger
2 teaspoons sugar
1½ teaspoons rice vinegar
½ teaspoon cornstarch

1 Submerge the bok choy in a large bowl of cold water, lift it out, and drain in a colander. Repeat, using fresh water, until no grit remains in the bottom of the bowl.

2 In a saucepan fitted with a steamer basket, bring 1 inch of water to a boil over high heat. Add the bok choy, reduce the heat to low, cover, and steam until tender, 4 to 5 minutes.

3 Meanwhile, combine the remaining ingredients in a small saucepan and stir until the cornstarch dissolves. Cook over medium heat, stirring constantly, until the mixture comes to a boil and thickens, 2 to 3 minutes.

4 To serve, arrange the bok choy on a serving platter and drizzle with the sauce. Serve at once.

Each serving: 5 g carb, 30 cal, 0 g fat, 0 g sat fat, 0 mg chol, 2 g fib, 2 g pro, 375 mg sod • Carb Choices: 0; Exchanges: 1 veg

Mushrooms

Sautéed Mixed Mushrooms with Rosemary QUICK

makes 4 servings

Almost any mixture of mushrooms or single type of mushroom works for this simple side dish. If you're using shiitake mushrooms, cut off the stems and discard, as they are too tough to eat. These are a welcome accompaniment to a broiled steak or serve them over polenta for a vegetarian dinner for two.

1 tablespoon extra virgin olive oil
½ cup minced shallots
2 garlic cloves, minced
1½ pounds mixed mushrooms (such as shiitake, cremini, or oyster), sliced
½ cup dry white wine
2 teaspoons minced fresh rosemary
½ teaspoon kosher salt
¼ teaspoon freshly ground pepper

1 Heat a large nonstick skillet over medium heat. Add the oil and tilt the pan to coat the bottom evenly. Add the shallots and cook, stirring often, until softened, 5 minutes. Add the garlic and cook, stirring constantly, until fragrant, 30 seconds.

2 Add the mushrooms and cook, stirring constantly, until the mushrooms are browned and start to give off their liquid, 5 minutes. Add the wine, rosemary, salt, and pepper and cook until the liquid is absorbed, about 3 minutes. Spoon the mushrooms into a serving dish and serve hot or warm.

Each serving: 11 g carb, 118 cal, 4 g fat, 1 g sat fat, 0 mg chol, 1 g fib, 5 g pro, 153 mg sod • Carb Choices: 1; Exchanges: 2 veg, ½ fat

Bacon-Basil Mushrooms [QUICK]

makes 4 servings

To accompany a grilled or broiled steak, these mushrooms are excellent. If you want to make them a few hours ahead, don't add the bacon or basil. When you're ready to serve, gently reheat the mushrooms and stir them in.

2 strips center-cut bacon
1 small red onion, cut in half and sliced
2 garlic cloves, minced
1½ pounds cremini mushrooms, sliced
¼ teaspoon kosher salt
¼ teaspoon freshly ground pepper
3 tablespoons chopped fresh basil

1 Cook the bacon in a large skillet over medium-high heat until crisp. Drain on paper towels and chop. Pour off and discard all but 2 teaspoons of the drippings.

2 Add the onion to the bacon drippings and cook, stirring often, until softened, about 5 minutes. Add the garlic and cook, stirring constantly, until fragrant, 30 seconds. Add the mushrooms and cook, stirring often, until the mushrooms are tender and most of the liquid has evaporated, about 8 minutes. Remove from the heat and stir in the bacon and the basil. Spoon the mushrooms into a serving dish and serve hot or warm.

Each serving: 9 g carb, 88 cal, 3 g fat, 1 g sat fat, 5 mg chol, 1 g fib, 5 g pro, 148 mg sod • Carb Choices: ½; Exchanges: 1 veg, ½ fat

Roasted Cremini Mushrooms with Thyme

makes 4 servings

Cremini mushrooms have deeper flavor than white mushrooms, but the white variety is a fine substitute in this recipe. Roasting concentrates the flavor of the mushrooms, so it's a delicious dish either way.

1½ pounds cremini or white mushrooms, left whole if small, quartered if large
1 tablespoon extra virgin olive oil
¾ teaspoon kosher salt
⅛ teaspoon freshly ground pepper
1 teaspoon sherry or red wine vinegar
1 teaspoon chopped fresh thyme

1 Preheat the oven to 425°F.

2 Place the mushrooms on a large rimmed baking sheet. Drizzle with the oil, sprinkle with the salt and pepper and toss to coat. Roast, stirring occasionally, until the mushrooms are tender and the liquid has evaporated, 30 to 35 minutes.

3 Spoon the mushrooms into a serving bowl. Add the vinegar and thyme and toss gently to coat. Spoon the mushrooms into a serving dish and serve hot, warm, or at room temperature.

Each serving: 7 g carb, 78 cal, 4 g fat, 1 g sat fat, 0 mg chol, 1 g fib, 4 g pro, 220 mg sod • Carb Choices: ½; Exchanges: 2 veg, ½ fat

Roasted Portobello Mushrooms with Balsamic Vinegar

makes 4 servings

I like to scrape out the dark gills on the underside of portobellos before cooking them. The gills turn black and have an undesirable slippery texture when cooked. And, if you're stuffing the mushrooms, it makes more room for whatever flavorful filling you are using.

4 large portobello mushrooms
1 tablespoon extra virgin olive oil
1 tablespoon chopped fresh Italian parsley
2 teaspoons balsamic vinegar
½ teaspoon kosher salt
⅛ teaspoon freshly ground pepper

1 Preheat the oven to 400°F.

2 Cut away and discard the tough stems of the mushrooms. Using a spoon, gently scrape away and discard the dark gills on the underside of each mushroom.

3 Place the mushrooms on a large rimmed baking sheet. Brush both sides of each mushroom with the oil. Roast, turning once, until the mushrooms are tender, 25 to 30 minutes.

4 Transfer the mushrooms to a cutting board and thinly slice. Place in a serving bowl. Add the parsley, vinegar, salt, and pepper and toss gently to coat. Serve hot, warm, or at room temperature.

Each serving: 6 g carb, 62 cal, 4 g fat, 1 g sat fat, 0 mg chol, 2 g fib, 3 g pro, 147 mg sod • Carb Choices: ½; Exchanges: 1 veg, ½ fat

Vegetable-Stuffed Portobello Mushrooms

makes 4 servings

At any time of year, I like to vary this recipe depending on what's fresh in the market. You can use any mixture of chopped yellow squash, zucchini, fresh fennel, or even cooked leftover vegetables to stuff the mushrooms. I do always use the tomato slices on the bottom, since they add such great flavor. Vary the cheese and the herb, too—you can't mess these up.

4 large portobello mushrooms
4 teaspoons extra virgin olive oil, divided
1 small red onion, chopped
1 small yellow bell pepper, chopped
1 small red bell pepper, chopped
2 garlic cloves, minced
½ teaspoon kosher salt
⅛ teaspoon freshly ground pepper
2 tablespoons chopped fresh basil or Italian parsley
2 plum tomatoes, thinly sliced
1 ounce shredded Gruyère or fontina (about ¼ cup)

1 Cut away and discard the tough stems of the mushrooms. Using a spoon, gently scrape away and discard the dark gills on the underside of each mushroom.

2 Heat a large nonstick skillet over medium-high heat. Add 2 teaspoons of the oil and tilt the pan to coat the bottom evenly. Add the mushrooms, cover, and cook, turning once, until tender, 6 to 8 minutes. Transfer the mushrooms, stem side up, to a medium rimmed baking sheet. Cover to keep warm.

3 Add the remaining 2 teaspoons oil to the same skillet. Add the onion, bell peppers, garlic, salt, and ground pepper and cook, stirring often, until the vegetables are softened, 8 minutes. Remove from the heat and stir in the basil.

4 Preheat the broiler.

5 Divide the tomato slices evenly inside the mushrooms. Spoon the vegetable mixture evenly on top of the tomatoes. Sprinkle with the Gruyère. Broil the mushrooms until the cheese melts, about 2 minutes. Serve at once.

Each serving: 10 g carb, 123 cal, 7 g fat, 2 g sat fat, 8 mg chol, 3 g fib, 5 g pro, 173 mg sod • Carb Choices: ½; Exchanges: 2 veg, 1 fat

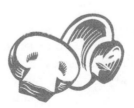

Grilled Mushrooms with Parmesan QUICK

makes 4 servings

Choose only firm-textured mushrooms for this recipe that will hold their shape on the grill. Cremini, portobello, white mushrooms, shiitakes, matsutake, and porcini are good choices. These are a delight to serve with whatever else you've got on the grill—chicken, steak, or pork chops.

1½ pounds mixed mushrooms (such as cremini, portobello, or white), left whole if small, thickly sliced if large

1 tablespoon plus ½ teaspoon extra virgin olive oil, divided

½ teaspoon kosher salt

⅛ teaspoon freshly ground pepper

½ ounce freshly shaved Parmesan (about ¼ cup)

1 Prepare the grill or heat a large grill pan over medium-high heat.

2 Place the mushrooms in a large bowl, drizzle with 1 tablespoon of the oil, and toss to coat. Brush the grill rack or grill pan with the remaining ½ teaspoon oil. Place the mushrooms on the grill rack or in the grill pan and grill, turning occasionally, until the mushrooms are tender and well browned, 8 to 10 minutes.

3 Return the mushrooms to the bowl, sprinkle with the salt and pepper, and toss to coat. Arrange the mushrooms on a serving platter and sprinkle with the Parmesan. Serve hot, warm, or at room temperature.

Each serving: 7 g carb, 98 cal, 5 g fat, 1 g sat fat, 3 mg chol, 1 g fib, 6 g pro, 204 mg sod • Carb Choices: ½; Exchanges: 2 veg, 1 fat

Shiitake Mushrooms with Ginger QUICK

makes 4 servings

Don't be tempted to add more oil or broth when you first place the mushrooms in the skillet. Within a minute or two, they start to exude their liquid and the mixture will become very moist. Serve these as a side dish with Asian-inspired beef, chicken, or fish entrées.

1½ pounds shiitake mushrooms

3 tablespoons Chicken Stock (page 149) or low-sodium chicken broth

2 tablespoons reduced-sodium soy sauce

1½ teaspoons rice vinegar

½ teaspoon cornstarch

½ teaspoon sugar

½ teaspoon chili-garlic paste

¼ teaspoon kosher salt

2 teaspoons canola oil

1 tablespoon minced fresh ginger

1 scallion, thinly sliced

1 Remove and discard the tough stems from the mushrooms and slice the caps.

2 Stir together the stock, soy sauce, vinegar, cornstarch, sugar, chili-garlic paste, and salt in a small bowl and set aside.

3 Heat a large wok or nonstick skillet over medium-high heat. Add the oil and tilt the pan to coat the bottom evenly. Add the ginger and cook, stirring constantly, until fragrant, 30 seconds.

4 Add the mushrooms and cook, stirring constantly, until softened, about 5 minutes. Stir the stock mixture and add to the skillet. Cook, stirring constantly, until the sauce comes to a boil and thickens slightly, 1 minute. Stir in the scallion. Spoon the mushrooms into a serving dish and serve at once.

Each serving: 15 g carb, 82 cal, 3 g fat, 0 g sat fat, 0 mg chol, 2 g fib, 2 g pro, 409 mg sod • Carb Choices: 1; Exchanges: 3 veg, ½ fat

Okra

Grilled Okra with Yogurt-Cilantro Sauce

makes 4 servings

Sprinkled with garam masala, an Indian spice blend of coriander, cumin, cardamom, cinnamon, and black pepper and grilled over a smoky fire, this recipe is a delight for okra lovers.

¼ cup fat-free Greek yogurt or strained yogurt (page 11)
1 small jalapeño, seeded and minced
1 tablespoon minced scallion
1 teaspoon fresh lime juice
1 tablespoon chopped fresh cilantro
Pinch plus ¼ teaspoon kosher salt, divided
12 ounces whole small okra
1½ teaspoons canola oil, divided
½ teaspoon garam masala

1 Stir together the yogurt, jalapeño, scallion, lime juice, cilantro, and the pinch of salt in a small bowl. Cover and refrigerate at least 30 minutes or up to 1 day.

2 Prepare the grill or heat a large grill pan over medium-high heat.

3 Combine the okra, 1 teaspoon of the oil, and the garam masala in a medium bowl and toss to coat. Brush the grill rack or grill pan with the remaining ½ teaspoon oil. Place the okra on the grill rack or in the grill pan and grill, turning often, until the okra is tender and well browned, about 15 minutes.

4 To serve, arrange the okra on a serving platter; sprinkle with the remaining ¼ teaspoon salt. Serve with the yogurt sauce.

Each serving: 6 g carb, 45 cal, 2 g fat, 0 g sat fat, 0 mg chol, 3 g fib, 2 g pro, 126 mg sod • Carb Choices: ½; Exchanges: 1 veg

Cajun Roasted Okra with Holy Trinity Salsa

makes 4 servings

The holy trinity of Cajun cooking that is the foundation of many recipes is bell peppers, celery, and onion. Here, combined with tomatoes, they make a fresh salsa for crisp roasted okra pods.

12 ounces whole small okra
2 teaspoons extra virgin olive oil
2 teaspoons no-salt Cajun seasoning
½ teaspoon kosher salt, divided
1 large tomato, chopped
¼ cup diced green or yellow bell pepper
¼ cup diced celery
2 tablespoons diced red onion
1 tablespoon chopped fresh Italian parsley
Pinch of ground cayenne

1 Preheat the oven to 425°F.

2 Place the okra on a large rimmed baking sheet. Drizzle with the oil, sprinkle with the Cajun seasoning and ¼ teaspoon of the salt, and toss to coat. Bake, stirring once, until the okra is lightly browned and tender, 20 to 25 minutes.

3 Meanwhile, stir together the tomato, bell pepper, celery, onion, parsley, remaining ¼ teaspoon salt, and the cayenne in a small bowl.

4 Arrange the okra on a serving platter. Spoon the salsa evenly over the okra. Serve hot or warm.

Each serving: 9 g carb, 59 cal, 3 g fat, 0 g sat fat, 0 mg chol, 3 g fib, 2 g pro, 155 mg sod • Carb Choices: ½; Exchanges: 2 veg, ½ fat

Unusual Onions

Sweet onions, cipolline or pearl onions, and leeks are a step above the more common members of the onion family. Braising, roasting, or grilling mellows the flavors of these already gentle onion cousins, turning them into rich and subtly sweet side dishes.

Once available only in the spring, different varieties of sweet onions are now available year round. In spring, look for Vidalias from Georgia and 1015s from Texas (named for the date they are planted) and in summer look for WallaWallas from Washington and NuMex Sweets from New Mexico. Myan Sweets and OsoSweets from South America are in abundance from fall through early spring. Maui onions from Hawaii are available almost all year round.

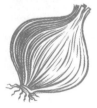

Onions

Crispy Oven-Fried Onion Rings

makes 4 servings

Be sure to use a sweet onion for this recipe, as a regular onion is too strong tasting. Serve them as an appetizer with Tomato Jam (page 599), as a side dish with a burger, or as a garnish on top of a grilled steak.

1 teaspoon plus 1 tablespoon canola oil, divided
2 tablespoons unbleached all-purpose flour
½ teaspoon salt
¼ teaspoon freshly ground pepper
⅛ teaspoon ground cayenne
2 large egg whites
2 tablespoons water
16 whole wheat or white Melba toasts, crumbled
2 large sweet onions

1 Preheat the oven to 400°F. Line 2 large rimmed baking sheets with foil. Place a wire rack in each baking sheet and brush each rack with ½ teaspoon of the oil.

2 Combine the flour, salt, pepper, and cayenne in a large resealable plastic bag. Place the egg whites and water in a shallow dish and beat lightly with a fork.

3 Place the Melba toasts in a food processor and process until fine crumbs form. Combine the Melba toast crumbs and the remaining 1 tablespoon oil in another shallow dish. Using your fingers, blend the oil evenly into the crumbs.

4 Cut the onions into ½-inch-thick slices and separate them into 24 large rings, reserving the smaller inner rings for another use.

5 Place the onion rings, a few at a time, into the plastic bag. Seal the bag and shake to coat the

onion rings. Dip the onion rings into the egg white mixture, then into the melba toast crumbs, pressing to adhere the crumbs.

6 Arrange the onion rings in a single layer on the racks. Bake until the onion rings are golden brown, 12 to 15 minutes (do not turn). Serve at once.

Each serving: 25 g carb, 165 cal, 5 g fat, 0 g sat fat, 0 mg chol, 2 g fib, 5 g pro, 493 mg sod • Carb Choices: 1½; Exchanges: 1 starch, 1 veg, 1 fat

Balsamic-Baked Sweet Onions

makes 4 servings

These are a perfect partner to any grilled or broiled steak. To put them over the top, sprinkle each onion slice with about ½ tablespoon of blue cheese just before serving. Use an inexpensive brand of balsamic vinegar for this recipe—the good stuff is not required here.

1 large sweet onion
2 teaspoons extra virgin olive oil
½ teaspoon kosher salt
⅛ teaspoon freshly ground pepper
¾ cup balsamic vinegar

1 Preheat the oven to 400°F.

2 Cut a thin slice off the stem and root end of the onion and discard. Peel the onion and cut into 4 slices.

3 Heat a large ovenproof skillet (large enough for the onion slices to fit in a single layer) over medium-high heat. Add the oil and tilt the pan to coat the bottom evenly. Sprinkle the onion slices with the salt and pepper and place in the skillet. Cook, carefully turning once with a wide spatula to prevent the rings from separating, until the onions are browned, about 4 minutes. Add the vinegar and bring to a boil. Transfer the skillet to the oven and bake, uncovered, turning once with a wide spatula, until the onions are tender, 40 to 45 minutes.

4 Arrange the onions on a serving platter, lifting them from the skillet with a wide spatula. Drizzle the onions with the liquid remaining in the skillet. Serve hot, warm, or at room temperature.

Each serving: 13 g carb, 77 cal, 3 g fat, 0 g sat fat, 0 mg chol, 1 g fib, 1 g pro, 158 mg sod • Carb Choices: 1; Exchanges: 1 veg, ½ fat

Grilled Sweet Onion Slices with Sherry Vinegar and Thyme QUICK

makes 4 servings

Serve this dish in summer with grilled steaks and make it indoors in a grill pan in winter to serve with meatloaf or roasted pork tenderloin.

1 large sweet onion
2½ teaspoons extra virgin olive oil, divided
2 teaspoons sherry vinegar or red wine vinegar
1 teaspoon chopped fresh thyme or
**   ¼ teaspoon dried thyme**
½ teaspoon kosher salt
Pinch of freshly ground pepper

1 Prepare the grill or heat a large grill pan over medium-high heat.

2 Cut a thin slice off the stem and root end of the onion and discard. Peel the onion and cut into 4 slices.

3 Brush the onion slices with 2 teaspoons of the oil. Brush the grill rack or grill pan with the remaining ½ teaspoon oil. Place the onions on the grill rack or in the grill pan and grill, turning once using a wide spatula to prevent the rings from separating, until the onions are tender, 8 to 10 minutes.

4 To serve, arrange the onions on a serving platter. Drizzle with the vinegar, sprinkle with the thyme, salt, and pepper. Serve hot, warm, or at room temperature.

Each serving: 6 g carb, 54 cal, 3 g fat, 0 g sat fat, 0 mg chol, 1 g fib, 1 g pro, 147 mg sod • Carb Choices: ½; Exchanges: 1 veg, ½ fat

Cipolline Onions with Wine and Rosemary

makes 4 servings

Cipolline are small button-shaped onions that originated in Italy. Cipolline are very sweet and mild flavored, but if they are not available, regular pearl onions are a fine substitute in this recipe.

1¼ pounds cipolline or pearl onions
2 teaspoons extra virgin olive oil
½ cup dry red wine
½ cup Chicken Stock (page 149) or low-sodium chicken broth
½ teaspoon kosher salt
2 teaspoons chopped fresh rosemary or thyme
⅛ teaspoon freshly ground pepper

1 Bring a medium saucepan of water to a boil over high heat. Add the onions and cook 1 minute. Drain in a colander and rinse with cold running water. Peel the onions (the skins will slip off easily after boiling).

2 Heat a medium nonstick skillet over medium heat. Add the oil and tilt the pan to coat the bottom evenly. Add the onions and cook, stirring often, until lightly browned, 5 minutes. Add the wine, stock, and salt and bring to a boil. Reduce the heat to low, cover, and simmer until the onions are tender, 30 to 35 minutes. If excess liquid remains in the pan, uncover and cook until most of the liquid evaporates. Stir in the rosemary and pepper. Spoon the onions into a serving dish and serve hot, warm, or at room temperature.

Each serving: 13 g carb, 100 cal, 2 g fat, 0 g sat fat, 1 mg chol, 3 g fib, 2 g pro, 158 mg sod • Carb Choices: 1; Exchanges: 2 veg, ½ fat

Leeks Braised in White Wine

makes 4 servings

I love the look of braised leeks that are simply cut in half lengthwise, but I can never get all the grit out of them unless I cut them into slices. This dish is a compromise: the leeks are cut into long slices for thorough washing and then braised in wine and olive oil. They make a nice accompaniment to fish or chicken.

4 medium leeks, cut in half lengthwise and sliced into 3-inch slices
1 tablespoon extra virgin olive oil
1 teaspoon kosher salt
½ cup dry white wine
1 teaspoon lemon juice
Pinch of freshly ground pepper

1 Submerge the sliced leeks in a large bowl of cold water, lift them out, and drain in a colander. Repeat, using fresh water, until no grit remains in the bottom of the bowl. Drain the leeks well.

2 Heat a large nonstick skillet over medium-high heat. Add the oil and tilt the pan to coat the bottom evenly. Add the leeks and salt and cook, stirring often, until the leeks are wilted, about 5 minutes. Add the wine and bring to a boil. Reduce the heat to low, cover, and simmer, stirring occasionally, until the leeks are very tender, about 30 minutes. Remove from the heat and stir in the lemon juice and pepper. Spoon the leeks into a serving dish and serve hot or warm.

Each serving: 13 g carb, 110 cal, 4 g fat, 1 g sat fat, 0 mg chol, 2 g fib, 1 g pro, 298 mg sod • Carb Choices: 1; Exchanges: 2 veg, ½ fat

Peas

Fresh English Peas

QUICK | HIGH FIBER

makes 4 servings

English peas are my favorite vegetable and this simple recipe is the best way I know to eat them. I cannot let the fleeting season of fresh peas pass without getting my fill, so I sometimes make these even for breakfast in early May. And, like fresh summer corn, peas must have butter.

**2 cups shelled fresh English peas
(about 2¼ pounds unshelled peas)**
2 teaspoons unsalted butter
½ teaspoon kosher salt

1 Bring a large saucepan of water to a boil over high heat. Add the peas, return to a boil, and cook just until the peas are tender, about 3 minutes. (Do not overcook.) Drain in a colander.

2 Spoon the peas into a serving bowl, add the butter and salt, and stir to combine. Serve at once.

Each serving: 14 g carb, 95 cal, 2 g fat, 1 g sat fat, 5 mg chol, 5 g fib, 5 g pro, 145 mg sod • Carb Choices: 1; Exchanges: 1 starch, ½ fat

English Pea Puree QUICK

makes 4 servings

This is a quick and elegant side dish that makes good use of frozen peas. If you have an abundance of fresh peas, by all means use them. You'll need about 2 cups of fresh peas (from about 2¼ pounds of unshelled peas).

1 (10-ounce) package frozen green peas
1 garlic clove, thinly sliced
1 teaspoon lemon juice
¼ cup water
**1 tablespoon coarsely chopped fresh mint or
Italian parsley (optional)**
2 teaspoons extra virgin olive oil
¾ teaspoon kosher salt

1 Bring a large saucepan of water to a boil over high heat. Add the peas and garlic and cook 3 minutes. Drain in a colander.

2 Place the pea mixture and the remaining ingredients in a food processor and process until smooth. Spoon the peas into a serving dish and serve hot or warm.

Each serving: 10 g carb, 77 cal, 3 g fat, 0 g sat fat, 0 mg chol, 3 g fib, 4 g pro, 290 mg sod • Carb Choices: ½; Exchanges: ½ starch, ½ fat

Sugar Snap Peas with Ginger and Orange QUICK

makes 4 servings

You barely have to get sugar snap peas warm in the water and they are crisp-tender. Take care not to overcook them or they will be mushy.

2 teaspoons grated fresh ginger
2 teaspoons unsalted butter
1 teaspoon grated orange zest
½ teaspoon kosher salt
1 pound fresh sugar snap peas, trimmed

1 Stir together the ginger, butter, orange zest, and salt in a medium serving bowl. Set aside.

2 Bring a large saucepan of water to a boil over high heat. Add the peas and cook until just crisp-tender, 1 minute. Drain in a colander.

3 Add the peas to the ginger mixture and toss gently to coat. Serve at once.

Each serving: 10 g carb, 71 cal, 2 g fat, 1 g sat fat, 5 mg chol, 3 g fib, 3 g pro, 154 mg sod • Carb Choices: ½; Exchanges: 2 veg, ½ fat

Potatoes

Buttermilk Mashed Potatoes QUICK

makes 4 servings

The secret to lump-free mashed potatoes is to make sure the potatoes are very tender before mashing them. For extra fluffy potatoes, beat them with an electric mixer—but don't overbeat or they will be gummy. Beat just until the potatoes are smooth.

1 pound Yukon Gold or baking potatoes, peeled and cut into 1-inch chunks
1 cup low-sodium vegetable or chicken broth
4 to 5 tablespoons low-fat buttermilk
2 teaspoons unsalted butter
½ teaspoon kosher salt
Pinch of freshly ground pepper

1 Place the potatoes and broth in a large saucepan and bring to a boil over high heat. Cover, reduce the heat to low, and simmer until the potatoes are fork-tender, about 15 minutes.

2 Drain the potatoes in a colander and return to the pan. Add 4 tablespoons of the buttermilk, the butter, salt, and pepper. Mash the potatoes with a potato masher to the desired consistency, adding the remaining 1 tablespoon buttermilk, if needed. Spoon the potatoes into a serving dish and serve at once.

Each serving: 22 g carb, 115 cal, 2 g fat, 2 g sat fat, 6 mg chol, 2 g fib, 3 g pro, 275 mg sod • Carb Choices: 1½; Exchanges: 1½ starch, ½ fat

HERB MASHED POTATOES QUICK : Follow the Buttermilk Mashed Potatoes recipe, above, adding 1 tablespoon chopped fresh parsley, basil, or tarragon, or 1 tablespoon minced fresh chives, with the buttermilk in step 2.

Each serving: 22 g carb, 115 cal, 2 g fat, 2 g sat fat, 6 mg chol, 2 g fib, 3 g pro, 275 mg sod • Carb Choices: 1½; Exchanges: 1½ starch, ½ fat

BLUE CHEESE AND CHIVE MASHED POTATOES QUICK : Follow the Buttermilk Mashed Potatoes recipe, at left, adding 2 tablespoons room-temperature crumbled blue cheese and 1 tablespoon minced fresh chives with the buttermilk in step 2.

Each serving: 22 g carb, 140 cal, 4 g fat, 3 g sat fat, 11 mg chol, 2 g fib, 4 g pro, 374 mg sod • Carb Choices: 1½; Exchanges: 1½ starch, ½ fat

Roasted Garlic Mashed Potatoes

makes 4 servings

Sweet roasted garlic is a wonderful partner to dress up ordinary mashed potatoes.

6 garlic cloves, unpeeled
1 pound Yukon Gold or baking potatoes, peeled and cut into 1-inch chunks
1 cup low-sodium vegetable or chicken broth
¼ cup plain low-fat yogurt
2 teaspoons unsalted butter
½ teaspoon kosher salt
Pinch of freshly ground pepper

1 Preheat the oven to 350°F.

2 Wrap the garlic cloves in a sheet of foil and place in a small baking dish. Bake until the garlic is very soft, about 30 minutes. Unwrap the garlic and let stand until cool enough to handle. Squeeze the garlic pulp from each clove into a small bowl.

3 Meanwhile, place the potatoes and broth in a large saucepan and bring to a boil over high heat. Cover, reduce the heat to low, and simmer until the potatoes are fork-tender, about 15 minutes.

4 Drain the potatoes in a colander and return to the pan. Add the garlic pulp, the yogurt, butter, salt, and pepper. Mash the potatoes with a potato masher to the desired consistency. Spoon the potatoes into a serving dish and serve at once.

Each serving: 23 g carb, 121 cal, 2 g fat, 1 g sat fat, 6 mg chol, 2 g fib, 3 g pro, 276 mg sod • Carb Choices: 1½; Exchanges: 1½ starch, ½ fat

Two-Potato Puree [QUICK]

makes 4 servings

Combining regular and sweet potatoes makes for an interesting dish that's not too sweet. Serve this with pork loin or chicken.

8 ounces Yukon Gold or baking potatoes, peeled and cut into 1-inch chunks

8 ounces sweet potatoes, peeled and cut into 1-inch chunks

4 to 5 tablespoons 1% low-fat milk

2 teaspoons unsalted butter

¾ teaspoon kosher salt

Pinch of freshly ground pepper

1 Place the potatoes in a large saucepan. Add water to cover and bring to a boil. Cover, reduce the heat to low, and simmer until the potatoes are fork-tender, about 15 minutes.

2 Drain the potatoes in a colander and return to the pan. Add 4 tablespoons of the milk, the butter, salt, and pepper. Mash the potatoes with a potato masher to the desired consistency, adding the remaining 1 tablespoon milk, if needed. Spoon the potatoes into a serving dish and serve at once.

Each serving: 18 g carb, 97 cal, 2 g fat, 1 g sat fat, 6 mg chol, 2 g fib, 2 g pro, 234 mg sod • Carb Choices: 1; Exchanges: 1 starch, ½ fat

Potato-Cauliflower Mash

[QUICK]

makes 8 servings

The mildly cabbagey flavor of cauliflower is a natural partner for neutral potatoes.

1 pound Yukon Gold or baking potatoes, peeled and cut into 1-inch chunks

1 pound cauliflower, cut into 1-inch florets (about 4 cups)

⅓ cup plain low-fat yogurt

½ teaspoon kosher salt

⅛ teaspoon freshly ground pepper

1 Place the potatoes and cauliflower in a large saucepan. Add water to cover and bring to a boil over high heat. Cover, reduce the heat to low, and simmer until the vegetables are fork-tender, about 15 minutes.

2 Drain the vegetables in a colander and return to the pan. Add the yogurt, salt, and pepper and mash with a potato masher to the desired consistency. Spoon the potatoes into a serving dish and serve at once.

Each serving: 11 g carb, 53 cal, 0 g fat, 0 g sat fat, 1 mg chol, 1 g fib, 2 g pro, 86 mg sod • Carb Choices: 1; Exchanges: 1 starch

Chile-Lime Oven Fries

makes 4 servings

Ancho chile and lime zest turn fries into a stellar side dish. Serve with burgers or fish.

2 medium baking potatoes (about 1 pound), well scrubbed

2 teaspoons canola oil

¼ teaspoon ancho chile powder or chili powder

¼ teaspoon ground cumin

¾ teaspoon kosher salt, divided

¼ teaspoon grated lime zest

1 Preheat the oven to 425°F.

2 Cut each potato into 8 wedges and place on a large rimmed baking sheet. Drizzle with the oil and sprinkle with the chile powder, cumin, and ¼ teaspoon of the salt. Turn to coat. Arrange the potatoes in a single layer.

3 Bake 25 minutes. Turn the wedges and bake until the potatoes are tender and well browned, 8 to 10 minutes longer.

4 Arrange the potatoes on a serving platter. Stir together the remaining ½ teaspoon salt and the lime zest in a small bowl and sprinkle over the potatoes. Serve at once.

Each serving: 20 g carb, 109 cal, 3 g fat, 0 g sat fat, 0 mg chol, 3 g fib, 2 g pro, 220 mg sod • Carb Choices: 1; Exchanges: 1 starch, ½ fat

Roasted Potatoes with Fresh Herbs and Lemon

makes 4 servings

If your market has a wide selection of baby potatoes, select several varieties to make this dish even more appealing. Try to choose potatoes that are nearly the same size so they will cook in the same amount of time.

1 pound baby or fingerling potatoes, well scrubbed and halved

2 teaspoons extra virgin olive oil

½ teaspoon kosher salt

⅛ teaspoon freshly ground pepper

2 teaspoons any combination minced fresh chives, Italian parsley, rosemary, or thyme

½ teaspoon grated lemon zest

1 tablespoon lemon juice

1 Preheat the oven to 425°F.

2 Place the potatoes on a large rimmed baking sheet. Drizzle with the oil, and sprinkle with the salt and pepper. Toss to coat. Arrange the potatoes in a single layer.

3 Roast, turning the potatoes once, until tender and browned, 30 to 35 minutes.

4 Transfer the potatoes to a serving platter, sprinkle with the herbs, lemon zest, and lemon juice, and toss to combine. Serve at once.

Each serving: 18 g carb, 101 cal, 3 g fat, 0 g sat fat, 0 mg chol, 2 g fib, 2 g pro, 147 mg sod • Carb Choices: 1; Exchanges: 1 starch, ½ fat

Rutabagas and Turnips

Roasted Rutabagas with Molasses

makes 4 servings

Just a touch of molasses makes all the difference in balancing the flavor of this dish. You can use maple syrup instead of molasses, if you wish.

1 pound rutabagas, peeled and cut into 2-inch pieces

2 teaspoons extra virgin olive oil

½ teaspoon kosher salt

Pinch of freshly ground pepper

2 teaspoons molasses

1 teaspoon chopped fresh rosemary

1 Preheat the oven to 425°F.

2 Place the rutabagas on a large rimmed baking sheet. Drizzle with the oil and sprinkle with the salt and pepper. Toss to coat. Arrange the rutabagas in a single layer.

3 Roast, turning the rutabagas once, until tender and browned, 35 to 40 minutes.

4 Transfer the rutabagas to a serving platter, drizzle with the molasses, sprinkle with the rosemary, and toss to combine. Serve hot or warm.

Each serving: 10 g carb, 65 cal, 2 g fat, 0 g sat fat, 0 mg chol, 2 g fib, 1 g pro, 161 mg sod • Carb Choices: ½; Exchanges: 2 veg, ½ fat

Rutabaga-Apple Puree

makes 4 servings

You would never believe an elegant side dish could be made from such common ingredients as rutabagas and apples. This lovely pairing makes a complementary match for roasted pork loin or chicken.

1 pound rutabagas, peeled and cut into 1-inch pieces

2 cups low-sodium vegetable or chicken broth

1 small Granny Smith apple, peeled, cored, and cut into wedges

2 teaspoons unsalted butter

2 teaspoons packed light brown sugar

¼ teaspoon kosher salt

Pinch of freshly ground pepper

1 Combine the rutabaga and broth in a medium saucepan and bring to a boil over high heat. Reduce the heat to low, cover, and simmer until almost tender, 30 to 35 minutes. Add the apple and simmer until tender, but not falling apart, about 8 minutes longer. Drain in a colander, reserving the cooking liquid.

2 Place the rutabaga mixture, butter, sugar, salt, and pepper in a food processor. Process until smooth, adding the reserved cooking liquid as needed to make a smooth puree. Spoon the puree into a serving dish and serve at once.

Each serving: 17 g carb, 90 cal, 2 g fat, 1 g sat fat, 5 mg chol, 3 g fib, 2 g pro, 320 mg sod • Carb Choices: 1; Exchanges: ½ carb, 2 veg, ½ fat

Roasted Turnips with Honey and Toasted Spices

makes 4 servings

This is a dish for people who don't like root vegetables. The toasted fennel and coriander complement the flavor of the turnips perfectly and a touch of honey smoothes out any bitterness.

½ teaspoon fennel seeds

½ teaspoon coriander seeds

6 whole black peppercorns

1½ pounds turnips, peeled and cut into ¾-inch pieces

2 teaspoons extra virgin olive oil

¾ teaspoon kosher salt

1 teaspoon honey

1 Preheat the oven to 425°F.

2 Place the fennel, coriander, and pepper in a small dry skillet over medium heat and toast, shaking the pan often, until the spices are fragrant, about 3 minutes. Transfer to a small dish and allow to cool. Place the spices in a mortar and crush with a pestle. Alternatively, place the spices in a small resealable plastic bag. Seal the bag, place on a cutting board, and crush using a meat mallet or the back of a large spoon.

3 Place the turnips on a large rimmed baking sheet. Drizzle with the oil and sprinkle with the toasted spices and the salt. Toss to coat. Arrange the turnips in a single layer.

4 Roast, turning the turnips once, until tender and browned, 35 to 40 minutes.

5 Transfer the turnips to a serving bowl, drizzle with the honey, and toss to coat. Serve hot or warm.

Each serving: 10 g carb, 65 cal, 3 g fat, 0 g sat fat, 0 mg chol, 3 g fib, 1 g pro, 302 mg sod • Carb Choices: ½; Exchanges: 2 veg, ½ fat

Summer Squash

Sautéed Zucchini with Cilantro and Lime QUICK

makes 4 servings

This simple 10-minute side dish is a summer staple at my house. Try it with fresh basil and lemon juice instead of the cilantro and lime juice. It's light, refreshing, and nutritious.

2 teaspoons extra virgin olive oil
1 garlic clove, minced
1 pound zucchini, halved lengthwise and sliced
1 tablespoon lime juice
½ teaspoon kosher salt
Pinch of freshly ground pepper
1 tablespoon chopped fresh cilantro

1 Heat a large nonstick skillet over medium-high heat. Add the oil and tilt the pan to coat the bottom evenly. Add the garlic and cook, stirring constantly, until fragrant, 30 seconds.

2 Add the zucchini and cook, stirring constantly, until crisp-tender, 3 minutes. Stir in the lime juice, salt, and pepper.

3 Spoon the zucchini onto a serving platter and sprinkle with the cilantro. Serve hot, warm, or at room temperature.

Each serving: 4 g carb, 39 cal, 2 g fat, 0 g sat fat, 0 mg chol, 1 g fib, 1 g pro, 143 mg sod • Carb Choices: 0; Exchanges: 1 veg, ½ fat

Summer Squash with Onion and Dill en Papillote

makes 4 servings

You can add halved cherry tomatoes, a medium chopped tomato, or thinly sliced bell pepper to the packets. You can also use aluminum foil to make the packets and cook them on a medium-high grill for 15 to 20 minutes.

1 pound zucchini, yellow squash, or pattypan squash (or combination), cut in half lengthwise and sliced
¼ cup thinly sliced red onion
1 tablespoon chopped fresh dill
2 teaspoons extra virgin olive oil
½ teaspoon kosher salt
½ teaspoon grated lemon zest
1 garlic clove, minced
Pinch of freshly ground pepper

1 Preheat the oven to 450°F.

2 Place all the ingredients in a large bowl and toss to combine.

3 Tear off four 24 x 12-inch pieces of parchment paper. Fold each piece in half crosswise and cut each one to make a rounded heart shape. Open a parchment "heart" and arrange one-quarter of the vegetable mixture in the middle of one side.

4 Beginning at the bottom end of each "heart," fold the edges of the parchment in overlapping 1-inch segments, crimping as you go, to form a tight seal. (You can also use aluminum foil to make the packets.)

5 Place the packages on a large rimmed baking sheet and bake until the vegetables are tender, 20 minutes. Place the packets on plates and serve at once. Use caution when opening the packets, since steam will escape. Serve at once.

Each serving: 5 g carb, 40 cal, 2 g fat, 0 g sat fat, 0 mg chol, 2 g fib, 1 g pro, 143 mg sod • Carb Choices: 0; Exchanges: 1 veg, ½ fat

Roasted Summer Squash Spears with Basil and Mint

makes 4 servings

A mix of zucchini and yellow squash makes a beautiful presentation for a summer meal. For a buffet, double the recipe and arrange the squash on a platter. Garnish with cherry tomatoes and mint and basil sprigs.

1 medium zucchini (about 8 ounces)

1 medium yellow summer squash (about 8 ounces)

2 teaspoons extra virgin olive oil

¼ teaspoon kosher salt

Pinch of freshly ground pepper

2 teaspoons lemon juice

1 tablespoon thinly sliced fresh basil leaves

2 teaspoons thinly sliced fresh mint leaves

1 Preheat the oven to 425°F.

2 Halve the zucchini and yellow squash crosswise and cut each half into quarters lengthwise. Place on a large rimmed baking sheet. Drizzle with the oil and sprinkle with the salt and pepper. Toss to coat. Arrange in a single layer.

3 Roast, turning the squash once, until tender and browned, 25 to 30 minutes.

4 Transfer the squash to a serving platter, drizzle with the lemon juice, and sprinkle with the basil and mint. Serve hot, warm, or at room temperature.

Each serving: 4 g carb, 37 cal, 2 g fat, 0 g sat fat, 0 mg chol, 1 g fib, 1 g pro, 73 mg sod • Carb Choices: 0; Exchanges: 1 veg, ½ fat

Grilled Summer Squash with Corn Vinaigrette

makes 4 servings

Serve the corn vinaigrette on almost any grilled or roasted summer vegetables, or drizzle it over a platter of beefsteak tomatoes.

1 small ear corn, kernels cut from the cob

1 tablespoon white wine vinegar

1 large garlic clove, crushed through a press

½ teaspoon Dijon mustard

¾ teaspoon kosher salt, divided

Pinch plus ⅛ teaspoon freshly ground pepper, divided

1 tablespoon plus 2½ teaspoons extra virgin olive oil, divided

2 teaspoons chopped fresh thyme

1 pound zucchini, yellow squash, or pattypan squash (or combination), cut into ½-inch slices

1 small red onion, cut into wedges through the root end

1 Bring a small saucepan of water to a boil over high heat. Add the corn kernels and cook 1 minute. Drain the corn in a colander and cool.

2 Whisk together the vinegar, garlic, mustard, ½ teaspoon of the salt, and the pinch of pepper in a small bowl. Slowly whisk in 1 tablespoon of the oil. Stir in ¼ cup of the cooked corn, reserving the remaining corn for another use. Stir in the thyme.

3 Prepare the grill or heat a large grill pan over medium-high heat.

4 Combine the squash, onion, 2 teaspoons of the remaining oil, the remaining ¼ teaspoon salt, and the remaining ⅛ teaspoon pepper in a large bowl and toss to coat. Brush the grill rack or the grill pan with the remaining ½ teaspoon oil. Place the vegetables on the grill rack or in the grill pan and grill, turning often, until the vegetables are tender and well browned, 6 to 8 minutes.

5 Arrange the squash and onions on a serving platter and drizzle with the vinaigrette. Serve hot, warm, or at room temperature.

Each serving: 7 g carb, 86 cal, 6 g fat, 1 g sat fat, 0 mg chol, 2 g fib, 2 g pro, 238 mg sod • Carb Choices: ½; Exchanges: 1 veg, 1 fat

Roasted Zucchini with Toasted Cumin and Basil

makes 4 servings

2 medium zucchini

2 teaspoons plus 1 tablespoon extra virgin olive oil, divided

½ teaspoon kosher salt, divided

¼ teaspoon cumin seeds

½ teaspoon grated lemon zest

2 teaspoons lemon juice

Pinch of freshly ground pepper

1 tablespoon chopped fresh basil

1 Preheat the oven to 425°F.

2 Halve the zucchini crosswise and cut each half into quarters lengthwise. Place on a large rimmed baking sheet. Drizzle with 2 teaspoons of the oil and sprinkle with ¼ teaspoon of the salt. Toss to coat. Arrange in a single layer.

3 Roast, turning the zucchini once, until tender and browned, 25 to 30 minutes.

4 Meanwhile, place the cumin in a small dry skillet over medium heat and toast, shaking the pan often, until the cumin is fragrant, about 3 minutes. Transfer to a small plate and allow to cool. Place the cumin in a mortar and crush with a pestle. Alternatively, place the cumin in a small resealable plastic bag. Seal the bag, place on a cutting board, and crush using a meat mallet or the back of a large spoon.

5 Place the cumin in a small bowl. Add the lemon zest, lemon juice, the remaining ¼ teaspoon salt, and the pepper and whisk to combine. Slowly whisk in the remaining 1 tablespoon oil.

6 Arrange the zucchini on a platter, drizzle with the oil mixture, and sprinkle with the basil. Serve hot, warm, or at room temperature.

Each serving: 4 g carb, 70 cal, 6 g fat, 1 g sat fat, 0 mg chol, 1 g fib, 1 g pro, 151 mg sod • Carb Choices: 0; Exchanges: 1 veg, 1 fat

Sweet Potatoes

Roasted Sweet Potatoes with Ginger and Lime

makes 4 servings

These potatoes, with their deliciously crisp caramelized crust, are a nice change from oven fries made with white potatoes. You can enjoy them plain if you wish, or with the ginger and lime.

2 medium sweet potatoes (about 1 pound)

2 teaspoons extra virgin olive oil

¼ teaspoon kosher salt

1 tablespoon lime juice

1 teaspoon grated fresh ginger

1 Preheat the oven to 425°F.

2 Peel the potatoes and cut each into 8 wedges. Place the potatoes on a large rimmed baking sheet. Drizzle with the oil and sprinkle with the salt. Toss to coat. Arrange in a single layer.

3 Roast, turning the potatoes once, until tender and browned, 30 to 35 minutes.

4 Stir together the lime juice and ginger in a small bowl. To serve, arrange the potatoes on a serving platter, drizzle with the lime mixture, and turn to coat. Serve hot or warm.

Each serving: 15 g carb, 84 cal, 2 g fat, 0 g sat fat, 0 mg chol, 2 g fib, 1 g pro, 95 mg sod • Carb Choices: 1; Exchanges: 1 starch, ½ fat

ROASTED SWEET POTATOES WITH HONEY AND ROSEMARY: Follow the Roasted Sweet Potatoes with Ginger and Lime recipe, above, through step 3. Stir together 1 teaspoon honey and 1 teaspoon grated fresh ginger. Drizzle over the potatoes and turn to coat.

Each serving: 16 g carb, 90 cal, 2 g fat, 0 g sat fat, 0 mg chol, 2 g fib, 1 g pro, 95 mg sod • Carb Choices: 1; Exchanges: 1 starch, ½ fat

Sweet Potato and Pear Puree [HIGH FIBER]

makes 4 servings

Fresh pear tempers the sweetness of the potatoes in this dish. Double the recipe for a Thanksgiving crowd. You can make it ahead and reheat in a nonstick pan over a low flame.

2 medium sweet potatoes (about 1 pound), peeled and cut into 2-inch pieces
1 cup apple cider or apple juice
1 very ripe Bartlett pear, peeled, cored, and chopped
2 teaspoons unsalted butter
¼ teaspoon kosher salt
Pinch of ground nutmeg

1 Combine the potatoes and the apple cider in a large saucepan and bring to a boil over high heat. Cover, reduce the heat to low, and simmer until the potatoes are almost tender, 20 minutes. Add the pear and cook until the potatoes and pear are very tender, about 5 minutes longer. Drain in a colander, reserving the cooking liquid.

2 Place the potato mixture, butter, salt, and nutmeg in a food processor. Process until smooth, adding the reserved cooking liquid as needed to make a smooth puree. Spoon the potatoes into a serving dish and serve at once.

Each serving: 28 g carb, 133 cal, 2 g fat, 1 g sat fat, 5 mg chol, 4 g fib, 2 g pro, 102 mg sod • Carb Choices: 2; Exchanges: 1 starch, 1 fruit, ½ fat

Sweet Potato Puree with Cranberries [QUICK]

makes 8 servings

Silky smooth sweet potatoes swirled with fresh cranberries makes the perfect Thanksgiving side dish.

4 medium sweet potatoes (about 2¼ pounds), peeled and cut into 1-inch pieces
¾ cup fresh cranberries
⅓ cup packed light brown sugar
3 tablespoons orange juice
½ teaspoon ground cinnamon
¼ teaspoon kosher salt
Pinch of ground cloves
½ teaspoon vanilla extract

1 In a saucepan fitted with a steamer basket, bring 1 inch of water to a boil over high heat. Add the potatoes, reduce the heat to low, cover, and steam until tender, about 15 minutes.

2 Meanwhile, combine the cranberries, sugar, orange juice, cinnamon, salt, and cloves in a small saucepan. Bring to a boil over high heat, reduce the heat to low, and simmer until the cranberries pop, about 5 minutes. Remove from the heat and stir in the vanilla.

3 Transfer the potatoes to a large bowl. Mash using a potato masher until smooth. Stir in the cranberry mixture. Serve at once.

Each serving: 26 g carb, 110 cal, 0 g fat, 0 g sat fat, 0 mg chol, 3 g fib, 2 g pro, 66 mg sod • Carb Choices: 2; Exchanges: 1 starch, 1 carb

Super Sweet Potatoes

Sweet potatoes are a must at Thanksgiving, but they are so delicious and nutritious, they should be enjoyed more often. A medium sweet potato (about 8 ounces) has 2 Carb Choices (30 grams of carbs) and just 125 calories. But it has all the vitamin A you need for a day and 5 grams of fiber—probably more than most people get in their breakfast cereal. And they're so sweet, it's almost like getting permission to eat dessert with your meal.

Tomatoes

Broiled Beefsteak Tomatoes with Basil and Parmesan QUICK

makes 4 servings

Make this recipe only with peak-of-summer tomatoes and serve them as a centerpiece to a summer vegetable plate, or as a side dish with sautéed fish fillets or pan-seared steaks.

2½ teaspoons extra virgin olive oil, divided
2 large beefsteak tomatoes, cut in half horizontally
½ teaspoon kosher salt
Pinch of freshly ground pepper
1 ounce freshly grated Parmesan (about ¼ cup)
1 tablespoon chopped fresh basil

1 Preheat the broiler. Brush a broiler pan with ½ teaspoon of the oil.

2 Brush the cut side of the tomatoes with the remaining 2 teaspoons oil and sprinkle with the salt and pepper. Place the tomatoes cut side up on the broiler pan and broil until the tomatoes begin to soften, about 6 minutes. Remove from the oven and sprinkle with the Parmesan. Broil until the cheese melts, 1 to 2 minutes longer.

3 Transfer the tomatoes to a serving platter and sprinkle with the basil. Serve hot, warm, or at room temperature.

Each serving: 3 g carb, 35 cal, 2 g fat, 1 g sat fat, 0 mg chol, 1 g fib, 1 g pro, 144 mg sod • Carb Choices: 0; Exchanges: 1 veg, ½ fat

Braised Plum Tomatoes

QUICK

makes 4 servings

You want the tomatoes to brown slightly, but you don't want to let the garlic burn, so watch these very carefully as they cook. They're ready in 5 minutes, so it's an easy task. You can use balsamic vinegar in this recipe, too, though it will darken the color of the tomatoes.

2 teaspoons extra virgin olive oil
1 garlic clove, minced
4 plum tomatoes, halved lengthwise
2 tablespoons sherry vinegar
½ teaspoon kosher salt
Pinch of freshly ground pepper
1 tablespoon chopped fresh basil or 2 teaspoons chopped fresh rosemary or thyme

1 Heat a large nonstick skillet over medium-high heat. Add the oil and tilt the pan to coat the bottom evenly. Add the garlic and cook, stirring constantly, until fragrant, 30 seconds.

2 Add the tomatoes, cut side down, and cook until lightly browned, 2 minutes. Turn the tomatoes. Add the vinegar and sprinkle with the salt and pepper. Reduce the heat to low, cover, and cook until the tomatoes are softened, 2 to 3 minutes.

3 Transfer the tomatoes to a serving dish. Drizzle with any juices remaining in the skillet and sprinkle with the basil. Serve hot, warm, or at room temperature.

Each serving: 3 g carb, 37 cal, 3 g fat, 0 g sat fat, 0 mg chol, 1 g fib, 1 g pro, 118 mg sod • Carb Choices: 0; Exchanges: 1 veg, ½ fat

Roasted Plum Tomatoes with Garlic and Capers

makes 4 servings

Roasting is the best way to coax flavor from plum tomatoes in the winter. These require no further attention once you get them in the oven, so they're almost an effortless side dish to make. You can double the recipe to have them on hand to serve with pasta. Slip them out of their skins, reheat gently in a nonstick skillet, and toss with hot pasta. Sprinkle with crumbled feta or grated Parmesan to finish the dish.

4 large plum tomatoes, halved lengthwise
2 teaspoons extra virgin olive oil
2 garlic cloves, minced
¼ teaspoon kosher salt
Pinch of freshly ground pepper
2 teaspoons capers, rinsed and drained

1 Preheat the oven to 400°F.

2 Place the tomatoes on a large rimmed baking sheet. Drizzle with the oil and turn to coat. Turn the tomatoes cut side up and sprinkle with the garlic, salt, and pepper. Roast until the tomatoes are soft and the bottoms are well browned, 40 to 45 minutes.

3 Transfer the tomatoes to a serving plate and sprinkle with the capers. Serve hot, warm, or at room temperature.

Each serving: 3 g carb, 37 cal, 3 g fat, 0 g sat fat, 0 mg chol, 1 g fib, 1 g pro, 118 mg sod • Carb Choices: 0; Exchanges: 1 veg, ½ fat

Blistered Cherry Tomatoes with Rosemary QUICK

makes 4 servings

Spiked with lemon zest and juice, these are ideal for serving with any simply prepared fish or shellfish dish. Or serve them over pasta or polenta for a vegetarian meal for two.

3 cups cherry tomatoes
2 teaspoons extra virgin olive oil
2 teaspoons chopped fresh rosemary
½ teaspoon grated lemon zest
2 teaspoons lemon juice
¼ teaspoon kosher salt
Pinch of freshly ground pepper

1 Preheat the oven to 425°F.

2 Place the tomatoes on a medium rimmed baking sheet. Drizzle with the oil and stir to coat. Roast until some of the tomatoes burst, 15 to 18 minutes.

3 Transfer the tomatoes and any pan juices to a serving bowl. Add the rosemary, lemon zest, lemon juice, salt, and pepper and stir to coat. Serve hot, warm, or at room temperature.

Each serving: 5 g carb, 42 cal, 3 g fat, 3 g sat fat, 0 mg chol, 1 g fib, 1 g pro, 76 mg sod • Carb Choices: 0; Exchanges: 1 veg, ½ fat

Oven-Fried Green Tomatoes

makes 4 servings

These were a staple when I was growing up in Kentucky. We'd have them in early summer before the tomatoes got ripe, then again in the fall before frost killed the tomato vines. Ours were fried, usually in bacon grease. This version uses ground Melba toasts as a coating—a great trick I learned from *Cooks* magazine—and bakes them on a rack in the oven. They're as crispy and flavorful as the ones I grew up eating, but a whole lot healthier.

1 tablespoon plus ½ teaspoon extra virgin olive oil, divided

12 whole wheat or white Melba toasts, crumbled

1 ounce freshly grated Parmesan (about ¼ cup)

¼ cup whole wheat flour

2 egg whites, lightly beaten

2 medium green tomatoes, each cut into four ½-inch slices

1 teaspoon kosher salt

⅛ teaspoon ground cayenne

1 Position an oven rack in the top third of the oven. Preheat the oven to 400°F. Line a large rimmed baking sheet with foil. Place a wire rack in the baking sheet and brush the rack with ½ teaspoon of the oil.

2 Place the Melba toasts in a food processor and process until fine crumbs form. Place the Melba toast crumbs, Parmesan, and remaining 1 tablespoon oil in another shallow dish. Using your fingers, blend the oil evenly into the crumb mixture. Place the flour in another shallow dish. Place the egg whites in another shallow dish.

3 Place the tomato slices in a large bowl and sprinkle with the salt and cayenne. Dip the tomato slices, one at a time, into the flour, then into the egg whites, then into the Melba toast crumb mixture, pressing to adhere the crumbs.

4 Arrange the tomato slices in a single layer on the rack. Bake until golden brown, 30 to 35 minutes (do not turn). Serve at once.

Each serving: 21 g carb, 143 cal, 4 g fat, 1 g sat fat, 0 mg chol, 3 g fib, 6 g pro, 440 mg sod • Carb Choices: 1½; Exchanges: 1 starch, 1 veg, 1 fat

Winter Squash

Roasted Acorn Squash with Ginger Butter

makes 4 servings

This simple fresh ginger butter pairs well with any winter squash or with sweet potatoes. Use a rasp grater such as a Microplane to make fast work of grating the ginger.

1 medium acorn squash (about 1¾ pounds)
2 teaspoons canola oil
1 tablespoon unsalted butter, softened
1 tablespoon grated fresh ginger
½ teaspoon kosher salt

1 Preheat the oven to 425°F.

2 Cut the squash in half vertically, remove the seeds, and cut each half into 2 wedges, leaving the peel intact.

3 Place the squash on a large rimmed baking sheet. Drizzle with the oil and turn to coat. Roast until the squash is tender, turning once, 35 to 40 minutes.

4 Meanwhile, stir together the butter, ginger, and salt in a small dish.

5 To serve, arrange the squash wedges skin side down on a serving platter and divide the butter mixture evenly among the wedges. Serve at once.

Each serving: 16 g carb, 107 cal, 5 g fat, 2 g sat fat, 8 mg chol, 2 g fib, 1 g pro, 145 mg sod • Carb Choices: 1; Exchanges: 1 starch, 1 fat

Masala-Roasted Acorn Squash

makes 4 servings

The warm spices in garam masala (coriander, cumin, cardamom, cinnamon, and black pepper) are delicious with winter squash. I've added some fresh ginger here, too, for an extra kick of flavor, but you can omit it and still have a delicious dish.

1 medium acorn squash (about 1¾ pounds)
2 teaspoons canola oil
2 teaspoons minced fresh ginger
2 garlic cloves, minced
1 teaspoon garam masala
½ teaspoon kosher salt
Lime wedges

1 Preheat the oven to 425°F.

2 Cut the squash in half vertically, remove the seeds, and cut each half into 4 wedges, leaving the peel intact.

3 Place the squash on a large rimmed baking sheet. Drizzle with the oil and turn to coat. Combine the ginger, garlic, garam masala, and salt in a small bowl. Sprinkle the squash with the ginger mixture.

4 Roast until the squash is tender, turning once, 35 to 40 minutes. Serve at once with the lime wedges.

Each serving: 16 g carb, 84 cal, 3 g fat, 0 g sat fat, 0 mg chol, 2 g fib, 1 g pro, 145 mg sod • Carb Choices: 1; Exchanges: 1 starch, ½ fat

Butternut Squash and Gruyère Gratin

makes 8 servings

Sliced butternut squash, layered with velvety caramelized onions and nutty Gruyère cheese is a comforting, yet sophisticated casserole for fall and winter. Serve it with roasted chicken or turkey breast, pork chops, or pork tenderloin.

5 teaspoons extra virgin olive oil, divided
2 large onions, thinly sliced
¾ teaspoon kosher salt, divided
1 tablespoon chopped fresh rosemary
¼ teaspoon freshly ground pepper
1 large butternut squash (about 3 pounds), peeled, seeded, and cut into ¼-inch slices
3 ounces shredded Gruyère (about ¾ cup), divided
¾ cup fresh whole wheat breadcrumbs

1 Heat a large nonstick skillet over medium heat. Add 2 teaspoons of the oil and tilt the pan to coat the bottom evenly. Add the onions and ¼ teaspoon of the salt and cook, stirring occasionally, until very soft and browned, about 25 minutes. Stir in the rosemary and pepper and set aside.

2 Preheat the oven to 350°F. Brush a shallow 3-quart baking dish with 1 teaspoon of the remaining oil. Place one-third of the squash slices in the dish and sprinkle with ¼ teaspoon of the remaining salt. Top the squash with half of the onion mixture. Top the onions with half of the Gruyère. Top the Gruyère with one-third of the squash slices and sprinkle with the remaining ¼ teaspoon salt. Spread the remaining onions over the squash. Sprinkle with the remaining half of the Gruyère. Top with the remaining one-third of the squash slices.

3 Cover and bake 30 minutes. Uncover and bake 20 more minutes. Stir together the breadcrumbs and the remaining 2 teaspoons oil. Sprinkle over the gratin and bake until the crumbs are browned, 10 minutes longer. Let stand 5 minutes before serving.

Each serving: 21 g carb, 150 cal, 6 g fat, 2 g sat fat, 12 mg chol, 3 g fib, 5 g pro, 176 mg sod • Carb Choices: 1½; Exchanges: 1½ starch, ½ high-fat protein

Roasted Butternut Squash with Goat Cheese HIGH FIBER

makes 4 servings

Sharp salty goat cheese is a delicious counterpoint to sweet caramelized squash.

1 medium butternut squash (about 2 pounds), peeled, seeded, and cut into 1-inch pieces
2 teaspoons extra virgin olive oil
½ teaspoon kosher salt
⅛ teaspoon freshly ground pepper
2 ounces goat cheese (about ½ cup), at room temperature
2 teaspoons chopped fresh thyme

1 Preheat the oven to 425°F.

2 Place the squash on a large rimmed baking sheet. Drizzle with the oil, sprinkle with the salt and pepper, and toss to coat. Roast, stirring once, until tender, 40 to 45 minutes.

3 Immediately transfer the squash to a serving platter. Using a knife and spoon, drop the goat cheese in small pieces on top of the squash. Sprinkle with the thyme and serve at once.

Each serving: 23 g carb, 158 cal, 7 g fat, 3 g sat fat, 11 mg chol, 4 g fib, 5 g pro, 221 mg sod • Carb Choices: 1½; Exchanges: 1½ starch, ½ high-fat protein, ½ fat

Butternut Squash Hash

HIGH FIBER

makes 4 servings

Watch the heat carefully when making this hash. If it starts to get too brown before it gets tender, turn the heat down and be patient.

2 teaspoons extra virgin olive oil
1 medium butternut squash (about 2 pounds), peeled, seeded, and cut into 1-inch pieces
1 medium red onion, halved and thinly sliced
½ teaspoon kosher salt
1 teaspoon chopped fresh sage or ¼ teaspoon dried sage, crumbled
⅛ teaspoon freshly ground pepper

1 Heat a large nonstick skillet over medium-high heat. Add the oil and tilt the pan to coat the bottom evenly.

2 Add the squash, onion, and salt and stir to coat. Cook, stirring occasionally, until the squash is lightly browned, about 5 minutes. Reduce the heat to medium, cover, and cook, stirring occasionally, until the squash is tender, 5 to 8 minutes longer. Stir in the sage and pepper. Spoon the hash into a serving bowl and serve at once.

Each serving: 25 g carb, 118 cal, 3 g fat, 0 g sat fat, 0 mg chol, 4 g fib, 2 g pro, 149 mg sod • Carb Choices: 1½; Exchanges: 1½ starch, ½ fat

Winter Squash Puree with Olive Oil and Rosemary

HIGH FIBER

makes 4 servings

Extra virgin olive oil and fresh rosemary are essential to this straightforward recipe. You can substitute fresh sage or thyme for the rosemary.

1 medium butternut, acorn, or sweet dumpling squash (about 2¼ pounds), halved lengthwise and seeded
2 teaspoons extra virgin olive oil
1 teaspoon minced fresh rosemary
Pinch of kosher salt

1 Preheat the oven to 425°F. Place the squash cut side up in a medium deep sided baking dish and add water to a depth of ½ inch. Cover and bake until very tender, 45 to 50 minutes. Let the squash stand until cool enough to handle and scoop out the flesh.

2 Heat a medium nonstick skillet over medium heat. Add the oil and tilt the pan to coat the bottom evenly. Add the rosemary and cook, stirring constantly, until fragrant, 30 seconds. Add the squash and salt and cook, stirring often, until heated through, 3 minutes. Spoon the squash into a serving dish and serve at once.

Each serving: 25 g carb, 117 cal, 3 g fat, 0 g sat fat, 0 mg chol, 4 g fib, 2 g pro, 26 mg sod • Carb Choices: 1½; Exchanges: 1½ starch, ½ fat

Roasted Delicata Squash with Sage and Garlic

HIGH FIBER

makes 4 servings

If your delicata squash is freshly harvested (press on the skin with your thumbnail, and if you can make a dent, it is tender), you can eat the skin, too, and you won't have to peel it.

1 delicata squash (about 2 pounds), peeled, seeded, and cut into 1-inch pieces
4 teaspoons extra virgin olive oil, divided
½ teaspoon kosher salt
2 garlic cloves, minced
2 teaspoons chopped fresh sage

1 Preheat the oven to 425°F.

2 Place the squash on a large rimmed baking sheet. Drizzle with 2 teaspoons of the oil, sprinkle with the salt, and toss to coat. Bake, stirring once, until the squash is browned and tender, 40 to 45 minutes.

3 Meanwhile, heat a small skillet over medium heat. Add the remaining 2 teaspoons oil and tilt to coat the bottom evenly. Add the garlic and cook, stirring constantly, until lightly browned, about 2 minutes. Transfer to a small dish.

4 Spoon the squash into a serving dish. Drizzle with the garlic mixture, sprinkle with the sage, and toss to combine. Serve hot or warm.

Each serving: 23 g carb, 131 cal, 5 g fat, 1 g sat fat, 0 mg chol, 7 g fib, 2 g pro, 146 mg sod • Carb Choices: 1; Exchanges: 1 starch, 1 fat

Mixed Vegetable Dishes

Corn and Bell Peppers with Thyme QUICK

makes 6 servings

You can think of this dish as a salsa, but served hot. Pair it with any summer entrée that needs a little dressing up: grilled shrimp or chicken, sautéed fish fillets, or broiled steaks.

2 teaspoons extra virgin olive oil
3 ears corn, kernels cut from the cob
1 small onion, diced
1 small red bell pepper, diced
2 garlic cloves, minced
½ cup low-sodium vegetable or chicken broth
1 teaspoon chopped fresh thyme
½ teaspoon kosher salt
⅛ teaspoon freshly ground pepper

1 Heat a large nonstick skillet over medium-high heat. Add the oil and tilt the pan to coat the bottom evenly. Add the corn, onion, bell pepper, and garlic and cook, stirring frequently, until the vegetables are softened, 5 minutes.

2 Add the broth, thyme, salt, and ground pepper and bring to a boil. Cook, stirring occasionally, until the vegetables are tender and most of the liquid has evaporated, 3 minutes longer. Spoon the vegetables into a serving dish and serve at once.

Each serving: 11 g carb, 64 cal, 2 g fat, 0 g sat fat, 0 mg chol, 2 g fib, 2 g pro, 113 mg sod • Carb Choices: ½; Exchanges: ½ starch, ½ fat

Summer Succotash QUICK

makes 6 servings

I've called this summer succotash, but it's almost as good in winter made with frozen corn and canned diced tomatoes. When you need a dish with a punch of color and flavors everyone will love, this is a home-style side dish that tastes like a treat.

2 teaspoons extra virgin olive oil
1 small red bell pepper, diced
1 small onion, diced
1 garlic clove, minced
1 large ear corn, kernels cut from the cob, or 1 cup frozen corn kernels
1 cup frozen baby lima beans
¼ cup water
½ teaspoon kosher salt
¼ teaspoon freshly ground pepper
1 large tomato, chopped
2 tablespoons chopped fresh Italian parsley
2 teaspoons lemon juice

1 Heat a large nonstick skillet over medium-high heat. Add the oil and tilt the pan to coat the bottom evenly. Add the bell pepper, onion, and garlic and cook, stirring frequently, until the vegetables are softened, 5 minutes.

2 Add the corn, lima beans, water, salt, and ground pepper and bring to a boil over high heat. Reduce the heat to low, cover, and simmer, stirring occasionally, until the vegetables are tender, 5 minutes. Stir in the tomato and cook just until heated through, 1 to 2 minutes. Remove from the heat and stir in the parsley and lemon juice. Spoon the succotash into a serving dish and serve hot or warm.

Each serving: 15 g carb, 85 cal, 2 g fat, 0 g sat fat, 0 mg chol, 3 g fib, 3 g pro, 114 mg sod • Carb Choices: 1; Exchanges: 1 starch

Carrots and Fennel Braised with White Wine and Garlic QUICK

makes 4 servings

This is a striking looking side dish, especially if you find a fennel bulb with the fronds attached and reserve some to chop and sprinkle over the dish just before serving. It goes nicely with grilled or sautéed seafood or chicken.

1 medium bulb fennel
2 teaspoons extra virgin olive oil
2 garlic cloves, minced
½ teaspoon fennel seeds
8 ounces carrots, peeled and cut into ½-inch-thick sticks
½ cup dry white wine
¾ teaspoon kosher salt
1 teaspoon lemon juice

1 Trim the tough outer stalks from the fennel. Cut the fennel bulb in half vertically and cut away and discard the core. Cut each half lengthwise into ¼-inch slices.

2 Heat a large nonstick skillet over medium heat. Add the oil and tilt the pan to coat the bottom evenly. Add the garlic and fennel seeds and cook, stirring constantly, until fragrant, 30 seconds. Add the fennel bulb, carrots, wine, and salt and bring to a boil over high heat. Reduce the heat to low, cover, and simmer until the vegetables are tender, 10 minutes. Uncover and cook until most of the liquid has evaporated, 2 minutes. Remove from the heat and stir in the lemon juice. Spoon the vegetables into a serving dish and serve at once.

Each serving: 10 g carb, 86 cal, 3 g fat, 0 g sat fat, 0 mg chol, 3 g fib, 1 g pro, 276 mg sod • Carb Choices: ½; Exchanges: 2 veg, ½ fat

Roasted Root Vegetables with Kale [HIGH FIBER]

makes 8 servings

When you come home with a bouquet of greens and an assortment of root vegetables, this is a wonderful dish to make. The greens (you can use mustard greens, beet greens, or Swiss chard instead of the kale) make a lush emerald bed for colorful roasted root vegetables. This side dish is all you'll need to serve with a roast pork loin to make a delicious fall meal.

2 medium sweet potatoes, peeled and cut into 1-inch pieces
2 large parsnips, peeled and cut into 1-inch pieces
2 large turnips, peeled and cut into 1-inch pieces
2 large carrots, peeled and cut into 1-inch pieces
2 teaspoons extra virgin olive oil
1 teaspoon kosher salt, divided
⅛ teaspoon freshly ground pepper
½ cup low-sodium vegetable or chicken broth
2 pounds kale, tough stems removed and leaves cut into ¼-inch slices
⅛ teaspoon crushed red pepper

1 Preheat the oven to 425°F.

2 Place the potatoes, parsnips, turnips, and carrots in a large, deep-sided roasting pan. Drizzle with the oil, sprinkle with ½ teaspoon of the salt and the pepper, and toss to coat.

3 Roast, stirring occasionally, until the vegetables are tender and lightly browned, 45 to 50 minutes.

4 Meanwhile, bring the broth and the remaining ½ teaspoon salt to a boil over medium-high heat in a large, deep-sided skillet. Add the kale in batches and cook, stirring constantly, until the kale is wilted, about 3 minutes. Stir in the crushed red pepper. Reduce the heat, cover, and simmer until the greens are tender, 15 to 20 minutes. If the greens are tender and excess liquid remains in the skillet, remove the cover and cook until most of liquid evaporates.

5 To serve, arrange the kale on a serving platter and spoon the roasted root vegetables on top. Serve hot or warm.

Each serving: 23 g carb, 125 cal, 2 g fat, 2 g sat fat, 0 mg chol, 5 g fib, 4 g pro, 256 mg sod • Carb Choices: 1½; Exchanges: ½ starch, 3 veg, ½ fat

Fruit and Honey–Roasted Vegetables [HIGH FIBER]

makes 6 servings

Tossing a colorful mix of roasted root vegetables with jewel-like dried fruits, a drizzle of honey, and a scattering of fresh thyme makes a stellar side dish.

2 medium sweet potatoes, peeled and cut into 1-inch pieces
2 medium turnips, peeled and cut into 1-inch pieces
2 large parsnips, peeled and cut into 1-inch pieces
2 teaspoons extra virgin olive oil
½ teaspoon kosher salt
¼ teaspoon freshly ground pepper
⅓ cup orange juice
1 tablespoon honey
¼ cup diced dried apricots
¼ cup dried cranberries
2 teaspoons minced fresh thyme or ½ teaspoon dried thyme

1 Preheat the oven to 425°F.

2 Place the potatoes, turnips, and parsnips in a large, deep-sided roasting pan. Drizzle with the oil, sprinkle with the salt and pepper, and toss to coat.

3 Roast, stirring occasionally, until the vegetables are tender and lightly browned, 45 to 50 minutes.

4 Meanwhile, combine the orange juice and honey in a small saucepan and bring just to a boil

over medium heat. Remove from the heat and stir in the apricots and cranberries. Cover and let stand while the vegetables roast.

5 Combine the roasted vegetables, the orange juice mixture, and the thyme in a large bowl and toss to coat. Serve hot or warm.

Each serving: 27 g carb, 126 cal, 2 g fat, 0 g sat fat, 0 mg chol, 4 g fib, 2 g pro, 137 mg sod • Carb Choices: 2; Exchanges: 1½ starch, ½ fruit

Roasted Broccoli and Cauliflower with Indian Spices

makes 4 servings

Contrasting green and white vegetables tossed with a warming spice mixture make this an unusually welcome accompaniment to weeknight dinners. If you'd like to give the dish more heat, add more cayenne at your own discretion.

2 teaspoons minced fresh ginger
1 garlic clove, minced
½ teaspoon ground cumin
½ teaspoon ground coriander
½ teaspoon kosher salt
Pinch of ground cayenne
2 cups broccoli florets
3 cups cauliflower florets
2 teaspoons extra virgin olive oil

1 Preheat the oven to 425°F.

2 Stir together the ginger, garlic, cumin, coriander, salt, and cayenne in a small dish. Place the broccoli and cauliflower on a large rimmed baking sheet. Drizzle with the oil, sprinkle with the ginger mixture, and toss to coat.

3 Arrange the vegetables in a single layer. Bake, stirring once, until the vegetables are browned, 25 to 30 minutes. Spoon the vegetables into a serving dish and serve at once.

Each serving: 6 g carb, 52 cal, 3 g fat, 0 g sat fat, 0 mg chol, 3 g fib, 3 g pro, 172 mg sod • Carb Choices: ½; Exchanges: 1 veg, ½ fat

Eggplant and Tomatoes with Herb Sauce QUICK | HIGH FIBER

makes 8 servings

This fresh minty sauce is addictive on grilled vegetables. It goes well with grilled chicken, shrimp, and fish, too.

4 plum tomatoes, halved lengthwise
1 medium eggplant (about 1½ pounds), cut into ½-inch slices
1 large red onion, cut into ½-inch slices
3 tablespoons plus ½ teaspoon extra virgin olive oil, divided
½ teaspoon kosher salt
¼ teaspoon freshly ground pepper
1½ cups fresh Italian parsley leaves
½ cup fresh mint leaves
2 tablespoons cold water
2 tablespoons thinly sliced scallions
1 tablespoon lemon juice
1 tablespoon capers, rinsed and drained
1 garlic clove, chopped
1 canned anchovy fillet, rinsed and chopped

1 Prepare the grill or heat a large grill pan over medium-high heat.

2 Brush the tomatoes, eggplant, and onion with 1 tablespoon of the oil. Brush the grill rack or grill pan with ½ teaspoon of the remaining oil. Place the vegetables on the grill rack or in the grill pan and grill, turning often, until the vegetables are browned, 3 to 4 minutes for the tomatoes and 8 to 10 minutes for the eggplant and onion. Arrange on a serving platter and sprinkle with the salt and pepper.

3 To make the sauce, combine the remaining 2 tablespoons of the oil and the remaining ingredients in a food processor and process until smooth. Spoon over the vegetables. Serve hot, warm, or at room temperature.

Each serving: 9 g carb, 92 cal, 6 g fat, 1 g sat fat, 0 mg chol, 4 g fib, 2 g pro, 132 mg sod • Carb Choices: ½; Exchanges: 2 veg, 1 fat

Summer Garden Vegetable Gratin [HIGH FIBER]

makes 8 servings

This gratin recipe is infinitely forgiving. Keep the total amount of vegetables about the same, but if you don't like eggplant, leave it out and add more zucchini (roast it first to add flavor and to decrease the moisture of the finished dish); use any kind of peppers you find at the market; and substitute your favorite herb for the basil.

2 tablespoons extra virgin olive oil, divided
1 medium eggplant (about 1½ pounds), peeled and sliced into ½-inch rounds
6 plum tomatoes, sliced
2 medium zucchini, halved lengthwise and sliced
1 yellow bell pepper, thinly sliced
1 red bell pepper, thinly sliced
1 small onion, halved and thinly sliced
2 garlic cloves, minced
2 tablespoons chopped fresh basil
1 teaspoon kosher salt
¼ teaspoon freshly ground pepper
½ cup plain dry breadcrumbs
2 ounces shredded Gruyère (about ½ cup)
1 ounce freshly grated Parmesan (about ¼ cup)

1 Preheat the oven to 400°F.

2 Brush a large rimmed baking sheet with ½ teaspoon of the oil. Brush the eggplant slices with 1 tablespoon of the remaining oil. Arrange the eggplant in a single layer on the baking sheet and bake, turning once, until tender and browned, 20 to 25 minutes. Reduce the oven temperature to 350°F.

3 Brush a shallow 3-quart baking dish with ½ teaspoon of the remaining oil. Combine the tomatoes, zucchini, bell peppers, onion, garlic, basil, salt, and ground pepper in a large bowl. Drizzle with the remaining 2 teaspoons olive oil and toss to coat. Add the eggplant slices and toss to combine. Arrange the vegetables in the baking dish.

4 Bake, uncovered, for 45 minutes. Remove from the oven. Stir together the breadcrumbs, Gruyère, and Parmesan in a medium bowl. Sprinkle over the vegetables and bake until the breadcrumb mixture is lightly browned, 15 minutes longer. Let the gratin stand 10 minutes before serving. Serve at once.

Each serving: 16 g carb, 148 cal, 7 g fat, 2 g sat fat, 0 mg chol, 5 g fib, 6 g pro, 433 mg sod • Carb Choices: 1; Exchanges: ½ carb, 2 veg, ½ high-fat protein, ½ fat

Stewed Okra and Tomatoes

makes 6 servings

This recipe is for okra lovers only, as the long cooking time actually plays up the slick texture of the pods. I think it's delicious.

2 teaspoons extra virgin olive oil
1 small onion, chopped
2 garlic cloves, minced
12 ounces okra, sliced
2 large tomatoes, chopped (about 1½ cups) or 1 (14½-ounce) can no-salt-added diced tomatoes
½ cup water
½ teaspoon kosher salt
Pinch of freshly ground pepper

1 Heat a medium saucepan over medium-high heat. Add the oil and tilt the pan to coat the bottom evenly. Add the onion and cook, stirring often, until softened, 5 minutes. Add the garlic and cook, stirring constantly, until fragrant, 30 seconds.

2 Add the okra, tomatoes, water, salt, and pepper and bring to a boil over high heat. Reduce the heat to low, cover, and simmer until the okra is tender and the mixture is thickened slightly, 15 to 20 minutes. Spoon the vegetables into a serving dish and serve at once.

Each serving: 8 g carb, 48 cal, 2 g fat, 0 g sat fat, 0 mg chol, 3 g fib, 2 g pro, 101 mg sod • Carb Choices: ½; Exchanges: 1 veg, ½ fat

Root Vegetable Hash with Brussels Sprouts

QUICK | HIGH FIBER

makes 4 servings

This is a pretty fall side dish to serve with roast meats or chicken. It's a good way to use up small amounts of vegetables you have on hand. Add or substitute leeks for the onion or red-skinned potatoes for the turnip. Don't use rutabaga in this recipe, as it takes much longer to cook than the other vegetables.

2 teaspoons extra virgin olive oil
1 medium turnip, peeled and chopped
1 parsnip, peeled and sliced
1 carrot, peeled and sliced
1 small red onion, halved and thinly sliced
¾ teaspoon kosher salt
Pinch of freshly ground pepper
1 cup Brussels sprouts, trimmed and quartered
1 garlic clove, minced

1 Heat a large nonstick skillet over medium-high heat. Add the oil and tilt the pan to coat the bottom evenly.

2 Add the turnip, parsnip, carrot, onion, salt, and pepper and stir to coat. Cook, stirring occasionally, until the vegetables are lightly browned, about 5 minutes. Reduce the heat to medium, cover, and cook, stirring occasionally, until the vegetables are almost tender, about 5 minutes. Add the Brussels sprouts and garlic, cover, and cook, stirring occasionally, until all the vegetables are tender, 3 to 5 minutes longer. Spoon the hash into a serving dish and serve hot or warm.

Each serving: 14 g carb, 83 cal, 3 g fat, 0 g sat fat, 0 mg chol, 4 g fib, 2 g pro, 347 mg sod • Carb Choices: 1; Exchanges: 3 veg, ½ fat

Asian Vegetable Stir-fry QUICK

makes 4 servings

Fresh bean sprouts lighten the look of this stir-fry and add a clean crunch. You can leave them out if you don't have them and the dish will still be delicious. Serve this over rice for a quick lunch or pair it with Lime-Marinated Grilled Pork Tenderloin (page 308) or Asian Barbecue Chicken (page 241).

⅓ cup Vegetable Stock (page 149) or
    low-sodium vegetable broth
2 tablespoons reduced-sodium soy sauce
2 teaspoons cornstarch
1 teaspoon Asian sesame oil
¼ teaspoon crushed red pepper
2 teaspoons canola oil
2 tablespoons minced fresh ginger
2 garlic cloves, minced
4 scallions, cut into 2-inch pieces
2 cups snow peas, trimmed
1 red bell pepper, thinly sliced
1 cup bean sprouts
¼ cup chopped fresh cilantro

1 Combine the stock, soy sauce, cornstarch, sesame oil, and crushed red pepper in a small bowl and stir until the cornstarch dissolves.

2 Heat a large wok or nonstick skillet over medium-high heat. Add the canola oil and tilt the pan to coat the bottom evenly. Add the ginger and garlic and cook, stirring constantly until fragrant, 30 seconds.

3 Add the scallions, snow peas, and bell pepper and cook, stirring constantly, until crisp-tender, 3 minutes. Stir in the stock mixture and cook until the sauce is thickened, 30 seconds. Remove from the heat and stir in the bean sprouts and cilantro. Spoon the vegetables into a serving dish and serve at once.

Each serving: 11 g carb, 88 cal, 4 g fat, 0 g sat fat, 0 mg chol, 3 g fib, 3 g pro, 321 mg sod • Carb Choices: 1; Exchanges: 2 veg, ½ fat

Breads

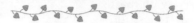

Quick Breads and Muffins

Zucchini-Carrot Bread

Apricot-Pecan Bread

Banana-Walnut Bread

Oatmeal-Raisin Bread

Pumpkin-Cranberry Bread

Southern Cornbread

Irish Soda Bread

Boston Brown Bread

Chocolate-Zucchini Muffins

Cherry-Almond Muffins

Pineapple-Carrot Muffins

Blueberry-Lemon Muffins

Banana-Berry Muffins

Moist Bran Muffins

Ginger-Pear Muffins with Almond Streusel

Cornmeal Muffins with Fresh Cranberries

Red Bell Pepper, Corn, and Basil Muffins

Cornmeal Muffins with Chiles and Cheese

Parmesan Muffins

Scones and Biscuits

Fresh Cranberry–Orange Scones

Gingerbread Scones

Oat Scones with Currants

Baking Powder Biscuits

Sweet Potato Biscuits

Griddle Cakes and Tortillas

Fresh Corn Griddle Cakes

Whole Wheat Flour Tortillas

Yeast Breads

Whole Wheat Bread

Parmesan-Rosemary Wheat Loaf

Dried Cherry Loaf Bread with Toasted Almonds

Chocolate Yeast Bread

Caraway Beer Bread

Yeast-Risen Cornmeal Loaf

Caramelized Onion and Thyme-Focaccia

Rosemary-Olive Focaccia

Onion-Rye Rolls

Crispy Poppy Seed Breadsticks

Stuffings

Dried Apricot–Pecan Stuffing

Pear and Walnut Stuffing

Chestnut Stuffing

Cornbread Stuffing with Sausage and Apples

Rye Stuffing with Roasted Carrots and Leeks

Multigrain Bread Stuffing with Mixed Mushrooms

Having diabetes doesn't mean you have to give up bread. But you do need to enjoy bread in sensible portions and always take into account the total carbohydrate in your meal. If your meal contains other carbohydrate-rich foods such as potatoes or pasta, the carbs can add up fast, so always be observant of serving sizes and the total carb count for the entire meal.

Most of the breads in this chapter are made with healthier high-fiber whole wheat flours that contain more vitamins, minerals, and antioxidants than their white counterparts. In many recipes, all-purpose flour is used in combination with whole wheat flour to give muffins and loaves a lighter texture and a more delicate flavor.

You'll find healthy versions of all your favorite breads, like Banana-Walnut Bread (page 505) and Moist Bran Muffins (page 513), along with some new treats to try like Ginger Pear Muffins with Almond Streusel (page 514), and Red Bell Pepper, Corn, and Basil Muffins (page 515) that are perfect with soup or chili. Whole Wheat Bread (page 522) is a terrific basic bread recipe with two versions to change up the flavors. Focaccia is one of my favorite breads to make (probably because it's so easy) and you'll find several versions here that taste better than those you'll get at any bakery.

You'll find great stuffing recipes in this chapter, too. Serve them not just at Thanksgiving, but any time of year as a side dish with a roasted chicken or pork loin.

Breads aren't off-limits when you have diabetes; just enjoy them wisely.

Quick Breads and Muffins

Zucchini-Carrot Bread

makes 16 servings

With the green and orange vegetables, this is a colorful bread to slice and serve for brunch or afternoon tea. The vegetables make the bread super-moist, but take time to squeeze the moisture from the shredded zucchini or the bread will be soggy.

1 teaspoon plus ⅓ cup canola oil, divided
Unbleached all-purpose flour for dusting the pan
1 cup coarsely shredded zucchini
2 cups whole wheat flour
¾ cup sugar
2 teaspoons baking powder
1½ teaspoons ground cinnamon
½ teaspoon baking soda
¼ teaspoon ground cloves
¼ teaspoon salt
½ cup low-fat buttermilk
2 large eggs
1 teaspoon vanilla extract
1 cup coarsely shredded carrots

1 Preheat the oven to 350°F. Brush an 8½ x 4½-inch loaf pan with 1 teaspoon of the oil. Dust the pan lightly with the all-purpose flour, shaking the pan to remove the excess.

2 Spread the zucchini onto several layers of paper towels, cover with additional paper towels, and roll up and press to remove the excess moisture. Let the zucchini stand 5 minutes, pressing occasionally.

3 Combine the whole wheat flour, sugar, baking powder, cinnamon, baking soda, cloves, and salt in a large bowl and whisk to mix well.

4 Combine the remaining ⅓ cup oil, the buttermilk, eggs, and vanilla in a medium bowl and whisk until smooth. Add the oil mixture to the flour mixture and stir just until moistened. Stir in the zucchini and the carrots.

5 Spoon the batter into the prepared pan and bake until a wooden toothpick inserted in the center of the loaf comes out clean, 1 hour to 1 hour 10 minutes.

6 Cool the bread in the pan on a wire rack for 10 minutes. Remove from the pan and cool completely on a wire rack before slicing. The bread can be stored in an airtight container at room temperature for up to 2 days or frozen for up to 3 months.

Each serving: 23 g carb, 158 cal, 6 g fat, 1 g sat fat, 27 mg chol, 2 g fib, 4 g pro, 148 mg sod • Carb Choices: 1 ½ carb, 1 fat

Apricot-Pecan Bread

makes 16 servings

Chopped dried apricots plumped in orange juice give this bread the look of jewels scattered throughout the slices. It makes a lovely hostess or welcome-to-the neighborhood gift.

1 to 1¼ cups orange juice, divided
1 cup chopped dried apricots
1 teaspoon plus ¼ cup canola oil, divided
1 cup unbleached all-purpose flour plus flour for dusting the pan
1 cup whole wheat flour
¾ cup sugar
2 teaspoons baking powder
¼ teaspoon salt
1 large egg
2 teaspoons grated orange zest
¼ cup pecans, toasted and chopped (page 4)

1 Place 1 cup of the orange juice in a medium saucepan and set over medium heat until hot but not boiling. Remove from the heat and stir in the apricots. Cover and let stand 30 minutes. Drain the apricots, reserving the juice. Place the juice in a glass measuring cup and add enough of the additional orange juice to make ¾ cup. Set aside.

2 Preheat the oven to 350°F. Brush an 8½ x 4½-inch loaf pan with 1 teaspoon of the oil. Dust the pan lightly with all-purpose flour, shaking the pan to remove the excess.

3 Combine the 1 cup all-purpose flour, whole wheat flour, sugar, baking powder, and salt in a large bowl and whisk to mix well.

4 Combine the reserved orange juice, the remaining ¼ cup oil, the egg, and orange zest in a medium bowl and whisk until smooth. Add the orange juice mixture to the flour mixture and stir just until moistened. Stir in the apricots and pecans.

5 Spoon the batter into the prepared pan and bake until a wooden toothpick inserted in the center of the loaf comes out clean, 1 hour to 1 hour 5 minutes.

6 Cool the bread in the pan on a wire rack for 10 minutes. Remove from the pan and cool completely on a wire rack before slicing. The bread can be stored in an airtight container at room temperature for up to 2 days or frozen for up to 3 months.

Each serving: 26 g carb, 163 cal, 6 g fat, 0 g sat fat, 13 mg chol, 2 g fib, 3 g pro, 92 mg sod • Carb Choices: 2; Exchanges: 2 carb, 1 fat

Banana-Walnut Bread

makes 16 servings

Laced with cinnamon and scattered with walnuts, this is a lower-calorie—yet still incredibly delicious—version of classic banana bread.

1 teaspoon plus ¼ cup canola oil, divided
1 cup unbleached all-purpose flour plus flour for dusting the pan
1 cup whole wheat flour
½ cup sugar
2 teaspoons baking powder
1 teaspoon ground cinnamon
½ teaspoon baking soda
¼ teaspoon salt
1 cup low-fat buttermilk
1 cup mashed ripe banana (about 2 medium bananas)
2 large eggs
2 teaspoons vanilla extract
⅓ cup walnuts, toasted and chopped (page 4)

1 Preheat the oven to 350°F. Brush an 8½ x 4½-inch loaf pan with 1 teaspoon of the oil. Dust the pan lightly with all-purpose flour, shaking the pan to remove the excess.

2 Combine the 1 cup all-purpose flour, whole wheat flour, sugar, baking powder, cinnamon, baking soda, and salt in a large bowl and whisk to mix well. Combine the remaining ¼ cup oil, the buttermilk, banana, eggs, and vanilla in a medium bowl and whisk until smooth. Add the oil mixture to the flour mixture and stir just until moistened. Stir in the walnuts.

3 Spoon the batter into the prepared pan and bake until a wooden toothpick inserted in the center of the loaf comes out clean, 55 minutes to 1 hour.

4 Cool the bread in the pan on a wire rack for 10 minutes. Remove from the pan and cool completely on a wire rack before slicing. The bread can be stored in an airtight container at room temperature for up to 2 days or frozen for up to 3 months.

Each serving: 22 g carb, 157 cal, 6 g fat, 1 g sat fat, 27 mg chol, 2 g fib, 4 g pro, 115 mg sod • Carb Choices: 1½; Exchanges: 1½ carb, 1 fat

Oatmeal-Raisin Bread

serves 18

Sprinkling oats over the top of this bread give a hint of what's inside. Slice the bread and toast it for breakfast or an afternoon snack. It's great spread with peanut butter.

½ cup skim milk

½ cup raisins

1 teaspoon plus ⅓ cup canola oil, divided

1 cup unbleached all-purpose flour plus flour for dusting the pan

2 cups whole wheat flour

1 cup plus 1 tablespoon old-fashioned rolled oats, divided

¾ cup packed light brown sugar

2 teaspoons baking powder

1 teaspoon baking soda

½ teaspoon salt

1½ cups plain low-fat yogurt

2 large eggs

1 Pour the milk into a small saucepan and set over medium heat until hot but not boiling. Remove from the heat and stir in the raisins. Cover and let stand 30 minutes.

2 Preheat the oven to 350°F. Brush a 9 x 5-inch loaf pan with 1 teaspoon of the oil. Dust the pan lightly with all-purpose flour, shaking the pan to remove the excess.

3 Combine 1 cup all-purpose flour, whole wheat flour, 1 cup of the oats, sugar, baking powder, baking soda, and salt in large bowl and whisk to mix well. Combine the remaining ⅓ cup of the oil, the yogurt, and eggs in a medium bowl and whisk until smooth. Add the oil mixture and the raisin mixture to the flour mixture and stir just until moistened.

4 Spoon the batter into the prepared pan and sprinkle the top with the remaining 1 tablespoon oats. Bake until a wooden toothpick inserted in the center of the loaf comes out clean, 1 hour to 1 hour 5 minutes.

5 Cool the bread in the pan on a wire rack for 10 minutes. Remove from the pan and cool completely on a wire rack before slicing. The bread can be stored in an airtight container at room temperature for up to 2 days or frozen for up to 3 months.

Each serving: 22 g carb, 147 cal, 6 g fat, 1 g sat fat, 25 mg chol, 1 g fib, 3 g pro, 143 mg sod • Carb Choices: 1½; Exchanges: 1½ carb, 1 fat

Pumpkin-Cranberry Bread

makes 16 servings

Pulsing the cranberries in a food processor creates a red-flecked bread that's perfect for holiday gift giving. Slices of the bread reheat beautifully in the microwave or toaster oven.

1 teaspoon plus ⅓ cup canola oil, divided

Unbleached all-purpose flour for dusting the pan

1 cup fresh cranberries or unthawed frozen cranberries

2 cups whole wheat flour

¾ cup sugar

2 teaspoons baking powder

2 teaspoons pumpkin pie spice

½ teaspoon baking soda

½ teaspoon salt

1 cup canned pumpkin (not pumpkin pie filling)

½ cup low-fat buttermilk

2 large eggs

2 teaspoons vanilla extract

1 Preheat the oven to 350°F. Brush a 8½ x 4½-inch loaf pan with 1 teaspoon of the oil. Dust the pan lightly with the all-purpose flour, shaking the pan to remove the excess.

2 Place the cranberries in a food processor and pulse 4 or 5 times or until coarsely chopped. Set aside.

3 Combine the whole wheat flour, sugar, baking powder, pumpkin pie spice, baking soda, and salt in a large bowl and whisk to mix well. Combine the remaining ⅓ cup oil, the pumpkin, buttermilk, eggs, and vanilla in a medium bowl and whisk until smooth. Add the pumpkin mixture and the cranberries to the flour mixture and stir just until moistened. (The batter will be very thick.)

4 Spoon the batter into the prepared pan and bake until a wooden toothpick inserted in the center of the loaf comes out clean, 50 to 55 minutes.

5 Cool the bread in the pan on a wire rack for 10 minutes. Remove from the pan and cool completely on a wire rack before slicing. The bread can be stored in an airtight container at room temperature for up to 2 days or frozen for up to 3 months.

Each serving: 24 g carb, 162 cal, 6 g fat, 1 g sat fat, 27 mg chol, 3 g fib, 4 g pro, 180 mg sod • Carb Choices: 1½; Exchanges: 1½ carb, 1 fat

Types of Flour

Regular whole wheat flour is made from ground hard red wheat kernels (also called wheat berries). It contains the entire kernel, which is made up of the bran layer (where the fiber is contained), the germ (which contains iron, vitamin A, and vitamin B), and the endosperm (which contains most of the protein). Use whole wheat flour alone or mixed with unbleached all-purpose flour for making yeast breads, quick breads, muffins, and all but the most delicate cakes.

Whole wheat pastry flour is the same as regular whole wheat flour, but is made from soft wheat, which contains less protein than hard wheat. It is an excellent flour for making light and flaky biscuits and scones, as well as pastry crusts and cookies.

White whole wheat flour is made from hard white wheat, rather than red wheat. It has a lighter color and a more delicate flavor than regular whole wheat. You can use it to replace all-purpose flour in any baked good except the most delicate cakes. It has virtually the same amount of fiber, vitamins, and calories as regular whole wheat flour. If you don't enjoy the robust flavor of regular whole wheat flour but want the nutritional benefits of whole wheat, give this flour a try.

Unbleached all-purpose white flour contains only the endosperm—the fiber-containing bran and vitamin-packed germ are removed. Combining it with whole wheat flour gives cakes and muffins a lighter texture and a more tender crumb. Unlike bleached all-purpose flour, unbleached flour has not been whitened with a chemical bleaching process. Unbleached flour has a minute amount more protein, which some exacting cooks find makes baked goods a bit tougher in texture. In my experience, I cannot tell the difference in texture, taste, or rising properties when using unbleached versus bleached flour. Bleaching of flour is not allowed in Europe.

Southern Cornbread QUICK

makes 12 servings

If you have a well-seasoned 10-inch cast iron skillet, use it for this bread. Brush the skillet with the oil, but don't dust it with flour or use parchment. Place the skillet in the oven to preheat, then carefully pour the batter into the hot skillet and bake as directed.

2 teaspoons plus 1 tablespoon canola oil, divided

½ cup unbleached all-purpose flour plus flour for dusting the pan

1½ cups fine-grind yellow cornmeal

1 tablespoon sugar

2 teaspoons baking powder

1 teaspoon baking soda

½ teaspoon salt

2 cups low-fat buttermilk

2 large eggs

1 Preheat the oven to 425°F. Brush an 8-inch square metal baking pan with 2 teaspoons of the oil. Dust the pan lightly with flour, shaking the pan to remove the excess. Line the bottom of the pan with parchment paper.

2 Combine the ½ cup flour, cornmeal, sugar, baking powder, baking soda, and salt in a large bowl and whisk to mix well. Combine the buttermilk, the remaining 1 tablespoon oil, and eggs in a medium bowl and whisk until smooth. Add the buttermilk mixture to the cornmeal mixture and stir just until moistened.

3 Spoon the batter into the prepared pan and bake until lightly browned, 25 to 30 minutes.

4 Cool the bread in the pan 5 minutes. Invert onto a rack and remove the parchment paper. Serve hot, warm, or at room temperature. Store in an airtight container at room temperature for up to 2 days or freeze for up to 3 months.

Each serving: 23 g carb, 148 cal, 4 g fat, 1 g sat fat, 38 mg chol, 1 g fib, 5 g pro, 334 mg sod • Carb Choices: 1½; Exchanges: 1½ starch, 1 fat

YANKEE CORNBREAD: Follow the Southern Cornbread recipe, at left, but use ½ cup sugar instead of 1 tablespoon and proceed as directed.

Each serving: 31 g carb, 176 cal, 4 g fat, 1 g sat fat, 38 mg chol, 1 g fib, 5 g pro, 332 mg sod • Carb Choices: 1½; Exchanges: 1½ starch, ½ carb, 1 fat

Storing and Freezing Breads

Unless you have a large family, most bread recipes make more than you can eat before the bread gets stale. Most quick breads, muffins, and yeast breads can be frozen for up to 3 months without affecting the quality of the bread.

Muffins, biscuits, and scones are the simplest to freeze. Just place them in a resealable freezer bag and freeze for up to 3 months.

For quick loaf breads or yeast breads, cut the loaves in half, into quarters, or into individual slices, depending on your needs. Place each portion of bread in an inexpensive plastic storage bag (the kind that come in a box on a roll are especially convenient) and seal with a twist tie or tie a knot in the bag. Place the portions in a resealable freezer bag and freeze. Thaw the portion you need at room temperature. Thawing in the microwave works in a pinch, but it can dry the bread out and make the edges tough.

To store quick breads or yeast breads for just a few days, store them at room temperature. Store quick breads in a resealable plastic bag and yeast breads in a paper bag to keep the crust crisp. Surprisingly, breads will get stale faster in the refrigerator than at room temperature.

Irish Soda Bread

makes 16 servings

This simple homey bread is good with almost anything. Toast it and serve it with eggs for breakfast, have it with afternoon tea, or enjoy it with a bowl of soup for dinner.

1 teaspoon canola oil
2 cups unbleached all-purpose flour plus flour for dusting the pan
2 cups whole wheat flour
1 tablespoon baking powder
1 tablespoon sugar
1 teaspoon salt
1½ teaspoons baking soda
1¾ cups low-fat buttermilk

1 Preheat the oven to 375°F. Brush a 9-inch round cake pan with the oil. Dust the pan lightly with all-purpose flour, shaking the pan to remove the excess.

2 Combine the 2 cups all-purpose flour, whole wheat flour, baking powder, sugar, salt, and baking soda in a large bowl and whisk to mix well. Add the buttermilk and stir just until a sticky dough forms. Transfer the dough to a lightly floured surface, sprinkle the dough lightly with flour, and using floured hands, knead until the dough is smooth, about 2 minutes.

3 Place the dough in the prepared pan and pat the dough to the edge of the pan. Bake until the top of the loaf is lightly browned and the loaf sounds hollow when tapped, 30 to 35 minutes.

4 Cool the bread in the pan on a wire rack for 5 minutes. Remove the loaf from the pan and cool completely on a wire rack before slicing. The bread can be stored in an airtight container at room temperature for up to 2 days or frozen for up to 3 months.

Each serving: 25 g carb, 128 cal, 1 g fat, 0 g sat fat, 2 mg chol, 2 g fib, 5 g pro, 368 mg sod • Carb Choices: 1½; Exchanges: 1½ starch

Boston Brown Bread

makes 16 servings

Moist and full of complex flavors from the blend of grains, molasses, and buttermilk, this bread is delicious with almost anything.

3 teaspoons canola oil, divided
¾ cup whole wheat flour
¾ cup rye flour
¾ cup fine-grind yellow cornmeal
1 teaspoon baking soda
½ teaspoon salt
1½ cups low-fat buttermilk
⅓ cup light or dark molasses (not blackstrap)
½ cup dried currants

1 Preheat the oven to 325°F. Brush an 8½ x 4½-inch loaf pan with 2 teaspoons of the oil.

2 Combine the whole wheat flour, rye flour, cornmeal, baking soda, and salt in a large bowl and whisk to mix well. Combine the buttermilk and molasses in a small bowl and whisk until smooth. Add the buttermilk mixture and the currants to the flour mixture and stir just until smooth.

3 Spoon the batter into the prepared pan. Brush one side of a 24-inch sheet of aluminum foil with the remaining 1 teaspoon oil. Wrap the pan tightly with the foil, leaving enough room for the bread to expand. Place the loaf pan in a deep baking dish and add boiling water to the baking dish to a depth of 2 inches. Carefully place the pans in the oven and bake until a wooden toothpick inserted in the center of the loaf comes out clean, about 1 hour 20 minutes.

4 Cool the bread in the pan on a wire rack for 10 minutes. Remove the loaf from the pan and cool completely on a wire rack before slicing. Serve warm or at room temperature. The bread can be stored in an airtight container at room temperature for up to 2 days or frozen for up to 3 months.

Each serving: 24 g carb, 120 cal, 2 g fat, 0 g sat fat, 1 mg chol, 2 g fib, 3 g pro, 183 mg sod • Carb Choices: 1½; Exchanges: 1½ starch

Chocolate-Zucchini Muffins QUICK

makes 18 servings

Cocoa in addition to chocolate chips in the batter makes these muffins irresistible. The zucchini adds moisture, but you can hardly tell it's there in the baked muffins.

2 cups coarsely shredded zucchini (1 medium zucchini)

2 cups whole wheat pastry flour or 2 cups unbleached all-purpose flour

½ cup sugar

¼ cup unsweetened cocoa

2 teaspoons baking powder

½ teaspoon baking soda

¼ teaspoon salt

1 cup low-fat buttermilk

2 tablespoons canola oil

1 large egg

1 teaspoon vanilla extract

½ cup semisweet mini chocolate chips

1 Preheat the oven to 350°F. Line 18 muffin tin cups with paper muffin liners.

2 Spread the zucchini onto several layers of paper towels, cover with additional paper towels, and roll up and press to remove the excess moisture. Let the zucchini stand 5 minutes, pressing occasionally.

3 Combine the flour, sugar, cocoa, baking powder, baking soda, and salt in a large bowl and whisk to mix well. Combine the buttermilk, oil, egg, and vanilla in a medium bowl and whisk until smooth. Add the buttermilk mixture to the flour mixture and stir just until moistened. Gently stir in the chocolate chips.

4 Spoon the batter evenly into the muffin cups. Bake until a toothpick inserted into the centers of the muffins comes out clean, 20 to 22 minutes.

5 Cool the muffins in the pan on a wire rack for 5 minutes. Remove the muffins from the pan and place on the rack. Serve hot, warm, or at room temperature. The muffins can be stored in an airtight container at room temperature for up to 2 days or frozen for up to 3 months.

Each serving: 21 g carb, 122 cal, 4 g fat, 1 g sat fat, 12 mg chol, 3 g fib, 3 g pro, 132 mg sod • Carb Choices: 1½; Exchanges: 1½ carb, ½ fat

Cherry-Almond Muffins

QUICK

makes 12 servings

The delicate texture of these muffins requires using either whole wheat pastry flour or all-purpose flour. Don't use regular whole wheat flour or the muffins will be too dense. If you use frozen cherries, don't thaw them first or their juices will color the batter.

2 teaspoons plus 2 tablespoons canola oil, divided

2 cups whole wheat pastry flour or 2 cups unbleached all-purpose flour

½ cup sugar

3½ ounces almond paste (about ⅓ cup, packed)

2 teaspoons baking powder

½ teaspoon baking soda

¼ teaspoon salt

1 cup plain fat-free yogurt

1 large egg

1 cup pitted fresh cherries or unthawed frozen unsweetened cherries, halved

2 tablespoons sliced almonds

1 Preheat the oven to 350°F. Brush a 12-cup muffin tin with 2 teaspoons of the oil or omit the oil and line the tin with paper muffin liners.

2 Combine the flour, sugar, almond paste, baking powder, baking soda, and salt in a food processor and process until the mixture is well

combined. Transfer to a large bowl. Combine the yogurt, remaining 2 tablespoons oil, and the egg in a medium bowl and whisk until smooth. Add the yogurt mixture to the flour mixture and stir just until moistened. Gently stir in the cherries.

3 Spoon the batter evenly into the muffin cups and sprinkle evenly with the almonds. Bake until a toothpick inserted into the centers of the muffins comes out clean, 22 to 25 minutes.

4 Cool the muffins in the pan on a wire rack for 5 minutes. Remove the muffins from the pan and place on the rack. Serve hot, warm, or at room temperature. The muffins can be stored in an airtight container at room temperature for up to 2 days or frozen for up to 3 months.

Each serving: 31 g carb, 201 cal, 7 g fat, 1 g sat fat, 18 mg chol, 3 g fib, 5 g pro, 192 mg sod • Carb Choices: 2; Exchanges: 2 carb, 1 fat

Pineapple-Carrot Muffins

QUICK

makes 12 servings

Reminiscent of carrot cake, these muffins are filled with wholesome ingredients. When you freeze them and reheat in the microwave, they taste almost fresh-baked.

2 teaspoons plus ⅓ cup canola oil, divided
2 cups whole wheat pastry flour or
    1 cup unbleached all-purpose flour
    and 1 cup whole wheat flour
½ cup sugar
2 teaspoons baking powder
¾ teaspoon ground cinnamon
¼ teaspoon salt
1 large egg
1 teaspoon vanilla extract
1 cup finely shredded carrots
1 (8-ounce) can crushed pineapple packed in
    juice, undrained
2 tablespoons unsalted shelled sunflower seeds

1 Preheat the oven to 350°F. Brush a 12-cup muffin tin with 2 teaspoons of the oil or omit the oil and line the tin with paper muffin liners.

2 Combine the flour, sugar, baking powder, cinnamon, and salt in a large bowl and whisk to mix well. Combine the remaining ⅓ cup oil, the egg, and vanilla in a small bowl and whisk until smooth. Add the oil mixture, carrots, and pineapple with juice to the flour mixture and stir just until moistened.

3 Spoon the batter evenly into the muffin cups and sprinkle evenly with the sunflower seeds. Bake until a toothpick inserted into the centers of the muffins comes out clean, 22 to 25 minutes.

4 Cool the muffins in the pan on a wire rack for 5 minutes. Remove the muffins from the pan and place on the rack. Serve hot, warm, or at room temperature. The muffins can be stored in an airtight container at room temperature for up to 2 days or frozen for up to 3 months.

Each serving: 28 g carb, 192 cal, 8 g fat, 1 g sat fat, 18 mg chol, 3 g fib, 3 g pro, 129 mg sod • Carb Choices: 2; Exchanges: 2 carb, 1½ fat

PINEAPPLE-CARROT-RAISIN MUFFINS QUICK
HIGH FIBER: Follow the recipe for Pineapple Carrot Muffins, at left, adding ⅓ cup raisins to the batter in step 2, and proceed as directed.

Each serving: 31 g carb, 204 cal, 8 g fat, 1 g sat fat, 18 mg chol, 4 g fib, 3 g pro, 129 mg sod • Carb Choices: 2; Exchanges: 2 carb, 1½ fat

Blueberry-Lemon Muffins

QUICK

makes 12 servings

The delicate flavor of these muffins would be overwhelmed by regular whole wheat flour; be sure to use one of the flours recommended here. If you need to dress the muffins up for a special meal or to give as a gift, drizzle them with Citrus Glaze (page 586).

2 teaspoons plus ⅓ cup canola oil, divided
2 cups white whole wheat flour, whole wheat pastry flour, or unbleached all-purpose flour
½ cup sugar
2 teaspoons baking powder
½ teaspoon baking soda
¼ teaspoon salt
1 large egg
¾ cup 1% low-fat milk
½ cup plain low-fat yogurt
2 teaspoons grated lemon zest
¾ cup fresh blueberries or unthawed frozen blueberries

1 Preheat the oven to 350°F. Brush a 12-cup muffin tin with 2 teaspoons of the oil or omit the oil and line the tin with paper muffin liners.

2 Combine the flour, sugar, baking powder, baking soda, and salt in a large bowl and whisk to mix well. Combine the remaining ⅓ cup oil, the egg, milk, yogurt, and lemon zest in a medium bowl and whisk until smooth. Add the egg mixture to the flour mixture and stir just until moistened. Gently stir in the blueberries.

3 Spoon the batter evenly into the muffin cups. Bake until a toothpick inserted into the centers of the muffins comes out clean, 25 to 28 minutes.

4 Cool the muffins in the pan on a wire rack for 5 minutes. Remove the muffins from the pan and place on the rack. Serve hot, warm, or at room temperature. The muffins can be stored in an airtight container at room temperature for up to 2 days or frozen for up to 3 months.

Each serving: 27 g carb, 192 cal, 8 g fat, 1 g sat fat, 19 mg chol, 3 g fib, 4 g pro, 187 mg sod • Carb Choices: 2; Exchanges: 2 carb, 1½ fat

Banana-Berry Muffins QUICK

makes 12 servings

These muffins taste like banana bread, but with the bright addition of berries. In the spring, try making these with ¾ cup chopped fresh strawberries instead of the blueberries.

2 teaspoons plus ¼ cup canola oil, divided
2 cups whole wheat pastry flour or
    1 cup unbleached all-purpose flour
    and 1 cup whole wheat flour
½ cup sugar
2 teaspoons baking powder
½ teaspoon baking soda
¼ teaspoon salt
¼ teaspoon ground nutmeg
¾ cup mashed ripe banana (1 large banana)
⅔ cup low-fat buttermilk
1 large egg
1 teaspoon vanilla extract
¾ cup fresh blueberries or raspberries or unthawed frozen unsweetened blueberries or raspberries

1 Preheat the oven to 350°F. Brush a 12-cup muffin tin with 2 teaspoons of the oil or omit the oil and line the tin with paper muffin liners.

2 Combine the flour, sugar, baking powder, baking soda, salt, and nutmeg in a large bowl and whisk to mix well. Combine the remaining ¼ cup oil, the banana, buttermilk, egg, and vanilla in a medium bowl and whisk until smooth. Add the oil mixture to the flour mixture and stir just until moistened. Gently stir in the blueberries.

3 Spoon the batter evenly into the muffin cups. Bake until a toothpick inserted into the centers of the muffins comes out clean, 22 to 25 minutes.

4 Cool the muffins in the pan on a wire rack for 5 minutes. Remove the muffins from the pan and place on the rack. Serve hot, warm, or at room temperature. The muffins can be stored in an airtight container at room temperature for up to 2 days or frozen for up to 3 months.

Each serving: 28 g carb, 181 cal, 6 g fat, 1 g sat fat, 18 mg chol, 3 g fib, 3 g pro, 189 mg sod • Carb Choices: 2; Exchanges: 2 carb, 1 fat

BANANA–CHOCOLATE CHIP MUFFINS: Follow the Banana-Berry Muffins recipe, at left, but omit the blueberries and nutmeg. Stir in ⅓ cup semisweet mini chocolate chips in step 2 and proceed with the recipe.

Each serving: 31 g carb, 210 cal, 8 g fat, 2 g sat fat, 18 mg chol, 3 g fib, 4 g pro, 188 mg sod • Carb Choices: 2; Exchanges: 2 carb, 1½ fat

Moist Bran Muffins QUICK

makes 12 servings

If you buy bran muffins in a bakery, they'll probably be at least twice the size of these— and have twice the carbs, fat, and calories. Making them at home is easy and this recipe makes muffins that are sweet enough to be a treat, yet won't blow your carb budget for breakfast or a snack. Unprocessed wheat bran is the outer coating of the wheat kernel. Sometimes called miller's bran, it is an excellent source of fiber. Sprinkle 2 tablespoons of it over your morning cereal and boost your fiber intake by 3 grams.

1 cup 1% low-fat milk
1 cup unprocessed wheat bran
2 teaspoons plus ¼ cup canola oil, divided
1 cup whole wheat flour
¼ cup packed light brown sugar
2 teaspoons baking powder
¾ teaspoon ground cinnamon
¼ teaspoon salt
2 large eggs
⅓ cup light or dark molasses (not blackstrap)
1 teaspoon vanilla extract

1 Pour the milk into a medium saucepan and set over medium heat until hot but not boiling. Remove from the heat and stir in the bran. Cover and let stand 10 minutes.

2 Meanwhile, preheat the oven to 350°F. Brush a 12-cup muffin tin with 2 teaspoons of the oil or omit the oil and line the tin with paper muffin liners.

3 Combine the flour, sugar, baking powder, cinnamon, and salt in a large bowl and whisk to mix well. Combine the remaining ¼ cup oil, the eggs, molasses, and vanilla in a medium bowl and whisk until smooth. Add the bran mixture to the oil mixture and stir to mix well. Add the bran mixture to the flour mixture and stir just until moistened. (The batter will be thin.)

4 Spoon the batter evenly into the muffin cups. Bake until a toothpick inserted into the centers of the muffins comes out clean, 20 to 22 minutes.

5 Cool the muffins in the pan on a wire rack for 5 minutes. Remove the muffins from the pan and place on the rack. Serve hot, warm, or at room temperature. The muffins can be stored in an airtight container at room temperature for up to 2 days or frozen for up to 3 months.

Each serving: 23 g carb, 157 cal, 6 g fat, 1 g sat fat, 36 mg chol, 3 g fib, 4 g pro, 142 mg sod • Carb Choices: 1½; Exchanges: 1½ carb, 1 fat

CARROT-BRAN MUFFINS QUICK HIGH FIBER : Follow the Moist Bran Muffins recipe, at left, adding 1 cup peeled finely shredded carrot along with the bran mixture in step 3. Proceed with the recipe.

Each serving: 24 g carb, 161 cal, 6 g fat, 1 g sat fat, 36 mg chol, 4 g fib, 4 g pro, 148 mg sod • Carb Choices: 1½; Exchanges: 1½ carb, 1 fat

PINEAPPLE-BRAN MUFFINS QUICK HIGH FIBER : Follow the Moist Bran Muffins recipe, at left, adding 1 (8-ounce) can crushed pineapple in juice, drained, along with the bran mixture in step 3. Proceed with the recipe.

Each serving: 26 g carb, 168 cal, 6 g fat, 1 g sat fat, 36 mg chol, 4 g fib, 4 g pro, 142 mg sod • Carb Choices: 2; Exchanges: 2 carb, 1 fat

Ginger-Pear Muffins with Almond Streusel QUICK

makes 12 servings

The crunchy streusel provides a textural contrast to the delicate muffins underneath. If you don't have almonds, you can make the streusel with pecans or walnuts. Instead of fresh ginger, you can use 1½ teaspoons ground ginger, stirring it into the flour mixture in step 3.

2 teaspoons canola oil

STREUSEL

2 tablespoons all-purpose flour
2 tablespoons light brown sugar
1 tablespoon cold unsalted butter, cut into small pieces
3 tablespoons chopped almonds

MUFFINS

1 cup whole wheat pastry flour or
    1 cup unbleached all-purpose flour
    and 1 cup whole wheat flour
½ cup sugar
2 teaspoons baking powder
½ teaspoon baking soda
¼ teaspoon salt
½ cup plain low-fat yogurt
¼ cup canola oil
2 large eggs
1 teaspoon grated fresh ginger
1 medium ripe pear, peeled, and coarsely shredded (about ½ cup)

1 Preheat the oven to 350°F. Brush a 12-cup muffin tin with the 2 teaspoons oil or omit the oil and line the tin with paper muffin liners.

2 To make the streusel, combine the flour, sugar, and butter in a small bowl and stir with a fork until the mixture is crumbly. Stir in the almonds and set aside.

3 To make the muffins, combine the flour, sugar, baking powder, baking soda, and salt in a large

bowl and whisk to mix well. Combine the yogurt, ¼ cup oil, eggs, and ginger in a medium bowl and whisk until smooth. Add the yogurt mixture and pear to the flour mixture and stir just until moistened.

4 Spoon the batter evenly into the muffin cups and sprinkle evenly with the streusel. Bake until a toothpick inserted into the centers of the muffins comes out clean, 25 to 28 minutes.

5 Cool the muffins in the pan on a wire rack for 5 minutes. Remove the muffins from the pan and place on the rack. Serve hot, warm, or at room temperature. The muffins can be stored in an airtight container at room temperature for up to 2 days.

Each serving: 30 g carb, 211 cal, 8 g fat, 1 g sat fat, 38 mg chol, 2 g fib, 5 g pro, 240 mg sod • Carb Choices: 2; Exchanges: 2 carb, 1½ fat

Cornmeal Muffins with Fresh Cranberries QUICK

makes 12 servings

When I was growing up in Kentucky, it would have been heresy to add sugar to a cornmeal muffin. They were a savory bread to be served with soup or chili. When I moved to New York, I discovered all sorts of sweet ways to use cornmeal. Fruit and cornmeal are a lovely pairing, as you'll see when you try these deliciously sweet muffins. This version is nice to enjoy during the fall and winter months, but in summer, you can replace the cranberries with blueberries and the orange zest with lemon zest.

2 teaspoons plus 2 tablespoons canola oil, divided
1 cup fine-grind yellow cornmeal
1 cup unbleached all-purpose flour
½ cup sugar
2 teaspoons baking powder
½ teaspoon baking soda

¼ teaspoon salt

1 cup low-fat buttermilk

1 large egg

2 teaspoons grated orange zest

½ teaspoon vanilla extract

¾ cup fresh cranberries or unthawed frozen cranberries

1 Preheat the oven to 375°F. Brush a 12-cup muffin tin with 2 teaspoons of the oil or omit the oil and line the tin with paper muffin liners.

2 Combine the cornmeal, flour, sugar, baking powder, baking soda, and salt in a large bowl and whisk to mix well. Combine the buttermilk, remaining 2 tablespoons oil, the egg, orange zest, and vanilla in a medium bowl and whisk until smooth. Add the buttermilk mixture to the cornmeal mixture and stir just until moistened. Gently stir in the cranberries.

3 Spoon the batter evenly into the muffin cups. Bake until a toothpick inserted into the centers of the muffins comes out clean, 25 to 28 minutes.

4 Cool the muffins in the pan on a wire rack for 5 minutes. Remove the muffins from the pan and place on the rack. Serve hot, warm, or at room temperature. The muffins can be stored in an airtight container at room temperature for up to 2 days or frozen for up to 3 months.

Each serving: 28 g carb, 165 cal, 4 g fat, 0 g sat fat, 19 mg chol, 1 g fib, 4 g pro, 200 mg sod • Carb Choices: 2; Exchanges: 2 carb, 1 fat

Red Bell Pepper, Corn, and Basil Muffins QUICK

makes 12 servings

A unique savory muffin like these can elevate a bowl of soup or chili to a special meal. Because of the high moisture content of the vegetables in both versions of this recipe, the muffins do not freeze well.

1 cup fine-grind yellow cornmeal

1 cup unbleached all-purpose flour

2 tablespoons sugar

2 teaspoons baking powder

½ teaspoon baking soda

½ teaspoon salt

¾ cup low-fat buttermilk

¼ cup canola oil

1 large egg

1 medium ear corn, kernels cut from the cob

½ cup red Roasted Bell Peppers (page 21) or roasted red peppers from a jar, diced

½ cup chopped fresh basil

1 Preheat the oven to 375°F. Line a 12-cup muffin tin with paper liners.

2 Combine the cornmeal, flour, sugar, baking powder, baking soda, and salt in a large bowl and whisk to mix well. Combine the buttermilk, oil, and egg in a medium bowl and whisk until smooth. Add the buttermilk mixture to the cornmeal mixture and stir just until moistened. Gently stir in the corn, roasted peppers, and basil.

3 Spoon the batter evenly into the muffin cups and bake 15 to 18 minutes or until the tops of the muffins are lightly browned.

4 Cool the muffins in the pan on a wire rack for 5 minutes. Remove the muffins from the pan and place on the rack. Serve hot or warm. The muffins are best on the day they are made.

Each serving: 23 g carb, 157 cal, 6 g fat, 1 g sat fat, 19 mg chol, 2 g fib, 4 g pro, 245 mg sod • Carb Choices: 1½; Exchanges: 1½ starch, 1 fat

CORN AND ZUCCHINI MUFFINS QUICK: Follow the Red Bell Pepper, Corn, and Basil Muffins recipe, at left, but replace the roasted pepper with 1 cup coarsely shredded zucchini and proceed with the recipe.

Each serving: 23 g carb, 157 cal, 6 g fat, 1 g sat fat, 19 mg chol, 2 g fib, 4 g pro, 245 mg sod • Carb Choices: 1½; Exchanges: 1½ starch, 1 fat

Cornmeal Muffins with Chiles and Cheese QUICK

makes 12 servings

Fresh from the oven, these slightly spicy muffins are a tasty partner for chili, soup, or a salad. Make sure you have a crowd when you make these, since they don't reheat very well.

1 cup fine-grind yellow cornmeal
1 cup unbleached all-purpose flour
2 teaspoons baking powder
½ teaspoon baking soda
½ teaspoon salt
½ teaspoon ground cayenne
¾ cup low-fat buttermilk
¼ cup canola oil
2 tablespoons honey
1 large egg
2 ounces shredded extra-sharp Cheddar cheese (about ½ cup)
1 (4½-ounce) can diced green chiles, drained
¼ cup thinly sliced scallions
¼ cup chopped fresh cilantro

1 Preheat the oven to 375°F. Line a 12-cup muffin tin with paper liners.

2 Combine the cornmeal, flour, baking powder, baking soda, salt, and cayenne in a large bowl and whisk to mix well. Combine the buttermilk, oil, honey, and egg in a medium bowl and whisk until smooth. Add the buttermilk mixture to the cornmeal mixture and stir just until moistened. Gently stir in the Cheddar, chiles, scallions, and cilantro.

3 Spoon the batter evenly into the muffin cups. Bake until a toothpick inserted into the centers of the muffins comes out clean, 15 to 18 minutes.

4 Cool the muffins in the pan on a wire rack for 5 minutes. Remove the muffins from the pan and place on the rack. Serve hot or warm. The muffins are best on the day they are made.

Each serving: 23 g carb, 172 cal, 7 g fat, 1 g sat fat, 24 mg chol, 1 g fib, 5 g pro, 286 mg sod • Carb Choices: 1½; Exchanges: 1½ starch, 1½ fat

Parmesan Muffins QUICK

makes 12 servings

Use good quality Parmesan cheese to make these muffins. Serve with soup, a salad, or instead of a roll with dinner.

2¼ cups whole wheat pastry flour or 1¼ cups unbleached all-purpose flour and 1 cup whole wheat flour
4 ounces freshly grated Parmesan (about 1 cup), preferably Parmigiano-Reggiano
2 tablespoons sugar
2 teaspoons baking powder
½ teaspoon baking soda
¼ teaspoon salt
¼ teaspoon freshly ground pepper
1½ cups 1% low-fat milk
¼ cup canola oil
1 large egg
1 tablespoon finely shredded Parmesan, preferably Parmigiano-Reggiano

1 Preheat the oven to 375°F. Line a 12-cup muffin tin with paper liners.

2 Combine the flour, grated Parmesan, sugar, baking powder, baking soda, salt, and pepper in a large bowl and whisk to mix well. Combine the milk, oil, and egg in a medium bowl and whisk until smooth. Add the milk mixture to the flour mixture and stir just until moistened.

3 Spoon the batter evenly into the muffin cups and sprinkle evenly with the shredded Parmesan. Bake until a toothpick inserted into the centers of the muffins comes out clean, 15 to 18 minutes.

4 Cool the muffins in the pan on a wire rack for 5 minutes. Remove the muffins from the pan and place on the rack. Serve hot, warm, or at room temperature. The muffins can be stored in an airtight container at room temperature for up to 2 days or frozen for up to 3 months.

Each serving: 21 g carb, 183 cal, 8 g fat, 2 g sat fat, 25 mg chol, 3 g fib, 7 g pro, 300 mg sod • Carb Choices: 1½; Exchanges: 1½ starch, 1½ fat

Scones and Biscuits

Fresh Cranberry–Orange Scones QUICK

makes 12 servings

Fresh cranberries are stirred into an orange-scented batter to make these tender scones. With all the versions here, you have options for fresh fruity scones at any time of year. Instead of the whole wheat pastry flour or white whole wheat, you can also use 1 cup of regular whole wheat flour and 1 cup of unbleached all-purpose flour.

2 cups whole wheat pastry flour or white whole wheat flour

2 teaspoons baking powder

½ teaspoon baking soda

¼ teaspoon salt

2 tablespoons cold unsalted butter, cut into small pieces

½ cup plus 2 teaspoons sugar, divided

¾ cup plain low-fat yogurt

2 teaspoons grated orange zest

1 cup fresh cranberries or unthawed frozen cranberries

1 Preheat the oven to 400°F. Line a large baking sheet with parchment paper.

2 Combine the flour, baking powder, baking soda, salt, and butter in a large bowl. Cut the butter into the dry ingredients using a pastry blender until the mixture resembles coarse meal. Stir in ½ cup of the sugar. Combine the yogurt and orange zest in a medium bowl and whisk until smooth. Add the yogurt mixture and the cranberries to the flour mixture and stir just until moistened.

3 Divide the dough in half and transfer to a lightly floured surface. Sprinkle the dough lightly with flour and pat each half into a 6-inch circle. Place each circle of dough onto the prepared baking sheet.

4 Cut each round into 6 wedges, but do not separate the wedges. Sprinkle the tops of the rounds with the remaining 2 teaspoons sugar. Bake until the tops are lightly browned, 18 to 20 minutes. Serve warm.

Each serving: 27 g carb, 140 cal, 3 g fat, 1 g sat fat, 6 mg chol, 3 g fib, 3 g pro, 154 mg sod • Carb Choices: 2; Exchanges: 2 carb, ½ fat

BLUEBERRY-LEMON SCONES QUICK: Follow the Fresh Cranberry–Orange Scones recipe, at left, but replace the cranberries with 1 cup fresh blueberries or unsweetened frozen blueberries and replace the grated orange zest with lemon zest and proceed as directed.

Each serving: 27 g carb, 143 cal, 3 g fat, 1 g sat fat, 6 mg chol, 3 g fib, 3 g pro, 153 mg sod • Carb Choices: 2; Exchanges: 2 carb, ½ fat

PEACH SCONES WITH ALMONDS QUICK: Follow the Fresh Cranberry–Orange Scones recipe, at left, but replace the cranberries with 1 cup chopped fresh peeled peaches. In addition to sprinkling with the sugar, sprinkle the tops of each of the rounds with 1 tablespoon sliced almonds just before baking.

Each serving: 27 g carb, 145 cal, 3 g fat, 1 g sat fat, 6 mg chol, 3 g fib, 3 g pro, 153 mg sod • Carb Choices: 2; Exchanges: 2 carb, ½ fat

Gingerbread Scones QUICK

makes 16 servings

These deliciously moist and fragrant scones are worth making for the aroma alone. The extra sprinkle of raw sugar on top gives them a nice crunch.

2 cups white whole wheat flour or regular whole wheat flour

2 teaspoons ground ginger

1 teaspoon ground cinnamon

½ teaspoon ground nutmeg

½ teaspoon ground cloves

2 teaspoons baking powder

½ teaspoon baking soda

¼ teaspoon salt

2 tablespoons cold unsalted butter, cut into small pieces

⅓ cup packed light brown sugar

⅔ cup low-fat buttermilk

2 tablespoons light or dark molasses (not blackstrap)

2 teaspoons turbinado (raw) sugar

1 Preheat the oven to 400°F. Line a large baking sheet with parchment paper.

2 Combine the flour, ginger, cinnamon, nutmeg, cloves, baking powder, baking soda, salt, and butter in a large bowl. Cut the butter into the dry ingredients using a pastry blender until the mixture resembles coarse meal. Stir in the brown sugar. Combine the buttermilk and molasses in a small bowl and whisk until smooth. Add the buttermilk mixture to the flour mixture and stir just until moistened.

3 Transfer the dough to a lightly floured surface. Pat the dough into a 6 x 8-inch rectangle. Cut the dough in half lengthwise and into quarters crosswise. Cut each resulting rectangle in half diagonally to make 2 wedges. Using a baker's bench scraper or a wide spatula, transfer the wedges to the prepared baking sheet. Sprinkle the wedges with the turbinado sugar. Bake until the tops are lightly browned, 12 to 15 minutes. Serve warm.

Each serving: 20 g carb, 102 cal, 2 g fat, 1 g sat fat, 4 mg chol, 2 g fib, 2 g pro, 121 mg sod • Carb Choices: 1; Exchanges: 1 carb, ½ fat

Oat Scones with Currants

QUICK

makes 16 servings

Ground oats in the batter give these scones a hearty texture and the currants are a sweet embellishment. Serve them with a smear of marmalade or jam.

¼ cup unsweetened apple juice

⅓ cup currants

¾ cup plus 1 tablespoon old-fashioned rolled oats

1½ cups white whole wheat flour or regular whole wheat flour

2 teaspoons baking powder

½ teaspoon baking soda

¼ teaspoon salt

2 tablespoons cold unsalted butter, cut into small pieces

¼ cup sugar

⅔ cup low-fat buttermilk

1 Pour the apple juice into a medium saucepan and set over medium heat until hot but not boiling. Remove from the heat and stir in the currants. Cover and let stand 30 minutes.

2 Preheat the oven to 400°F. Line a large baking sheet with parchment paper.

3 Place the oats in a food processor and process until finely ground. Combine the ground oats, flour, baking powder, baking soda, salt, and butter in a large bowl. Cut the butter into the dry ingredients using a pastry blender until the mixture resembles coarse meal. Stir in the sugar. Add the buttermilk and the currant mixture to the flour mixture and stir just until moistened.

4 Transfer the dough to a lightly floured surface. Pat the dough into a 6 x 8-inch rectangle. Cut the dough in half lengthwise and into quarters crosswise. Cut each resulting rectangle in half diagonally to make 2 wedges. Using a baker's bench scraper or a wide spatula, transfer the wedges to the prepared baking sheet. Bake until the tops are lightly browned, 12 to 15 minutes. Serve warm.

Each serving: 18 g carb, 98 cal, 2 g fat, 1 g sat fat, 4 mg chol, 2 g fib, 3 g pro, 118 mg sod • Carb Choices: 1; Exchanges: 1 starch

Baking Powder Biscuits QUICK

makes 12 servings

A blend of white whole wheat and all-purpose flours makes the highest-rising and lightest-textured biscuits, but you can make these using all whole wheat flour or all whole wheat pastry flour with delicious results. It's quicker to cut the butter into the flour using a food processor, but cutting it in with a pastry blender makes the pieces of butter bigger, resulting in a flakier biscuit.

1 cup white whole wheat flour or regular whole wheat flour

½ cup unbleached all-purpose flour

1½ teaspoons baking powder

¼ teaspoon baking soda

½ teaspoon salt

3 tablespoons cold unsalted butter, cut into small pieces

⅔ cup low-fat buttermilk

1 Preheat the oven to 400°F. Position an oven rack in the top third of the oven.

2 Combine the whole wheat flour, all-purpose flour, baking powder, baking soda, salt, and butter in a large bowl. Cut the butter into the dry ingredients using a pastry blender until the mixture resembles coarse meal. Stir in the buttermilk.

3 Transfer the dough to a lightly floured surface and knead 6 to 8 times until the dough holds together. Pat the dough to a ½-inch thickness and cut into rounds with a 2-inch biscuit cutter. Gather the dough scraps and repeat the patting and cutting to make a total of 12 biscuits.

4 Place the biscuits on an ungreased baking sheet. Bake in the top third of the oven until the tops of the biscuits are lightly browned, 10 to 12 minutes. Serve hot or warm.

Each serving: 12 g carb, 85 cal, 3 g fat, 2 g sat fat, 8 mg chol, 1 g fib, 2 g pro, 189 mg sod • Carb Choices: 1; Exchanges: 1 starch, ½ fat

CHEDDAR-SAGE BISCUITS QUICK : Follow the Baking Powder Biscuits recipe, at left, stirring in ½ cup finely shredded extra-sharp white Cheddar cheese and 2 teaspoons minced fresh sage with the flours in step 2, and proceed as directed.

Each serving: 12 g carb, 103 cal, 5 g fat, 3 g sat fat, 13 mg chol, 1 g fib, 4 g pro, 219 mg sod • Carb Choices: 1; Exchanges: 1 starch, 1 fat

HERB BISCUITS QUICK : Follow the Baking Powder Biscuits recipe, at left, stirring in 2 tablespoons of one or more of minced fresh basil or dill or 2 teaspoons minced fresh tarragon, oregano, rosemary, or thyme with the flours in step 2, and proceed as directed.

Each serving: 12 g carb, 85 cal, 3 g fat, 2 g sat fat, 8 mg chol, 1 g fib, 2 g pro, 189 mg sod • Carb Choices: 1; Exchanges: 1 starch, ½ fat

Sweet Potato Biscuits

serves 18

These biscuits are a natural with a holiday ham, but you can serve them as a special treat with brunch any time of year. They also make great hors d'oeuvres: cut the biscuits using a 1-inch biscuit cutter and bake as directed. Split the tiny biscuits, fill them with thinly sliced ham, and watch them disappear.

1 large sweet potato, peeled and cut into
    ½-inch cubes (about 1¼ cups)

¼ cup sugar

¼ cup plain low-fat yogurt

2 tablespoons unsalted butter, softened

2 cups whole wheat pastry flour or 1 cup
    unbleached all-purpose flour and 1 cup
    whole wheat flour

2 teaspoons baking powder

½ teaspoon baking soda

½ teaspoon salt

½ cup low-fat buttermilk

1 Place the potato in a large saucepan and add water to cover. Bring to a boil over high heat, reduce the heat to low, and simmer until tender, about 15 minutes.

2 Drain the potato in a colander and transfer to a medium bowl. Add the sugar, yogurt, and butter and mash the mixture with a potato masher until smooth. Let cool slightly.

3 Preheat the oven to 400°F. Position an oven rack in the top third of the oven.

4 Combine the flour, baking powder, baking soda, and salt in a large bowl and whisk to mix well. Add the potato mixture and the buttermilk and stir just until a moist dough forms.

5 Transfer the dough to a lightly floured surface and knead 6 to 8 times until the dough holds together. Pat the dough to a ¾-inch thickness and cut into rounds with a 2-inch biscuit cutter. Gather the dough scraps and repeat the patting and cutting to make a total of 18 biscuits.

6 Place the biscuits on an ungreased baking sheet. Bake in the top third of the oven until the tops are lightly browned, 10 to 12 minutes. Serve hot or warm.

Each serving: 15 g carb, 84 cal, 2 g fat, 1 g sat fat, 4 mg chol, 2 g fib, 2 g pro, 159 mg sod • Carb Choices: 1; Exchanges: 1 starch

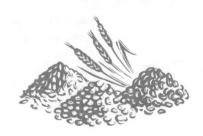

Griddle Cakes and Tortillas

Fresh Corn Griddle Cakes

QUICK

makes 10 servings

Crispy on the outside and moist on the inside, these are perfect to serve with a summer vegetable plate, a salad, or soup. You can make them in winter, too. Use ¾ cup of frozen thawed corn kernels instead of the fresh corn.

1 cup fine-grind yellow cornmeal
½ cup whole wheat flour
1½ teaspoons baking powder
¼ teaspoon salt
1 cup low-fat buttermilk
1 large egg
1 tablespoon plus 1 teaspoon canola oil, divided
1 medium ear corn, kernels cut from the cob
2 ounces shredded extra-sharp Cheddar cheese (about ½ cup)

1 Combine the cornmeal, flour, baking powder, and salt in a large bowl and stir to mix well. Combine the buttermilk, egg, and 1 tablespoon of the oil in a small bowl and whisk until smooth. Add the buttermilk mixture, corn, and Cheddar to the cornmeal mixture and stir until a smooth batter forms.

2 Heat a large nonstick griddle or large nonstick skillet over medium heat. Brush with ½ teaspoon of the remaining oil using a silicone brush. Spoon the batter by scant ¼ cup measures onto the griddle, spreading the batter into 3-inch rounds. Cook until well browned, 2 to 3 minutes on each side. Repeat the procedure with the remaining ½ teaspoon oil and remaining batter to make 10 griddle cakes. Serve warm.

Each serving: 21 g carb, 152 cal, 5 g fat, 1 g sat fat, 29 mg chol, 2 g fib, 6 g pro, 215 mg sod • Carb Choices: 1½; Exchanges: 1½ starch, 1 fat

GRIDDLE CAKES WITH JALAPEÑO AND CILANTRO: Follow the Fresh Corn Griddle Cakes recipe, at left, stirring in 1 jalapeño, seeded and minced, and 2 tablespoons chopped fresh cilantro with the corn. Proceed as directed.

Each serving: 21 g carb, 153 cal, 5 g fat, 1 g sat fat, 29 mg chol, 2 g fib, 6 g pro, 215 mg sod • Carb Choices: 1½; Exchanges: 1½ starch, 1 fat

Whole Wheat Flour Tortillas

makes 12 servings

These tortillas are a lot of effort to make, but try them sometime when you're having a special Mexican-themed meal. They make the best soft tacos ever.

2 cups whole wheat flour
1 teaspoon salt
¾ teaspoon baking powder
⅔ to ¾ cup hot water
2 tablespoons canola oil

1 Combine the flour, salt, and baking powder in a large bowl and whisk to mix well. Add ⅔ cup of the water and the oil and stir until the dough is moistened, adding the additional water, 1 tablespoon at a time, as needed, to form a stiff dough. Cover the dough and let stand 30 minutes.

2 Divide the dough into 12 equal pieces. Roll each piece on a lightly floured surface into an 8-inch round.

3 Heat a large nonstick skillet over medium-high heat. Working with one tortilla at a time, place a tortilla in the skillet and cook until puffed and well browned, 1½ to 2 minutes on each side. Place the tortillas on a plate under a towel to keep warm while making the remaining tortillas. The tortillas are best within 2 hours.

Each serving: 16 g carb, 101 cal, 3 g fat, 0 g sat fat, 0 mg chol, 3 g fib, 3 g pro, 219 mg sod • Carb Choices: 1; Exchanges: 1 starch, ½ fat

Yeast Breads

Whole Wheat Bread

makes 16 servings

This bread uses all whole wheat flour, resulting in a dense loaf that is hearty and full of earthy wheat flavor. For a lighter-textured loaf, replace 1 cup of the whole wheat flour with 1 cup of unbleached all-purpose flour.

1 cup lukewarm water

1 package active dry yeast

2 tablespoons honey

2¼ to 2½ cups whole wheat flour

2 tablespoons plus 1 teaspoon canola oil, divided

1 teaspoon salt

1 Combine the water and yeast in a large bowl and stir until the yeast dissolves. Let stand 5 minutes. Stir in the honey. Add 2¼ cups of the flour, 2 tablespoons of the oil, and the salt and stir until a soft dough forms.

2 Turn the dough out onto a lightly floured surface. Knead until smooth and elastic, about 8 minutes. Add enough of the remaining ¼ cup flour, 1 tablespoon at a time, to prevent the dough from sticking to your hands. (Alternatively, knead the dough for 5 minutes at low speed with an electric mixer using a dough hook, adding enough of the remaining ¼ cup flour, 1 tablespoon at a time, to make a smooth dough.)

3 Brush a large bowl with the remaining 1 teaspoon oil. Place the dough in the bowl and turn to coat the top. Cover and let rise in a warm place (85°F), free from drafts, until doubled in size, about 1 hour.

4 Line a medium baking sheet with parchment paper. Shape the dough into a 6-inch round loaf and place on the prepared pan. Cover loosely with lightly oiled plastic wrap and let rise in a warm place (85°F), free from drafts, until doubled in size, about 45 minutes.

5 Preheat the oven to 350°F. Remove the plastic wrap and bake the loaf 20 minutes. Cover loosely with foil and bake until the loaf is golden brown and sounds hollow when tapped, about 10 minutes longer.

6 Remove the loaf from the pan and cool completely on a wire rack. Slice using a serrated knife. The bread can be stored inside a paper bag at room temperature for up to 2 days or frozen for up to 3 months.

Each serving: 16 g carb, 95 cal, 2 g fat, 0 g sat fat, 0 mg chol, 2 g fib, 3 g pro, 146 mg sod • Carb Choices: 1; Exchanges: 1 starch, ½ fat

SEEDED WHEAT BREAD: Follow the Whole Wheat Bread recipe, at left, adding ⅓ cup toasted sunflower seeds (page 4) and 2 teaspoons toasted sesame seeds (page 4) with the other ingredients in step 1, and proceed with the recipe.

Each serving: 16 g carb, 112 cal, 4 g fat, 0 g sat fat, 0 mg chol, 3 g fib, 4 g pro, 146 mg sod • Carb Choices: 1; Exchanges: 1 starch, ½ fat

RAISIN-WALNUT BREAD: Follow the Whole Wheat Bread recipe, at left, adding ½ cup golden raisins and ¼ cup walnuts, toasted and chopped (page 4), with the other ingredients in step 1, and proceed with the recipe.

Each serving: 20 g carb, 121 cal, 4 g fat, 0 g sat fat, 0 mg chol, 3 g fib, 4 g pro, 146 mg sod • Carb Choices: 1; Exchanges: 1 starch, ½ fat

Parmesan-Rosemary Wheat Loaf

makes 16 servings

Aromatic and moist, this bread has so much flavor on its own, it will turn a boring chicken breast or an ordinary slice of cheese into a great sandwich. If you don't eat bread often, you can cut this loaf in half and freeze it to enjoy later.

1 cup lukewarm water
1 package active dry yeast
2¼ to 2½ cups whole wheat flour
2 ounces freshly grated Parmesan
    (about ½ cup)
2 tablespoons plus 1 teaspoon canola oil,
    divided
1 tablespoon sugar
1 tablespoon chopped fresh rosemary
1 teaspoon salt
⅛ teaspoon freshly ground pepper

1 Combine the water and yeast in a large bowl and stir until the yeast dissolves. Let stand 5 minutes. Add 2¼ cups of the flour, the Parmesan, 2 tablespoons of the oil, the sugar, rosemary, salt, and pepper and stir until a soft dough forms.

2 Turn the dough out onto a lightly floured surface. Knead until smooth and elastic, about 8 minutes. Add enough of the remaining ¼ cup flour, 1 tablespoon at a time, to prevent the dough from sticking to your hands. (Alternatively, knead the dough for 5 minutes at low speed with an electric mixer using a dough hook, adding enough of the remaining ¼ cup flour, 1 tablespoon at a time, to make a smooth dough.)

3 Brush a large bowl with the remaining 1 teaspoon oil. Place the dough in the bowl and turn to coat the top. Cover and let rise in a warm place (85°F), free from drafts, until doubled in size, about 1 hour.

4 Line a 9 x 5-inch loaf pan with parchment paper. Place the dough in the prepared pan. Cover loosely with lightly oiled plastic wrap and let rise in a warm place (85°F), free from drafts, until doubled in size, about 45 minutes.

5 Preheat the oven to 350°F. Remove the plastic wrap and bake the loaf 20 minutes. Cover loosely with foil and bake until the loaf is golden brown and sounds hollow when tapped, about 10 minutes longer.

6 Cool the bread in the pan on a wire rack for 10 minutes. Remove from the pan and cool completely on a wire rack. Slice using a serrated knife. The bread can be stored inside a paper bag at room temperature for up to 2 days or frozen for up to 3 months.

Each serving: 15 g carb, 101 cal, 3 g fat, 1 g sat fat, 2 mg chol, 2 g fib, 4 g pro, 184 mg sod • Carb Choices: 1; Exchanges: 1 starch, ½ fat

Instant Yeast

If you make yeast breads frequently, instant yeast is worth keeping on hand. It can be added to dry ingredients without first dissolving it in water, as you must do when using regular yeast or quick-rising yeast. It's also much more economical than the yeast that comes in single-use packages. Look for it in natural foods stores or baking supply stores. Instant yeast can be stored in an airtight container in the freezer for up to a year. When using it in a recipe that calls for packaged yeast, use 2½ teaspoons instant yeast and skip the step of dissolving the yeast in liquid.

Dried Cherry Loaf Bread with Toasted Almonds

makes 16 servings

Because it's just slightly sweet, you can serve this nutty loaf at breakfast or afternoon tea, or with a salad at lunch. With the crimson cherries scattered throughout, slices of this bread make a dramatic presentation at a special brunch or tea.

1 cup lukewarm water
1 package active dry yeast
2 tablespoons plus 1 teaspoon canola oil, divided
¼ teaspoon almond extract
2¼ to 2½ cups whole wheat flour
½ cup dried cherries
¼ cup slivered almonds, toasted (page 4)
2 tablespoons sugar
1 teaspoon salt

1 Combine the water and yeast in a large bowl and stir until the yeast dissolves. Let stand 5 minutes. Stir in 2 tablespoons of the oil and the almond extract. Add 2¼ cups of the flour, the cherries, almonds, sugar, and salt and stir until a soft dough forms.

2 Turn the dough out onto a lightly floured surface. Knead until smooth and elastic, about 8 minutes. Add enough of the remaining ¼ cup flour, 1 tablespoon at a time, to prevent the dough from sticking to your hands. (Alternatively, knead the dough for 5 minutes at low speed with an electric mixer using a dough hook, adding enough of the remaining ¼ cup flour, 1 tablespoon at a time, to make a smooth dough.)

3 Brush a large bowl with the remaining 1 teaspoon oil. Place the dough in the bowl and turn to coat the top. Cover and let rise in a warm place (85°F), free from drafts, until doubled in size, about 1 hour.

4 Line a medium baking sheet with parchment paper. Shape the dough into a 12 x 3-inch loaf and place on the prepared pan. Cover loosely

with lightly oiled plastic wrap and let rise in a warm place (85°F), free from drafts, until doubled in size, about 45 minutes.

5 Preheat the oven to 350°F. Remove the plastic wrap and bake the loaf 20 minutes. Cover loosely with foil and bake until the loaf is golden brown and sounds hollow when tapped, about 10 minutes longer.

6 Remove the loaf from the pan and cool completely on a wire rack. Slice using a serrated knife. The bread can be stored inside a paper bag at room temperature for up to 2 days or frozen for up to 3 months.

Each serving: 19 g carb, 130 cal, 4 g fat, 0 g sat fat, 0 mg chol, 3 g fib, 4 g pro, 146 mg sod • Carb Choices: 1; Exchanges: 1 starch, ½ fat

Chocolate Yeast Bread

makes 24 servings

If you're partial to the combination of peanut butter and chocolate, use this bread for a peanut butter sandwich—it's pure heaven. This recipe makes two loaves, but the bread freezes well and it makes a very welcome gift.

½ cup lukewarm water
1 package active dry yeast
1 cup 1% low-fat milk
1 large egg, at room temperature
½ cup unsweetened cocoa
⅓ cup granulated sugar
1¼ teaspoons salt
2 tablespoons plus 1 teaspoon canola oil, divided
4¼ to 4½ cups white whole wheat flour or unbleached all-purpose flour
8 ounces semisweet chocolate, chopped
4 teaspoons turbinado (raw) sugar

1 Combine the water and yeast in a large bowl and stir until the yeast dissolves. Let stand 5 minutes. Add the milk, egg, cocoa, granulated sugar, salt, and 2 tablespoons of the oil and whisk until the mixture is smooth. Add 2 cups of

the flour and stir until well combined. Add 2¼ cups of the remaining flour and stir until a soft dough forms.

2 Turn the dough out onto a lightly floured surface. Knead until smooth and elastic, about 8 minutes. Add enough of the remaining ¼ cup flour, 1 tablespoon at a time, to prevent the dough from sticking to your hands. (Alternatively, knead the dough for 5 minutes at low speed with an electric mixer using a dough hook, adding enough of the remaining ¼ cup flour, 1 tablespoon at a time, to make a smooth dough.) Add the chocolate during the last minute of kneading.

3 Brush a large bowl with the remaining 1 teaspoon oil. Place the dough in the bowl and turn to coat the top. Cover and let rise in a warm place (85°F), free from drafts, until doubled in size, about 1 hour.

4 Line a large baking sheet with parchment paper. Divide the dough in half and shape into two 6-inch round loaves and place on the prepared pan. Cover loosely with lightly oiled plastic wrap and let rise in a warm place (85°F), free from drafts, until doubled in size, about 45 minutes.

5 Preheat the oven to 375°F. Remove the plastic wrap and sprinkle the loaves evenly with the turbinado sugar. Bake until the loaves sound hollow when tapped, 25 to 30 minutes.

6 Remove the loaf from the pan and cool completely on a wire rack. Slice using a serrated knife. The bread can be stored inside a paper bag at room temperature for up to 2 days or frozen for up to 3 months.

Each serving: 28 g carb, 162 cal, 5 g fat, 2 g sat fat, 9 mg chol, 3 g fib, 5 g pro, 131 mg sod • Carb Choices: 2; Exchanges: 1½ starch, ½ carb, 1 fat

Caraway Beer Bread HIGH FIBER

makes 16 servings

Beer gives this bread an especially fermented yeasty flavor. Serve it with soup or use it for making cheese or roast beef sandwiches. If you are not a fan of caraway, omit the caraway seeds.

12 ounces pale lager beer, at room temperature
1 package active dry yeast
3½ to 3¾ cups whole wheat flour
2 teaspoons caraway seeds
1 teaspoon salt
1 teaspoon canola oil

1 Combine the beer and yeast in a large bowl and stir until the yeast dissolves. Let stand 5 minutes. Add 3½ cups of the flour, the caraway seeds, and salt and stir until a soft dough forms.

2 Turn the dough out onto a lightly floured surface. Knead until smooth and elastic, about 8 minutes. Add enough of the remaining ¼ cup flour, 1 tablespoon at a time, to prevent the dough from sticking to your hands. (Alternatively, knead the dough for 5 minutes at low speed with an electric mixer using a dough hook, adding enough of the remaining ¼ cup flour, 1 tablespoon at a time, to make a smooth dough.)

3 Brush a large bowl with the oil. Place the dough in the bowl and turn to coat the top. Cover and let rise in a warm place (85°F), free from drafts, until doubled in size, about 1 hour.

4 Line a medium baking sheet with parchment paper. Shape the dough into an 8-inch round loaf and place on the prepared baking sheet. Cover loosely with lightly oiled plastic wrap and let rise in a warm place (85°F), free from drafts, until doubled in size, about 45 minutes.

5 Preheat the oven to 400°F. Remove the plastic wrap and bake until the loaf is golden brown, 20 to 25 minutes.

6 Remove the loaf from the pan and cool completely on a wire rack. Slice using a serrated knife. The bread can be stored inside a paper bag at room temperature for up to 2 days or frozen for up to 3 months.

Note: To bake the bread in a loaf pan, line a 9 x 5-inch loaf pan with parchment paper. Place the dough in the pan and let rise as directed in step 4. Proceed with baking as directed.

Each serving: 22 g carb, 118 cal, 1 g fat, 0 g sat fat, 0 mg chol, 4 g fib, 5 g pro, 147 mg sod • Carb Choices: 1½; Exchanges: 1½ starch

Yeast-Risen Cornmeal Loaf

makes 12 servings

This bread has a fine soft center with a delicately crispy crust and just a hint of corn flavor. The slices look like biscotti, so they add an interesting shape to a bread basket. It's just as good with a smear of jam as it is with a bowl of soup.

¾ cup lukewarm water
1 package active dry yeast
1¼ to 1½ cups unbleached all-purpose flour
½ cup fine-grind yellow cornmeal plus
    cornmeal for dusting pan
1 teaspoon salt
1 teaspoon canola oil

1 Combine the water and yeast in a large bowl and stir until the yeast dissolves. Let stand 5 minutes. Add 1¼ cups of the flour, the cornmeal, and salt and stir until a soft dough forms.

2 Turn the dough out onto a lightly floured surface. Knead until smooth and elastic, about 8 minutes. Add enough of the remaining ¼ cup flour, 1 tablespoon at a time, to prevent the dough from sticking to your hands. (Alternatively, knead the dough for 5 minutes at low speed with an electric mixer using a dough hook, adding enough of the remaining ¼ cup flour, 1 tablespoon at a time, to make a smooth dough.)

3 Brush a large bowl with the oil. Place the dough in the bowl and turn to coat the top. Cover and let rise in a warm place (85°F), free from drafts, until doubled in size, about 1 hour.

4 Line a large baking sheet with parchment paper and dust the parchment lightly with cornmeal. Shape the dough into a 12 x 4-inch rectangle and place on the prepared baking sheet. Cover loosely with lightly oiled plastic wrap and let rise in a warm place (85°F), free from drafts, until doubled in size, about 45 minutes.

5 Preheat the oven to 400°F. Remove the plastic wrap and bake until the loaf is golden brown and sounds hollow when tapped, 20 to 25 minutes.

6 Remove the loaf from the pan and cool completely on a wire rack. Slice using a serrated knife. The bread can be stored inside a paper bag at room temperature for up to 2 days or frozen for up to 3 months.

Each serving: 16 g carb, 80 cal, 1 g fat, 0 g sat fat, 0 mg chol, 1 g fib, 2 g pro, 197 mg sod • Carb Choices: 1; Exchanges: 1 starch

Caramelized Onion and Thyme-Focaccia

makes 15 servings

Even if you've never made homemade bread, you can make focaccia. It's foolproof and will win you so many compliments, you may become a frequent baker. You cook the caramelized onions while the dough rises in this recipe, but if you wish, you can make them a day ahead of time.

1 cup lukewarm water
1 package active dry yeast
1¼ cups unbleached all-purpose flour, divided
1 cup whole wheat flour
¾ teaspoon table salt
4 teaspoons extra virgin olive oil, divided
2 large onions, halved and thinly sliced
¼ teaspoon kosher salt
1 tablespoon minced fresh thyme or
    1 teaspoon dried thyme
¼ teaspoon freshly ground pepper

1 Combine the water and yeast in a large bowl and stir until the yeast dissolves. Let stand 5 minutes. Add 1 cup of the all-purpose flour, the whole wheat flour, and table salt and stir until a soft dough forms.

2 Turn the dough out onto a lightly floured surface. Knead until smooth and elastic, about

8 minutes. Add enough of the remaining ¼ cup all-purpose flour, 1 tablespoon at a time, to prevent the dough from sticking to your hands. (Alternatively, knead the dough for 5 minutes at low speed with an electric mixer using a dough hook, adding enough of the remaining ¼ cup all-purpose flour, 1 tablespoon at a time, to make a smooth dough.)

3 Brush a large bowl with 1 teaspoon of the oil. Place the dough in the bowl and turn to coat the top. Cover and let rise in a warm place (85°F), free from drafts, until doubled in size, about 1 hour.

4 Meanwhile, make the onions. Heat a large nonstick skillet over medium-low heat. Add 2 teaspoons of the remaining oil and tilt the pan to coat the bottom evenly. Add the onions and the kosher salt and cook, covered, stirring occasionally, until the onions are very tender, about 30 minutes. Increase the heat to medium-high, uncover, and cook, stirring often, until the onions are golden brown and most of the liquid has evaporated, 8 to 10 minutes longer. Stir in the thyme and pepper. Transfer the onion mixture to a plate and let cool to room temperature.

5 Brush a 15 x 10-inch jellyroll pan or large rimmed baking sheet with the remaining 1 teaspoon oil. Place the dough into the pan and pat to evenly cover the pan. If you have trouble stretching the dough, let it rest 5 minutes, then try again.

6 Top the dough evenly with the onion mixture. Cover loosely with lightly oiled plastic wrap and let rise in a warm place (85°F), free from drafts, until doubled in size, about 45 minutes.

7 Preheat the oven to 400°F. Remove the plastic wrap and bake until the focaccia is lightly browned, 25 to 30 minutes. Transfer the focaccia to a cutting board and cut into 15 pieces. Serve warm or at room temperature. The bread is best the day it is made.

Each serving: 16 g carb, 91 cal, 2 g fat, 0 g sat fat, 0 mg chol, 2 g fib, 3 g pro, 168 mg sod • Carb Choices: 1; Exchanges: 1 starch

Rosemary-Olive Focaccia

makes 15 servings

Serve this bread to accompany soups or stews or use it to make open-face sandwiches. You can also cut it into small squares and top with thinly sliced Gruyère or fontina cheese to serve as an hors d'oeuvre.

1 cup lukewarm water
1 package active dry yeast
1¼ cups unbleached all-purpose flour, divided
1 cup whole wheat flour
¾ teaspoon salt
2 teaspoons extra virgin olive oil, divided
⅓ cup Kalamata olives, pitted and sliced
2 teaspoons chopped fresh rosemary or
½ teaspoon crumbled dried rosemary

1 Combine the water and yeast in a large bowl and stir until the yeast dissolves. Let stand 5 minutes. Add 1 cup of the all-purpose flour, the whole wheat flour, and salt and stir until a soft dough forms.

2 Turn the dough out onto a lightly floured surface. Knead until smooth and elastic, about 8 minutes. Add enough of the remaining ¼ cup all-purpose flour, 1 tablespoon at a time, to prevent the dough from sticking to your hands. (Alternatively, knead the dough for 5 minutes at low speed with an electric mixer using a dough hook, adding enough of the remaining ¼ cup all-purpose flour, 1 tablespoon at a time, to make a smooth dough.)

3 Brush a large bowl with 1 teaspoon of the oil. Place the dough in the bowl and turn to coat the top. Cover and let rise in a warm place (85°F), free from drafts, until doubled in size, about 1 hour.

4 Brush a 15 x 10-inch jellyroll pan or large rimmed baking sheet with the remaining 1 teaspoon oil. Place the dough into the pan and pat to evenly

continues on next page

cover the pan. If you have trouble stretching the dough, let it rest 5 minutes, then try again.

5 Sprinkle the dough evenly with the olives and rosemary. Cover loosely with lightly oiled plastic wrap and let rise in a warm place (85°F), free from drafts, until doubled in size, about 45 minutes.

6 Preheat the oven to 400°F. Remove the plastic wrap and bake until the focaccia is lightly browned, 25 to 30 minutes. Transfer the focaccia to a cutting board and cut into 15 pieces. Serve warm or at room temperature. The bread is best the day it is made.

Each serving: 14 g carb, 78 cal, 1 g fat, 0 g sat fat, 0 mg chol, 1 g fib, 3 g pro, 149 mg sod • Carb Choices: 1; Exchanges: 1 starch

RED PEPPER–ASIAGO FOCACCIA: Follow the Rosemary-Olive Focaccia recipe, page 527, through step 4. In step 5, sprinkle the dough with ½ cup red Roasted Bell peppers (page 21) or roasted red peppers from a jar, thinly sliced, and ½ cup finely shredded Asiago cheese. Proceed with the recipe.

Each serving: 14 g carb, 94 cal, 3 g fat, 1 g sat fat, 3 mg chol, 2 g fib, 4 g pro, 193 mg sod • Carb Choices: 1; Exchanges: 1 starch, ½ fat

Onion-Rye Rolls

makes 16 servings

Take care to finely chop the onion for this recipe because you want the pieces to be small inside the rolls. If you like garlic, add a couple cloves of minced garlic when you cook the onion.

3 teaspoons extra virgin olive oil, divided
1 cup finely chopped onion
1 cup lukewarm water
1 package active dry yeast
2 cups rye flour
1 to 1¼ cups unbleached all-purpose flour, divided
1 tablespoon sugar
1 teaspoon salt

1 Heat a medium nonstick skillet over medium heat. Add 2 teaspoons of the oil and tilt the pan to coat the bottom evenly. Add the onion, cover, and cook, stirring occasionally, until the onion is tender and lightly browned, about 10 minutes. Transfer the onion to a bowl and let stand to cool to room temperature.

2 Combine the water and yeast in a large bowl and stir until the yeast dissolves. Let stand 5 minutes. Add the cooled onion, the rye flour, 1 cup of the all-purpose flour, the sugar, and salt and stir until a soft dough forms.

3 Turn the dough out onto a lightly floured surface. Knead until smooth and elastic, about 8 minutes. Add enough of the remaining ¼ cup all-purpose flour, 1 tablespoon at a time, to prevent the dough from sticking to your hands. (Alternatively, knead the dough for 5 minutes at low speed with an electric mixer using a dough hook, adding enough of the remaining ¼ cup all-purpose flour, 1 tablespoon at a time, to make a smooth dough.)

4 Brush a large bowl with the remaining 1 teaspoon oil. Place the dough in the bowl and turn to coat the top. Cover and let rise in a warm place (85°F), free from drafts, until doubled in size, about 1 hour.

5 Line a large baking sheet with parchment paper. Divide the dough into 16 pieces and shape each piece into a ball. Place the balls onto the prepared baking sheet. Cover loosely with lightly oiled plastic wrap and let rise in a warm place (85°F), free from drafts, until doubled in size, about 45 minutes.

6 Preheat the oven to 400°F. Remove the plastic wrap and bake the rolls until lightly browned, 15 to 18 minutes. Transfer to wire racks to cool. Serve warm or at room temperature. The rolls can be stored inside a paper bag at room temperature for up to 2 days or frozen for up to 3 months.

Each serving: 17 g carb, 84 cal, 1 g fat, 0 g sat fat, 0 mg chol, 2 g fib, 2 g pro, 146 mg sod • Carb Choices: 1; Exchanges: 1 starch

Crispy Poppy Seed Breadsticks

makes 64

For a special meal, these are worth the effort for the dramatic presentation they make in a vase or a glass on your dining table. Don't stress about making the breadsticks exactly the same length or getting them twisted evenly—the irregularities are part of their charm.

1 cup lukewarm water

1 package active dry yeast

2¾ to 3 cups unbleached all-purpose flour, divided

2 tablespoons poppy seeds

¾ teaspoon salt

1 teaspoon canola oil

Yellow cornmeal

1 Combine the water and yeast in a large bowl and stir until the yeast dissolves. Let stand 5 minutes. Add 2¾ cups of the flour, the poppy seeds, and salt and stir until a soft dough forms.

2 Turn the dough out onto a lightly floured surface. Knead until smooth and elastic, about 8 minutes. Add enough of the remaining ¼ cup flour, 1 tablespoon at a time, to prevent the dough from sticking to your hands. (Alternatively, knead the dough for 5 minutes at low speed with an electric mixer using a dough hook, adding enough of the remaining ¼ cup flour, 1 tablespoon at a time, to make a smooth dough.)

3 Brush a large bowl with the oil. Place the dough in the bowl and turn to coat the top. Cover and let rise in a warm place (85°F), free from drafts, until doubled in size, about 1 hour.

4 Preheat the oven to 375°F. Line 2 large baking sheets with parchment paper.

5 Divide the dough into 4 pieces. Working with one piece at a time (keep the remaining dough covered to prevent drying), place the dough on a work surface lightly dusted with cornmeal. Roll the dough into a 12 x 6-inch rectangle. Cut the dough into 16 (12-inch) strips. Place the strips on the prepared baking sheets. Holding each strip by the ends, gently twist the strips. Repeat with the remaining dough. (Unless you have a large oven and a lot of pans, you'll need to bake two pans at a time.)

6 Bake until the breadsticks are crisp and lightly browned, 10 to 12 minutes. Transfer to wire racks to cool completely. The breadsticks can be stored inside an airtight container at room temperature for up to 3 days. If the breadsticks soften, bake them in a 350°F oven for 3 to 5 minutes to recrisp them.

Each serving (4 breadsticks): 18 g carb, 91 cal, 1 g fat, 0 g sat fat, 0 mg chol, 1 g fib, 3 g pro, 110 mg sod • Carb Choices: 1; Exchanges: 1 starch

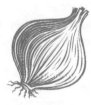

Stuffings

Dried Apricot–Pecan Stuffing [HIGH FIBER]

makes 8 servings

You can make this, or any of the stuffing recipes in this section, ahead of time. To do so, cool the stuffing to room temperature and refrigerate, covered, up to 1 day. Let it stand at room temperature for 30 minutes, then bake as directed. The fruit and nuts in this dish pair beautifully with roast chicken or turkey or pork tenderloin.

6 cups ½-inch whole wheat bread cubes
3 teaspoons extra virgin olive oil, divided
1 small onion, diced
1 carrot, peeled and diced
1 stalk celery, diced
1½ cups Chicken Stock (page 149) or low-sodium chicken broth, divided
½ cup dried apricots, chopped
½ teaspoon dried thyme leaves
¼ teaspoon kosher salt
⅛ freshly ground pepper
⅓ cup pecans, toasted and chopped (page 4)
2 tablespoons chopped fresh Italian parsley

1 Preheat the oven to 350°F. Place the bread cubes in a single layer on a large rimmed baking sheet. Bake, stirring once, until the cubes are lightly toasted, 12 to 15 minutes. Set aside. Maintain the oven temperature.

2 Brush a 2-quart baking dish with 1 teaspoon of the oil.

3 Heat a large nonstick skillet over medium heat. Add the remaining 2 teaspoons oil and tilt the pan to coat the bottom evenly. Add the onion, carrot, and celery and cook, stirring often, until the vegetables are softened, 8 minutes. Stir in ½ cup of the stock, the apricots, thyme, salt, and pepper and bring to a boil. Reduce the heat to low and simmer until the apricots are slightly softened, about 2 minutes.

4 Transfer the vegetable mixture to a large bowl and stir in the toasted bread cubes, pecans, and parsley. Add the remaining 1 cup stock and stir until the stock is absorbed.

5 Spoon the stuffing into the prepared baking dish, cover with foil, and bake 20 minutes. Uncover and bake until the top of the stuffing is lightly browned, about 15 minutes longer. Serve at once.

Each serving: 18 g carb, 140 cal, 6 g fat, 1 g sat fat, 1 mg chol, 6 g fib, 4 g pro, 157 mg sod • Carb Choices: 1; Exchanges: 1 starch, 1 fat

Pear and Walnut Stuffing

[HIGH FIBER]

makes 8 servings

Toasting your own bread for stuffing means that you can choose which herbs and seasonings to use and you can have big rustic pieces of bread in your stuffing. Making your own means less sodium, too, since most prepared stuffing cubes have a lot of added salt. Pears in this stuffing add an unexpected flavor and texture, but you can use Granny Smith or Gala apples instead of the pears in this stuffing if you wish.

6 cups ½-inch whole grain bread cubes
3 teaspoons extra virgin olive oil, divided
1 small onion, diced
1 carrot, peeled and diced
1 stalk celery, diced
2 large ripe pears (about 1 pound), peeled, cored, and chopped
2 teaspoons chopped fresh thyme or ½ teaspoon dried thyme
¼ teaspoon kosher salt
⅛ teaspoon freshly ground pepper
⅓ cup walnuts, toasted and chopped (page 4)
1½ cups Chicken Stock (page 149) or low-sodium chicken broth

1 Preheat the oven to 350°F. Place the bread cubes in a single layer on a large rimmed baking sheet. Bake, stirring once, until the cubes are lightly toasted, 12 to 15 minutes. Set aside. Maintain the oven temperature.

2 Brush a 2-quart baking dish with 1 teaspoon of the oil.

3 Heat a large nonstick skillet over medium heat. Add the remaining 2 teaspoons oil and tilt the pan to coat the bottom evenly. Add the onion, carrot, and celery and cook, stirring often, until the vegetables are softened, 8 minutes. Stir in the pears and cook, stirring occasionally, until they begin to soften, 5 minutes. Stir in the thyme, salt, and pepper. Transfer the vegetable mixture to a large bowl and stir in the bread cubes and walnuts. Add the stock and stir until the stock is absorbed.

4 Spoon the stuffing into the prepared baking dish, cover with foil, and bake 20 minutes. Uncover and bake until the top of the stuffing is lightly browned, about 15 minutes longer. Serve at once.

Each serving: 22 g carb, 153 cal, 6 g fat, 1 g sat fat, 1 mg chol, 8 g fib, 4 g pro, 157 mg sod • Carb Choices: 1½; Exchanges: 1 starch, ½ fruit, 1 fat

Chestnut Stuffing

makes 8 servings

A holiday tradition in many families, this stuffing is superb with a roasted turkey or chicken. Using peeled vacuum-packed chestnuts makes it a snap to make.

6 cups ½-inch whole wheat sourdough bread cubes
3 teaspoons extra virgin olive oil, divided
1 medium onion, diced
1 stalk celery, diced
2 teaspoons chopped fresh sage or 1 teaspoon crumbled dried sage
¼ teaspoon kosher salt
⅛ teaspoons freshly ground pepper
1 cup vacuum-packed toasted chestnuts (about 5 ounces), chopped
1½ cups Chicken Stock (page 149) or low-sodium chicken broth

1 Preheat the oven to 350°F. Place the bread cubes in a single layer on a large rimmed baking sheet. Bake, stirring once, until the cubes are lightly toasted, 12 to 15 minutes. Set aside. Maintain the oven temperature.

2 Brush a 2-quart baking dish with 1 teaspoon of the oil.

3 Heat a large nonstick skillet over medium heat. Add the remaining 2 teaspoons oil and tilt the pan to coat the bottom evenly. Add the onion and celery and cook, stirring often, until the vegetables are softened, 8 minutes. Stir in the sage, salt, and pepper. Transfer the mixture to a large bowl and stir in the toasted bread cubes and chestnuts. Add the stock and stir until it is absorbed.

4 Spoon the stuffing into the prepared baking dish, cover with foil, and bake 20 minutes. Uncover and bake until the top of the stuffing is lightly browned, about 15 minutes longer. Serve at once.

Each serving: 27 g carb, 165 cal, 3 g fat, 0 g sat fat, 1 mg chol, 3 g fib, 5 g pro, 225 mg sod • Carb Choices: 2; Exchanges: 2 starch, ½ fat

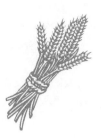

Cornbread Stuffing with Sausage and Apples

makes 8 servings

Depending on the brand you use, Italian turkey sausage will add a hint or a wallop of fennel and garlic flavor to this stuffing. Don't fuss over which sausage to use—you can even make it with turkey breakfast sausage with delicious results. Check the label if you are using purchased cornbread cubes as many brands have a lot of added sugar and sodium.

6 cups ½-inch Southern Cornbread cubes (page 508) or purchased cornbread cubes

3 teaspoons extra virgin olive oil, divided

2 ounces mild Italian turkey sausage, crumbled

1 medium onion, diced

2 stalks celery, diced

2 Granny Smith apples, peeled, cored, and chopped

1½ teaspoons crumbled dried sage

⅛ teaspoons freshly ground pepper

2 tablespoons chopped fresh Italian parsley

1½ cups Chicken Stock (page 149) or low-sodium chicken broth

1 Preheat the oven to 350°F. Place the bread cubes in a single layer on a large rimmed baking sheet. Bake, stirring once, until the cubes are lightly toasted, 20 to 25 minutes. Set aside. Maintain the oven temperature.

2 Brush a 2-quart baking dish with 1 teaspoon of the oil.

3 Heat a large nonstick skillet over medium heat. Add the remaining 2 teaspoons oil and tilt the pan to coat the bottom evenly. Add the sausage, onion, and celery and cook, stirring often, until the sausage is browned, 5 minutes. Stir in the apples and cook, stirring occasionally, until they begin to soften, 5 minutes. Stir in the sage and pepper. Transfer the mixture to a large bowl and stir in the bread cubes and parsley. Add the stock and stir until it is absorbed.

4 Spoon the stuffing into the prepared baking dish, cover with foil, and bake 20 minutes. Uncover and bake until the top of the stuffing is lightly browned, about 15 minutes longer. Serve at once.

Each serving: 24 g carb, 174 cal, 6 g fat, 1 g sat fat, 33 mg chol, 2 g fib, 6 g pro, 402 mg sod • Carb Choices: 1½; Exchanges: 1 starch, ½ fruit, 1 fat

Rye Stuffing with Roasted Carrots and Leeks HIGH FIBER

makes 8 servings

Roasting the vegetables for this stuffing adds an extra step, but it's worth it for the sweet caramelized flavor. If you don't have leeks, use a large sweet onion instead. Quarter the onion lengthwise, then cut it into ½-inch slices and proceed with the recipe.

3 medium leeks, halved lengthwise and sliced

3 medium carrots, peeled, halved lengthwise, and cut into ½-inch slices

5 teaspoons extra virgin olive oil, divided

½ teaspoon kosher salt, divided

6 cups ½-inch rye bread cubes

2 tablespoons chopped fresh Italian parsley

⅛ teaspoon freshly ground pepper

1½ cups Chicken Stock (page 149) or low-sodium chicken broth

1 Preheat the oven to 425°F.

2 Submerge the sliced leeks in a large bowl of water, lift them out, and drain in a colander. Repeat, using fresh water, until no grit remains in the bottom of the bowl. Drain the leeks well.

3 Place the carrots and leeks on 2 separate rimmed baking sheets. Drizzle each vegetable with 2 teaspoons of the oil, sprinkle each with ⅛ teaspoon of the salt, and toss to coat. Arrange the vegetables in a single layer on the baking pans. Bake, stirring once, until the vegetables are tender and lightly browned, about 20 minutes for the leeks and about 25 minutes for the carrots. Remove from the oven and set aside. Reduce the oven temperature to 350°F.

4 Place the bread cubes in a single layer on a large rimmed baking sheet. Bake, stirring once, until the cubes are lightly toasted, 12 to 15 minutes. Set aside. Maintain the oven temperature.

5 Brush a 2-quart baking dish with the remaining 1 teaspoon of the oil. Combine the toasted bread cubes, the roasted carrots and leeks, the parsley, the remaining ¼ teaspoon salt, and the pepper in a large bowl. Add the stock and stir until it is absorbed.

6 Spoon the stuffing into the prepared baking dish, cover with foil, and bake 20 minutes. Uncover and bake until the top of the stuffing is lightly browned, about 15 minutes longer. Serve at once.

Each serving: 22 g carb, 140 cal, 4 g fat, 1 g sat fat, 1 mg chol, 6 g fib, 5 g pro, 200 mg sod • Carb Choices: 1½; Exchanges: 1½ starch, ½ fat

Multigrain Bread Stuffing with Mixed Mushrooms

HIGH FIBER

makes 8 servings

Adding the soaking liquid from the mushrooms to the stuffing infuses the bread with woodsy mushroom flavor. This stuffing is especially good with a roasted pork loin.

1 cup water

½ ounce dried porcini mushrooms

6 cups ½-inch multigrain bread cubes

3 teaspoons extra virgin olive oil, divided

2 medium leeks, halved lengthwise and thinly sliced

6 ounces shiitake mushrooms, stemmed and thinly sliced

6 ounces cremini mushrooms, thinly sliced

1 tablespoon chopped fresh thyme or 1½ teaspoons dried thyme

¼ teaspoon kosher salt

⅛ teaspoons freshly ground pepper

1 cup Chicken Stock (page 149) or low-sodium chicken broth

1 Bring the water to a boil in a small saucepan over high heat. Remove from the heat, add the porcini mushrooms, cover, and let stand 30 minutes.

2 Meanwhile, preheat the oven to 350°F. Place the bread cubes in a single layer on a large rimmed baking sheet. Bake, stirring once, until the cubes are lightly toasted, 12 to 15 minutes. Set aside. Maintain the oven temperature.

3 Brush a 2-quart baking dish with 1 teaspoon of the oil.

4 Place a coffee filter in a fine wire mesh strainer and place over a bowl. Pour the mushroom mixture through the filter. Finely chop the mushrooms and reserve the mushroom soaking liquid.

5 Submerge the sliced leeks in a large bowl of water, lift them out, and drain in a colander. Repeat, using fresh water, until no grit remains in the bottom of the bowl. Drain the leeks well.

6 Heat a large nonstick skillet over medium heat. Add the remaining 2 teaspoons oil and tilt the pan to coat the bottom evenly. Add the shiitake and cremini mushrooms and the leeks and cook, stirring often, until the mushrooms are tender and most of the liquid has evaporated, 8 minutes. Stir in the thyme, salt, and pepper. Transfer the mixture to a large bowl and stir in the toasted bread cubes, soaked porcini mushrooms, reserved mushroom soaking liquid, and stock.

7 Spoon the stuffing into the prepared baking dish, cover with foil, and bake 20 minutes. Uncover and bake until the top of the stuffing is lightly browned, about 15 minutes longer. Serve at once.

Each serving: 22 g carb, 119 cal, 3 g fat, 0 g sat fat, 1 mg chol, 7 g fib, 6 g pro, 164 mg sod • Carb Choices: 1½; Exchanges: 1 starch, 1 veg, ½ fat

Desserts

Fruit Desserts

Apple-Walnut Crisp

Blueberry-Nectarine Crisp
with Cornmeal-Pecan
Topping

Southern Peach Cobbler

Cherry Clafouti

Strawberry Shortcakes

Double-Berry Napoleons

Fruit-and-Nut-Stuffed Baked
Apples

Pears Poached in
Vanilla-Anise Syrup

Poached Apricots with
Raspberry-Ginger Sauce

Yogurt-and-Brown
Sugar–Glazed Fruit

Roasted Peaches

Roasted Pears with
Yogurt and Honey

Fruit-Filled Meringues with
Custard Sauce

Chilled Nectarine Soup with
Toasted Almonds

Pies and Tarts

Pastry Crust

Graham Cracker Crust

Streusel-Topped Apple Pie

Lemon Meringue Pie

Pumpkin Pie

Pecan Pie

Strawberry Pie

Lemon Chiffon Pie

Chocolate-Raspberry
Chiffon Pie

Vanilla Cream Pie

Coconut Cream Pie

Strawberry-Yogurt Pie

Fresh Berry Tart

Peach-Blueberry Crostata

Ginger-Plum Crostata

Apricot-Almond Crostata

Puddings and Custards

Vanilla Pudding

Rich Chocolate Pudding

Banana Pudding

Chocolate Mousse

Crème Brûlée

Flan

Pumpkin Flan

Panna Cotta

Pumpkin Panna Cotta

Rice Pudding

Tapioca Pudding

Raisin Bread Pudding

Blueberry-Lemon
Bread Pudding

Cakes

Classic White Cake

White Layer Cake with
Fluffy White Frosting

Raspberry-Lemon
Layer Cake

Chocolate Cake

Chocolate Layer Cake with
Fluffy White Frosting

Carrot Cake with
Cream Cheese Glaze

Moist Yogurt Cake

Pineapple Upside-Down
Cake

Chiffon Cake

Sour Cream Pound Cake

Angel Food Cake

Gingerbread Bundt Cake

Apple-Spice Cake

Cornmeal–Olive Oil Cake

Blueberry–Poppy Seed
Coffee Cake

Spiced Fruitcake

Raspberry Pudding Cake

Chocolate Pudding Cake

New York–Style Cheesecake

Fresh Fruit Trifle

Tiramisù Layer Cake

Chocolate Soufflé

Cookies and Bars

Sugar Cookies

Classic Chocolate Chippers

Oatmeal-Raisin Cookies

Cut-Out Cookies

Peanut Butter Cookies

Almond Cookies

Almond Biscotti

Cranberry-Orange Biscotti

Meringue Cookies

Chocolate Brownies

Shortbread

Lemon Bars

Chewy Cranberry-Spice
Bars

Frozen Desserts

Raspberry Granita

Cantaloupe Sorbet

Red Grapefruit Sorbet

Chocolate Sorbet

Melon Pops

Frozen Yogurt

Dessert Sauces, Frostings, and Glazes

Light Whipped Cream

Vanilla Glaze

Citrus Glaze

Espresso Glaze

Fluffy White Frosting

Cream Cheese Frosting

Rich Chocolate Sauce

Raspberry Sauce

Strawberry Sauce

Whole Blueberry Sauce

Creamy Custard Sauce

Zabaglione

Rhubarb–Vanilla Bean Compote

Lemon Curd

Orange-Ricotta Cream

Desserts are one of the small pleasures of life, bringing a festive meal to a memorable end or turning an afternoon cup of tea with a friend into something special. People with diabetes can and should treat themselves to desserts, but not without planning and attention to carbs and calories.

To enjoy a sweet treat when you have diabetes means that you need to incorporate the carbohydrates from the dessert into your meal plan, not just add it to the carbs you've already eaten. If you've allotted 45 grams of carbs for dinner and you've had two slices of bread and a serving of mashed potatoes, you've spent your carbs for the meal before you get to dessert. Thinking ahead and planning for dessert means better blood glucose control and more opportunities for treating yourself to foods you love. If you know you want dessert at the end of the meal, skip the bread so that you can have a slice of pie. Always read the nutrition information on recipes and food labels to make sure you know the total carbohydrate in a serving so that you can make even substitutions when you do have dessert.

When you have a sweet, not only do you need to mind the carbs, but the calories, too. Most people with diabetes are overweight and are trying to lose a few (or more) pounds. All desserts—even those, like most of the sweets in this chapter, made with fresh fruits and whole wheat flour—are high in calories for the amount of nutrients they contain. Desserts are calorie dense—a small wedge of cake can have 150 calories or more. Compared to less calorie-dense foods—like fruits and vegetables—desserts don't give you a sense of fullness. Because of the refined flour, sugar, and fat they contain, a small portion of dessert is the calorie equivalent of a much larger portion of fruits or vegetables. For 150 calories you could eat a bowl piled high with spinach or blueberries.

Because they are high in calories and relatively low in nutrients—a fancy way of saying "empty calories"—moderation and portion control are essential. Desserts are not intended for every meal. When you do treat yourself to an occasional dessert, pay attention to the number of servings the recipe makes and adjust the numbers of the nutritional analysis accordingly if you eat more.

All the sweets in this chapter are made with natural ingredients. You won't find artificial sweeteners, margarine, or fat-free versions of any foods. The recipes use real sugar—just a smaller amount of it—to make treats that are a little less sweet than is common. From my own experience and from tasters who have provided feedback on these recipes, the flavors of the ingredients in less sweet desserts come through more than in cloying, sugar-packed desserts that only taste "sweet." In these recipes, the delicate flavor of vanilla shines through, you can discern all the spices in a cake or a pie, and fresh peak-season fruits taste marvelous.

After years of creating desserts sweetened with artificial sweeteners, I can say that there is no comparison between a dessert made with a chemical sweetener and one made with real sugar. Sugar makes a birthday cake rise to a height worthy of celebration, gives after-school cookies a crisp brown edge, makes brownies so tender they melt in your mouth, and gives cheesecakes and custards a balance of flavor that you never achieve using artificial sweetener.

As for margarine and laboratory-created fat-free versions of sour cream and cream cheese, they have no flavor and an ingredient list of unrecognizable substances. Using these artificial ingredients in foods that you regard as a treat and will enjoy with friends and family on special occasions seems more like a punishment than a pleasure.

A modest serving of a real dessert is infinitely more flavorful and enjoyable—and better for your health—than a huge serving of an artificial food product. When you treat yourself, do it with something luscious and satisfying, not something cooked up in a laboratory.

The desserts in this chapter are lightened and made healthier by using less sugar, eggs, and butter or oil than would be used in a traditional recipe. Where possible, I've used a mixture of whole wheat and white flour or used whole wheat pastry flour to add nutrients and increase fiber. You'll find lots of recipes here that use low-fat buttermilk. It is essential in low-sugar, low-fat baking to make cakes tender.

Using these tricks, I've created desserts that are healthful, natural, and fresh—worthy of the special occasions when you do take pleasure in a dessert. Enjoy them in moderation and in good health.

Fruit Desserts

Apple-Walnut Crisp

makes 8 servings

This homey crisp is so easy to make, you'll want to serve it several times during peak apple season. You can make it with pears instead of apples, too. Serve the crisp with a spoonful of Light Whipped Cream (page 586) for a special treat.

1 teaspoon canola oil
½ cup old-fashioned rolled oats
¼ cup packed light brown sugar
2 tablespoons cold unsalted butter, cut into small pieces
½ teaspoon ground cinnamon
¼ cup chopped walnuts
6 large Granny Smith apples (about 2½ pounds), peeled and sliced (about 6 cups)
2 tablespoons unbleached all-purpose flour
2 teaspoons grated lemon zest

1 Preheat the oven to 350°F. Brush an 8-inch square baking dish with the oil.

2 Combine the oats, sugar, butter, and cinnamon in a medium bowl. Using your fingers, blend the butter evenly into the oat mixture. Add the walnuts and set aside.

3 Combine the apples, flour, and lemon zest in a large bowl and toss to combine. Spoon the apple mixture into the prepared dish. Sprinkle the oat mixture over the apples.

4 Bake until the topping is lightly browned and the fruit is bubbly around the edges, 30 to 35 minutes. Let stand 10 minutes before serving. Serve warm.

Each serving: 23 g carb, 145 cal, 6 g fat, 2 g sat fat, 8 mg chol, 2 g fib, 2 g pro, 3 mg sod • Carb Choices: 1½; Exchanges: 1 carb, ½ fruit, 1 fat

APPLE-CRANBERRY CRISP: Follow the Apple-Walnut Crisp recipe, at left, but reduce the apples to 5 cups and add 1 cup fresh cranberries or unthawed frozen cranberries in step 3. Proceed with the recipe.

Each serving: 22 g carb, 144 cal, 6 g fat, 2 g sat fat, 8 mg chol, 2 g fib, 2 g pro, 4 mg sod • Carb Choices: 1½; Exchanges: 1 carb, ½ fruit, 1 fat

Blueberry-Nectarine Crisp with Cornmeal-Pecan Topping

makes 8 servings

The unusual cornmeal and pecan topping gives this dessert a Southern flair. Being a lazy cook, I like to make it with nectarines because you don't have to peel them first. It's just as good with fresh peeled peaches or with thawed frozen peaches.

1 teaspoon canola oil

¼ cup yellow cornmeal

¼ cup packed light brown sugar

2 tablespoons cold unsalted butter, cut into small pieces

½ teaspoon ground cinnamon

¼ cup chopped pecans

3 cups fresh blueberries or unthawed frozen blueberries

3 medium nectarines (about 1¼ pounds), pitted and sliced (about 3 cups)

2 tablespoons unbleached all-purpose flour

2 teaspoons grated lemon zest

1 Preheat the oven to 350°F. Brush an 8-inch square baking dish with the oil.

2 Combine the cornmeal, sugar, butter, and cinnamon in a medium bowl. Using your fingers, blend the butter evenly into the cornmeal mixture. Add the pecans and set aside.

3 Combine the blueberries, nectarines, flour, and lemon zest in a large bowl and toss to combine. Spoon the blueberry mixture into the prepared dish. Sprinkle the cornmeal topping mixture over the blueberry mixture.

4 Bake until the topping is lightly browned and the fruit is bubbly around the edges, 25 to 30 minutes. Let stand 10 minutes before serving. Serve warm.

Each serving: 26 g carb, 160 cal, 7 g fat, 2 g sat fat, 8 mg chol, 3 g fib, 2 g pro, 5 mg sod • Carb Choices: 2; Exchanges: 1½ carb, ½ fruit, 1 fat

Grilled Fruit

Grilling fruit is an easy and delicious way to serve dessert at summer and fall cookouts. You can grill almost any fruit. To prepare the fruit, cut peaches, nectarines, plums, or apricots in half and remove the pits. For apples and pears, core and quarter them, if small, or cut into eighths if large. Peel and core pineapple, then cut into slices or wedges. Toss the fruit with a couple teaspoons of canola oil and place on a medium-high grill. Grill, turning once, until the fruit begins to soften and is lightly browned, 5 to 8 minutes. Serve the fruit plain, or with low-fat frozen yogurt, or drizzled with Raspberry Sauce (page 588).

Southern Peach Cobbler

HIGH FIBER

makes 8 servings

A cobbler is a fruit dessert that is either topped with pastry dough or as in this version, biscuit dough. This one uses a traditional Southern buttermilk batter that bakes up tender and slightly tangy. To substitute frozen unsweetened sliced peaches in this recipe, use two 16-ounce packages and thaw and drain the peaches well.

1 teaspoon canola oil

FILLING

¼ cup sugar

2 tablespoons whole wheat pastry flour or unbleached all-purpose flour

½ teaspoon ground cinnamon

1 teaspoon grated lemon zest

6 medium fresh peaches (about 2½ pounds), peeled and sliced (about 6 cups) or frozen (thawed) and drained

TOPPING

¾ cup whole wheat pastry flour or unbleached all-purpose flour

¼ cup sugar plus 1 tablespoon sugar, divided

½ teaspoon baking powder

½ teaspoon baking soda

⅛ teaspoon salt

2 tablespoons cold unsalted butter, cut into small pieces

½ cup low-fat buttermilk

1 Preheat the oven to 425°F. Brush a shallow 2-quart baking dish with the oil.

2 To make the filling, combine the sugar, flour, cinnamon, and lemon zest in a large bowl and stir to mix well. Add the peaches and toss to coat. Transfer to the prepared baking dish. Bake until the fruit is bubbly around the edges, 15 to 20 minutes.

3 Meanwhile, make the topping. Combine the flour, ¼ cup of the sugar, baking powder, baking soda, and salt in a medium bowl. Add the butter, and using a pastry blender, cut in the butter until the mixture resembles coarse meal. Add the buttermilk and stir just until the ingredients are moistened.

4 Remove the baking dish from the oven and drop the dough by 2 tablespoon measures onto the peach mixture. Sprinkle the topping with the remaining 1 tablespoon sugar. Return the cobbler to the oven and bake until the topping is lightly browned, 15 to 20 minutes. Serve warm.

Each serving: 37 g carb, 190 cal, 4 g fat, 2 g sat fat, 8 mg chol, 4 g fib, 3 g pro, 157 mg sod • Carb Choices: 2½; Exchanges: 1½ carb, 1 fruit, ½ fat

BLACKBERRY-PEACH COBBLER: Follow the Southern Peach Cobbler recipe, at left, reducing the peaches to 4 cups and adding 2 cups fresh blueberries or frozen unthawed blackberries with the peaches in step 2.

Each serving: 37 g carb, 189 cal, 4 g fat, 2 g sat fat, 8 mg chol, 5 g fib, 3 g pro, 158 mg sod • Carb Choices: 2½; Exchanges: 1½ carb, 1 fruit, ½ fat

APPLE COBBLER: Follow the Southern Peach Cobbler recipe, at left, substituting 2 pounds Granny Smith apples, peeled, cored, and sliced (about 6 cups), for the peaches, and proceed as directed.

Each serving: 36 g carb, 180 cal, 4 g fat, 2 g sat fat, 8 mg chol, 3 g fib, 2 g pro, 157 mg sod • Carb Choices: 2½; Exchanges: 2 carb, ½ fruit, ½ fat

Cherry Clafouti

makes 8 servings

Clafouti is a rustic French dessert made by topping fresh fruit with a simple batter and baking. It's a homey comforting dessert that you can make from basic pantry staples. If you enjoy the flavor combination of almond and cherries, omit the nutmeg and vanilla extract in this recipe and add ¼ teaspoon almond extract.

1 teaspoon canola oil

2 cups pitted fresh cherries or frozen cherries, thawed and drained

¾ cup unbleached all-purpose flour

½ cup granulated sugar

1 teaspoon baking powder

½ teaspoon baking soda

¼ teaspoon ground nutmeg

¼ teaspoon salt

¾ cup low-fat buttermilk

¼ cup plain low-fat yogurt

1 large egg

2 teaspoons vanilla extract

1 teaspoon confectioners' sugar

1 Preheat the oven to 350°F. Brush a deep-dish glass pie plate with the oil. Place the cherries in the prepared dish.

2 Combine the flour, granulated sugar, baking powder, baking soda, nutmeg, and salt in a large bowl and whisk to mix well. Combine the buttermilk, yogurt, egg, and vanilla in a medium bowl and whisk until smooth. Add the buttermilk mixture to the flour mixture and stir until the batter is smooth. Pour the batter evenly over the cherries.

3 Bake until the top is lightly browned, 30 to 35 minutes. Cool on a wire rack 10 minutes. Sprinkle with the confectioners' sugar and cut into wedges. Serve warm.

Each serving: 28 g carb, 143 cal, 2 g fat, 0 g sat fat, 28 mg chol, 1 g fib, 4 g pro, 241 mg sod • Carb Choices: 2; Exchanges: 2 carb

APPLE CLAFOUTI: Follow the Cherry Clafouti recipe, at left, substituting 2 cups chopped peeled apple for the cherries. Proceed with the recipe.

Each serving: 27 g carb, 135 cal, 2 g fat, 0 g sat fat, 28 mg chol, 1 g fib, 3 g pro, 241 mg sod • Carb Choices: 2; Exchanges: 2 carb

Strawberry Shortcakes

HIGH FIBER

makes 8 servings

I make this dessert at least once every year in early spring. Flaky sugar-topped biscuits, split and filled with the first strawberries of the season, and topped with whipped cream—it's a delightful finish to any meal. If you're lucky enough to get local strawberries, which are usually tiny in comparison to the supermarket variety, leave them whole for an especially pretty presentation.

BISCUITS

1 cup whole wheat pastry flour or unbleached all-purpose flour

¼ cup plus 1 teaspoon sugar, divided

1 teaspoon baking powder

¼ teaspoon baking soda

⅛ teaspoon salt

2 tablespoons cold unsalted butter, cut into small pieces

½ cup low-fat buttermilk

FILLING

3 pints fresh strawberries, sliced (about 6 cups), divided

1 tablespoon sugar

8 tablespoons Light Whipped Cream (page 586)

1 Preheat the oven to 425°F. Position an oven rack in the top third of the oven.

2 To make the biscuits, combine the flour, ¼ cup of the sugar, baking powder, baking soda, and salt in a large bowl and stir to mix well. Add the butter and cut into the dry ingredients using a pastry blender until the mixture resembles coarse meal. Stir in the buttermilk.

continues on next page

3 Transfer the dough to a lightly floured surface and knead 6 to 8 times until the dough holds together. Pat the dough to a ½-inch thickness and cut with a 2-inch biscuit cutter. Gather the dough scraps and repeat the patting and cutting to make a total of 8 biscuits. Sprinkle the tops of the biscuits evenly with the remaining 1 teaspoon sugar. Place on an ungreased baking sheet. Bake in the top third of the oven until the bottoms are lightly browned, 10 to 12 minutes. Transfer to a wire rack to cool.

4 Meanwhile, to make the filling, place 2 cups of the strawberries and the sugar in a medium bowl and mash using a potato masher. Add the remaining strawberries and toss to coat. Let stand at room temperature, stirring occasionally, about 10 minutes.

5 To assemble, split the biscuits in half horizontally and place the bottoms on each of 8 serving plates. Top evenly with the filling mixture. Top with the biscuit tops and dollop each one with 1 tablespoon of the whipped cream. Serve at once.

Each serving: 31 g carb, 185 cal, 6 g fat, 3 g sat fat, 16 mg chol, 4 g fib, 4 g pro, 149 mg sod • Carb Choices: 2; Exchanges: 1½ carb, ½ fruit, 1 fat

PEACH MELBA SHORTCAKES HIGH FIBER : Follow the Strawberry Shortcakes recipe, page 541, omitting the strawberries. Mash 2 cups raspberries with the sugar in step 4. Add 4 cups sliced fresh peaches or frozen thawed peaches to the raspberry mixture and toss to coat. Assemble the shortcakes as directed.

Each serving: 34 g carb, 194 cal, 6 g fat, 3 g sat fat, 16 mg chol, 5 g fib, 4 g pro, 148 mg sod • Carb Choices: 2; Exchanges: 1½ carb, ½ fruit, 1 fat

Double-Berry Napoleons

makes 4 servings

In this recipe, healthful low-carb wonton wrappers stand in for the usual puff pastry used to make fruit napoleons. With their crisp texture and delicate taste, they let the flavor of the fresh berries shine through. You can bake the wonton wrappers a day ahead and store at room temperature in an airtight container and make the Raspberry Sauce (page 588) a day ahead and store refrigerated. Then, it only takes a few minutes to assemble these desserts. Choose the smallest blueberries you can find to make this dessert.

12 wonton wrappers
2 teaspoons canola oil
2 cups fresh blueberries
1 recipe Raspberry Sauce (page 588)
1 teaspoon confectioners' sugar

1 Preheat the oven to 375°F.

2 Brush both sides of each wonton wrapper with the oil. Arrange the wrappers in a single layer on a large baking sheet. Bake until golden brown, 7 to 9 minutes. Transfer the wrappers to a wire rack to cool.

3 To assemble, place one wonton wrapper on each of 4 large serving plates. Arrange about ¼ cup blueberries on each wrapper and drizzle with 1 tablespoon of the sauce. Repeat the layering with another wonton wrapper and the remaining blueberries. Drizzle each napoleon with another 1 tablespoon of the sauce. Top with the remaining wonton wrappers. Drizzle the remaining sauce evenly on the serving plates. Sprinkle the napoleons with the sugar and serve at once.

Each serving: 36 g carb, 182 cal, 3 g fat, 0 g sat fat, 2 mg chol, 1 g fib, 4 g pro, 139 mg sod • Carb choices: 2½; Exchanges: 1 starch, ½ carb, 1 fruit, ½ fat

Fruit-and-Nut-Stuffed Baked Apples HIGH FIBER

makes 4 servings

These comforting apples make an autumnal finish to a casual meal. You can make them ahead of time, too—though they won't look as good as when freshly baked. Refrigerate the baked apples, and bring them to room temperature before serving.

1 teaspoon canola oil
½ cup dried cranberries
2 tablespoons chopped walnuts
½ teaspoon ground cinnamon
4 medium Granny Smith or Rome apples
½ cup apple cider or unsweetened apple juice
½ cup water
2 teaspoons unbleached all-purpose flour

1 Preheat the oven to 350°F. Brush an 8-inch square glass baking dish with the oil.

2 Combine the cranberries, walnuts, and cinnamon in a small bowl and toss to coat. Set aside.

3 Core the apples, cutting to, but not through, the bottoms. Cut away 1 inch of the peel from the tops of the apples. Divide the cranberry mixture evenly among the apples, pressing the mixture into each cavity. Arrange the apples upright in the prepared baking dish.

4 Combine the apple cider, water, and flour in a medium bowl and whisk until smooth. Pour over the apples.

5 Bake, uncovered, basting twice, until the apples are tender, 40 to 45 minutes.

6 To serve, place the apples in shallow bowls and drizzle evenly with the sauce. Serve hot, warm, or at room temperature.

Each serving: 37 g carb, 175 cal, 4 g fat, 0 g sat fat, 0 mg chol, 5 g fib, 1 g pro, 5 mg sod • Carb Choices: 2½; Exchanges: 2½ fruit

Pears Poached in Vanilla-Anise Syrup

Bosc pears have a firmer flesh than other pears, making them suitable for recipes such as this one where the pears need to hold their shape after cooking. Instead of the vanilla bean, you can use 1 teaspoon vanilla extract. This is a great make-ahead dessert, since these actually taste better the day after they are made.

4 medium Bosc pears
2 cups Riesling or Gewürztraminer
3 tablespoons sugar
½ vanilla bean, split
2 whole star anise

1 Peel the pears, leaving the stems intact. If necessary, cut a thin slice off the bottom of each pear so they will sit upright.

2 Combine the Riesling, sugar, vanilla bean, and star anise in a large saucepan or Dutch oven and bring to a boil over high heat. Carefully place the pears in the saucepan. Reduce the heat to low, cover, and simmer until the pears are tender when pierced with a knife, 10 to 15 minutes. Transfer the pears to a plate with a slotted spoon and cool to room temperature.

3 Meanwhile, increase the heat to medium-high and boil the cooking liquid, uncovered, until reduced to about 1 cup, 15 to 20 minutes. Remove and discard the vanilla bean and star anise. Serve the pears with the syrup at room temperature or chilled.

Each serving: 39 g carb, 232 cal, 1 g fat, 0 g sat fat, 0 mg chol, 1 g fib, 1 g pro, 0 mg sod • Carb Choices: 2½; Exchanges: 1 carb, 1½ fruit

Poached Apricots with Raspberry-Ginger Sauce QUICK

makes 6 servings

These golden apricots in a rosy raspberry sauce are a celebration of summer—and they take less than 15 minutes to make.

½ cup water
¼ cup sugar
1 tablespoon grated fresh ginger
6 large apricots, halved and pitted
½ cup fresh raspberries or unthawed frozen raspberries

1 Combine the water, sugar, and ginger in a small saucepan and bring to a boil over high heat. Add the apricots, reduce the heat to low, cover, and simmer until the apricots are just tender, about 3 minutes.

2 Transfer the apricots to serving dishes using a slotted spoon. Add the raspberries to the skillet and simmer just until the raspberries are softened, about 2 minutes. Spoon the raspberry-ginger sauce evenly over the apricots. Serve warm.

Each serving: 19 g carb, 88 cal, 1 g fat, 0 g sat fat, 0 mg chol, 2 g fib, 1 g pro, 0 mg sod • Carb Choices: 1; Exchanges: ½ carb, ½ fruit

Yogurt-and-Brown-Sugar-Glazed Fruit QUICK

makes 4 servings

You can use any soft stone fruit (try pitted and sliced peaches, nectarines, or apricots or pitted cherries) or berries (try raspberries or sliced strawberries) for this simple summer dessert. The tangy yogurt and just a touch of caramelized sugar create a dessert that really lets the flavor of the fruit shine through.

4 large plums, pitted and quartered
1 cup fresh blueberries or frozen unsweetened blueberries, thawed
⅓ cup plain low-fat yogurt
1 teaspoon vanilla extract
2 tablespoons light brown sugar

1 Preheat the broiler.

2 Place the plums and blueberries in a shallow flameproof baking pan and toss to combine.

3 Stir together the yogurt and vanilla in a small bowl. Spoon the mixture over the fruit and sprinkle with the sugar.

4 Broil until the fruit is warmed and the sugar is lightly browned, about 5 minutes. Serve at once.

Each serving: 24 g carb, 103 cal, 0 g fat, 0 g sat fat, 1 mg chol, 2 g fib, 2 g pro, 17 mg sod • Carb Choices: 1½; Exchanges: ½ carb, 1 fruit

Roasted Peaches QUICK

makes 4 servings

You can use the same procedure to make roasted nectarines or roasted apricots (shorten the roasting time for apricots to 20 to 25 minutes). Serve the roasted fruit plain, or drizzled with Creamy Custard Sauce (page 588) or Raspberry Sauce (page 588).

2 teaspoons canola oil
4 medium peaches, halved and pitted
1 tablespoon sugar

1 Preheat the oven to 400°F. Brush a large rimmed baking sheet with the oil.

2 Place the peaches cut side up in the pan and sprinkle with the sugar. Roast, without turning, until the peaches are softened and lightly browned, 25 to 30 minutes. Serve warm or at room temperature.

Each serving: 18 g carb, 94 cal, 3 g fat, 0 g sat fat, 0 mg chol, 2 g fib, 1 g pro, 0 mg sod • Carb Choices: 1; Exchanges: 1 fruit, ½ fat

Roasted Pears with Yogurt and Honey QUICK

makes 4 servings

In Greek restaurants, you often see yogurt drizzled with honey and sprinkled with walnuts offered as a simple dessert. This version adds lightly spiced roasted pears to the mix for a fruity dessert that is light, fresh, and effortless to make.

3 teaspoons canola oil, divided
2 medium pears, each cut into 8 wedges
⅛ teaspoon ground cinnamon
1⅓ cups plain low-fat Greek yogurt or strained yogurt (page 11)
4 teaspoons honey
2 tablespoons walnuts, toasted and chopped (page 4)

1 Preheat the oven to 400°F. Brush a large rimmed baking sheet with 2 teaspoons of the oil.

2 Place the pears in a medium bowl. Drizzle with the remaining 1 teaspoon oil, sprinkle with the cinnamon, and toss to coat. Arrange the pears cut side down in a single layer on the prepared baking sheet and roast, turning once, until lightly browned and tender, 25 to 30 minutes. Let the pears stand to cool slightly.

3 To serve, spoon ⅓ cup of the yogurt into each of 4 bowls. Arrange the pears evenly around the yogurt. Drizzle evenly with the honey, sprinkle with the walnuts, and serve at once.

Each serving: 22 g carb, 171 cal, 7 g fat, 1 g sat fat, 5 mg chol, 3 g fib, 7 g pro, 26 mg sod • Carb Choices: 1½; Exchanges: ½ carb, 1 fruit, 1 fat

Fruit-Filled Meringues with Custard Sauce

makes 6 servings

Use the colorful blend of fruit in this recipe or try whatever looks best at the market. The crisp meringue shells and creamy sauce make a stellar dessert of almost any fresh fruit or berries.

Meringue Cookies (page 580; see step 1)
2 large ripe kiwi, peeled and chopped
1 cup quartered fresh strawberries
1 cup fresh blueberries
Creamy Custard Sauce (page 588)

1 Prepare Meringue Cookies (page 580) according to the instructions, but place the beaten egg white mixture on the prepared pan and use the back of a spoon to spread it into six 4-inch circles, creating indentations in the center of each one. Proceed with the recipe as directed.

2 Combine the kiwi, strawberries, and blueberries in a medium bowl and toss to mix well.

3 To assemble, place a baked meringue on each of 6 plates. Top each meringue with about ½ cup of the fruit mixture. Drizzle evenly with the sauce and serve at once.

Each serving: 39 g carb, 194 cal, 2 g fat, 1 g sat fat, 71 mg chol, 2 g fib, 5 g pro, 79 mg sod • Carb Choices: 2½; Exchanges: 2 carb, ½ fruit

Chilled Nectarine Soup with Toasted Almonds HIGH FIBER

makes 4 servings

This soup, which is only slightly sweet, can be served as a refreshing finish to a meal or as a starter as well. I like to keep this in the refrigerator in the summer and sip it from a glass for an afternoon treat.

2 pounds nectarines, peeled and sliced (about 5 cups)
1 cup Riesling or Gewürztraminer
1 (3-inch) cinnamon stick
2 tablespoons honey
2 teaspoons lemon juice
⅛ teaspoon almond extract
4 tablespoons sliced almonds, toasted (page 4)

1 Combine the nectarines, Riesling, and cinnamon stick in a medium saucepan and bring to a boil over high heat. Reduce the heat to low, cover, and simmer until the nectarines are tender, about 10 minutes. Let stand to cool to room temperature.

2 Remove and discard the cinnamon stick. Place the mixture in batches in a blender or food processor and process until smooth. Transfer to a large bowl. Stir in the honey, lemon juice, and almond extract. Cover and refrigerate until chilled, at least 2 hours and up to 1 day. Add cold water a few tablespoons at a time, if necessary, to adjust the consistency of the soup.

3 Ladle into 4 bowls, sprinkle evenly with the almonds, and serve at once.

Each serving: 34 g carb, 206 cal, 4 g fat, 0 g sat fat, 0 mg chol, 4 g fib, 4 g pro, 0 mg sod • Carb Choices: 2½; Exchanges: 1 carb, 1½ fruit

Pies and Tarts

Pastry Crust QUICK

makes 1 (9-inch) crust

This is a simple crust to make and the dough is easy to shape. There's no need to chill the dough before baking, although if you do need to make it ahead, you can wrap it and refrigerate it for a day. Let the dough stand at room temperature 10 to 15 minutes before rolling it out.

1 cup whole wheat pastry flour or unbleached all-purpose flour
¼ cup unbleached all-purpose flour
1 tablespoon sugar
¼ teaspoon salt
4 tablespoons (½ stick) cold unsalted butter, cut into small pieces
3 to 4 tablespoons cold water

1 Combine the flours, sugar, and salt in a food processor and pulse until well mixed. Add the butter and process until evenly incorporated.

2 Add 3 tablespoons of the water and pulse to combine. Add the remaining water, 1 teaspoon at a time, pulsing after each addition, until the dough holds together in your fingers, but is not sticky. Follow each recipe to shape and bake the dough.

Each serving (1/12 of crust): 10 g carb, 82 cal, 4 g fat, 2 g sat fat, 10 mg chol, 1 g fib, 1 g pro, 49 mg sod • Carb Choices: ½; Exchanges: ½ carb, ½ fat

Graham Cracker Crust QUICK

makes 1 (9-inch) crust

You can make a chocolate version of this crust by using chocolate graham crackers instead of the regular ones.

9 reduced-fat graham crackers, crumbled
1 tablespoon sugar
2 tablespoons unsalted butter, melted and cooled
1 large egg white

1 Preheat the oven to 350°F.

2 Place the graham crackers and sugar in a food processor and process until finely ground. Add the butter and egg white and pulse until the crumbs are moist, 6 to 8 times.

3 Press the mixture into the bottom and up the side of a 9-inch glass pie plate. Bake until the crust is lightly browned, 10 to 12 minutes. Cool completely on a wire rack before using.

Each serving (1/12 of crust): 10 carb, 67 cal, 2 g fat, 1 g sat fat, 5 mg chol, 0 g fib, 1 g pro, 76 mg sod • Carb Choices: 1/2; Exchanges: 1/2 carb, 1/2 fat

Streusel-Topped Apple Pie

makes 12 servings

This streusel-topped pie is like a cross between a pie and a crisp. The topping adds crunch and contrast to the tender spiced apples underneath. If you have nuts on hand, add a few tablespoons of chopped walnuts or pecans to the topping.

1 recipe Pastry Crust (page 546)

FILLING

6 medium Granny Smith apples (about 2¼ pounds), peeled, cored, and sliced ¼ inch thick

1 tablespoon lemon juice

½ cup sugar

3 tablespoons unbleached all-purpose flour

½ teaspoon ground cinnamon

TOPPING

¼ cup unbleached all-purpose flour

¼ cup packed light brown sugar

⅛ teaspoon ground cinnamon

2 tablespoons cold unsalted butter, cut into small pieces

1 Preheat the oven to 375°F.

2 Place the pastry dough between two sheets of wax paper. Roll the dough into a 12-inch circle. Remove the top layer of wax paper and place the dough, with the wax paper facing up, into a 9-inch glass pie plate. Starting from edge of the dough, gently remove the wax paper. Fold the overhanging dough under and crimp the edge decoratively. Cover and refrigerate while preparing the filling and topping.

3 To make the filling, combine the apples, lemon juice, sugar, flour, and cinnamon in a large bowl and toss to coat.

4 To make the topping, combine the flour, sugar, cinnamon, and butter and blend using your fingertips until the mixture is crumbly.

5 Spoon the filling into the prepared crust. Sprinkle the topping evenly over the filling. To prevent over-browning, loosely cover the edge of the pie with foil. Place the pie plate on a rimmed baking sheet. Bake 50 minutes. Remove the foil and bake until the apples are tender and the crust is browned, 15 to 20 minutes longer. Cool completely on a wire rack before serving.

Each serving: 35 g carb, 197 cal, 6 g fat, 4 g sat fat, 15 mg chol, 3 g fib, 2 g pro, 52 mg sod • Carb Choices: 2; Exchanges: 1½ carb, ½ fruit, 1 fat

STREUSEL-TOPPED CHERRY PIE: Follow the Streusel-Topped Apple Pie recipe, at left, but use 6 cups pitted fresh sweet cherries instead of the apples. Replace the flour with ¼ cup cornstarch and proceed with the recipe.

Each serving: 39 g carb, 212 cal, 6 g fat, 4 g sat fat, 15 mg chol, 3 g fib, 2 g pro, 51 mg sod • Carb Choices: 2½; Exchanges: 2 carb, ½ fruit, 1 fat

STREUSEL-TOPPED BLUEBERRY PIE: Follow the Streusel-Topped Apple Pie recipe, at left, but use 5 cups fresh blueberries and proceed with the recipe. If using frozen blueberries, thaw and drain them first.

Each serving: 37 g carb, 204 cal, 6 g fat, 4 g sat fat, 15 mg chol, 3 g fib, 2 g pro, 52 mg sod • Carb Choices: 2½; Exchanges: 1½ carb, 1 fruit, 1 fat

Lemon Meringue Pie

makes 12 servings

Made with fewer egg yolks and a little less sugar, this version of the classic American pie is as sweet and tart as any version you grew up with. Make it in the morning if you're planning on serving it for dinner. It needs time to cool and then chill. If made a day ahead, the meringue will begin to weep.

1 recipe Pastry Crust (page 546)

FILLING

¾ cup sugar

¼ cup cornstarch

1¾ cups water

2 large egg yolks

½ cup lemon juice

2 teaspoons grated lemon zest

MERINGUE

4 large egg whites

½ teaspoon cream of tartar

½ teaspoon vanilla extract

¼ cup sugar

1 Preheat the oven to 400°F.

2 Place the pastry dough between two sheets of wax paper. Roll the dough into a 12-inch circle. Remove the top layer of wax paper and place the dough, with the wax paper facing up, into a 9-inch glass pie plate. Starting from the edge of the dough, gently remove the wax paper. Fold the overhanging dough under and crimp the edge decoratively.

3 Prick the bottom of the crust all over with a fork. Line the crust with parchment paper and fill with pie weights or dried beans. Bake 20 minutes. Remove the parchment and weights and bake until the crust is lightly browned, 5 to 8 minutes. Reduce the oven temperature to 350°F.

4 Meanwhile, to make the filling, combine the sugar, cornstarch, water, and egg yolks in a medium heavy-bottomed saucepan and whisk until the cornstarch dissolves. Cook over medium heat, whisking constantly, until the mixture comes to a boil and thickens, about 8 minutes.

5 Remove from the heat and stir in the lemon juice and lemon zest. Keep the filling warm while preparing the meringue.

6 To make the meringue, combine the egg whites and cream of tartar in a large bowl and beat at medium speed until foamy. Beat in the vanilla. Gradually add the sugar and beat at high speed until stiff peaks form.

7 Spoon the filling into the crust. Spread the meringue evenly over the filling, mounding in the center and spreading to seal the edge. Bake until the meringue is lightly browned, 15 minutes. Cool completely on a wire rack. Refrigerate 4 hours or until firm. The pie is best on the day it is made.

Each serving: 31 g carb, 175 cal, 5 g fat, 3 g sat fat, 44 mg chol, 2 g fib, 3 g pro, 69 mg sod • Carb Choices: 2; Exchanges: 2 carb, 1 fat

Pumpkin Pie

makes 12 servings

When I see people at the supermarket on the day before Thanksgiving with a factory-made pumpkin pie in their cart, I feel sorry for them. If they only knew how easy—and how much better tasting—the homemade version is, they would surely bake their own. Even if you've never made a pie before, you will have success with this one. If you don't have the spices for this pie, you can substitute 1 teaspoon of pumpkin pie spice for the cinnamon, allspice, and cloves.

1 recipe Pastry Crust (page 546)

1 (15-ounce) can pumpkin (not pumpkin pie filling)

½ cup fat-free evaporated milk

¾ cup packed light brown sugar

2 large eggs

1 teaspoon vanilla extract

½ teaspoon ground cinnamon

¼ teaspoon allspice

⅛ teaspoon cloves

1 Preheat the oven to 425°F.

2 Place the pastry dough between two sheets of wax paper. Roll the dough into a 12-inch circle. Remove the top layer of wax paper and place the dough, with the wax paper facing up, into a 9-inch glass pie plate. Starting from the edge of the dough, gently remove the wax paper. Fold the overhanging dough under and crimp the edge decoratively.

3 Combine the pumpkin, milk, sugar, eggs, vanilla, cinnamon, allspice, and cloves in a large bowl and whisk until smooth. Pour into the prepared crust.

4 Bake 15 minutes. Reduce the oven temperature to 350°F and bake until the filling is set, 35 to 40 minutes. Cover the edge of the crust with foil, if necessary, to prevent overbrowning. Cool completely on a wire rack before serving. The pie is best on the day it is made.

Each serving: 28 g carb, 168 cal, 5 g fat, 3 g sat fat, 45 mg chol, 2 g fib, 3 g pro, 81 mg sod • Carb Choices: 2; Exchanges: 2 carb, 1 fat

SWEET POTATO PIE: Follow the recipe for Pumpkin Pie, at left, but substitute 1¾ cups mashed sweet potato for the pumpkin. Before preparing the filling, place the potato and the evaporated milk in a food processor and process until smooth. Proceed with the recipe as directed.

Each serving: 34 g carb, 192 cal, 5 g fat, 3 g sat fat, 45 mg chol, 3 g fib, 4 g pro, 92 mg sod • Carb Choices: 2; Exchanges: 2 carb, 1 fat

Pecan Pie

makes 12 servings

Delicious enough to be a special treat for your Thanksgiving dessert table, this recipe is a much lighter version of typical pecan pies. As the pie bakes, it puffs up and creates a few cracks, but don't panic—they will disappear as the pie cools.

1 recipe Pastry Crust (page 546)

¾ cup light corn syrup

½ cup packed light brown sugar

2 large eggs

1 large egg white

3 tablespoons unbleached all-purpose flour

1 tablespoon unsalted butter, melted

1 teaspoon vanilla extract

Pinch of salt

¾ cup pecans, toasted and coarsely chopped (page 4)

1 Preheat the oven to 350°F.

2 Place the pastry dough between two sheets of wax paper. Roll the dough into a 12-inch circle. Remove the top layer of wax paper and place the dough, with the wax paper facing up, into a 9-inch glass pie plate. Starting from the edge of the dough, gently remove the wax paper. Fold the overhanging dough under and crimp the edge decoratively.

3 Whisk together the corn syrup, sugar, eggs, egg white, flour, butter, vanilla, and salt in a medium bowl until smooth. Stir in the pecans. Pour the filling into the prepared crust. Bake until the crust is browned and the filling is almost set, 40 to 45 minutes.

4 Cool the pie completely on a wire rack before slicing. The pie is best the day it is made.

Each serving: 38 g carb, 251 cal, 11 g fat, 4 g sat fat, 48 mg chol, 2 g fib, 3 g pro, 94 mg sod • Carb Choices: 2½; Exchanges: 2½ carb, 2 fat

Strawberry Pie

makes 12 servings

In this recipe, fresh strawberries are lightly coated in a strawberry sauce that doubles the great taste of this pie. Topped with slightly tangy Light Whipped Cream (page 586), it is a springtime delight.

8 cups halved (or quartered if large) fresh strawberries
¼ cup sugar
3 tablespoons cornstarch
½ cup water
1 tablespoon lemon juice
1 recipe Graham Cracker Crust (page 546)
12 tablespoons Light Whipped Cream (page 586)

1 Place 6 cups of the strawberries in a large bowl and set aside. Place the remaining 2 cups berries in a food processor and process until smooth.

2 Combine the pureed strawberries, sugar, cornstarch, and water in a medium saucepan and whisk until smooth. Cook over medium-high heat, stirring constantly, until the mixture comes to a boil and thickens, about 5 minutes. Remove from the heat and stir in the lemon juice.

3 Pour the hot mixture over the strawberries. Working quickly, toss the berries to coat and transfer into the prepared crust. Refrigerate until set, about 3 hours. The pie is best on the day it is made. Top each slice with 1 tablespoon of the whipped cream.

Each serving: 26 g carb, 152 cal, 5 g fat, 2 g sat fat, 12 mg chol, 3 g fib, 3 g pro, 82 mg sod • Carb Choices: 2; Exchanges: 1½ carb, ½ fruit, 1 fat

Lemon Chiffon Pie

makes 12 servings

This pie is as light as air, yet packed with fresh fruit flavor. It's perfect to serve after a warm weather lunch or dinner. The Key lime version is a special treat, but if you don't have access to these hard-to-find fruits, you can make it with regular limes.

¾ cup water
1 envelope unflavored gelatin
¾ cup sugar, divided
2 large egg yolks
1 teaspoon grated lemon zest
½ cup lemon juice
4 large egg whites
¼ teaspoon cream of tartar
1 recipe Graham Cracker Crust (page 546)

1 Place the water in a medium saucepan, sprinkle with the gelatin, and let stand 2 minutes to soften. Add ¼ cup of the sugar, egg yolks, lemon zest, and lemon juice and whisk until smooth. Cook over medium heat, stirring constantly, until the mixture thickens and coats the back of a spoon (do not boil). Transfer to a large bowl.

2 Refrigerate, stirring every 15 minutes, until thickened, but not set, 45 minutes to 1 hour.

3 Place the egg whites and cream of tartar in a large bowl and beat at high speed with an electric mixer until soft peaks form. Gradually beat in the remaining ½ cup sugar, beating until stiff peaks form. Fold the egg white mixture into the lemon mixture in three additions, mixing until no white streaks remain.

4 Spoon the filling into the prepared crust. Refrigerate 4 hours or until firm. The pie is best on the day it is made.

Each serving: 24 g carb, 135 cal, 3 g fat, 1 g sat fat, 39 mg chol, 0 g fib, 3 g pro, 96 mg sod • Carb Choices: 1½; Exchanges: 1½ carb, ½ fat

KEY LIME CHIFFON PIE: Follow the Lemon Chiffon Pie recipe, at left, substituting Key lime zest and juice for the lemon zest and juice. Proceed with the recipe as directed.

Each serving: 24 g carb, 135 cal, 3 g fat, 1 g sat fat, 39 mg chol, 0 g fib, 3 g pro, 96 mg sod • Carb Choices: 1½; Exchanges: 1½ carb, ½ fat

Chocolate-Raspberry Chiffon Pie

makes 12 servings

The contrast of red raspberries and dark chocolate in this pie creates a stunning dessert.

¾ cup water

1 envelope unflavored gelatin

¾ cup sugar, divided

2 large egg yolks

1 (10-ounce) package frozen unsweetened raspberries, thawed

4 large egg whites

¼ teaspoon cream of tartar

1 recipe Graham Cracker Crust (page 546), prepared using chocolate graham crackers

12 tablespoons Rich Chocolate Sauce (page 587)

1 Place the water in a medium saucepan, sprinkle with the gelatin, and let stand 2 minutes to soften. Add ¼ cup of the sugar and the egg yolks and whisk until smooth. Cook over medium heat, stirring constantly, until the mixture thickens and coats the back of a spoon (do not boil). Transfer to a large bowl.

2 Place the raspberries in a food processor and process until smooth. Stir the raspberry puree into the gelatin mixture. Refrigerate, stirring every 15 minutes, until thickened, but not set, 45 minutes to 1 hour.

3 Place the egg whites and cream of tartar in a large bowl and beat at high speed with an electric mixer until soft peaks form. Gradually beat in

the remaining ½ cup sugar, beating until stiff peaks form. Fold the egg white mixture into the raspberry mixture in three additions, mixing until no white streaks remain.

4 Spoon the filling into the prepared crust. Refrigerate 4 hours or until firm. Serve each slice of pie drizzled with 1 tablespoon of the sauce. The pie is best on the day it is made.

Each serving: 33 g carb, 241 cal, 6 g fat, 3 g sat fat, 40 mg chol, 3 g fib, 5 g pro, 102 mg sod • Carb Choices: 2; Exchanges: 2 carb, 1 fat

Vanilla Cream Pie

makes 12 servings

You can top the vanilla version of this pie with fresh berries just before serving. Instead of the pastry, make any of these pies using a baked Graham Cracker Crust (page 546).

1 recipe Pastry Crust (page 546)

2 cups 1% low-fat milk

1 large egg

½ cup sugar

3 tablespoons cornstarch

Pinch of salt

2 teaspoons vanilla extract

1 Preheat the oven to 400°F.

2 Place the pastry dough between two sheets of wax paper. Roll the dough into a 12-inch circle. Remove the top layer of wax paper and place the dough, with the wax paper facing up, into a 9-inch glass pie plate. Starting from the edge of the dough, gently remove the wax paper. Fold the overhanging dough under and crimp the edge decoratively. Prick the bottom of the crust all over with a fork. Line the crust with parchment paper and fill with pie weights or dried beans. Bake 20 minutes. Remove the parchment and weights and bake until the crust is lightly browned, 5 to 8 minutes. Cool completely on a wire rack.

continues on next page

3 Meanwhile, to make the filling, combine the milk, egg, sugar, cornstarch, and salt in a medium saucepan. Cook over medium heat, whisking constantly, until the mixture comes to a boil and thickens, about 8 minutes. Stir in the vanilla.

4 Spoon the hot filling into the crust. Place a sheet of wax paper directly on the filling and refrigerate 4 hours or until firm. The pie is best on the day it is made.

Each serving: 23 g carb, 147 cal, 5 g fat, 3 g sat fat, 30 mg chol, 1 g fib, 3 g pro, 85 mg sod • Carb Choices: 1½; Exchanges: 1½ carb, 1 fat

CHOCOLATE PIE: Follow the Vanilla Cream Pie recipe, page 551, adding ⅓ cup unsweetened cocoa to the milk mixture in step 3. Proceed with the recipe as directed.

Each serving: 24 g carb, 152 cal, 5 g fat, 3 g sat fat, 30 mg chol, 2 g fib, 4 g pro, 85 mg sod • Carb Choices: 1½; Exchanges: 1½ carb, 1 fat

BANANA CREAM PIE: Follow the Vanilla Cream Pie recipe, page 551, through step 2. Spoon half of the filling into the prepared crust and top with 1 large banana, sliced. Spoon the remaining filling over the banana and proceed with the recipe as directed.

Each serving: 25 g carb, 156 cal, 5 g fat, 3 g sat fat, 30 mg chol, 2 g fib, 3 g pro, 85 mg sod • Carb Choices: 1½; Exchanges: 1½ carb, 1 fat

Coconut Cream Pie

makes 12 servings

Traditional coconut cream pie can have enough fat and calories for an entire meal. This healthful version uses low-fat milk with coconut milk and extract to give rich flavor with much less fat. Toasting the coconut before adding it to the filling also heightens the flavor.

½ cup flaked sweetened coconut
1 recipe Pastry Crust (page 546)
1½ cups 1% low-fat milk
½ cup reduced-fat coconut milk
1 large egg
½ cup sugar
3 tablespoons cornstarch
Pinch of salt
½ teaspoon coconut extract

1 Preheat the oven to 350°F.

2 Place the coconut in a small baking pan and bake, stirring once, until lightly toasted, 6 to 8 minutes. Transfer to a plate to cool.

3 Increase the oven temperature to 400°F.

4 Place the pastry dough between two sheets of wax paper. Roll the dough into a 12-inch circle. Remove the top layer of wax paper and place the dough, with the wax paper facing up, into a 9-inch glass pie plate. Starting from the edge of the dough, gently remove the wax paper. Fold the overhanging dough under and crimp the edge decoratively. Prick the bottom of the crust all over with a fork. Line the crust with parchment paper and fill with pie weights or dried beans. Bake 20 minutes. Remove the parchment and weights and bake until the crust is lightly browned, 5 to 8 minutes. Cool completely on a wire rack.

5 Combine the milk, coconut milk, egg, sugar, cornstarch, and salt in a medium saucepan. Cook over medium heat, whisking constantly, until the mixture comes to a boil and thickens, about 8 minutes. Stir in the reserved toasted coconut and the coconut extract.

6 Spoon the hot filling into the crust. Place a sheet of wax paper directly on the filling and refrigerate 4 hours or until firm. The pie is best on the day it is made.

Each serving: 24 g carb, 167 cal, 7 g fat, 4 g sat fat, 29 mg chol, 2 g fib, 3 g pro, 93 mg sod • Carb Choices: 1½; Exchanges: 1½ carb, 1 fat

Strawberry-Yogurt Pie

makes 10 servings

If your car automatically turns when you see a u-pick strawberry sign on the highway, keep this simple and satisfying pie in mind the next time you bring home too many fresh berries. Using frozen berries for the filling makes the recipe almost effortless, but you can substitute 2 cups whole fresh strawberries for frozen strawberries.

¼ cup water
1 envelope unflavored gelatin
½ cup sugar
2 cups whole unsweetened frozen strawberries, thawed
1 cup plain low-fat yogurt
1 teaspoon grated lemon zest
1 recipe Graham Cracker Crust (page 546)
2½ cups sliced fresh strawberries

1 Place the water in a medium saucepan, sprinkle with the gelatin and let stand 2 minutes to soften. Stir in the sugar. Cook over medium heat, stirring constantly, until the gelatin dissolves, about 1 minute (do not boil). Transfer to a medium bowl.

2 Place the thawed frozen strawberries in a food processor and process until smooth. Add the puréed strawberries, yogurt, and lemon zest to the sugar mixture and whisk until smooth. Spoon the filling into the prepared crust. Refrigerate 4 hours or until firm. Serve each slice with ¼ cup of the sliced fresh strawberries. The pie is best on the day it is made.

Each serving: 28 g carb, 149 cal, 3 g fat, 1 g sat fat, 6 mg chol, 2 g fib, 4 g pro, 94 mg sod • Carb choices: 2; Exchanges: 1½ carb, 1 fruit, ½ fat

Fresh Berry Tart

makes 10 servings

1 recipe Pastry Crust (page 546)
⅓ cup sugar
2 tablespoons cornstarch
3 cups fresh blueberries or raspberries
1 tablespoon cold water
¼ cup apricot preserves

1 Place the pastry dough between two sheets of wax paper. Roll the dough into a 12-inch circle. Remove the top layer of wax paper and place the dough, with the wax paper facing up, into a 9-inch tart pan with a removable bottom. Starting from the edge of the dough, gently remove the wax paper. Trim the dough to fit the pan. Cover and refrigerate 1 hour.

2 Preheat the oven to 400°F.

3 Prick the bottom of the crust all over with a fork. Line the crust with parchment paper and fill with pie weights or dried beans. Bake 20 minutes. Remove the parchment and weights and bake until the crust is lightly browned, 5 to 8 minutes. Cool completely on a wire rack. Reduce the oven temperature to 350°F.

4 Combine the sugar and cornstarch in a large bowl and stir to mix well. Add the berries and toss to coat. Sprinkle with the water and toss to combine (a few white lumps will remain). Spoon into the prepared crust.

5 Bake until the filling begins to bubble around the edge, 45 to 50 minutes. Cool the tart completely on a wire rack.

6 Place the preserves in a small saucepan and melt over low heat. Strain the preserves through a fine wire mesh strainer, discarding the solids. Brush the top of the tart with the strained preserves. The tart is best the day it is made.

Each serving: 31 g carb, 171 cal, 5 g fat, 3 g sat fat, 12 mg chol, 3 g fib, 2 g pro, 59 mg sod • Carb Choices: 2; Exchanges: 1½ carb, ½ fruit, 1 fat

Peach-Blueberry Crostata

makes 10 servings

You don't have to fuss with fitting the pastry dough into a pie plate, so this rustic crostata is really easy to make. Just a sprinkle of cinnamon and lemon zest lets the fresh fruit show at its best.

1 recipe Pastry Crust (page 546)
1 pound peaches, peeled, pitted, and sliced (about 3 cups)
½ cup fresh blueberries or unthawed frozen blueberries
¼ cup plus 2 teaspoons sugar, divided
¼ cup unbleached all-purpose flour
1 teaspoon grated lemon zest
¼ teaspoon ground cinnamon
2 teaspoons unsalted butter, melted

1 Preheat the oven to 400°F.

2 Place the pastry dough between two sheets of parchment paper. Roll the dough into a 12-inch circle. Set aside, leaving the dough between the parchment paper to prevent it from drying out.

3 Combine the peaches, blueberries, ¼ cup of the sugar, the flour, lemon zest, and cinnamon in a large bowl and toss to coat. Transfer the dough inside the parchment paper sheets onto a large baking sheet. Remove the top layer of parchment.

4 Mound the fruit mixture in the center of the dough. Carefully fold the dough up and over the edge of the filling, pleating as necessary. Brush the dough with the melted butter and sprinkle with the remaining 2 teaspoons sugar. Bake until the fruit is bubbly and the crust is browned, 30 to 35 minutes. Serve warm or at room temperature. The crostata is best the day it is made.

Each serving: 27 g carb, 163 cal, 6 g fat, 3 g sat fat, 14 mg chol, 3 g fib, 2 g pro, 59 mg sod • Carb Choices: 2; Exchanges: 1½ carb, ½ fruit, 1 fat

Ginger-Plum Crostata

makes 10 servings

Dark purple Italian prune plums are the sweetest variety and an excellent choice for this recipe, but you can use any variety. The crystallized ginger adds a peppery bite, but if you don't have any on hand, add ½ teaspoon ground ginger instead.

1 recipe Pastry Crust (page 546)
1¼ pounds plums, pitted and sliced
¼ cup plus 2 teaspoons sugar, divided
¼ cup unbleached all-purpose flour
2 tablespoons minced crystallized ginger
2 teaspoons unsalted butter, melted

1 Preheat the oven to 400°F.

2 Place the pastry dough between two sheets of parchment paper. Roll the dough into a 12-inch circle. Set aside, leaving the dough between the parchment paper to prevent it from drying out.

3 Combine the plums, ¼ cup of the sugar, the flour, and ginger in a large bowl and toss to coat. Transfer the dough inside the parchment paper sheets onto a large baking sheet. Remove the top layer of parchment.

4 Mound the plum mixture in the center of the dough. Carefully fold the dough up and over the edge of the filling, pleating as necessary. Brush the dough with the melted butter and sprinkle with the remaining 2 teaspoons sugar. Bake until the plums are bubbly and the crust is browned, 30 to 35 minutes. Serve warm or at room temperature. The crostata is best the day it is made.

Each serving: 27 g carb, 165 cal, 6 g fat, 3 g sat fat, 14 mg chol, 3 g fib, 2 g pro, 59 mg sod • Carb Choices: 2; Exchanges: 1½ carb, ½ fruit, 1 fat

Apricot-Almond Crostata

makes 10 servings

Soft yellow apricots and toasted sliced almonds make a striking and fragrant pairing for a crostata. Make sure the apricots you choose are ripe—they should give slightly when pressed gently.

1 recipe Pastry Crust (page 546)
1¼ pounds apricots, pitted and sliced
¼ cup plus 2 teaspoons sugar, divided
¼ cup unbleached all-purpose flour
1 teaspoon grated lemon zest
⅛ teaspoon almond extract
2 teaspoons unsalted butter, melted
2 tablespoons sliced almonds

1 Preheat the oven to 400°F.

2 Place the pastry dough between two sheets of parchment paper. Roll the dough into a 12-inch circle. Set aside, leaving the dough between the parchment paper to prevent it from drying out.

3 Combine the apricots, ¼ cup of the sugar, the flour, lemon zest, and almond extract in a large bowl and toss to coat. Transfer the dough inside the parchment paper sheets onto a large baking sheet. Remove the top layer of parchment.

4 Mound the apricot mixture in the center of the dough. Carefully fold the dough up and over the edge of the filling, pleating as necessary. Brush the dough with the melted butter. Sprinkle with the almonds, then with the remaining 2 teaspoons sugar. Bake until the apricots are bubbly and the crust is browned, 30 to 35 minutes. Serve warm or at room temperature. The crostata is best the day it is made.

Each serving: 27 g carb, 171 cal, 6 g fat, 3 g sat fat, 14 mg chol, 3 g fib, 3 g pro, 59 mg sod • Carb Choices: 2; Exchanges: 1½ carb, ½ fruit, 1 fat

Puddings and Custards

Vanilla Pudding QUICK

makes 4 servings

Pudding is so quick and easy to make from the most basic of inexpensive pantry ingredients, there's no reason to ever buy premade pudding. The touch of butter at the end really enhances the flavor of this silky pudding.

2 cups 1% low-fat milk
1 large egg
⅓ cup sugar
3 tablespoons cornstarch
Pinch of salt
2 teaspoons vanilla extract
1 teaspoon unsalted butter

1 Combine the milk, egg, sugar, cornstarch, and salt in a medium saucepan and whisk until smooth. Cook over medium heat, whisking constantly, until the mixture comes to a boil and thickens, about 8 minutes.

2 Remove from the heat and stir in the vanilla and butter. Transfer to a serving bowl and cool slightly to serve warm, or cover the surface of the pudding with wax paper to prevent a skin from forming and chill before serving.

Each serving: 29 g carb, 171 cal, 3 g fat, 2 g sat fat, 61 mg chol, 0 g fib, 6 g pro, 145 mg sod • Carb Choices: 2; Exchanges: 2 carb

Rich Chocolate Pudding QUICK

makes 4 servings

Cocoa and semisweet chocolate make this pudding a super-rich chocolaty treat. Adults in need of a spoonful of comfort will find this dessert as enjoyable as the kids will.

2 cups 1% low-fat milk
1 large egg
⅓ cup sugar
¼ cup unsweetened cocoa
3 tablespoons cornstarch
Pinch of salt
1 ounce semisweet chocolate, chopped
2 teaspoons vanilla extract
1 teaspoon unsalted butter

1 Combine the milk, egg, sugar, cocoa, cornstarch, and salt in a medium saucepan and whisk until smooth. Cook over medium heat, whisking constantly, until the mixture comes to a boil and thickens, about 8 minutes.

2 Remove from the heat and add the chocolate, vanilla, and butter, stirring until the chocolate melts. Transfer to a serving bowl and cool slightly to serve warm, or cover the surface of the pudding with wax paper to prevent a skin from forming and chill before serving.

Each serving: 37 g carb, 227 cal, 6 g fat, 4 g sat fat, 60 mg chol, 2 g fib, 8 g pro, 127 mg sod • Carb Choices: 2½; Exchanges: 2½ carb

Banana Pudding

makes 8 servings

This is a crowd-pleasing dessert, perfect for a reunion or a potluck. The baked meringue on top makes a pretty presentation, but if you're short on time, you can skip this step and leave the top plain or sprinkle it with a few crumbled vanilla wafers. Without the meringue, there is no need to bake the pudding.

3 cups 1% low-fat milk
2 large eggs
½ cup plus 2 tablespoons sugar, divided
¼ cup cornstarch
Pinch of salt
2 teaspoons vanilla extract
2 medium ripe bananas, sliced
20 reduced-fat vanilla wafers
3 large egg whites
¼ teaspoon cream of tartar

1 Preheat the oven to 325°F.

2 Combine the milk, eggs, ½ cup of the sugar, the cornstarch, and salt in a medium saucepan and whisk until smooth. Cook over medium heat, whisking constantly, until the mixture comes to a boil and thickens, about 8 minutes.

3 Remove the pudding from the heat and stir in the vanilla.

4 Arrange one-third of the banana slices in the bottom of a 1½-quart soufflé or deep-sided baking dish. Spread 1 cup of the pudding over the banana slices. Arrange 10 of the wafers on top of the pudding. Top with one-third of the banana slices and spread another cup of the pudding over the bananas. Top with the remaining 10 wafers. Top the wafers with the remaining banana slices and pudding.

5 To make the meringue, combine the egg whites and cream of tartar in a large bowl and beat at high speed until foamy. Gradually add the remaining 2 tablespoons sugar, beating until stiff peaks form. Spread the meringue evenly over the pudding. Bake until the meringue is lightly browned, 25 to 30 minutes.

6 Cool the pudding to room temperature, then refrigerate at least 2 hours. The pudding tastes best on the day it is made.

Each serving: 38 g carb, 203 cal, 3 g fat, 1 g sat fat, 57 mg chol, 1 g fib, 7 g pro, 132 mg sod • Carb Choices: 2½; Exchanges: 2½ carb

Chocolate Mousse

makes 8 servings

The rich flavor of this light and airy mousse belies its healthy nutrient profile. Don't be daunted by beating the egg white mixture in the double boiler—it's easy to do with a handheld electric mixer and there's a delicious reward at the end.

½ cup unsweetened cocoa
⅓ cup boiling water
½ teaspoon vanilla extract
⅔ sugar
5 large egg whites
¼ teaspoon cream of tartar

1 Combine the cocoa and boiling water in a large bowl and whisk until smooth. Whisk in the vanilla. Set aside.

2 Combine the sugar, egg whites, and cream of tartar in the top of a double boiler. Place over simmering (not boiling) water and beat at high speed with a handheld electric mixer until soft peaks form, about 5 minutes.

3 Remove from the heat. Fold the egg white mixture into the cocoa mixture in three additions, stirring until no white streaks remain. Refrigerate the mousse, covered, until chilled, at least 2 hours and up to overnight, before serving.

Each serving: 20 g carb, 88 cal, 1 g fat, 0 g sat fat, 0 mg chol, 2 g fib, 3 g pro, 36 mg sod • Carb Choices: 1; Exchanges: 1 carb

Crème Brûlée

makes 8 servings

Crème brûlée is an ideal dessert to serve when you're entertaining. You have to make it a day ahead so that the custard can set. Then, when it's time to serve dessert, just a quick run under the broiler and you're ready to offer your guests the easiest and most impressive dessert there is.

3 cups 1% low-fat milk
2 large eggs
2 large egg whites
½ cup granulated sugar
1 tablespoon vanilla extract
¼ cup packed light brown sugar

1 Preheat the oven to 325°F.

2 Whisk together the milk, eggs, egg whites, granulated sugar, and vanilla in a large bowl. Divide the mixture evenly among eight 6-ounce crème brûlée dishes or custard cups. Place the cups inside a roasting pan and add water to the pan halfway up the sides of the dishes.

3 Bake until the custards are almost set but still soft in the centers, 45 to 50 minutes. Carefully remove the custards from the water bath and cool completely on wire racks. Refrigerate the custards, covered, until chilled, 4 hours or overnight.

4 To serve, preheat the broiler. Sprinkle the brown sugar evenly over each custard and arrange the custards on a large baking sheet. Broil until the sugar melts, rotating the baking sheet as needed, about 2 minutes. Let stand 5 minutes before serving.

Each serving: 24 g carb, 139 cal, 2 g fat, 1 g sat fat, 57 mg chol, 0 g fib, 6 g pro, 74 mg sod • Carb Choices: 1½; Exchanges: 1½ carb

ALMOND CRÈME BRÛLÉE: Follow the Crème Brûlée recipe, at left, but add 2 tablespoons almond liqueur to the milk mixture in step 2 and proceed with the recipe.

Each serving: 25 g carb, 147 cal, 2 g fat, 1 g sat fat, 57 mg chol, 0 g fib, 6 g pro, 75 mg sod • Carb Choices: 1½; Exchanges: 1 carb, ½ reduced-fat milk, ½ fat

Flan

makes 12 servings

Be sure to unmold this flan onto a plate with a rim—you don't want to lose any of the caramel syrup that pools in the bottom of the pan.

1 teaspoon canola oil
½ cup granulated sugar
2 tablespoons water
2 (12-ounce) cans fat-free evaporated milk
½ cup packed light brown sugar
3 large eggs
2 large egg whites
1 teaspoon vanilla extract

1 Preheat the oven to 350°F. Brush the inside rim of a 9-inch round cake pan with the oil, leaving the bottom of the pan uncoated.

2 Stir together the granulated sugar and water in a medium saucepan. Cook over medium heat, stirring constantly, until the sugar dissolves, about 3 minutes. Continue cooking, without stirring, until the mixture turns golden, about 6 minutes longer. Carefully pour the sugar mixture into the prepared pan, tilting the pan to coat the bottom (the pan will be hot after pouring in the caramel).

3 Whisk together the evaporated milk, brown sugar, eggs, egg whites, and vanilla in a large bowl. Pour into the cake pan. Place the cake pan inside a large roasting pan and add hot water to the pan halfway up the side of the cake pan.

4 Bake until a knife inserted in the edge of the flan comes out clean and flan is still soft in the center, 45 to 50 minutes. Carefully remove the flan from the water bath and cool on a wire rack for 1 hour. Refrigerate the flan, covered, overnight.

5 To serve, run a small spatula around the edge of the flan and invert onto a rimmed serving plate to avoid spilling the syrup.

Each serving: 25 g carb, 137 cal, 2 g fat, 0 g sat fat, 53 mg chol, 0 g fib, 6 g pro, 101 mg sod • Carb Choices: 1½; Exchanges: 1½ carb

Pumpkin Flan

makes 12 servings

If making a pie crust for a pumpkin pie is too overwhelming, here's your answer to a nearly effortless Thanksgiving dessert. You have to make this flan a day ahead so that the syrup has time to form, but all you have to do when you're ready to serve is invert it onto a rimmed plate.

1 teaspoon canola oil
½ cup granulated sugar
2 tablespoons water
1 (12-ounce) can fat-free evaporated milk
1 (15-ounce) can pumpkin (not pumpkin pie filling)
½ cup packed light brown sugar
1 teaspoon pumpkin pie spice
3 large eggs
2 large egg whites
1 teaspoon vanilla extract

1 Preheat the oven to 350°F. Brush the inside rim of a 9-inch round cake pan with the oil, leaving the bottom of the pan uncoated.

2 Stir together the granulated sugar and water in a medium saucepan. Cook over medium heat, stirring constantly, until the sugar dissolves, about 3 minutes. Continue cooking, without stirring, until the mixture turns golden, about 6 minutes longer. Carefully pour the sugar mixture into the prepared pan, tilting the pan to coat the bottom (the pan will be hot after pouring in the caramel).

3 Whisk together the evaporated milk, pumpkin, brown sugar, pumpkin pie spice, eggs, egg whites, and vanilla in a large bowl. Pour into the cake pan. Place the cake pan inside a large roasting pan and add hot water to the pan halfway up the side of the cake pan.

4 Bake until a knife inserted in the edge of the flan comes out clean and the flan is still soft in the center, 1 hour 20 minutes. Carefully remove the flan from the water bath and cool on a wire rack for 1 hour. Refrigerate the flan, covered, overnight.

5 To serve, run a small spatula around the edge of the flan and invert onto a rimmed serving plate to avoid spilling the syrup.

Each serving: 24 g carb, 126 cal, 2 g fat, 0 g sat fat, 53 mg chol, 1 g fib, 4 g pro, 68 mg sod • Carb Choices: 1½; Exchanges: 1½ carb

Panna Cotta

makes 6 servings

This cool and creamy panna cotta is a blank slate for whatever you're craving. Serve the individual custards with any fresh berries that are in season or you can drizzle them with Raspberry Sauce (page 588), Strawberry Sauce (page 588), or Creamy Custard Sauce (page 588). Instead of the vanilla, you can flavor the panna cotta with 2 tablespoons hazelnut, almond, or orange liqueur.

2 teaspoons canola oil
3 cups 2% low-fat milk, divided
1 tablespoon unflavored gelatin
½ cup sugar
1 tablespoon vanilla extract

1 Brush six 6-ounce ramekins or custard cups with the oil.

2 Place 1½ cups of the milk in a medium saucepan. Sprinkle with the gelatin and let stand 2 minutes to soften. Add the sugar and cook over medium heat, stirring constantly, until the mixture thickens and coats the back of a spoon (do not boil). Remove from the heat and stir in the remaining 1½ cups milk and the vanilla. Divide the mixture among the prepared ramekins. Refrigerate the custards, covered, overnight.

3 To serve, loosen the edge of each panna cotta with a knife and invert the ramekins onto individual plates.

Each serving: 23 g carb, 149 cal, 4 g fat, 2 g sat fat, 10 mg chol, 0 g fib, 5 g pro, 53 mg sod • Carb Choices: 1½; Exchanges: 1½ carb

Pumpkin Panna Cotta

makes 6 servings

More elegant than pie—and easier, too—this panna cotta is a welcome option to serve at a small Thanksgiving dinner or any fall get-together.

2 teaspoons canola oil
2 cups 1% low-fat milk
1½ teaspoons unflavored gelatin
½ cup packed light brown sugar
1 (15-ounce) can pumpkin (not pumpkin pie filling)
½ teaspoon pumpkin pie spice
¼ teaspoon vanilla extract

1 Brush six 8-ounce ramekins or custard cups with the oil.

2 Place the milk in a medium saucepan. Sprinkle with the gelatin and let stand 2 minutes to soften. Add the sugar and cook over medium heat, stirring constantly, until the mixture thickens and coats the back of a spoon (do not boil). Remove from the heat and stir in the pumpkin, pumpkin pie spice, and vanilla.

3 Pour the mixture through a fine wire mesh strainer into a clean bowl. Discard the solids. Divide the mixture among the prepared ramekins. Refrigerate the custards, covered, overnight.

4 To serve, loosen the edge of each panna cotta with a knife and invert the ramekins onto individual plates.

Each serving: 28 g carb, 151 cal, 3 g fat, 1 g sat fat, 3 mg chol, 0 g fib, 5 g pro, 61 mg sod • Carb choices: 2; Exchanges: ½ starch, 1½ carb

Rice Pudding

makes 8 servings

Rice pudding is a great example of the simplest ingredients coming together to make a dish that tastes divine. It is the ultimate in creamy comfort food. Try the berry version below for a fresh and colorful take on this classic dessert.

5 cups 1% low-fat milk
1 cup medium- or short-grain rice
⅓ cup sugar
½ teaspoon ground cinnamon (optional)
½ teaspoon salt
2 teaspoons vanilla extract

1 Combine the milk, rice, sugar, cinnamon, if using, and salt in a large saucepan and bring to a boil over medium-high heat. Reduce the heat to low and simmer, uncovered, stirring often, until the rice is tender and most of the milk is absorbed, 20 to 25 minutes. As the pudding thickens, stir it more often to prevent sticking. Remove from the heat and stir in the vanilla.

2 Transfer to a serving bowl and cool slightly to serve warm, or refrigerate the pudding, covered, until chilled, 4 hours or overnight.

Each serving: 36 g carb, 189 cal, 2 g fat, 1 g sat fat, 8 mg chol, 1 g fib, 7 g pro, 213 mg sod • Carb Choices: 2½; Exchanges: 2½ carb

BERRY RICE PUDDING: Prepare the Rice Pudding recipe, above, as directed. Place 3 cups fresh raspberries or strawberries in a medium bowl and mash with a fork until coarsely crushed. Spoon the pudding into serving bowls and swirl about 2 tablespoons of the crushed berries into each serving.

Each serving: 41 g carb, 213 cal, 2 g fat, 1 g sat fat, 8 mg chol, 4 g fib, 7 g pro, 213 mg sod • Carb Choices: 3; Exchanges: 3 carb

Tapioca Pudding

makes 4 servings

Even creamier and more delicate than rice pudding, tapioca pudding is an old-fashioned treat. Be sure to buy "minute" tapioca, which only needs to cook a short time.

2 cups 1% low-fat milk
1 large egg
⅓ cup sugar
3 tablespoons minute tapioca
⅛ teaspoon salt
1 teaspoon vanilla extract

1 Combine the milk, egg, sugar, tapioca, and salt in a medium saucepan and stir to mix well. Let stand 5 minutes.

2 Cook the milk mixture over medium heat, stirring constantly, until the mixture comes to a boil, about 6 minutes. Remove from the heat and stir in the vanilla. Transfer the pudding to a medium bowl and place a sheet of wax paper on the surface of the pudding to prevent a skin from forming. Cool to room temperature. Stir the pudding and refrigerate, covered, until chilled, 4 hours or overnight.

Each serving: 31 g carb, 173 cal, 2 g fat, 1 g sat fat, 59 mg chol, 0 g fib, 6 g pro, 144 mg sod • Carb Choices: 2; Exchanges: 2 carb

COCONUT TAPIOCA PUDDING: Follow the Tapioca Pudding recipe, above, replacing 1 cup of the milk with 1 cup reduced-fat coconut milk, and proceed with the recipe.

Each serving: 30 g carb, 182 cal, 5 g fat, 4 g sat fat, 56 mg chol, 0 g fib, 4 g pro, 142 mg sod • Carb Choices: 2; Exchanges: 2 carb

Raisin Bread Pudding

makes 8 servings

You probably have all the ingredients to make this homey and comforting bread pudding in your pantry. White bread gives the pudding a more delicate flavor and texture, but you can substitute whole grain bread if you wish, or make it with raisin bread and omit the raisins.

1 teaspoon canola oil
1¼ cups 1% low-fat milk
½ cup packed dark brown sugar
2 large eggs
1 teaspoon vanilla extract
½ teaspoon ground cinnamon
⅛ teaspoon ground nutmeg
6 cups ½-inch French bread cubes
   (about 9 ounces)
¼ cup raisins

1 Preheat the oven to 350°F. Brush a 1½-quart baking dish with the oil and set aside.

2 Whisk together the milk, sugar, eggs, vanilla, cinnamon, and nutmeg in a large bowl. Add the bread and raisins and stir to combine. Let the mixture stand, stirring occasionally, until almost all the liquid is absorbed, 15 to 20 minutes.

3 Spoon the mixture into the prepared dish. Place the baking dish inside a large roasting pan and add hot water to the pan halfway up the sides of the baking dish.

4 Bake until the top of the pudding is lightly browned and the custard is set, about 50 minutes. Carefully remove the baking dish from the roasting pan. Serve warm.

Each serving: 38 g carb, 200 cal, 3 g fat, 1 g sat fat, 55 mg chol, 1 g fib, 7 g pro, 248 mg sod • Carb Choices: 2½; Exchanges: 2½ carb

Blueberry-Lemon Bread Pudding

makes 8 servings

If you haven't tried dried blueberries, this fancied-up bread pudding is a good excuse to buy some. They are so intensely flavored, it only takes a few to flavor a dish. They're delicious in oatmeal, sprinkled over cereal, or as a snack. Whole wheat bread is healthier, but I like to make an exception here and use white bread for this refined pudding.

1 teaspoon canola oil
1¼ cups 1% low-fat milk
½ cup sugar
2 large eggs
2 teaspoons grated lemon zest
1 teaspoon vanilla extract
6 cups ½-inch French bread cubes
   (about 9 ounces)
¼ cup dried blueberries

1 Preheat the oven to 350°F. Brush a 1½-quart baking dish with the oil and set aside.

2 Whisk together the milk, sugar, eggs, lemon zest, and vanilla in a large bowl. Add the bread and the blueberries and stir to combine. Let the mixture stand, stirring occasionally, until almost all the liquid is absorbed, 15 to 20 minutes.

3 Spoon the mixture into the prepared dish. Place the baking dish inside a large roasting pan and add hot water to the pan halfway up the sides of the baking dish.

4 Bake until the top of the pudding is lightly browned and the custard is set, about 50 minutes. Carefully remove the baking dish from the roasting pan. Serve warm.

Each serving: 36 g carb, 198 cal, 3 g fat, 1 g sat fat, 55 mg chol, 2 g fib, 7 g pro, 243 mg sod • Carb Choices: 2½; Exchanges: 2½ carb

Cakes

Classic White Cake `QUICK`

makes 16 servings

Make this classic sheet cake for bake sales, birthday parties, and holiday celebrations. In this recipe, the cake is simply sprinkled with confectioners' sugar, but if you need to dress it up, frost it with Fluffy White Frosting (page 587) or Cream Cheese Frosting (page 587), or drizzle it with melted chocolate.

2 teaspoons plus ½ cup (1 stick) unsalted
    butter, softened, divided
2 cups cake flour
2 teaspoons baking powder
½ teaspoon baking soda
¼ teaspoon salt
⅔ cup granulated sugar
2 large eggs
2 teaspoons vanilla extract
1⅓ cup low-fat buttermilk
2 teaspoons confectioners' sugar

1 Preheat the oven to 350°F. Line the bottom of a 13 x 9-inch cake pan with parchment paper. Brush the sides of the pan with 2 teaspoons of the butter.

2 Combine the flour, baking powder, baking soda, and salt in a medium bowl and whisk to mix well.

3 Place the remaining ½ cup butter in a large bowl and beat at medium speed with an electric mixer until fluffy. Gradually beat in the granulated sugar. Beat in the eggs one at a time. Beat in the vanilla. Add the flour mixture and the buttermilk alternately to the butter mixture, beginning and ending with the flour mixture, beating well after each addition.

4 Spoon the batter into the prepared pan, smoothing the top. Bake until a wooden toothpick inserted in the center comes out clean, 22 to 24 minutes. Cool the cake in the pan on a wire rack for 10 minutes. Remove from the pan and cool completely, right side up, on a wire rack. Sprinkle the top of the cake with the confectioners' sugar. The cake can be covered in an airtight container and stored at room temperature for up to 3 days.

Each serving: 21 g carb, 156 cal, 7 g fat, 4 g sat fat, 44 mg chol, 0 g fib, 3 g pro, 157 mg sod • Carb Choices: 1½; Exchanges: 1½ carb, 1 fat

Note: To make cupcakes, spoon the batter into 24 paper-lined muffin cups and bake 18 to 20 minutes. Frost with Fluffy White Frosting (page 587), if desired.

White Layer Cake with Fluffy White Frosting

makes 16 servings

When an event calls for a dessert worthy of candles, this buttery layer cake covered in a cloud of fluffy frosting will please everyone. It will be as welcome at a children's birthday celebration as it is at a retirement party.

1 recipe Classic White Cake (at left)
1 recipe Fluffy White Frosting (page 587)

1 Prepare the cake, baking the cake in round cake pans. To do so, line two 8- or 9-inch round cake pans with parchment paper. Brush the sides of the pans with the 2 teaspoons butter. Spoon the batter evenly into the pans. Bake 8-inch cakes for 22 minutes and 9-inch cakes for 20 minutes.

2 Cool the cakes in the pans on a wire rack for 10 minutes. Remove from the pans and cool completely on a wire rack. Spread the frosting between the layers and on the sides and top of the cake.

Each serving: 27 g carb, 182 cal, 7 g fat, 4 g sat fat, 44 mg chol, 0 g fib, 3 g pro, 164 mg sod • Carb Choices: 2; Exchanges: 2 carb, 1 fat

Raspberry-Lemon Layer Cake

makes 16 servings

There's a wonderful raspberry surprise inside this simple yet sophisticated cake. The tart jam and lemony glaze temper the sweetness of the cake perfectly. For an attractive presentation, serve each slice with a handful of fresh raspberries.

1 recipe Classic White Cake (page 562)
½ cup seedless raspberry jam, at room temperature
1 recipe Citrus Glaze (page 586), prepared using lemon juice

1 Prepare the cake recipe, baking the cake in round cake pans. To do so, line two 8- or 9-inch round cake pans with parchment paper. Brush the sides of the pans with the 2 teaspoons butter. Spoon the batter evenly into the pans. Bake 8-inch cakes for 22 minutes and 9-inch cakes for 20 minutes.

2 Cool the cakes in the pans on a wire rack for 10 minutes. Remove from the pans and cool completely on a wire rack. Spread the raspberry jam between the layers. Drizzle the glaze over the top of the cake, allowing the glaze to drip down the sides of the cake.

Each serving: 35 g carb, 210 cal, 7 g fat, 4 g sat fat, 44 mg chol, 0 g fib, 3 g pro, 157 mg sod • Carb Choices: 2; Exchanges: 2 carb, 1½ fat

Preparing Pans for Baking

Inverting a cake onto a cooling rack to discover that half the cake remains in the pan is one of the most disappointing kitchen disasters. However, if pans are prepared properly, this will never happen to you.

When the directions call for a pan to be brushed with oil or with softened butter, use a silicone brush so that you are able to use less oil or butter. Brush the oil or butter into the corners of the pan and all the way to the top of the edge of the pan. If you are using a Bundt pan with a fancy design, take care to brush each of the tiny crevices of the design to ensure your finished cake looks as decorative as the pan.

If the recipe directs you to flour the pan, first brush it thoroughly with oil or butter. Then take about a heaping tablespoon of flour, and, holding the pan over the sink to catch any spills, sprinkle the flour onto the edge and bottom of the pan as evenly as you can. Tilt the pan and shake it to coat the entire surface with flour. Still holding the pan over the sink, turn it upside down and lightly tap the pan to release the excess flour. Cakes can have white spots of flour if you leave any large bits of flour in the pan.

When lining a pan with parchment paper, tear off the parchment and place it in the pan. Run the tip of a small knife around the bottom of the pan to cut the paper to size. Take the paper out, then brush the side of the pan with oil or butter and return the paper to the pan.

Chocolate Cake QUICK

makes 16 servings

Serve this versatile sheet cake as a simple sweet for any get-together or turn it into cupcakes for a bake sale. I love the combination of chocolate and cream cheese. If you do, too, try it frosted with Cream Cheese Frosting (page 587).

¾ cup unsweetened cocoa
¾ cup boiling water
2 teaspoons plus ½ cup (1 stick) unsalted
    butter, softened, divided
2 cups cake flour
2 teaspoons baking powder
½ teaspoon baking soda
¼ teaspoon salt
1⅓ cups granulated sugar
2 large eggs
¾ cup plain low-fat yogurt
2 teaspoons vanilla extract
2 teaspoons confectioners' sugar

1 Combine the cocoa and water in a medium bowl and whisk until smooth. Cool to room temperature.

2 Preheat the oven to 350°F. Line the bottom of a 13 x 9-inch cake pan with parchment paper. Brush the sides of the pan with 2 teaspoons of the butter.

3 Combine the flour, baking powder, baking soda, and salt in a medium bowl and whisk to mix well.

4 Place the remaining ½ cup butter in a large bowl and beat at medium speed with an electric mixer until fluffy. Gradually beat in the granulated sugar. Beat in the eggs one at a time. Add about one-third of the flour mixture and beat until smooth. Beat in the yogurt. Add another third of the flour mixture and beat until smooth. Beat in the cocoa mixture and vanilla. Add the remaining flour mixture and beat until smooth.

5 Spoon the batter into the prepared pan, smoothing the top. Bake until a wooden toothpick inserted in the center comes out clean, 25 to 28 minutes. Cool the cake in the pan on a wire rack for 10 minutes. Remove from the pan and cool completely, right side up, on a wire rack. Sprinkle the top of the cake with the confectioners' sugar. The cake can be covered in an airtight container and stored at room temperature for up to 3 days.

Each serving: 32 g carb, 196 cal, 8 g fat, 5 g sat fat, 43 mg chol, 2 g fib, 3 g pro, 144 mg sod • Carb Choices: 2; Exchanges: 2 carb, 1½ fat

Note: To make cupcakes, spoon the batter in 24 paper-lined muffin cups and bake 18 to 20 minutes. Frost with Fluffy White Frosting (page 587), if desired.

Chocolate Layer Cake with Fluffy White Frosting

makes 16 servings

This is a lovely birthday or celebration cake for anyone who loves chocolate. With the frothy white frosting on the outside, its rich dark secret is hidden until you cut into the cake.

1 recipe Chocolate Cake (at left)
1 recipe Fluffy White Frosting (page 587)

1 Prepare the cake recipe, baking the cake in round cake pans. To do so, line two 8- or 9-inch round cake pans with parchment paper. Brush the sides of the pans with the 2 teaspoons butter. Spoon the batter evenly into the pans. Bake 8-inch cakes for 25 minutes and 9-inch cakes for 23 minutes.

2 Cool the cakes in the pans on a wire rack for 10 minutes. Remove from the pans and cool completely on a wire rack. Spread the frosting between the layers and on the sides and top of the cake.

Each serving: 38 g carb, 222 cal, 8 g fat, 5 g sat fat, 43 mg chol, 2 g fib, 4 g pro, 151 mg sod • Carb Choices: 2½; Exchanges: 2½ carb, 1½ fat

Carrot Cake with Cream Cheese Glaze

makes 16 servings

Moist and lightly spiced, this old-fashioned cake never goes out of style. Baked in a Bundt pan, this one is drizzled with a light cream cheese glaze, rather than being covered in a heavy frosting. The cake is also delicious drizzled with the orange version of Citrus Glaze (page 586).

CAKE

2 teaspoons plus ¼ cup canola oil, divided

1¼ cups unbleached all-purpose flour plus flour for dusting the pan

1 cup sugar

¾ cup whole wheat flour

2 teaspoons baking powder

1 teaspoon ground cinnamon

½ teaspoon baking soda

¼ teaspoon salt

½ cup low-fat buttermilk

2 large eggs

2 teaspoons vanilla extract

2 cups coarsely shredded carrots

GLAZE

½ cup reduced-fat cream cheese, softened

½ cup confectioners' sugar

2 to 3 tablespoons 1% low-fat milk

½ teaspoon vanilla extract

1 To make the cake, preheat the oven to 350°F. Brush a 10- or 12-cup Bundt pan with 2 teaspoons of the oil. Dust the pan lightly with all-purpose flour, shaking the pan to remove the excess.

2 Combine the 1¼ cups all-purpose flour, sugar, whole wheat flour, baking powder, cinnamon, baking soda, and salt in a large bowl and whisk to mix well. Combine the buttermilk, the remaining ¼ cup oil, the eggs, and vanilla in a medium bowl and whisk until smooth. Add the buttermilk mixture to the flour mixture and stir just until moistened. Stir in the carrots.

3 Spoon the batter into the prepared pan and bake until a wooden toothpick inserted in the center of the loaf comes out clean, 40 to 45 minutes.

4 Cool the cake in the pan on a wire rack for 10 minutes. Remove from the pan and cool completely on a wire rack.

5 To make the glaze, combine the cream cheese, sugar, 2 tablespoons of the milk, and the vanilla in a medium bowl. Beat at medium speed with an electric mixer until smooth. Gradually beat in the remaining 1 tablespoon milk, a few drops at a time, to reach drizzling consistency. Drizzle the glaze over the cooled cake. The cake can be refrigerated, covered, for up to 3 days. Bring to room temperature before serving.

Each serving: 30 g carb, 191 cal, 6 g fat, 1 g sat fat, 31 mg chol, 1 g fib, 4 g pro, 176 mg sod • Carb Choices: 2; Exchanges: 2 carb, 1 fat

Moist Yogurt Cake QUICK

makes 10 servings

This simple little single-layer cake is just the thing to make to serve with Strawberry Sauce (page 588), Rhubarb-Ginger Compote (page 589), or a drizzle of Rich Chocolate Sauce (page 587). It's also nice with a handful of fresh berries alongside.

1 teaspoon plus 4 tablespoons (½ stick)
      unsalted butter, softened, divided
1 cup unbleached all-purpose flour
1 teaspoon baking powder
¼ teaspoon baking soda
¼ teaspoon salt
⅓ cup granulated sugar
1 large egg
1 teaspoon vanilla extract
⅔ cup plain low-fat yogurt
1 teaspoon confectioners' sugar

1 Preheat the oven to 350°F. Line the bottom of an 8-inch round cake pan with parchment paper. Brush the side of the pan with 1 teaspoon of the butter.

2 Combine the flour, baking powder, baking soda, and salt in a medium bowl and whisk to mix well.

3 Place the remaining 4 tablespoons butter in a large bowl and beat at medium speed with an electric mixer until fluffy. Gradually beat in the granulated sugar. Beat in the egg and vanilla. Add the flour mixture and the yogurt alternately to the butter mixture, beginning and ending with the flour mixture, beating well after each addition.

4 Spoon the batter into the prepared pan, smoothing the top. Bake until a wooden toothpick inserted in the center comes out clean, 20 to 22 minutes. Cool the cake in the pan on a wire rack for 10 minutes. Remove from the pan and cool completely, right side up, on a wire rack. Sprinkle the top of the cake with the confectioners' sugar. The cake can be covered in an airtight container and stored at room temperature for up to 3 days.

Each serving: 17 g carb, 129 cal, 6 g fat, 3 g sat fat, 35 mg chol, 0 g fib, 2 g pro, 149 mg sod • Carb Choices: 1; Exchanges: 1 carb, 1 fat

Pineapple Upside-Down Cake QUICK

makes 10 servings

This classic cake has been around for years for a reason—it's simple to make from ordinary supermarket ingredients and it's delicious. There's something about the combination of sturdy tart-tasting pineapple and delicate sweet cake that appeals to almost everyone.

1 teaspoon plus 4 tablespoons (½ stick)
      unsalted butter, softened, divided
1 tablespoon unsalted butter, melted
1 (20-ounce) can unsweetened pineapple slices
1 cup unbleached all-purpose flour
1 teaspoon baking powder
¼ teaspoon baking soda
¼ teaspoon salt
⅓ cup sugar
1 large egg
1 teaspoon vanilla extract
⅔ cup plain low-fat yogurt

1 Place an oven rack on the lowest rung of the oven. Preheat the oven to 350°F.

2 Brush the side of an 8-inch round cake pan with 1 teaspoon of the softened butter. Add the melted butter to the pan and tilt to coat the bottom.

3 Drain the pineapple slices, reserving 4 of the pineapple slices and the juice for another use. Blot the remaining 6 pineapple slices dry with paper towels. Place 1 slice in the center of the pan. Cut the remaining 5 slices in half and arrange around the center slice.

4 Combine the flour, baking powder, baking soda, and salt in a medium bowl and whisk to mix well.

5 Place the remaining 4 tablespoons softened butter in a large bowl and beat at medium speed with an electric mixer until fluffy. Gradually beat in the sugar. Beat in the egg and vanilla. Add the flour mixture and the yogurt alternately to the butter mixture, beginning and ending with the flour mixture, beating well after each addition.

6 Spoon the batter over the pineapple slices, smoothing the top. Bake on the rack on the lowest rung of the oven until the top of the cake is lightly browned, 25 to 30 minutes. Immediately invert the cake onto a serving platter. Serve the cake warm or at room temperature. The cake can be covered in an airtight container and stored at room temperature for up to 3 days.

Each serving: 22 g carb, 156 cal, 7 g fat, 4 g sat fat, 38 mg chol, 1 g fib, 2 g pro, 152 mg sod • Carb Choices: 1½; Exchanges: 1½ carb, 1 fat

Chiffon Cake

makes 16 servings

Chiffon cake is made with oil instead of butter, which makes it free of saturated fat, but also gives the cake a delicate flavor and a fine crumb. Instead of sprinkling this cake with powdered sugar, you can drizzle it with Citrus Glaze (page 586), Espresso Glaze (page 586), or serve it with Rich Chocolate Sauce (page 587) or Creamy Custard Sauce (page 588).

2 cups cake flour

1 cup granulated sugar, divided

2 teaspoons baking powder

¼ teaspoon salt

5 large eggs, separated

¾ cup water

½ cup canola oil

2 teaspoons grated lemon zest

2 teaspoons vanilla extract

½ teaspoon cream of tartar

1 teaspoon confectioners' sugar

1 Preheat the oven to 325°F. Have an ungreased 10-inch tube pan with a removable bottom ready.

2 Combine the flour, ¾ cup of the granulated sugar, the baking powder, and salt in a medium bowl. Place the egg yolks, water, oil, lemon zest, and vanilla in a large mixing bowl.

3 Place the egg whites and cream of tartar in another large mixing bowl and beat at high speed with an electric mixer until foamy. Gradually beat in the remaining ¼ cup granulated sugar, beating until stiff peaks form. Do not wash the beaters.

4 Beat the egg yolk mixture at medium speed with an electric mixer until smooth. Add the flour mixture and beat just until combined. Fold the egg white mixture into the egg yolk mixture in three additions, mixing until no white streaks remain.

5 Spoon the batter into the tube pan. Bake until a wooden toothpick inserted into the center of the cake comes out clean, 50 to 55 minutes. Invert the cake pan and cool the cake completely. Run a thin metal spatula around the edge of the cake to loosen. Invert onto a serving platter and sprinkle with the confectioners' sugar. The cake can be covered in an airtight container and stored at room temperature for up to 3 days.

Each serving: 24 g carb, 185 cal, 9 g fat, 1 g sat fat, 66 mg chol, 0 g fib, 3 g pro, 108 mg sod • Carb Choices: 1½; Exchanges: 1½ carb, 1½ fat

Sour Cream Pound Cake

makes 16 servings

You'd never guess this is a light pound cake. It has an intense buttery flavor, a fine crumb, and a crust with just the right amount of crunch.

1 teaspoon plus 4 tablespoons (½ stick)
    unsalted butter, softened, divided
2 cups cake flour plus flour for dusting the pan
2 teaspoons baking powder
½ teaspoon baking soda
¼ teaspoon salt
1 cup sugar
2 large eggs
1 cup reduced-fat sour cream
1 tablespoon vanilla extract

1 Preheat the oven to 350°F. Brush an 8½ x 4½-inch loaf pan with 1 teaspoon of the butter. Dust the pan lightly with flour, shaking the pan to remove the excess.

2 Combine the 2 cups flour, baking powder, baking soda, and salt in a medium bowl and whisk to mix well.

3 Place the remaining 4 tablespoons butter in a large mixing bowl and beat at medium speed with an electric mixer until fluffy. Gradually beat in the sugar. Beat in the eggs one at a time. Add the sour cream and vanilla and beat until smooth. Add the flour mixture and beat at low speed just until smooth.

4 Spoon the batter into the pan and bake until a wooden toothpick inserted in the center of the loaf comes out clean, 50 to 55 minutes.

5 Cool the cake in the pan on a wire rack for 10 minutes. Remove from the pan and cool completely on a wire rack before slicing. The cake can be covered in an airtight container and stored at room temperature for up to 3 days.

Each serving: 25 g carb, 157 cal, 6 g fat, 3 g sat fat, 40 mg chol, 0 g fib, 2 g pro, 141 mg sod • Carb Choices: 1½; Exchanges: 1½ carb, 1 fat

LEMON POUND CAKE: Follow the Sour Cream Pound Cake recipe, at left, substituting 1 teaspoon lemon extract for the vanilla extract and adding 2 teaspoons grated lemon zest in step 3. Proceed with the recipe.

Each serving: 25 g carb, 156 cal, 6 g fat, 3 g sat fat, 40 mg chol, 0 g fib, 2 g pro, 141 mg sod • Carb Choices: 1½; Exchanges: 1½ carb, 1 fat

CHOCOLATE CHIP POUND CAKE: Follow the Sour Cream Pound Cake recipe, at left, stirring in ½ cup semisweet mini chocolate chips with the flour mixture in step 3. Proceed with the recipe.

Each serving: 28 g carb, 183 cal, 7 g fat, 4 g sat fat, 40 mg chol, 1 g fib, 2 g pro, 142 mg sod • Carb Choices: 2; Exchanges: 2 carb, 1½ fat

Angel Food Cake

makes 16 servings

Angel food cake is a fun recipe for children to help out with. Separating the eggs, watching the egg whites change from a pale liquid to a bright white cloud, and then tasting the puffy white cake—it's kitchen magic even for adults.

1 cup cake flour
⅛ teaspoon salt
1½ cups sugar, divided
12 large egg whites
½ teaspoon cream of tartar
1 teaspoon vanilla extract

1 Preheat the oven to 350°F. Have an ungreased 10-inch tube pan ready.

2 Sift the flour and salt into a medium bowl. Stir in ½ cup of the sugar.

3 Combine the egg whites and cream of tartar in a large bowl. Beat at medium speed with an electric mixer until foamy. Beat in the vanilla. Beat in the remaining 1 cup of sugar, 2 tablespoons at a time, beating at high speed until stiff peaks form.

4 Add the flour mixture to the egg white mixture in four additions, stirring until no white streaks appear. Pour the batter into the pan.

5 Bake until a wooden toothpick inserted in the center comes out clean, 20 to 25 minutes. Invert the cake pan and cool the cake completely. Loosen the cake from the sides of the pan with a thin metal spatula and invert onto a serving platter. Slice using a serrated knife. The cake can be stored in an airtight container at room temperature for up to 2 days.

Each serving: 25 g carb, 111 cal, 0 g fat, 0 g sat fat, 0 mg chol, 0 g fib, 3 g pro, 60 mg sod • Carb Choices: 1½; Exchanges: 1½ carb

CHOCOLATE ANGEL FOOD CAKE: Follow the Angel Food Cake recipe, at left, adding ¼ cup unsweetened cocoa with the flour in step 2. Proceed with the recipe.

Each serving: 25 g carb, 114 cal, 0 g fat, 0 g sat fat, 0 mg chol, 1 g fib, 3 g pro, 60 mg sod • Carb Choices: 1½; Exchanges:1½ carb

CITRUS ANGEL FOOD CAKE: Follow the Angel Food Cake recipe, at left, substituting 2 teaspoons grated lemon zest and 1 teaspoon lemon extract for the vanilla extract in step 3. Proceed with the recipe.

Each serving: 25 g carb, 112 cal, 0 g fat, 0 g sat fat, 0 mg chol, 0 g fib, 3 g pro, 60 mg sod • Carb Choices: 1½; Exchanges: 1½ carb

Gingerbread Bundt Cake

makes 16 servings

Both my sister and I adore gingerbread. When we go on vacation together, we always order gingerbread if it's on any restaurant menu. I've played with gingerbread recipes for years and have refined this one to the perfect level of sweetness and spice. To dress this cake up, sprinkle the cooled cake with confectioners' sugar or drizzle it with lemon or orange versions of Citrus Glaze (page 586) or serve it with a dollop of Lemon Curd (page 590).

2 teaspoons plus ⅓ cup canola oil, divided

1½ cups unbleached all-purpose flour plus flour for dusting the pan

1 cup whole wheat flour

1 tablespoon ground ginger

2 teaspoons baking powder

1 teaspoon baking soda

1 teaspoon ground cinnamon

½ teaspoon ground cloves

¼ teaspoon salt

½ cup packed light brown sugar

¾ cup light or dark molasses (not blackstrap)

1 large egg

1 cup hot water

1 Preheat the oven to 350°F. Brush a 10- or 12-cup Bundt pan with 2 teaspoons of the oil. Dust the pan lightly with all-purpose flour, shaking the pan to remove the excess.

2 Combine the 1½ cups all-purpose flour, whole wheat flour, ginger, baking powder, baking soda, cinnamon, cloves, and salt in a large bowl and whisk to mix well.

3 Combine the sugar, remaining ⅓ cup oil, molasses, and egg in a large bowl and beat at medium speed until smooth. Beat in the flour mixture alternately with the hot water, at low speed, in three additions, beating until smooth after each addition.

4 Spoon the batter into the prepared pan and bake until a wooden toothpick inserted in the center of the cake comes out clean, 35 to 40 minutes. Cool the cake in the pan on a wire rack for 10 minutes. Remove from the pan and cool completely on a wire rack before slicing. The cake can be covered in an airtight container and stored at room temperature for up to 3 days.

Each serving: 32 g carb, 187 cal, 6 g fat, 0 g sat fat, 13 mg chol, 1 g fib, 2 g pro, 179 mg sod • Carb Choices: 2; Exchanges: 2 carb, 1 fat

Apple-Spice Cake

makes 16 servings

The shredded apple in this cake not only adds flavor, but it keeps the cake especially moist. Any variety of apple works in this recipe.

2 teaspoons plus ⅓ cup canola oil, divided
1¼ cups unbleached all-purpose flour plus flour for dusting pan
¾ cup whole wheat flour
2 teaspoons baking powder
1 teaspoon baking soda
1 teaspoon ground cinnamon
½ teaspoon ground allspice
¼ teaspoon salt
½ cup granulated sugar
½ cup packed light brown sugar
½ cup plain low-fat yogurt
2 large eggs
2 large apples, peeled, cored, and coarsely shredded (about 1¼ cups)

1 Preheat the oven to 350°F. Brush a 10- or 12-cup Bundt pan with 2 teaspoons of the oil. Dust the pan lightly with all-purpose flour, shaking the pan to remove the excess.

2 Combine the 1¼ cups all-purpose flour, whole wheat flour, baking powder, baking soda, cinnamon, allspice, and salt in a large bowl and whisk to mix well.

3 Combine the granulated sugar, brown sugar, the remaining ⅓ cup oil, the yogurt, and eggs in a medium bowl and whisk until smooth. Add the sugar mixture to the flour mixture and stir just until the batter is moist. Stir in the apples.

4 Spoon the batter into the prepared pan and bake until a wooden toothpick inserted in the center of the cake comes out clean, 40 to 45 minutes. Cool the cake in the pan on a wire rack for 10 minutes. Remove from the pan and cool completely on a wire rack before slicing. The cake can be covered in an airtight container and stored at room temperature for up to 3 days.

Each serving: 27 g carb, 172 cal, 6 g fat, 1 g sat fat, 27 mg chol, 1 g fib, 3 g pro, 182 mg sod • Carb Choices: 2; Exchanges: 2 carb, 1 fat

Cornmeal–Olive Oil Cake

makes 12 servings

This Italian-inspired cornmeal cake is delicious on its own, or serve it with Rhubarb–Vanilla Bean Compote (page 589), Raspberry Sauce (page 588), or Strawberry Sauce (page 588).

1 teaspoon plus ½ cup extra virgin olive oil, divided
1 cup yellow cornmeal
1 cup sugar
¾ cup unbleached all-purpose flour
⅔ cup plain low-fat yogurt
½ teaspoon baking soda
¼ teaspoon salt
2 large eggs
1 tablespoon grated orange zest

1 Preheat the oven to 350°F. Line the bottom of an 8-inch round cake pan with parchment paper. Brush the side of the pan with 1 teaspoon of the oil.

2 Combine the remaining ½ cup oil and the remaining ingredients in a large bowl and beat at medium speed with an electric mixer until the batter is smooth, about 2 minutes.

3 Spoon the batter into the prepared pan. Bake until a wooden toothpick inserted in the center comes out clean, 35 to 40 minutes. Cool the cake in the pan on a wire rack for 10 minutes. Run a thin-bladed knife around the edge of the cake and remove from the pan. Cool completely, right side up, on a wire rack. The cake can be covered in an airtight container and stored at room temperature for up to 3 days.

Each serving: 34 g carb, 251 cal, 11 g fat, 2 g sat fat, 36 mg chol, 1 g fib, 4 g pro, 127 mg sod • Carb Choices: 2; Exchanges: 2 carb, 2 fat

Blueberry–Poppy Seed Coffee Cake

makes 12 servings

This not-too-sweet cake is perfect for brunch or afternoon tea. You can make it with raspberries instead of blueberries or for a more tart version, use fresh cranberries.

1 teaspoon plus ¼ cup canola oil, divided
1 cup whole wheat flour
¾ cup sugar
½ cup unbleached all-purpose flour
1 tablespoon poppy seeds
1 teaspoon baking powder
½ teaspoon baking soda
¼ teaspoon salt
¾ cup low-fat buttermilk
1 large egg
1 teaspoon vanilla extract
2 teaspoons grated orange zest
1 cup fresh blueberries or unthawed frozen unsweetened blueberries

1 Preheat the oven to 350°F. Line the bottom of an 8-inch round cake pan with parchment paper. Brush the side of the pan with 1 teaspoon of the oil.

2 Combine the whole wheat flour, sugar, all-purpose flour, poppy seeds, baking powder, baking soda, and salt in a large bowl and whisk to mix well.

3 Combine the buttermilk, remaining ¼ cup oil, the egg, vanilla, and orange zest in a medium bowl and whisk until smooth. Add the buttermilk mixture to the flour mixture, stirring just until moistened. Spread half of the batter into the prepared pan. Top with the blueberries. Dollop the remaining batter over the blueberries, leaving some of the berries uncovered. Bake until the top is lightly browned, 35 to 40 minutes.

4 Cool the cake in the pan on a wire rack for 10 minutes. Run a thin-bladed knife around the edge of the cake and remove from the pan. Serve the cake warm or at room temperature. The cake is best on the day it is made.

Each serving: 27 g carb, 174 cal, 6 g fat, 1 g sat fat, 19 mg chol, 2 g fib, 3 g pro, 109 mg sod • Carb Choices: 2; Exchanges: 2 carb, 1 fat

Spiced Fruitcake

makes 16 servings

This light-textured cake is not as dense as most fruitcakes. Even those who aren't fond of the traditional holiday sweet might enjoy this lightened version.

2 teaspoons plus ½ cup (1 stick) unsalted butter, softened, divided
2 cups unbleached all-purpose flour plus flour for dusting the pan
2 teaspoons baking powder
½ teaspoon baking soda
1 teaspoon ground cinnamon
½ teaspoon ground allspice
¼ teaspoon ground nutmeg
¼ teaspoon ground cloves
¼ teaspoon salt
¾ cup sugar
2 large eggs
1 tablespoon grated orange zest
2 teaspoons vanilla extract
½ cup low-fat buttermilk
1½ cups mixed dried fruits (such as raisins, currants, cranberries, cherries, or chopped apples, apricots, or pears)
½ cup walnuts or pecans, toasted and chopped (page 4)

1 Preheat the oven to 350°F. Brush an 8½ x 4½-inch loaf pan with 2 teaspoons of the butter. Dust the pan lightly with flour, shaking the pan to remove the excess.

continues on next page

2 Combine the 2 cups flour, baking powder, baking soda, cinnamon, allspice, nutmeg, cloves, and salt in a large bowl and whisk to mix well.

3 Place the remaining ½ cup butter in a large bowl and beat at medium speed with an electric mixer until fluffy. Gradually beat in the sugar. Beat in the eggs, orange zest, and vanilla. Add the flour mixture and the buttermilk alternately to the butter mixture, beginning and ending with the flour mixture, beating well after each addition. Stir in the dried fruits and walnuts.

4 Spoon the batter into the prepared pan. Bake until a wooden toothpick inserted in the center comes out clean, 50 to 55 minutes.

5 Cool the cake in the pan on a wire rack for 10 minutes. Remove from the pan and cool completely on a wire rack before slicing. The cake can be stored in an airtight container at room temperature for up to a week.

Each serving: 32 g carb, 224 cal, 9 g fat, 4 g sat fat, 43 mg chol, 2 g fib, 4 g pro, 128 mg sod • Carb Choices: 2; Exchanges: 1½ carb, ½ fruit, 2 fat

Raspberry Pudding Cake

makes 10 servings

You can have your cake and pudding, too, with this soft, spoonable dessert. The edge of the cake is firm and turns lightly brown and the center stays gooey and soft.

1 teaspoon plus 2 tablespoons canola oil, divided
½ cup granulated sugar
¼ cup unbleached all-purpose flour
Pinch of salt
1 cup 1% low-fat buttermilk
2 teaspoons grated orange zest
¼ cup orange juice
1 large egg yolk
2 large egg whites
1 cup fresh raspberries
1 teaspoon confectioners' sugar

1 Preheat the oven to 350°F. Line the bottom of a 9-inch round cake pan with parchment paper. Brush the side of the pan with 1 teaspoon of the oil.

2 Combine the granulated sugar, flour, salt, buttermilk, orange zest, orange juice, egg yolk, and remaining 2 tablespoons oil in a medium bowl and whisk until the batter is smooth.

3 Place the egg whites in a medium bowl and beat at high speed with an electric mixer until stiff peaks form. Fold the egg whites into the batter in three additions, stirring until no white streaks appear. Gently stir in the raspberries. Spoon the batter into the prepared pan.

4 Place the cake pan in a large roasting pan and add hot water to the roasting pan halfway up the sides of the cake pan. Bake until the cake springs back when touched in the center and tiny cracks appear on the surface, about 35 minutes.

5 Cool the cake in the pan on a wire rack for 10 minutes. Sprinkle the top of the cake with the confectioners' sugar. Serve warm from the pan.

Each serving: 16 g carb, 108 cal, 4 g fat, 1 g sat fat, 22 mg chol, 1 g fib, 2 g pro, 54 mg sod • Carb Choices: 1; Exchanges: 1 carb, ½ fat

Chocolate Pudding Cake

makes 12 servings

The texture of this cake is soft and gooey, so serve it with a spoon.

1 teaspoon unsalted butter, softened
1 cup unbleached all-purpose flour
1¼ cups sugar, divided
⅓ cup plus 3 tablespoons unsweetened cocoa, divided
2 teaspoons baking powder
⅛ teaspoon salt
½ cup 1% low-fat milk
4 tablespoons (½ stick) unsalted butter, melted and cooled
2 teaspoons vanilla extract
1½ cups boiling water

1 Preheat the oven to 375°F. Brush an 8-inch square glass baking dish with the softened butter.

2 Combine the flour, 1 cup of the sugar, ⅓ cup of the cocoa, the baking powder, and salt in a medium bowl and whisk to mix well. Combine the milk, melted butter, and vanilla in a small bowl and stir to mix well. Add the milk mixture to the flour mixture and stir until smooth. Spread the batter into the prepared dish.

3 Combine the remaining ¼ cup sugar and remaining 3 tablespoons cocoa in a small bowl and stir to mix well. Sprinkle the mixture over the batter in the baking dish. Pour the boiling water over the batter (do not stir).

4 Bake until the cake springs back slightly when touched in the center, 25 to 30 minutes. Cool 10 minutes before serving. Serve the cake warm.

Each serving: 30 g carb, 165 cal, 5 g fat, 3 g sat fat, 11 mg chol, 1 g fib, 2 g pro, 97 mg sod • Carb Choices: 2; Exchanges: 2 carb, 1 fat

New York–Style Cheesecake

makes 12 servings

Creamy and sweet with a touch of tang from the cottage cheese, this light cheesecake is good enough to please to the most discerning of cheesecake lovers.

1 recipe Graham Cracker Crust (page 546)
1 (16-ounce) container 1% low-fat cottage cheese
1 (8-ounce) package reduced-fat cream cheese, softened
½ cup reduced-fat sour cream
3 tablespoons unbleached all-purpose flour
1 cup sugar
3 large eggs
2 teaspoons vanilla extract
½ teaspoon grated lemon zest

1 Prepare the crust as directed, but bake in a 9-Inch springform pan instead of a pie plate.

2 Preheat the oven to 325°F.

3 If the cottage cheese has excess liquid, place it in a fine wire mesh strainer and drain (brands vary in the amount of liquid). Place the cottage cheese in a food processor. Add the cream cheese, sour cream, and flour and process until the mixture is smooth, stopping to scrape down the sides, about 2 minutes. Add the sugar, eggs, vanilla, and lemon zest and pulse until combined.

4 Pour the mixture into the prepared crust. Place the springform pan on a baking sheet and bake until the edges of the cheesecake are set and the center remains soft, 1 hour. Place the cheesecake on a wire rack and immediately run a thin-bladed knife around the edge of the cake to release it from the side of the pan and prevent cracking as it cools. Cool completely on a wire rack. Cover and refrigerate 8 hours before slicing. The cheesecake can be refrigerated, covered, for up to 3 days.

Each serving: 31 g carb, 245 cal, 9 g fat, 5 g sat fat, 77 mg chol, 0 g fib, 10 g pro, 331 mg sod • Carb Choices: 2; Exchanges: 2 carb, 2 fat

RASPBERRY-TOPPED CHEESECAKE: Follow the New York–Style Cheesecake recipe, at left. Before refrigerating the cake, spread the top with ⅓ cup seedless raspberry jam and arrange 2½ cups fresh raspberries decoratively on top of the cake.

Each serving: 40 g carb, 281 cal, 9 g fat, 5 g sat fat, 77 mg chol, 2 g fib, 10 g pro, 332 mg sod • Carb Choices: 2½; Exchanges: 2½ carb, 2 fat

CHOCOLATE CHEESECAKE: Follow the New York–Style Cheesecake recipe, at left, omitting the lemon zest. Add 3 ounces semisweet chocolate, melted and cooled, with the sugar in step 3. Proceed with the recipe.

Each serving: 35 g carb, 281 cal, 11 g fat, 7 g sat fat, 77 mg chol, 0 g fib, 10 g pro, 331 mg sod • Carb Choices: 2; Exchanges: 2 carb, 2½ fat

Fresh Fruit Trifle

makes 16 servings

Using homemade yogurt cake makes this trifle a special treat, but if you're rushed for time, substitute 5 cups of cubed purchased angel food cake or pound cake. Vary the fruits depending on what looks best at the market and always make the trifle in a clear bowl to show off the colorful fruits.

2 large oranges
1 Moist Yogurt Cake (page 566), prepared, cooled, and cut into 1-inch cubes
2 recipes Vanilla Pudding (page 555), prepared and cooled to room temperature
2 cups sliced fresh strawberries
1 medium banana, sliced
2 tablespoons flaked sweetened coconut

1 Cut a thin slice from the top and bottom of the oranges, exposing the flesh. Stand each orange upright, and using a sharp knife, thickly cut off the peel, following the contour of the fruit and removing all the white pith and membrane. Holding each orange over a bowl, carefully cut along both sides of each section to free it from the membrane. Discard any seeds and let the sections fall into the bowl.

2 To assemble the trifle, arrange one-third of the cake cubes in a 4-quart trifle bowl, top with one-third of the pudding, one-third of the oranges, one-third of the strawberries, and one-third of the banana slices. Repeat the layering twice with the remaining ingredients. Sprinkle the trifle with the coconut. Serve the trifle at room temperature or chilled. The trifle tastes best on the day it is made.

Each serving: 35 g carb, 202 cal, 5 g fat, 3 g sat fat, 51 mg chol, 1 g fib, 5 g pro, 167 mg sod • Carb Choices: 2; Exchanges: 2 carb, ½ fruit, 1 fat

Tiramisù Layer Cake

makes 10 servings

This version of tiramisù skips the mascarpone cheese and uses a light sour cream custard instead. Slice the cake while it is cold because the custard softens as it comes to room temperature.

1½ cups 1% low-fat milk
1 large egg
½ cup sugar
2 tablespoons cornstarch
Pinch of salt
¼ cup reduced-fat sour cream
2 tablespoons sweet Marsala wine
2 tablespoons brewed espresso or strong coffee, cooled
1 recipe Moist Yogurt Cake (page 566), see note at right for baking instructions
1 teaspoon unsweetened cocoa

1 Combine the milk, egg, sugar, cornstarch, and salt in a medium saucepan and whisk until smooth. Cook over medium heat, whisking constantly, until the mixture comes to a boil and thickens, about 8 minutes.

2 Remove from the heat and stir in the sour cream. Transfer to a medium bowl and cover the surface of the custard with wax paper to prevent a skin from forming. Cool to room temperature.

3 To assemble the tiramisù, line a 9 x 5-inch loaf pan with plastic wrap, leaving a 4-inch overhang on each side.

4 Combine the Marsala and espresso in a small bowl.

5 Using a serrated knife, carefully cut the cake horizontally into three layers, using a long metal spatula to transfer the layers to a work surface. Brush the cut side of the top and bottom layers and one side of the center layer with the espresso mixture. Place the bottom layer of the

cake in the pan and top with half of the custard. Place the center cake layer over the custard. Top the center cake layer with the remaining half of the custard. Place the top layer of the cake over the custard.

6 Cover and refrigerate 8 hours or overnight. Lift the cake from the pan using the overhanging sides of plastic wrap and sprinkle the top of the cake with cocoa. Carefully transfer the cake to a serving plate. Serve the cake chilled and slice using a serrated knife. The cake tastes best within 24 hours.

Each serving: 32 g carb, 211 cal, 7 g fat, 4 g sat fat, 60 mg chol, 0 g fib, 4 g pro, 193 mg sod • Carb Choices: 2; Exchanges: 2 carb, 1½ fat

Note: For the Tiramisù Layer Cake, bake the Moist Yogurt Cake in a 9 x 5-inch loaf pan. To do so, omit the pan preparation instructions in step 1 and brush the loaf pan with 2 teaspoons unsalted butter, softened. Dust the pan lightly with unbleached all-purpose flour, shaking the pan to remove the excess. Proceed with the recipe as directed, keeping the baking time the same. This makes a squat cake (about 1½ inches tall), perfect for the tiramisù, but not tall enough to serve on its own.

Chocolate Soufflé

makes 10 servings

How soufflés got their reputation of being difficult to make will be a mystery to you when you actually make one. They are so simple and foolproof to prepare, yet a soufflé impresses like no other sweet.

¾ cup 1% low-fat milk

¾ cup granulated sugar

½ cup unsweetened cocoa

3 tablespoons unbleached all-purpose flour

¼ teaspoon salt

3 large eggs, separated

2 teaspoons vanilla extract

1 teaspoon unsalted butter, softened

1 large egg white

⅛ teaspoon cream of tartar

1 teaspoon confectioners' sugar

1 Combine the milk, granulated sugar, cocoa, flour, and salt in a medium saucepan and whisk until smooth. Cook over medium heat, whisking constantly, until the mixture comes to a boil and thickens, about 5 minutes. Transfer the mixture to a large bowl and let stand 15 minutes to cool slightly. Whisk in the egg yolks and vanilla.

2 Preheat the oven to 350°F. Brush a 1½-quart round baking dish with the butter.

3 Place the egg whites and cream of tartar in a large bowl and beat at high speed with an electric mixer until stiff peaks form. Fold the egg white mixture into the chocolate mixture in three additions, mixing until no white streaks remain.

4 Spoon the batter into the prepared baking dish. Bake until the soufflé is puffed and set, 35 to 40 minutes. Sprinkle the soufflé with the confectioners' sugar and serve at once.

Each serving: 20 g carb, 113 cal, 3 g fat, 1 g sat fat, 65 mg chol, 1 g fib, 4 g pro, 94 mg sod • Carb Choices: 1; Exchanges: 1 carb, ½ fat

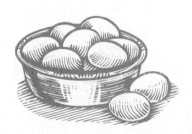

Cookies and Bars

Sugar Cookies `QUICK`

makes 24

Modest and satisfying, these are the cookies that remind you of a treat at Grandma's house, an after-school snack, or tea with an elderly aunt. There's a reason they are timeless—they are simply delicious.

¾ cup whole wheat pastry flour or unbleached all-purpose flour
¼ teaspoon baking soda
Pinch of salt
4 tablespoons (½ stick) unsalted butter, softened
⅓ cup plus 2 tablespoons sugar, divided
1 large egg
½ teaspoon vanilla extract

1 Preheat the oven to 350°F. Line 2 baking sheets with parchment paper.

2 Combine the flour, baking soda, and salt in a medium bowl and whisk to mix well.

3 Place the butter in a large bowl and beat at medium speed with an electric mixer until fluffy. Gradually beat in ⅓ cup of the sugar. Beat in the egg and vanilla. Add the flour mixture and beat at low speed just until blended. Shape 24 level tablespoonfuls of dough into balls.

4 Place the remaining 2 tablespoons sugar in a small bowl. Roll each ball in the sugar and place 2 inches apart onto the prepared baking sheets. Bake until the edges of the cookies are lightly browned, about 8 minutes. Cool the cookies on the baking sheets for 2 minutes. Transfer to wire racks to cool completely. The cookies can be stored in an airtight container at room temperature for up to 3 days.

Each serving (2 cookies): 13 g carb, 97 cal, 4 g fat, 3 g sat fat, 28 mg chol, 1 g fib, 1 g pro, 45 mg sod • Carb Choices: 1; Exchanges: 1 carb, ½ fat

CITRUS SUGAR COOKIES: Follow the Sugar Cookies recipe, at left, adding 2 tablespoons fresh lemon or lime juice and 2 teaspoons grated lemon or lime zest with the egg in step 3. Proceed as directed.

Each serving (2 cookies): 14 g carb, 98 cal, 4 g fat, 3 g sat fat, 28 mg chol, 1 g fib, 1 g pro, 45 mg sod • Carb Choices: 1; Exchanges: 1 carb, ½ fat

Classic Chocolate Chippers `QUICK`

makes 36

For a more sophisticated chocolate cookie, use 4 ounces of chopped dark chocolate instead of the chocolate chips.

½ cup unbleached all-purpose flour
½ cup whole wheat flour
¼ teaspoon baking soda
¼ teaspoon salt
4 tablespoons (½ stick) unsalted butter, softened
½ cup granulated sugar
½ cup packed light brown sugar
1 large egg
1 teaspoon vanilla extract
½ cup semisweet chocolate chips

1 Preheat the oven to 350°F. Line 2 baking sheets with parchment paper.

2 Combine the all-purpose flour, whole wheat flour, baking soda, and salt in a medium bowl and whisk to mix well.

3 Place the butter in a large bowl and beat at medium speed with an electric mixer until fluffy. Gradually beat in the sugars. Beat in the egg and vanilla. Add the flour mixture and beat at low speed just until blended. Stir in the chocolate chips.

4 Drop the batter by level tablespoonfuls 2 inches apart onto the prepared baking sheets. Bake until the edges of the cookies are lightly browned, 10 to 12 minutes. Cool the cookies on the baking sheets for 2 minutes. Transfer to wire racks to cool completely. The cookies can be stored in an airtight container at room temperature for up to 3 days.

Each serving (1 cookie): 10 g carb, 63 cal, 2 g fat, 1 g sat fat, 9 mg chol, 0 g fib, 1 g pro, 28 mg sod • Carb Choices: ½; Exchanges: ½ carb, ½ fat

WALNUT–CHOCOLATE CHIPPERS QUICK : Follow the Classic Chocolate Chippers recipe, at left, stirring in ⅓ cup walnuts, toasted and chopped (page 4), with the chocolate chips in step 3. Proceed as directed.

Each serving (1 cookie): 10 g carb, 71 cal, 3 g fat, 1 g sat fat, 9 mg chol, 1 g fib, 1 g pro, 28 mg sod • Carb Choices: ½; Exchanges: ½ carb, ½ fat

Oatmeal-Raisin Cookies

QUICK

makes 24

Crisp on the outside and soft and chewy in the center, these are classic oatmeal cookies. If your crowd doesn't like raisins, use dried cranberries, dried blueberries, or coarsely chopped dried cherries instead.

½ cup unbleached all-purpose flour
½ cup whole wheat flour
¼ teaspoon ground cinnamon
¼ teaspoon baking soda
¼ teaspoon salt
4 tablespoons (½ stick) unsalted butter, softened
¾ cup packed light brown sugar
1 large egg
1 teaspoon vanilla extract
1 cup old-fashioned rolled oats
½ cup dark raisins

1 Preheat the oven to 350°F. Line 2 baking sheets with parchment paper.

2 Combine the all-purpose flour, whole wheat flour, cinnamon, baking soda, and salt in a medium bowl and whisk to mix well.

3 Place the butter in a large bowl and beat at medium speed with an electric mixer until fluffy. Gradually beat in the sugar. Beat in the egg and vanilla. Add the flour mixture and beat at low speed just until blended. Stir in the oats and raisins.

4 Drop the batter by level tablespoonfuls 2 inches apart onto the prepared baking sheets. Bake until the edges of the cookies are lightly browned, 10 to 12 minutes. Cool the cookies on the baking sheets for 2 minutes. Transfer to racks to cool completely. The cookies can be stored in an airtight container at room temperature for up to 3 days.

Each serving (1 cookie): 15 g carb, 85 cal, 2 g fat, 1 g sat fat, 14 mg chol, 1 g fib, 2 g pro, 44 mg sod • Carb Choices: 1; Exchanges: 1 carb, ½ fat

OATMEAL–CHOCOLATE CHIP COOKIES QUICK : Follow the Oatmeal Cookies recipe, at left, replacing the raisins with ½ cup mini semisweet chocolate chips. Proceed as directed.

Each serving (1 cookie): 15 g carb, 94 cal, 3 g fat, 2 g sat fat, 14 mg chol, 1 g fib, 2 g pro, 44 mg sod • Carb Choices: 1; Exchanges: 1 carb, ½ fat

Cut-Out Cookies

makes 24

Use this recipe when you want to make shaped cookies for any holiday or celebration. You can top them with Vanilla Glaze (page 586) if you wish. For a festive look, add a drop or two of food coloring to the recipe when preparing the glaze.

1½ cups unbleached all-purpose flour

¼ teaspoon baking soda

⅛ teaspoon salt

4 tablespoons (½ stick) unsalted butter, softened

⅓ cup sugar

1 large egg

1 teaspoon vanilla extract or ½ teaspoon almond extract

1 Combine the flour, baking soda, and salt in a medium bowl and whisk to mix well.

2 Place the butter in a large bowl and beat at medium speed with an electric mixer until fluffy. Gradually beat in the sugar. Beat in the egg and vanilla. Add the flour mixture and beat at low speed just until blended.

3 Divide the dough in half. Place each half between two sheets of parchment paper and roll to a ¼-inch thickness. Place the dough on a baking sheet and refrigerate 1 hour.

4 Preheat the oven to 375°F. Line 2 baking sheets with parchment paper.

5 Cut the dough into the desired shapes using 1½-inch cookie cutters. Transfer the cookies to the prepared baking sheets. Bake until the edges are lightly browned, 8 to 10 minutes. Cool the cookies on the baking sheets for 2 minutes. Transfer to racks to cool completely. The cookies can be stored in an airtight container at room temperature for up to 3 days.

Note: To make additional cookies, gather the scraps from the cut-out cookies and reroll the dough as directed in step 3.

Each serving (2 cookies): 16 g carb, 112 cal, 4 g fat, 3 g sat fat, 28 mg chol, 0 g fib, 2 g pro, 66 mg sod • Carb Choices: 1; Exchanges: 1 carb, ½ fat

Peanut Butter Cookies QUICK

makes 36

To make these even peanuttier, use chunky peanut butter or add about ¼ cup chopped dry-roasted peanuts to the batter.

¾ cup unbleached all-purpose flour

¾ cup whole wheat flour

¼ teaspoon baking soda

¼ teaspoon salt

½ cup creamy natural peanut butter

4 tablespoons (½ stick) unsalted butter, softened

¾ cup packed light brown sugar

1 large egg

1 teaspoon vanilla extract

1 Preheat the oven to 350°F. Line 2 baking sheets with parchment paper.

2 Combine the all-purpose flour, whole wheat flour, baking soda, and salt in a medium bowl and whisk to mix well.

3 Place the peanut butter and butter in a large bowl and beat at medium speed with an electric mixer until fluffy. Gradually beat in the sugar. Beat in the egg and vanilla. Add the flour mixture and beat at low speed just until blended. Shape 36 level tablespoonfuls of the dough into balls.

4 Place 2 inches apart onto the prepared baking sheets. Press each ball with a fork to flatten. Bake until the bottoms of the cookies are lightly browned, 10 to 12 minutes. Cool the cookies on the baking sheets for 2 minutes. Transfer to wire racks to cool completely. The cookies can be stored in an airtight container at room temperature for up to 3 days.

Each serving (2 cookies): 18 g carb, 143 cal, 6 g fat, 2 g sat fat, 18 mg chol, 1 g fib, 3 g pro, 84 mg sod • Carb Choices: 1; Exchanges: 1 carb, 1 fat

Almond Cookies

makes 24

These plain-looking cookies are simply bursting with almond flavor.

1 cup slivered almonds
½ cup (1 stick) unsalted butter, softened
⅓ cup confectioners' sugar
1 large egg yolk
½ teaspoon almond extract
1 cup unbleached all-purpose flour
¼ teaspoon salt
24 whole almonds

1 Place the slivered almonds in a food processor and process until finely ground.

2 Place the butter in a large bowl and beat at medium speed with an electric mixer until fluffy. Gradually beat in the sugar. Beat in the egg yolk and almond extract.

3 Add the flour, the ground almonds, and salt and beat at low speed just until blended. Cover and refrigerate until chilled, about 2 hours.

4 Preheat the oven to 325°F. Line 2 baking sheets with parchment paper.

5 Shape 24 level tablespoonfuls of the dough into balls. Place 1½ inches apart onto the prepared baking sheets. Place a whole almond in the center of each ball, pressing to flatten the dough slightly.

6 Bake until the bottoms of the cookies are lightly browned, about 15 minutes. Cool on baking sheets 2 minutes. Transfer to racks to cool completely. Store in an airtight container at room temperature for up to 3 days.

Each serving (1 cookie): 7 g carb, 94 cal, 7 g fat, 3 g sat fat, 19 mg chol, 1 g fib, 2 g pro, 25 mg sod • Carb choices: ½; Exchanges: ½ carb, 1 fat

Almond Biscotti

makes 16

These crunchy biscotti are easy to make from pantry ingredients. They keep for a week, so they're nice to have on hand for a treat with an afternoon cup of tea. You can substitute any kind of chopped nuts for the almonds. If you do, replace the almond extract with 1 teaspoon vanilla extract.

1½ cups white whole wheat flour or unbleached all-purpose flour
½ cup sugar
1 teaspoon baking powder
⅛ teaspoon salt
4 tablespoons (½ stick) unsalted butter, melted and cooled
2 tablespoons 2% low-fat milk
1 large egg
¼ teaspoon almond extract
⅓ cup slivered almonds

1 Preheat the oven to 350°F. Line a large baking sheet with parchment paper.

2 Combine the flour, sugar, baking powder, and salt in a large bowl and whisk to mix well. Combine the butter, milk, egg, and almond extract in a medium bowl and whisk until smooth.

3 Add the butter mixture to the flour mixture and stir until moistened. Stir in the almonds. Place the dough on the baking sheet, press into a 12-inch log, and flatten it slightly.

4 Bake until the top is lightly browned, 25 to 30 minutes. Remove from the baking sheet and transfer to a wire rack. Let cool until just slightly warm, about 20 minutes.

5 Reduce the oven temperature to 325°F. Cut the log diagonally into 16 (¾-inch) slices using a serrated knife. Place on a parchment-lined baking sheet and bake 15 minutes. Turn the biscotti and bake until lightly browned, 10 to 15 minutes longer. Remove from the baking sheet and transfer to a wire rack to cool completely. The biscotti can be stored in an airtight container at room temperature for up to 1 week.

Each serving (1 cookie): 16 g carb, 109 cal, 5 g fat, 2 g sat fat, 21 mg chol, 2 g fib, 2 g pro, 31 mg sod • Carb Choices: 1; Exchanges: 1 carb, 1 fat

Cranberry-Orange Biscotti

makes 16

During the winter holidays, these biscotti are thoughtful and festive treats to keep on hand for unexpected guests or to give as a gift.

1½ cups white whole wheat flour or unbleached all-purpose flour
½ cup sugar
1 teaspoon baking powder
¼ teaspoon ground cinnamon
⅛ teaspoon salt
4 tablespoons (½ stick) unsalted butter, melted and cooled
2 tablespoons 2% low-fat milk
1 large egg
1 teaspoon grated orange zest
1 teaspoon vanilla extract
¼ cup dried cranberries

1 Preheat the oven to 350°F. Line a large baking sheet with parchment paper.

2 Combine the flour, sugar, baking powder, cinnamon, and salt in a large bowl and whisk to mix well. Combine the butter, milk, egg, orange zest, and vanilla in a medium bowl and whisk until smooth.

3 Add the butter mixture to the flour mixture and stir just until moistened. Stir in the cranberries. Place the dough on the prepared baking sheet, press into a 12-inch log, and press on the log to flatten it slightly.

4 Bake until the top is lightly browned, 25 to 30 minutes. Remove from the baking sheet and transfer to a wire rack. Let cool until just slightly warm, about 20 minutes.

5 Reduce the oven temperature to 325°F.

6 Cut the log diagonally into 16 (¾-inch) slices using a serrated knife. Place on a parchment-lined baking sheet and bake 15 minutes. Turn the biscotti and bake until lightly browned, 10 to 15 minutes longer. Remove from the baking sheet and transfer to a wire rack to cool completely. The biscotti can be stored in an airtight container at room temperature for up to 1 week.

Each serving (1 cookie): 17 g carb, 103 cal, 3 g fat, 2 g sat fat, 21 mg chol, 2 g fib, 2 g pro, 31 mg sod • Carb Choices: 1; Exchanges: 1 carb, ½ fat

Meringue Cookies

makes 18

Crisp and crunchy, these snow-white cookies are a treat on their own or serve them to dress up a simple bowl of berries or ice cream.

3 large egg whites
¼ teaspoon cream of tartar
1 teaspoon vanilla extract
½ cup sugar

1 Preheat the oven to 225°F. Line 2 baking sheets with parchment paper.

2 Combine the egg whites and cream of tartar in a medium bowl and beat at medium speed with an electric mixer until foamy. Beat in the vanilla. Gradually add the sugar and beat at high speed until stiff peaks form.

3 Drop the mixture by rounded tablespoonfuls 1½ inches apart onto the prepared baking sheets. Bake the meringues for 1 hour 15 minutes. Turn off the oven, leaving the meringues inside until completely dry, about 3 hours. The cookies can be stored in an airtight container at room temperature for up to 2 days.

Each serving (1 cookie): 6 g carb, 25 cal, 0 g fat, 0 g sat fat, 0 mg chol, 0 g fib, 1 g pro, 9 mg sod • Carb Choices: ½; Exchanges: ½ carb

CHOCOLATE MERINGUE COOKIES: Follow the Meringue Cookies recipe, above, sifting together the sugar and 2 tablespoons unsweetened cocoa before adding the sugar to the egg white mixture in step 2. Proceed as directed.

Each serving (1 cookie): 6 g carb, 27 cal, 0 g fat, 0 g sat fat, 0 mg chol, 0 g fib, 1 g pro, 9 mg sod • Carb Choices: ½; Exchanges: ½ carb

Chocolate Brownies QUICK

makes 16 servings

Moist, rich, and fudgey, these treats are everything a brownie should be. The addition of espresso amplifies the flavor of the chocolate.

1 teaspoon plus ½ cup (1 stick) unsalted butter, softened, divided
½ cup unbleached all-purpose flour
½ cup unsweetened cocoa
½ teaspoon baking powder
¼ teaspoon salt
1 tablespoon hot water
½ teaspoon instant espresso granules
1 cup sugar
2 egg whites
1 large egg
1 teaspoon vanilla extract

1 Preheat the oven to 350°F. Line an 8-inch square metal baking pan with foil, allowing the foil to extend over the rim of the pan by 2 inches. Brush the foil with 1 teaspoon of the butter.

2 Combine the flour, cocoa, baking powder, and salt in a medium bowl and whisk to mix well.

3 Combine the hot water and espresso granules in a small dish and stir until the espresso dissolves.

4 Place the remaining ½ cup butter in a large bowl and beat at medium speed with an electric mixer until fluffy. Gradually beat in the sugar. Beat in the egg whites, egg, vanilla, and espresso mixture. Add the flour mixture and beat at low speed just until the batter is moistened.

5 Spoon the batter into the prepared pan and spread evenly. Bake until a wooden toothpick inserted into the center comes out clean, 20 to 23 minutes. (Be careful not to overbake. The center of the brownies should still be soft.) Cool completely in pan on a wire rack. Lift from the pan using the foil overhang as handles. Cut into 16 squares. The brownies can be stored in an airtight container at room temperature for up to 3 days.

Each serving (1 square): 17 g carb, 127 cal, 7 g fat, 4 g sat fat, 29 mg chol, 1 g fib, 2 g pro, 62 mg sod • Carb Choices: 1; Exchanges: 1 carb, 1 fat

CHOCOLATE-WALNUT BROWNIES: Follow the Chocolate Brownies recipe, at left, adding ⅓ cup walnuts, toasted and chopped (page 4), with the flour mixture in step 4. Proceed as directed.

Each serving (1 square): 17 g carb, 142 cal, 8 g fat, 4 g sat fat, 29 mg chol, 1 g fib, 2 g pro, 62 mg sod • Carb Choices: 1; Exchanges: 1 carb, 1½ fat

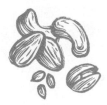

Shortbread QUICK

makes 24 servings

Don't even think about making this recipe with margarine. Shortbread is all about the butter, though this recipe does reduce the usual amount by using some canola oil. Enjoy a small square with a cup of tea or coffee and savor every buttery bite.

1 teaspoon plus ½ cup (1 stick) unsalted butter, softened, divided
2 cups unbleached all-purpose flour
¼ cup cornstarch
¼ teaspoon salt
½ cup canola oil
½ cup sugar
2 teaspoons vanilla extract

1 Preheat the oven to 350°F. Line an 8-inch square metal baking pan with foil, allowing the foil to extend over the rim of the pan by 2 inches. Brush the foil with 1 teaspoon of the butter.

2 Combine the flour, cornstarch, and salt in a medium bowl and whisk to mix well.

3 Place the remaining ½ cup butter in a large bowl and beat at medium speed with an electric mixer until fluffy. With the mixer running, slowly beat in the oil. Gradually beat in the sugar. Beat in the vanilla. Add the flour mixture and beat at low speed just until well mixed.

4 Spread the dough evenly into the prepared pan. Bake until the edges of the shortbread are lightly browned, 25 to 30 minutes (do not overbake). Cool in the pan on a wire rack for 5 minutes, then cut the shortbread into 24 squares in the pan. Cool the shortbread completely in the pan on a wire rack. The shortbread can be stored in an airtight container at room temperature for up to 1 week.

Each serving (1 square): 13 g carb, 136 cal, 9 g fat, 3 g sat fat, 10 mg chol, 0 g fib, 1 g pro, 25 mg sod • Carb choices: 1; Exchanges: 1 carb, 1½ fat

Lemon Bars

makes 16 servings

To turn these simple bars into a pretty treat for a party, cut them into squares and top each square with a fresh raspberry, then dust lightly with confectioners' sugar.

CRUST
1 teaspoon plus 4 tablespoons (½ stick) unsalted butter, softened, divided
¼ cup sugar
1 cup whole wheat pastry flour or unbleached all-purpose flour
⅛ teaspoon salt

FILLING
2 large egg whites
1 large egg
⅔ cup sugar
2 teaspoons grated lemon zest
⅓ cup lemon juice
2 tablespoons unbleached all-purpose flour
½ teaspoon baking powder
⅛ teaspoon salt

1 Preheat the oven to 350°F. Line an 8-inch square metal baking pan with foil, allowing the foil to extend over the rim of the pan by 2 inches. Brush the foil with 1 teaspoon of the butter.

2 To make the crust, place the remaining 4 tablespoons butter in a medium bowl and beat at medium speed with an electric mixer until fluffy. Gradually beat in the sugar. Add the flour and salt and beat just until blended. Press the dough into the bottom of the prepared pan.

3 Bake until browned, 15 minutes. Maintain oven temperature. Cool the crust on a wire rack.

4 Meanwhile, to make the filling, whisk together all the filling ingredients in a medium bowl until smooth. Pour the filling over the crust and bake until the filling is set, 20 to 25 minutes.

5 Cool completely in the pan on a wire rack. Lift from the pan using the foil overhang as handles. Cut into 16 squares. The bars can be stored in an airtight container at room temperature for up to 3 days.

Each serving (1 square): 10 g carb, 80 cal, 4 g fat, 2 g sat fat, 22 mg chol, 1 g fib, 2 g pro, 61 mg sod • Carb Choices: ½; Exchanges: ½ carb, ½ fat

Chewy Cranberry-Spice Bars

makes 24 servings

These bars have a moist cakey bottom layer topped with a creamy layer of dried cranberries and yogurt. They're quicker to make than most bar cookies, since the bottom layer does not have to be prebaked.

CRUST

2 teaspoons unsalted butter, softened

1 cup old-fashioned rolled oats

1 cup whole wheat pastry flour or unbleached all-purpose flour

½ cup sugar

½ teaspoon baking soda

½ teaspoon ground cinnamon

⅛ teaspoon salt

4 tablespoons (½ stick) unsalted butter, melted and cooled

⅓ cup orange juice

FILLING

1 cup dried cranberries

¾ cup plain low-fat yogurt

½ cup sugar

1 large egg

2 tablespoons whole wheat pastry flour or unbleached all-purpose flour

1 teaspoon vanilla extract

1 teaspoon grated orange zest

1 Preheat the oven to 325°F. Line an 11 x 7-inch metal baking pan with foil, allowing foil to extend over the rim of the pan by 2 inches. Brush the foil with the softened butter.

2 To make the crust, place the oats in a food processor and process until coarsely ground. Transfer to a large bowl. Add the flour, sugar, baking soda, cinnamon, and salt and stir to mix well. Drizzle with the melted butter and orange juice and stir just until moistened. Place ½ cup of the oat mixture in a small bowl and set aside. Press the remaining oat mixture into the bottom of the prepared pan (the mixture will be sticky).

3 To make the filling, combine all the filling ingredients in a medium bowl and stir to mix well. Spread the filling over the crust. Using your fingers, separate the reserved oat mixture into small pieces and drop evenly over the filling. Bake until the topping is lightly browned, about 40 minutes.

4 Cool completely in the pan on a wire rack. Lift from the pan using the foil overhang as handles. Cut into 24 squares using a serrated knife. The bars can be covered in an airtight container and stored at room temperature for up to 2 days.

Each serving: 20 g carb, 108 cal, 3 g fat, 2 g sat fat, 15 mg chol, 1 g fib, 2 g pro, 47 mg sod • Carb Choices: 1; Exchanges: 1 carb, ½ fat

Frozen Desserts

Raspberry Granita

makes 6 servings

Refreshing and summery, this granita makes a cool finish to a hot weather meal. Serve the granita on its own, or place a Meringue Cookie (page 580) or an Almond Biscotti (page 579) alongside.

1 cup water
⅓ cup sugar
1 (12-ounce) package frozen unsweetened raspberries, thawed
1 tablespoon lemon juice

1 Cook the water and sugar in a small saucepan over medium heat, until the sugar dissolves. Cool to room temperature.

2 Place the raspberries and lemon juice in a food processor and process until smooth. Press the mixture through a fine wire mesh strainer, discarding the solids. Combine the sugar syrup and the raspberry mixture in a shallow glass baking dish and stir to mix well.

3 Freeze, stirring every 15 minutes, until the granita is almost firm, about 2 hours. Freeze without stirring until firm, 2 hours or overnight.

4 When ready to serve, let stand at room temperature 10 minutes. Scrape the granita with a fork to break it into crystals. Serve at once. The granita can be frozen for 1 week.

Each serving: 16 g carb, 63 cal, 0 g fat, 0 g sat fat, 0 mg chol, 1 g fib, 0 g pro, 7 mg sod • Carb Choices: 1; Exchanges: 1 carb

BLACKBERRY-GINGER GRANITA: Follow the Raspberry Granita recipe, above, substituting blackberries for the raspberries. Add 1 teaspoon fresh grated ginger with the lemon juice in step 2. Proceed with the recipe.

Each serving: 17 g carb, 69 cal, 0 g fat, 0 g sat fat, 0 mg chol, 1 g fib, 0 g pro, 8 mg sod • Carb Choices: 1; Exchanges: 1 carb

Cantaloupe Sorbet

makes 4 servings

Choose a melon at the peak of ripeness for this sorbet. You can make the sorbet with honeydew melon, too.

1¼ cups water
⅓ cup sugar
2 cups chopped cantaloupe
2 teaspoons lime juice

1 Stir together the water and sugar in a small saucepan. Cook over medium heat, stirring often, until the sugar dissolves, about 3 minutes. Let stand to cool to room temperature.

2 Combine the sugar syrup, cantaloupe, and lime juice in a food processor and process until smooth. Refrigerate until chilled, 2 hours.

3 Transfer to an ice cream maker and freeze according to manufacturer's instructions. Transfer to an airtight container and freeze overnight. Let stand at room temperature 10 minutes before serving. The sorbet can be frozen for 1 week.

Each serving: 23 g carb, 92 cal, 0 g fat, 0 g sat fat, 0 mg chol, 1 g fib, 1 g pro, 13 mg sod • Carb Choices: 1½; Exchanges: 1 carb, ½ fruit

Red Grapefruit Sorbet

makes 6 servings

Tart, sweet, and gorgeously pink, this sorbet refreshes after a heavy meal. With just two ingredients, its flavor belies its simplicity.

3 cups freshly squeezed red grapefruit juice, divided
⅔ cup sugar

1 Stir together ½ cup of the grapefruit juice and the sugar in a small saucepan. Cook over medium heat, stirring often, until the sugar dissolves, about 3 minutes. Pour the sugar mixture into a medium bowl, add the remaining 2½ cups grapefruit juice, and cover, and refrigerate until chilled, about 2 hours.

2 Transfer to an ice cream maker and freeze according to manufacturer's instructions

3 Transfer to an airtight container and freeze overnight. The sorbet can be frozen, covered, for up to 1 week.

Each serving: 34 g carb, 134 cal, 0 g fat, 0 g sat fat, 0 mg chol, 0 g fib, 1 g pro, 1 mg sod • Carb choices: 2; Exchanges: 1 carb, 1 fruit

Chocolate Sorbet

makes 6 servings

This sorbet tastes so rich, you only need a tiny scoop to satisfy your sweet tooth.

1¾ **cups water**
⅔ **cup sugar**
½ **cup unsweetened cocoa**
1 **teaspoon vanilla extract**

1 Whisk together the water, sugar, and cocoa in a medium saucepan. Cook over medium heat, whisking constantly, until the mixture comes to a boil, about 5 minutes. Remove from the heat and let cool to room temperature. Stir in the vanilla. Cover and refrigerate until chilled, about 2 hours.

2 Transfer to an ice cream maker and freeze according to manufacturer's instructions.

3 Transfer to an airtight container and freeze overnight. The sorbet can be frozen, covered, for up to 1 week.

Each serving: 26 g carb, 104 cal, 1 g fat, 1 g sat fat, 0 mg chol, 2 g fib, 1 g pro, 2 mg sod • Carb Choices: 2; Exchanges: 2 carb

Melon Pops

makes 6 servings

You can make these easy and refreshing pops not only with melon, but with any fresh summer fruit. Keep a batch in the freezer all summer long for a healthful low-carb treat. Try them with peeled peaches, nectarines, or mangoes, or any kind of fresh berries.

3 **cups 1-inch cubes seedless watermelon, cantaloupe, and honeydew melon**
2 **tablespoons lime juice**

1 Combine the melon and lime juice in a food processor and process until smooth. Pour the mixture into 6 freezer pop molds or into small paper cups.

2 Freeze 1½ hours or until almost firm. Insert popsicle sticks in the center of each cup and freeze 6 hours or until firm. The popsicles can be frozen for up to 1 week.

Each serving: 7 g carb, 28 cal, 0 g fat, 0 g sat fat, 0 mg chol, 1 g fib, 1 g pro, 13 mg sod • Carb Choices: ½; Exchanges: ½ fruit

Frozen Yogurt

makes 8 servings

This delicious yogurt tastes nothing like what you buy at the supermarket. It's just sweet enough that the natural tang of the yogurt comes through. After the yogurt has processed in the ice cream maker, stir in some fresh raspberries, strawberries, or blackberries.

1 **cup 1% low-fat milk**
¾ **cup sugar**
2 **cups plain low-fat yogurt**
½ **teaspoon vanilla extract**

1 Stir together the milk and sugar in a small saucepan. Cook over medium heat, stirring often, until the sugar dissolves, about 3 minutes (do not boil). Transfer to a small bowl and let cool to room temperature. Refrigerate, covered, until chilled, about 2 hours.

2 Whisk together the milk mixture, yogurt, and vanilla in a medium bowl until smooth. Spoon the mixture into an ice cream maker and freeze according to manufacturer's instructions. Transfer to an airtight container and freeze overnight. The yogurt can be frozen, covered, for up to 1 week.

Each serving: 25 g carb, 125 cal, 1 g fat, 1 g sat fat, 5 mg chol, 0 g fib, 4 g pro, 56 mg sod • Carb Choices: 1½; Exchanges: 1½ carb

Dessert Sauces, Frostings, and Glazes

Light Whipped Cream QUICK

makes ¾ cup

If the artificial taste of commercial low-fat whipped "creams" are not to your liking, try this natural version.

¼ cup whipping cream
1 tablespoon confectioners' sugar
½ cup plain low-fat Greek yogurt or strained yogurt (page 11)

1 Combine the cream and sugar in a medium bowl. Beat at high speed with an electric mixer until stiff peaks form.

2 Place the yogurt in a medium bowl. Gently fold the whipped cream mixture into the yogurt in three additions. The cream can be refrigerated, covered, for up to 3 days.

Each serving (1 tablespoon): 1 g carb, 26 cal, 2 g fat, 1 g sat fat, 7 mg chol, 0 g fib, 1 g pro, 5 mg sod • Carb Choices: 0; Exchanges: ½ fat

Vanilla Glaze QUICK

makes ⅓ cup

This glaze is just the thing to dress up almost any dessert that needs a little drizzle of flavor.

1 cup confectioners' sugar
1 to 2 tablespoons 1% low-fat milk
1 teaspoon vanilla extract

1 Combine the sugar, 2 teaspoons of the milk, and the vanilla in a medium bowl. Stir until smooth.

2 Add the remaining milk, a few drops at a time, until a drizzling consistency is reached. Immediately drizzle over cakes, cupcakes, or cookies.

Each serving (about 1 teaspoon): 8 g carb, 30 cal, 0 g fat, 0 g sat fat, 0 mg chol, 0 g fib, 0 g pro, 1 mg sod • Carb Choices: ½; Exchanges: ½ carb

Citrus Glaze QUICK

makes ⅓ cup

Made with lemon, lime, or orange juice, this glaze adds tart-sweet flavor to all kinds of baked desserts. To add even more flavor, you can add ½ teaspoon of grated citrus zest to the glaze.

1 cup confectioners' sugar
1 to 2 tablespoons lemon, lime, or orange juice

1 Combine the confectioners' sugar and 1 tablespoon of the juice in a medium bowl. Stir until smooth.

2 Add the remaining juice, a few drops at a time, until a drizzling consistency is reached. Immediately drizzle over cakes, cupcakes, or cookies.

Each serving (about 1 teaspoon): 8 g carb, 29 cal, 0 g fat, 0 g sat fat, 0 mg chol, 0 g fib, 0 g pro, 0 mg sod • Carb Choices: ½; Exchanges: ½ carb

Espresso Glaze QUICK

makes ⅓ cup

If you love coffee-flavored desserts, drizzle this glaze over Moist Yogurt Cake (page 566) or Classic White Cake (page 562).

1 tablespoon hot water
1 teaspoon instant espresso granules
1 cup confectioners' sugar
1 teaspoon vanilla extract

Combine the water and espresso granules in a medium bowl and stir until the espresso dissolves. Add the sugar and vanilla. Stir until smooth, adding additional water a few drops at a time, if necessary, until a drizzling consistency is reached. Immediately drizzle over cakes, cupcakes, or cookies.

Each serving (about 1 teaspoon): 8 g carb, 30 cal, 0 g fat, 0 g sat fat, 0 mg chol, 0 g fib, 0 g pro, 0 mg sod • Carb Choices: ½; Exchanges: ½ carb

Fluffy White Frosting QUICK

makes 2½ cups

This classic melt-in-your-mouth white frosting is sometimes called 7-minute frosting, because you have to beat it for 7 minutes for the stiff peaks to form.

½ cup sugar
2 tablespoons water
⅛ teaspoon cream of tartar
2 large egg whites
½ teaspoon vanilla extract

1 Combine the sugar, water, cream of tartar, and egg whites in the top of a double boiler and place over barely simmering water.

2 Beat at high speed with a handheld electric mixer until stiff peaks form, about 7 minutes. Beat in the vanilla. Makes enough to frost a 13 x 9-inch sheet cake, an 8- or 9-inch layer cake, or 24 cupcakes.

Each serving (2½ tablespoons): 6 g carb, 27 cal, 0 g fat, 0 g sat fat, 0 mg chol, 0 g fib, 0 g pro, 7 mg sod • Carb Choices: ½; Exchanges: ½ carb

Cream Cheese Frosting

QUICK

makes 2 cups

Using reduced-fat cream cheese and no butter makes this version of the classic frosting healthy enough for an occasional treat.

8 ounces reduced-fat cream cheese, softened
1 teaspoon vanilla extract
3 cups confectioners' sugar, sifted

Place the cream cheese in a large bowl and beat at medium speed with an electric mixer until fluffy. Beat in the vanilla. Add the sugar and beat just until smooth (do not overbeat or the frosting will thin). Makes enough to frost a 13 x 9-inch sheet cake, an 8- or 9-inch layer cake, or 24 cupcakes.

Each serving (2 tablespoons): 23 g carb, 121 cal, 3 g fat, 2 g sat fat, 8 mg chol, 0 g fib, 2 g pro, 42 mg sod • Carb Choices: 1½; Exchanges: 1½ carb, ½ fat

Rich Chocolate Sauce QUICK

makes 1¼ cups

With two kinds of chocolate, this sauce is a chocolate lover's dream. It thickens in the refrigerator, so gently reheat it before serving.

1 cup 1% low-fat milk
½ cup sugar
½ cup unsweetened cocoa
2 ounces unsweetened chocolate, chopped
1 teaspoon vanilla extract

1 Combine the milk, sugar, and cocoa in a medium saucepan and whisk until smooth. Cook over medium heat, stirring often, until the mixture comes to a simmer.

2 Remove from the heat and stir in the unsweetened chocolate and vanilla, stirring until the chocolate melts. Serve warm or at room temperature. The sauce can be refrigerated, covered, for up to a week. Gently reheat in a saucepan over low heat or microwave for 1 to 1½ minutes before serving.

Each serving (1 tablespoon): 8 g carb, 44 cal, 2 g fat, 1 g sat fat, 1 mg chol, 1 g fib, 1 g pro, 7 mg sod • Carb Choices: ½; Exchanges: ½ carb

Raspberry Sauce [QUICK]

makes 1 cup

Serve this brilliant red sauce with any kind of plain cake, drizzle it over fresh fruit or ice cream, or swirl it into plain low-fat yogurt.

1 (12-ounce) package frozen unsweetened
    raspberries, thawed
1 tablespoon sugar
2 teaspoons lemon juice

1 Combine all the ingredients in a food processor and process until smooth.

2 Place the mixture in a fine wire mesh strainer over a medium bowl. Press the mixture through the strainer, discarding the solids. The sauce can be refrigerated, covered, for up to a week.

Each serving (2 tablespoons): 8 g carb, 33 cal, 0 g fat, 0 g sat fat, 0 mg chol, 0 g fib, 1 g pro, 1 mg sod • Carb Choices: ½; Exchanges: ½ carb

Strawberry Sauce [QUICK]

makes 1½ cups

When you make this sauce with fresh local strawberries, taste the puree before you add the sugar. The berries may be so naturally sweet that you won't need to use it.

2 cups sliced fresh strawberries
¼ cup water
2 tablespoons sugar
2 teaspoons lemon juice

1 Combine all the ingredients in a food processor and process until smooth.

2 Place the mixture in a fine wire mesh strainer over a medium bowl. Press the mixture through the strainer, discarding the solids. The sauce can be refrigerated, covered, for up to a week.

Each serving (2 tablespoons): 4 g carb, 17 cal, 0 g fat, 0 g sat fat, 0 mg chol, 0 g fib, 0 g pro, 0 mg sod • Carb Choices: 0

Whole Blueberry Sauce [QUICK]

makes 2 cups

Adding more berries after the sauce has cooked gives this a chunky look and a burst of fresh blueberry flavor. Serve it on anything from ice cream to waffles.

3 cups fresh blueberries, divided
¾ cup water
⅓ cup sugar
½ teaspoon vanilla extract

1 Combine 2 cups of the blueberries, the water, and sugar in a medium saucepan. Bring to a boil over high heat. Reduce the heat to low and simmer, uncovered, until the blueberries are soft and the sauce is slightly thickened, about 10 minutes.

2 Remove from the heat and stir in the remaining 1 cup blueberries and the vanilla. Serve the sauce warm or at room temperature. The sauce can be refrigerated, covered, for up to a week.

Each serving (2 tablespoons): 8 g carb, 32 cal, 0 g fat, 0 g sat fat, 0 mg chol, 1 g fib, 0 g pro, 0 mg sod • Carb Choices: ½; Exchanges: ½ carb

Creamy Custard Sauce

makes 1½ cups

A puddle of this custard sauce on a plate will elevate the simplest cake or tart, or even a brownie, to a special dessert.

1¼ cups 1% low-fat milk
2 large egg yolks
⅓ cup sugar
1 tablespoon cornstarch
Pinch of salt
¼ teaspoon vanilla extract

1 Combine the milk, egg yolks, sugar, cornstarch, and salt in a medium saucepan. Cook over medium heat, whisking constantly, until the sauce comes to a boil and thickens, about 5 minutes.

2 Remove from the heat and whisk in the vanilla. Pour into a serving bowl and let cool slightly to serve warm. To serve chilled, place a sheet of wax paper on the surface of the sauce to prevent a skin from forming. Let the sauce cool to room temperature. The sauce can be refrigerated, covered, for up to 3 days.

Each serving (2 tablespoons): 9 g carb, 53 cal, 1 g fat, 1 g sat fat, 42 mg chol, 0 g fib, 2 g pro, 30 mg sod • Carb Choices: ½; Exchanges: ½ carb

Zabaglione `QUICK`

makes 6 servings

Serve this ethereal custard over any fresh fruit or berries, pound cake, chiffon cake, or angel food cake. Before you begin to make the custard, have the fruit or cake you will serve it with placed on serving plates. Part of the appeal of zabaglione is the frothiness it has as soon as it comes off the stove.

¼ cup sugar
4 large egg yolks
¼ cup fruit- or nut-flavored liqueur (such as orange, raspberry, hazelnut, or almond)

1 Combine the sugar and egg yolks in the top of a double boiler and whisk to mix well. Whisk in the liqueur. Place over simmering (not boiling) water and beat at high speed with a handheld electric mixer until soft peaks form, about 5 minutes.

2 Spoon the custard over fruit, berries, or cake and serve at once.

Each serving: 13 g carb, 109 cal, 3 g fat, 1 g sat fat, 137 mg chol, 0 g fib, 2 g pro, 6 mg sod • Carb Choices: 1; Exchanges: 1 carb

Rhubarb–Vanilla Bean Compote

makes 8 servings

Rhubarb characteristically falls apart when it is cooked. In this recipe, the rhubarb is added to a hot sugar syrup and then removed from the heat. It's the best method I've found for keeping the pretty slices somewhat intact. Serve the compote over ice cream, frozen yogurt, pound cake, or angel food cake.

¾ cup water
½ cup sugar
12 ounces rhubarb, trimmed and cut into ½-inch slices (about 2½ cups)
½ vanilla bean or ½ teaspoon vanilla extract

1 Combine the water and sugar in a small saucepan and bring to a boil over high heat. Add the rhubarb and return to a boil. Remove from the heat. Scrape the seeds from the vanilla bean and add the seeds and the pod to the rhubarb mixture.

2 Cover and let stand to cool to room temperature. Refrigerate the compote, covered, until chilled, 2 hours or up to 5 days. Discard the vanilla bean pod before serving.

Each serving (¼ cup): 14 g carb, 55 cal, 0 g fat, 0 g sat fat, 0 mg chol, 1 g fib, 0 g pro, 1 mg sod • Carb Choices: 1; Exchanges: 1 carb

RHUBARB-GINGER COMPOTE: Follow the Rhubarb–Vanilla Bean Compote recipe, above, substituting 1 teaspoon grated fresh ginger for the vanilla bean.

Each serving: 14 g carb, 55 cal, 0 g fat, 0 g sat fat, 0 mg chol, 1 g fib, 0 g pro, 1 mg sod • Carb Choices: 1; Exchanges: 1 carb

Lemon Curd

makes 2½ cups

Serve this sweet-tart curd with biscuits, scones, or angel food cake. You can spoon the hot curd into a prepared, baked, and cooled Graham Cracker Crust (page 546), for a delicious lemon pie. Cover the surface of the curd with wax paper and let cool to room temperature. Then refrigerate until chilled before slicing the pie.

1½ cups water
½ cup lemon juice
2 large egg yolks
1 cup sugar
¼ cup cornstarch
Pinch of salt
1 tablespoon unsalted butter
1 tablespoon grated lemon zest

1 Combine the water, lemon juice, egg yolks, sugar, cornstarch, and salt in a large saucepan and whisk until smooth. Cook over medium heat, whisking constantly, until the mixture comes to a boil and thickens, about 6 minutes.

2 Remove from the heat and stir in the butter and lemon zest. Spoon into a medium bowl and cover the surface of the curd with wax paper to prevent a skin from forming. Cool to room temperature. Refrigerate until chilled, at least 2 hours and up to a week.

Each serving (¼ cup): 24 g carb, 114 cal, 2 g fat, 1 g sat fat, 44 mg chol, 0 g fib, 1 g pro, 17 mg sod • Carb Choices: 1½; Exchanges: 1½ carb, ½ fat

Orange-Ricotta Cream

makes ½ cup

Ricotta cheese is not just for lasagna. When pureed with just a bit of sugar, it turns into a creamy sauce that's refreshingly pleasant as an accompaniment to any fresh fruit, pound cake, or angel food cake.

½ cup part-skim ricotta cheese
1 tablespoon sugar
½ teaspoon grated orange zest

Combine the ricotta and sugar in a food processor and process until smooth. Transfer to a small bowl and stir in the orange zest. Cover and refrigerate until chilled, at least 1 hour and up to 3 days.

Each serving (2 tablespoons): 5 g carb, 55 cal, 2 g fat, 2 g sat fat, 10 mg chol, 0 g fib, 4 g pro, 39 mg sod • Carb choices: 0; Exchanges: ½ lean protein

Sauces, Condiments, and Seasonings

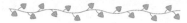

Sauces

Marinara Sauce

Romesco Sauce

Chimichurri Sauce

Yogurt Tartar Sauce

Peanut Sauce

Asian Dipping Sauce

Sweet Soy-Lemon
Dipping Sauce

Smoky Red Pepper–Orange
Sauce

Tomatillo Sauce

Creamy Avocado Sauce

Condiments

Basil Pesto

Cilantro Pesto

Mint Pesto

Asian Pesto

Scallion-Spinach Pesto

Tapenade

Tomato Jam

Julia's Fig Chutney

Tangerine-Ginger
Cranberry Sauce

Dried Cranberry Chutney

Pear Butter

Fresh Strawberry Jam

15-Minute Clementine
Marmalade

Seasonings

Pepper-Spice Seasoning

Indian Spice Rub

Sweet-and-Spicy BBQ Rub

Citrus Spice Rub

Cilantro-Ginger Rub

Herb-Seasoned Salt

How you season a dish or what you serve to accompany it can make the difference between a boring meal and a brilliant one. Sauces and condiments are a busy cook's dream. If all you've got time to make for dinner is plain baked fish or sautéed chicken breasts, a fresh salsa that you prepare in 5 minutes or a spoonful of tapenade or chutney that you've got stashed in the refrigerator can make your meal sing.

If you're in a weeknight meal rut, a seasoning rub that takes just a couple of minutes to stir together can turn standbys like chicken breasts, pork chops, salmon fillets, and shrimp into something special. The seasonings in this chapter are accompanied by suggested uses, but those are simply guidelines and you should experiment to add sparkle to the weeknight dishes you cook most often.

There are even a few treats in this chapter that you can bring out at breakfast. If you love marmalade, but don't get excited about hours of stirring, 15-Minute Clementine Marmalade (page 601) will be a revelation. Thin-skinned clementines soften quickly and taste fresh from the tree since they cook in such a short time. Pear Butter (page 600) and Fresh Strawberry Jam (page 601) take a little longer, but all they require is an occasional stir.

All the sauces, condiments, and seasonings in this chapter are meant to make good-for-you foods taste fantastic. Don't be afraid of flavor—it could be the big obstacle that's standing between you and a healthy diet.

Sauces

Marinara Sauce QUICK

makes 3 cups

In about 30 minutes, using basic pantry ingredients, you can make homemade marinara sauce that tastes fresher than purchased pasta sauce and has less sodium and none of the added sugars. If you have fresh basil, omit the dried herbs and stir in 2 tablespoons of fresh chopped basil during the last 5 minutes of cooking.

2 teaspoons extra virgin olive oil
1 small onion, chopped
2 garlic cloves, minced
1 (28-ounce) can no-salt-added whole
   tomatoes, undrained and chopped
½ teaspoon dried oregano
½ teaspoon dried basil
¼ teaspoon kosher salt
⅛ teaspoon freshly ground pepper

1 Heat a large deep-sided skillet over medium heat. Add the oil and tilt the pan to coat the bottom evenly. Add the onion and cook, stirring occasionally until softened, 5 minutes. Add the garlic and cook, stirring constantly, until fragrant, 30 seconds.

2 Stir in the tomatoes and their juices, the oregano, basil, salt, and pepper and bring to a boil over high heat. Reduce the heat to low, cover, and simmer 15 minutes. Uncover and simmer until the sauce is slightly thickened, 5 minutes longer. The sauce can be refrigerated, covered, for up to 4 days.

Each serving (½ cup): 7 g carb, 43 cal, 2 g fat, 0 g sat fat, 0 mg chol, 2 g fib, 1 g pro, 64 mg sod • Carb Choices: ½; 1 veg

Romesco Sauce QUICK

makes 1 cup

This traditional Spanish sauce is great with grilled shrimp, salmon, steaks, pork chops, or lamb. It's terrific with grilled or roasted vegetables, too.

1 cup red Roasted Bell Peppers (page 21) or
   roasted red peppers from a jar, chopped
¼ cup slivered almonds, toasted (page 4)
2 tablespoons chopped fresh Italian parsley
1 tablespoon extra virgin olive oil
1 garlic clove, minced
1 teaspoon sherry vinegar or red wine vinegar
1 teaspoon paprika or smoked paprika
¼ teaspoon kosher salt
Pinch of ground cayenne

Place all the ingredients in a food processor and pulse until a chunky sauce forms. The sauce can be refrigerated, covered, for up to 4 days.

Each serving (2 tablespoons): 2 g carb, 42 cal, 4 g fat, 0 g sat fat, 0 mg chol, 1 g fib, 1 g pro, 36 mg sod • Carb Choices: 0; Exchanges: ½ fat

Chimichurri Sauce QUICK

makes ¾ cup

Traditionally served with grilled meats and sausages in Argentinean cooking, chimichurri is also excellent on any grilled meat, shrimp, or vegetable kebabs or with grilled salmon or tuna.

1 cup loosely packed fresh Italian parsley leaves
2 garlic cloves, chopped
½ jalapeño, seeded and chopped
¼ cup extra virgin olive oil
3 tablespoons water
2 tablespoons red wine vinegar
¼ teaspoon kosher salt
⅛ teaspoon crushed red pepper

Place all the ingredients in a blender or food processor and process until smooth. The sauce can be refrigerated, covered, for up to 4 days.

Each serving (1 tablespoon): 1 g carb, 45 cal, 5 g fat, 1 g sat fat, 0 mg chol, 0 g fib, 0 g pro, 26 mg sod • Carb Choices: 0; Exchanges: 1 fat

Yogurt Tartar Sauce QUICK

makes ½ cup

Any baked, grilled, or oven-fried shrimp or fish is fabulous with this sauce. Spoon it over sliced tomatoes or steamed and chilled asparagus (or both together) for an easy and appealing salad.

¼ cup mayonnaise
¼ cup plain low-fat yogurt
1 tablespoon finely minced scallion, white part only
1 tablespoon minced fresh Italian parsley
2 teaspoons sweet pickle relish
2 teaspoons lemon juice
½ teaspoon Dijon mustard
⅛ teaspoon kosher salt

Stir together all the ingredients in a small bowl. The sauce can be refrigerated, covered, for up to 3 days.

Each serving (1 tablespoon): 1 g carb, 58 cal, 6 g fat, 1 g sat fat, 3 mg chol, 0 g fib, 0 g pro, 79 mg sod • Carb Choices: 0; Exchanges: 1 fat

Peanut Sauce QUICK

makes ½ cup

Drizzle this sauce over grilled chicken, beef, or shrimp kebabs. Or you can toss it with pasta and vegetables to make a pasta salad. Most kids love this sauce as a dip with fresh vegetables and you can leave out the chili-garlic paste or use less when making this for the little ones.

⅓ cup water
¼ cup natural creamy peanut butter
2 tablespoons rice vinegar
1 tablespoon reduced-sodium soy sauce
1 tablespoon light brown sugar
1 garlic clove, minced
1 teaspoon chili-garlic paste
½ teaspoon grated fresh ginger

1 Whisk together all the ingredients in a small saucepan until smooth. Set over medium heat and cook, whisking often, until the sauce just comes to a boil.

2 Transfer to a bowl to cool. The sauce can be refrigerated, covered, for up to 4 days. Bring to room temperature before serving.

Each serving (1 tablespoon): 4 g carb, 58 cal, 4 g fat, 1 g sat fat, 0 mg chol, 1 g fib, 2 g pro, 107 mg sod • Carb Choices: 0; Exchanges: 1 fat

Asian Dipping Sauce QUICK

makes ⅓ cup

Fish sauce gives this dipping sauce its characteristic flavor, but you can substitute soy sauce if you prefer. Serve it with grilled seafood, steamed dumplings, or fresh raw vegetables. It also makes a delicious dressing for a pasta and vegetable salad.

2 tablespoons Asian fish sauce
2 tablespoons lime juice
2 tablespoons cold water
1 teaspoon sugar
1 garlic clove, crushed through a press
½ jalapeño or other small hot chile, minced

Combine all the ingredients in a small bowl and stir until the sugar dissolves. The sauce can be refrigerated, covered, for up to 4 days.

Each serving (scant 1 tablespoon): 1 g carb, 5 cal, 0 g fat, 0 g sat fat, 0 mg chol, 0 g fib, 0 g pro, 348 mg sod • Carb Choices: 0

Sweet Soy-Lemon Dipping Sauce QUICK

makes ¼ cup

A touch of sweetness makes this a nice sauce to accompany rich-tasting salmon or scallops. It's also good drizzled on grilled shrimp or chicken or as a dressing for a cucumber and onion salad.

1 teaspoon grated lemon zest
3 tablespoons lemon juice
1 tablespoon honey
1 tablespoon minced fresh cilantro
2 teaspoons reduced-sodium soy sauce
¼ teaspoon chili-garlic paste

Combine all the ingredients in a small bowl and stir until smooth. Serve at once.

Each serving (1 tablespoon): 6 g carb, 21 cal, 0 g fat, 0 g sat fat, 0 mg chol, 0 g fib, 0 g pro, 101 mg sod • Carb Choices: ½; Exchanges: ½ carb

Smoky Red Pepper–Orange Sauce QUICK

makes 1¼ cups

Bell peppers and orange may sound like an odd combination, but it works in this recipe. Serve this slightly sweet and tangy sauce as a dip for fresh vegetables or drizzle it over grilled chicken, shrimp kebabs, or baked salmon.

1 large red Roasted Bell Pepper (page 21) or
    1 cup roasted red peppers from a jar, chopped
⅓ cup frozen orange juice concentrate, thawed
1 tablespoon extra virgin olive oil
1 tablespoon lime juice
½ teaspoon minced chipotle in adobo sauce
½ teaspoon ground cumin
¼ teaspoon kosher salt

Combine all the ingredients in a food processor and process until smooth. Serve at once, or cover and refrigerate for up to 4 days.

Each serving (2 tablespoons): 5 g carb, 34 cal, 2 g fat, 0 g sat fat, 0 mg chol, 0 g fib, 0 g pro, 47 mg sod • Carb Choices: 0

Tomatillo Sauce QUICK

makes 2 cups

Spoon this tart green sauce over baked fish, grilled shrimp or salmon, grilled steaks, tacos, burritos, or enchiladas, or serve it as a dip with baked tortilla chips or fresh vegetables.

1 pound tomatillos, husks removed
1 cup Vegetable Stock (page 149) or
    low-sodium vegetable broth
2 jalapeños, halved lengthwise and seeded
2 garlic cloves, sliced
½ cup loosely packed fresh cilantro leaves
⅓ cup thinly sliced scallions
2 tablespoons lime juice
2 teaspoons honey
1 teaspoon canola oil
¾ teaspoon kosher salt

1 Combine the tomatillos, stock, jalapeños, and garlic in a small saucepan and bring to a boil over high heat. Cover, reduce the heat, and simmer until the tomatillos are very tender, 12 to 15 minutes. Drain and let cool slightly.

2 Transfer the tomatillo mixture to a food processor. Add the cilantro, scallions, lime juice, honey, oil, and salt and process until smooth. Serve at once or cover and refrigerate for up to 4 days. Bring to room temperature before serving.

Each serving (¼ cup): 6 g carb, 35 cal, 1 g fat, 0 g sat fat, 0 mg chol, 1 g fib, 1 g pro, 120 mg sod • Carb Choices: ½; Exchanges: 1 veg

Creamy Avocado Sauce QUICK

makes ⅔ cup

The only problem with this vibrant green sauce is that it starts browning quickly after you blend it together, so you can't make it ahead. But it only takes 5 minutes to make, so the browning is not too much of a setback. Serve it with any Tex-Mex dish, with grilled fish or chicken, or with beef kebabs. It provides a cooling counterpoint when drizzled over a bowl of chili, too.

½ ripe avocado, peeled, pitted, and chopped
½ cup plain low-fat yogurt
¼ cup loosely packed fresh cilantro leaves
2 teaspoons lime juice
¼ teaspoon kosher salt

Place all the ingredients in a food processor or blender and process until smooth. Serve at once.

Each serving (generous 2 tablespoons): 5 g carb, 60 cal, 4 g fat, 1 g sat fat, 2 mg chol, 2 g fib, 2 g pro, 94 mg sod • Carb Choices: ½; Exchanges: ½ carb, 1 fat

Condiments

Basil Pesto [QUICK]

makes ½ cup

What doesn't taste better with basil pesto? It's such a versatile condiment to have on hand to dress up plain grilled steak, seafood, or vegetables. You can stir it into cooked rice or other grains to make an ordinary side dish special, try it as a sandwich spread, or toss it with pasta and vegetables for a fresh and light vegetarian dinner.

¼ cup pine nuts, toasted (page 4)
1 cup tightly packed fresh basil leaves
1 ounce freshly grated Parmesan (about ¼ cup)
3 tablespoons extra-virgin olive oil
1 tablespoon lemon juice
1 small garlic clove, chopped
¼ teaspoon kosher salt

Combine all the ingredients in a food processor and process until the mixture is finely chopped. The sauce can be refrigerated, with the surface covered with plastic wrap, for up to 4 days.

Each serving (1 tablespoon): 1 g carb, 89 cal, 9 g fat, 1 g sat fat, 2 mg chol, 0 g fib, 2 g pro, 74 mg sod • Carb Choices: 0; Exchanges: 2 fat

Cilantro Pesto [QUICK]

makes ½ cup

Stir this pesto into rice to serve with a Tex-Mex meal, spread it onto tortillas before filling them when you make quesadillas or add a spoonful to ground beef to make flavorful burgers.

¼ cup slivered almonds, toasted (page 4)
1 cup tightly packed fresh cilantro leaves
1 ounce freshly grated Parmesan (about ¼ cup)
3 tablespoons canola oil

1 tablespoon lime juice
1 small garlic clove, chopped
½ teaspoon ground cumin
¼ teaspoon kosher salt
⅛ teaspoon ground cayenne

Combine all the ingredients in a food processor and process until the mixture is finely chopped. The sauce can be refrigerated, with the surface covered with plastic wrap, for up to 4 days.

Each serving (1 tablespoon): 1 g carb, 78 cal, 8 g fat, 1 g sat fat, 2 mg chol, 0 g fib, 2 g pro, 74 mg sod • Carb Choices: 0; Exchanges: 2 fat

Mint Pesto [QUICK]

makes ½ cup

Naturally, it's a perfect accompaniment to lamb chops or leg of lamb, but this pesto also makes a deliciously unusual addition to pasta or potato salad or spooned on top of fresh sliced cucumbers or tomatoes.

¼ cup pecans, toasted (page 4)
½ cup tightly packed fresh mint leaves
½ cup tightly packed fresh Italian parsley leaves
1 ounce freshly grated Parmesan (about ¼ cup)
3 tablespoons extra-virgin olive oil
1 tablespoon lemon juice
1 small garlic clove, chopped
¼ teaspoon kosher salt

Combine all the ingredients in a food processor and process until the mixture is finely chopped. The sauce can be refrigerated, with the surface covered with plastic wrap, for up to 4 days.

Each serving (1 tablespoon): 1 g carb, 85 cal, 8 g fat, 1 g sat fat, 2 mg chol, 0 g fib, 1 g pro, 76 mg sod • Carb Choices: 0; Exchanges: 2 fat

Asian Pesto QUICK

makes ½ cup

Serve this with tofu, fish or shellfish, grilled or broiled chicken, or steamed or grilled vegetables. Mix in a few tablespoons with ground beef to put an Asian spin on burgers or meatloaf.

¼ cup slivered almonds, toasted (page 4)
½ cup tightly packed fresh cilantro leaves
½ cup tightly packed fresh basil leaves
1 ounce freshly grated Parmesan (about ¼ cup)
2 tablespoons cold water
1 tablespoon extra-virgin olive oil
1 tablespoon lime juice
1 tablespoon reduced-sodium soy sauce
1 small garlic clove, chopped
¼ teaspoon Asian sesame oil
¼ teaspoon kosher salt

Combine all the ingredients in a food processor and pulse until the mixture is finely chopped. The sauce can be refrigerated, with the surface covered with plastic wrap, for up to 4 days.

Each serving (1 tablespoon): 1 g carb, 51 cal, 4 g fat, 1 g sat fat, 2 mg chol, 1 g fib, 2 g pro, 150 mg sod • Carb Choices: 0; Exchanges: 1 fat

Scallion-Spinach Pesto QUICK

makes ½ cup

This pesto is great with any type of grilled seafood. I also like to put a spoonful inside a baked potato. Or add it to potato or pasta salad or deviled eggs, or mix it with plain low-fat yogurt to make a sandwich spread.

1 cup loosely packed fresh baby spinach
½ cup thinly sliced scallions
¼ cup pine nuts, toasted (page 4)
1 ounce freshly grated Parmesan (about ¼ cup)
1 garlic clove, chopped
2 tablespoons extra virgin olive oil
1 tablespoon cold water
2 teaspoons lemon juice
¼ teaspoon kosher salt

Combine all the ingredients in a food processor and pulse until the mixture is finely chopped. The sauce can be refrigerated, with the surface covered with plastic wrap, for up to 4 days.

Each serving (1 tablespoon): 2 g carb, 54 cal, 5 g fat, 1 g sat fat, 2 mg chol, 0 g fib, 2 g pro, 78 mg sod • Carb Choices: 0; Exchanges: 1 fat

Tapenade QUICK

makes ½ cup

This classic French olive spread is perfect to pair with grilled or roasted lamb, grilled or pan-seared tuna or shrimp, or sliced beefsteak tomatoes. Spread it on thin slices of toasted whole wheat baguette as an appetizer, toss it with pasta and fresh tomatoes to make a summer salad, or use it as a sandwich spread. If you want to use Kalamata olives to make the tapenade (they are easier to find) use a well-rounded ½ cup of them instead of the niçoise olives.

½ cup niçoise olives, pitted
2 tablespoons chopped fresh Italian parsley
1 tablespoon capers, rinsed and drained
2 canned anchovy fillets, drained
2 teaspoons grated lemon zest
2 teaspoons lemon juice
1 small garlic clove, minced
⅛ teaspoon freshly ground pepper
2 tablespoons extra virgin olive oil

Combine all the ingredients except the oil in a food processor and pulse until finely chopped. Add the oil and pulse to combine. The tapenade can be refrigerated, covered, for up to a week.

Each serving (1 tablespoon): 1 g carb, 58 cal, 6 g fat, 1 g sat fat, 1 mg chol, 0 g fib, 0 g pro, 206 mg sod • Carb Choices: 0; Exchanges: 1 fat

MINT TAPENADE QUICK: Follow the Tapenade recipe, above, substituting 2 tablespoons whole fresh mint leaves for the parsley leaves.

Each serving (1 tablespoon): 1 g carb, 58 cal, 6 g fat, 1 g sat fat, 1 mg chol, 0 g fib, 0 g pro, 206 mg sod • Carb Choices: 0; Exchanges: 1 fat

GREEN OLIVE TAPENADE QUICK : Follow the Tapenade recipe, at left, substituting ½ cup picholine or other brine-cured green olives for the niçoise olives and 2 tablespoons whole fresh mint leaves for the parsley leaves.

Each serving (1 tablespoon): 2 g carb, 49 cal, 4 g fat, 1 g sat fat, 1 mg chol, 0 g fib, 0 g pro, 234 mg sod • Carb Choices: 0; Exchanges: 1 fat

Tomato Jam

makes 2¼ cups

This jam is a delicious way to use a bumper crop of end-of-season tomatoes. It's terrific with grilled steaks, pork chops, tuna, salmon, or shrimp. It makes a great stand in for mayonnaise as a sandwich spread, too.

6 large tomatoes (about 4 pounds)
⅓ cup packed light brown sugar
⅓ cup finely minced onion
2 garlic cloves, minced
1 jalapeño, minced, reserving half the seeds
¼ teaspoon kosher salt
¼ cup chopped fresh cilantro
3 tablespoons lime juice

1 Bring a large pot of water to a boil over high heat. Carefully add the tomatoes and cook for 1 minute. Transfer the tomatoes to a colander using a slotted spoon. Rinse with cold running water until cool enough to handle. Peel and core the tomatoes and cut them into wedges. Place the tomatoes, in batches, in a food processor and pulse until a chunky puree forms. Transfer the tomatoes to a large saucepan.

2 Add the sugar, onion, garlic, jalapeño with seeds, and salt. Bring the mixture to a boil. Reduce the heat and simmer, uncovered, stirring occasionally, until the mixture thickens, 45 minutes to 1 hour (stir more often as the mixture thickens). Transfer the jam to a bowl and let stand to cool to room temperature. Stir in the cilantro and lime juice. The jam can be refrigerated,

covered, for up to 4 days. Bring to room temperature before serving

Each serving (generous ¼ cup): 19 g carb, 78 cal, 0 g fat, 0 g sat fat, 0 mg chol, 3 g fib, 2 g pro, 50 mg sod • Carb Choices: 1; Exchanges: ½ carb, 1 veg

Julia's Fig Chutney

makes 4 cups

My friend Julia has a Brown Turkey fig tree in her backyard and uses her harvest to make a batch of this chutney every year in late summer. You can make the chutney with any variety of fresh figs, though. Serve this sweet and spicy condiment with roasted or grilled pork loin or pork chops, or roast chicken or turkey breast, or do as Julia does and stir a spoonful of it into your favorite chicken salad recipe.

1¾ cups apple cider vinegar
1 cup packed light brown sugar
⅓ cup chopped crystallized ginger
1½ teaspoons mustard seeds
1 teaspoon kosher salt
½ teaspoon grated lemon zest
¼ teaspoon ground cinnamon
¼ teaspoon ground coriander
¼ teaspoon crushed red pepper
⅛ teaspoon ground cloves
2 pounds fresh figs, stemmed and chopped

1 Combine all the ingredients except the figs in a large saucepan. Bring to a boil over high heat, reduce the heat to low, and simmer, uncovered, until the liquid is reduced by two-thirds, about 30 minutes.

2 Add the figs and simmer, uncovered, stirring occasionally, until the chutney is thickened, about 1 hour (stir more often as the mixture thickens). Transfer the chutney to a bowl and let stand to cool to room temperature. The chutney can be refrigerated, covered, for up to 1 month.

Each serving (2 tablespoons): 13 g carb, 54 cal, 0 g fat, 0 g sat fat, 0 mg chol, 1 g fib, 0 g pro, 39 mg sod • Carb Choices: 1; Exchanges: 1 carb

Tangerine-Ginger Cranberry Sauce

makes 2½ cups

This sauce is so easy and delicious that you will never serve cranberry sauce from a can again. If you don't like ginger, or want a simpler sauce, you can omit it.

1 small tangerine, cut into wedges and seeded (do not peel)
1 (12-ounce) package fresh cranberries or unthawed frozen cranberries
¾ cup packed light brown sugar
⅓ cup crystallized ginger, finely chopped
½ cup tangerine or orange juice

1 Place the tangerine in a food processor and pulse until finely chopped.

2 Combine the chopped tangerine, the cranberries, sugar, ginger, and tangerine juice in a medium saucepan. Bring to a boil over high heat. Reduce the heat to low and simmer, uncovered, stirring occasionally, until most of the cranberries pop, 8 to 10 minutes.

3 Transfer the sauce to a bowl and let stand to cool to room temperature. The sauce can be refrigerated, covered, for up to 4 days. Bring to room temperature before serving.

Each serving (2 tablespoons): 13 g carb, 51 cal, 0 g fat, 0 g sat fat, 0 mg chol, 1 g fib, 0 g pro, 4 mg sod • Carb Choices: 1; Exchanges: 1 carb

Dried Cranberry Chutney

makes 2¾ cups

Serve this chutney instead of fresh cranberry sauce with the Thanksgiving turkey. It's also great on a ham or turkey sandwich, and surprisingly, with baked sweet potatoes or winter squash.

2 cups dried cranberries
1 cup packed light brown sugar
1 cup unsweetened cranberry juice
½ cup diced onion
½ cup white wine vinegar
¼ cup minced fresh ginger
½ teaspoon ground cinnamon
¼ teaspoon ground cloves
⅛ teaspoon ground cayenne
2 teaspoons grated orange zest

1 Combine all the ingredients except the orange zest in a large saucepan. Bring to a boil over high heat, reduce the heat to low, and simmer, uncovered, stirring occasionally, until the chutney is thickened, about 35 minutes (stir more often as the mixture thickens).

2 Transfer the chutney to a bowl and let stand to cool to room temperature. Stir in the orange zest. The chutney can be refrigerated, covered, for up to 1 month.

Each serving (2 tablespoons): 20 g carb, 77 cal, 0 g fat, 0 g sat fat, 0 mg chol, 1 g fib, 0 g pro, 6 mg sod • Carb Choices: 1; Exchanges: 1 carb

Pear Butter

makes 1½ cups

If apple butter is a favorite, try this pear version. If you have whole nutmeg, grate it fresh for this recipe. Serve the butter on toast, biscuits, pancakes, or waffles. It's also a flavorful substitute for jelly on a peanut butter sandwich.

2½ pounds ripe pears, peeled, cored, and coarsely chopped
½ cup sugar
1 teaspoon grated fresh ginger
⅛ teaspoon ground nutmeg
½ teaspoon grated lemon zest
1 tablespoon lemon juice

1 Place the pears in a food processor and process until smooth. Transfer the puree to a medium saucepan. Add the sugar, ginger, and nutmeg and bring to a boil over high heat.

2 Reduce the heat to low and simmer, uncovered, stirring occasionally, until the mixture is very thick, about 45 minutes (stir more often as the mixture thickens). Remove from the heat and stir in the lemon zest and lemon juice.

3 Transfer the pear butter to a bowl and let stand to cool to room temperature. The butter can be refrigerated in an airtight container for up to 2 weeks.

Each serving (2 tablespoons): 23 g carb, 90 cal, 1 g fat, 0 g sat fat, 0 mg chol, 0 g fib, 1 g pro, 0 mg sod • Carb Choices: 1½; Exchanges: ½ carb, 1 fruit

Fresh Strawberry Jam

makes 2 cups

Strawberry jam is unbelievably simple to make, and when you make it with fresh local strawberries, it is bursting with flavor.

3 pints fresh strawberries (about 2 pounds), hulled
¾ cup sugar
1 teaspoon lemon juice

1 Place the strawberries in a food processor and pulse to form a chunky puree. (You will have about 3½ cups of strawberry puree.) Transfer the puree to a medium saucepan. Add the sugar and bring to a boil over high heat.

2 Reduce the heat to low and simmer, uncovered, stirring often, until the jam is very thick, 35 to 40 minutes (stir more often as the mixture thickens). Remove from the heat and stir in the lemon juice.

3 Transfer to a bowl and let stand to cool to room temperature. The jam will thicken as it cools. The jam can be refrigerated in an airtight container for up to 2 weeks.

Each serving (2 tablespoons): 13 g carb, 53 cal, 0 g fat, 0 g sat fat, 0 mg chol, 1 g fib, 0 g pro, 1 mg sod • Carb Choices: 1; Exchanges: 1 carb

15-Minute Clementine Marmalade QUICK

makes 1½ cups

Thin-skinned clementines make a delicious marmalade. Though you rarely find a seed in clementines, check for seeds before chopping the fruit. Because this marmalade has no pectin, it has a softer texture and does not form a gel like traditional marmalades. And because it cooks for such a short time, the fresh flavor of the clementines is incredible.

6 clementines, quartered and seeded (about 1¼ pounds)
1 cup sugar

1 Place the clementines in a food processor and process until finely chopped. (You will have about 2 cups of chopped clementines.) Transfer the clementines to a medium saucepan. Add the sugar and bring to a boil over high heat.

2 Reduce the heat to low and simmer, uncovered, stirring often, until the marmalade is very thick, 15 minutes (stir more often as the mixture thickens).

3 Transfer the marmalade to a bowl and let stand to cool to room temperature. The marmalade can be refrigerated in an airtight container for up to 2 weeks.

Each serving (2 tablespoons): 22 g carb, 87 cal, 0 g fat, 0 g sat fat, 0 mg chol, 1 g fib, 0 g pro, 0 mg sod • Carb Choices: 1½; Exchanges: 1 carb, ½ fruit

Seasonings

Pepper-Spice Seasoning QUICK

makes 1½ teaspoons

Sprinkle this flavorful all-purpose seasoning over steaks, burgers, tuna, chicken, or pork before grilling, sautéing, or baking. It makes enough to season 1 pound of food.

½ teaspoon kosher salt
½ teaspoon ground cumin
¼ teaspoon ground coriander
⅛ teaspoon freshly ground black pepper
⅛ teaspoon ground white pepper
Pinch of ground cayenne

Stir together all the ingredients in a small bowl.

Each serving (¼ of rub): 0 g carb, 2 cal, 0 g fat, 0 g sat fat, 0 mg chol, 0 g fib, 0 g pro, 141 mg sod • Carb Choices: 0

Indian Spice Rub QUICK

makes 1½ teaspoons

Use this rub to add Indian-inspired flavor to grilled or broiled lamb, chicken, or salmon. Stir the rub into ½ cup of plain fat-free yogurt and use it as a marinade for chicken. The rub makes enough to season 1 pound of food.

½ teaspoon kosher salt
¼ teaspoon ground cumin
¼ teaspoon ground coriander
⅛ teaspoon ground cinnamon
⅛ teaspoon ground cardamom
⅛ teaspoon freshly ground pepper
Pinch of ground cayenne

Stir together all the ingredients in a small bowl.

Each serving (¼ of rub): 0 g carb, 1 cal, 0 g fat, 0 g sat fat, 0 mg chol, 0 g fib, 0 g pro, 140 mg sod • Carb Choices: 0

Sweet-and-Spicy BBQ Rub QUICK

makes about 1 tablespoon

This rub gives food the flavor of barbecue, even if you're cooking your pork chops, chicken, or shrimp indoors. If you don't have chipotle chile powder on hand, you can add smoky flavor with 1 teaspoon of smoked paprika instead. If you use paprika, add a little more cayenne to compensate for the heat in the missing chipotle powder. The rub makes enough to season 1 pound of food.

1 teaspoon chili powder
1 teaspoon light brown sugar
½ teaspoon ground cumin
½ teaspoon kosher salt
⅛ teaspoon chipotle chile powder
⅛ teaspoon freshly ground pepper

Stir together all the ingredients in a small bowl.

Each serving (¼ of rub): 2 g carb, 9 cal, 0 g fat, 0 g sat fat, 0 mg chol, 0 g fib, 0 g pro, 157 mg sod • Carb Choices: 0

Citrus Spice Rub QUICK

makes about 2 teaspoons

Rub this seasoning over steaks, chicken, fish fillets, scallops, or shrimp before grilling or broiling. It also makes a great seasoning for rubbing under the skin of a whole chicken before roasting. If you have time, let meat or poultry stand for about an hour in the refrigerator after applying the rub and let seafood stand for 30 minutes. The rub makes enough to season 1 pound of food.

2 teaspoons extra virgin olive oil
2 teaspoons grated lemon zest
1 teaspoon grated lime zest
1 garlic clove, crushed through a press
1 teaspoon ground cumin
1 teaspoon ground coriander
1 teaspoon paprika
½ teaspoon kosher salt
⅛ teaspoon freshly ground pepper

Stir together all the ingredients in a small bowl.

Each serving (¼ of rub): 1 g carb, 27 cal, 3 g fat, 0 g sat fat, 0 mg chol, 1 g fib, 0 g pro, 142 mg sod • Carb Choices: 0; Exchanges: ½ fat

Cilantro-Ginger Rub QUICK

makes about ⅓ cup

Asian flavors enliven this wet rub, which is superb on grilled pork tenderloin, flank steak, chicken breast, or shrimp. Rub it on just before grilling, or if you have time, cover and refrigerate meats for an hour or two and shrimp for 30 minutes. The rub makes enough to season 1 pound of food.

½ cup fresh cilantro leaves
¼ cup sliced scallions
2 garlic cloves, chopped
1 tablespoon chopped fresh ginger
1 jalapeño, seeded and chopped
1 tablespoon lime juice
2 teaspoons canola oil
¼ teaspoon Asian sesame oil
½ teaspoon kosher salt
½ teaspoon chili-garlic paste

Combine all the ingredients in a food processor and process until finely chopped.

Each serving (¼ of rub): 2 g carb, 31 cal, 3 g fat, 0 g sat fat, 0 mg chol, 0 g fib, 0 g pro, 169 mg sod • Carb Choices: 0; Exchanges: ½ fat

Herb-Seasoned Salt QUICK

makes 1½ tablespoons

You can change the herb in this salt to suit your mood, your menu, or what's in your garden. Sprinkle the salt over grilled, baked, or sautéed chicken, steak, pork chops, fish, or shrimp or steamed or grilled vegetables. Stir the ingredients together just before you use them, since the salt starts to break down the herbs almost immediately. The salt makes enough to season 4 portions.

1 tablespoon chopped fresh basil, cilantro, or Italian parsley or 1½ teaspoons chopped fresh rosemary, sage, or tarragon
1 teaspoon freshly grated lemon zest
½ teaspoon kosher salt or flaked sea salt (such as Maldon)
⅛ teaspoon freshly ground pepper

Stir together all the ingredients in a small bowl.

Each serving (¼ of seasoned salt): 0 g carb, 1 cal, 0 g fat, 0 g sat fat, 0 mg chol, 0 g fib, 0 g pro, 140 mg sod • Carb Choices: 0

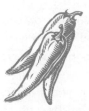

Beverages

Raspberry-Pear Smoothies

Kiwi-Apple Smoothies

Peach-Almond Smoothies

Citrus-Ginger Sparkler

Cucumber-Mint Cooler

Grapefruit-Hibiscus Cooler

Fresh Spicy
Tomato Juice

Watermelon
Agua Fresca

Vegetable Water

Herb Water

Berry Water

Americans get on average about 20 percent of their daily calories from beverages. If you're consuming 1,800 calories, that translates into 360 calories a day. Fancy coffee drinks, sports drinks, gourmet sodas, and ordinary soft drinks all add extra calories that collect on our waistlines but contribute little else toward good nutrition. As a person with diabetes, kicking the habit of these empty-calorie beverages is a must, if you haven't already.

Even if your beverage of choice is sweetened with artificial sweeteners, rethink these drinks. There are conflicting studies, but some researchers have found a correlation between consumption of diet sodas and other artificially sweetened foods and weight gain, impaired kidney function, and greater risk for developing type 2 diabetes and metabolic syndrome (the combination of high amounts of abdominal fat, high blood pressure, high cholesterol and triglycerides, and insulin resistance).

If you're trying to train your taste buds to enjoy foods that are less sweet overall, then drinking diet soda is probably not helping you reach this goal. If you're accustomed to drinking artificially sweetened drinks that taste extremely sweet, you'll expect this level of sweetness in other foods. This makes it harder for your taste buds to accept unsweetened fruits, unsweetened or lightly sweetened whole grain cereals, unsweetened yogurt, and other healthful foods.

When there are hundreds of beverage options that have none of the potential risks or the extra calories, drinking sugary or artificially sweetened beverages seems unwise. The lowest-calorie, best-tasting, most-economical, good-for-your-health beverage is as close as your kitchen tap.

If you find plain water boring, there are endless ways to dress it up. The obvious is to enjoy it with a wedge of lemon, lime, orange, or tangerine. Why not add a tablespoon or two of fruit juice or fruit nectar to a glass of water to add a light fruit flavor? Always check the label, but this small amount of juice or nectar will almost always add less than 5 grams of carbs to your water.

And think beyond adding ordinary orange juice or grapefruit juice. Check out the bottled and canned juice section as well as the refrigerated beverage section of your supermarket. You will find apricot, guava, mango, peach, pear, papaya, passion fruit, pineapple, strawberry, and unsweetened cranberry juices and nectars in most large supermarkets. In addition to using water, try flavoring club soda with juices for a fizzy treat.

At the end of this chapter you'll find recipes for making flavored waters. These recipes are as simple as pureeing an ingredient (that you probably already have in your kitchen) in the blender with water, then straining and chilling the water. Keep one of these flavored waters in the refrigerator at all times—they are a refreshing and flavorful thirst quencher.

Another carb- and calorie-free beverage is tea, both hot and cold. If you think you don't like tea, try different types until you find one you enjoy. There are hundreds of kinds of teas, both with and without caffeine, so it may take a while, but you'll surely find many teas that suit your taste. As someone who stopped sweetening my tea—both with sugar and artificial sweeteners—a few years ago, I can say that if you're trying to switch to unsweetened tea, you'll probably hate it for the first week. When I first made the change, I thought it was dreadful. After about a week, I started to really taste and enjoy the flavor of the tea, and not just the sweetness that I was accustomed to.

There are some great-tasting smoothies in this chapter, which do have carbs and calories, but they also have the nutrients contained in the fruit, yogurt, or milk that they're made from. They make a nutritious and refreshing midmorning or midafternoon snack. Beverages are an essential part of everyone's day. So drink up, but drink smart.

3 Ways to Brew Iced Tea

Iced tea is a simple-to-make beverage to have on hand, especially during the warm months, to quench thirst without adding carbohydrates or calories. Here are three foolproof ways to make smooth-tasting clear iced tea:

Boiling water method: Bring 2 cups of water to a boil in a small saucepan. Add 8 tea bags and let stand 5 to 10 minutes, depending on the type of tea. Check the instructions on the box; herbal teas generally need to brew longer than other types of tea. Remove and discard the tea bags. Pour the tea into a 2-quart pitcher and add 6 cups of cold water. Serve over ice.

Room temperature method: Fill a 2-quart pitcher with water and add 8 tea bags. Let stand at room temperature for 4 to 6 hours, depending on the type of tea and the strength you prefer. If you put the pitcher in a sunny window or outside in the sun (don't forget to cover the pitcher if you take it outside), it will brew in about half the time. Remove and discard the tea bags and serve over ice.

Refrigerator method: Fill a 2-quart pitcher with water and add 8 tea bags. Cover and refrigerate 8 hours. Remove and discard the tea bags and serve over ice.

Raspberry-Pear Smoothies `QUICK` `HIGH FIBER`

makes 2 servings

Smoothies are a nourishing treat to enjoy for breakfast, a snack, or an after-workout refresher. As a bonus, this one has some fiber from the raspberries and the unpeeled pear.

1½ cups unthawed frozen unsweetened raspberries
1 small ripe pear, cored and cut into chunks
1 cup ice cubes
⅓ cup orange juice

Combine all the ingredients in a blender and process until smooth, about 2 minutes.

Each serving: 15 g carb, 60 cal, 0 g fat, 0 g sat fat, 0 mg chol, 4 g fib, 1 g pro, 1 mg sod • Carb Choices: 1; Exchanges: 1 fruit

Kiwi-Apple Smoothies `QUICK`

makes 4 servings

Bright green and flecked with black kiwi seeds, this smoothie looks as good as it tastes. If the kiwis are not ripe, they can be quite tart, so make sure the kiwis you use yield to light pressure when gently squeezed.

2 medium ripe kiwis, peeled and chopped
1 small Granny Smith apple, cored and chopped
1 cup ice cubes
⅓ cup unsweetened apple juice
2 teaspoons honey

Combine all the ingredients in a blender and process until smooth, about 2 minutes.

Each serving: 14 g carb, 56 cal, 0 g fat, 0 g sat fat, 0 mg chol, 1 g fib, 1 g pro, 2 mg sod • Carb Choices: 1; Exchanges: 1 fruit

Peach-Almond Smoothies `QUICK`

makes 4 servings

Use this recipe as a blueprint for making any smoothie by switching the frozen fruit. Use blueberries, strawberries, raspberries, or cherries. If you don't want to use almond milk, use skim milk and add ¼ teaspoon almond extract.

2 cups unthawed frozen unsweetened sliced peaches
1 (6-ounce) container plain low-fat yogurt (generous ½ cup)
1½ cups unsweetened almond milk
1 tablespoon honey

Combine all the ingredients in a blender and process until smooth.

Each serving: 22 g carb, 112 cal, 2 g fat, 1 g sat fat, 3 mg chol, 1 g fib, 3 g pro, 87 mg sod • Carb Choices: 1½; Exchanges: 1 carb, ½ fruit

Citrus-Ginger Sparkler

makes 6 servings

Freshly squeezed juice and a hint of ginger give this drink bright flavor with a touch of sweetness. It's a healthful drink option to serve when you entertain. Those who wish can add a shot of vodka for a little kick.

2½ cups freshly squeezed orange juice
⅓ cup freshly squeezed lime juice
2 teaspoons grated fresh ginger
3 cups club soda, chilled
6 thin lime slices

Combine the orange juice, lime juice, and ginger in a large pitcher. Refrigerate until chilled, at least 2 hours and up to 1 day. Stir in the club soda just before serving. Serve over ice and garnish each serving with a lime slice.

Each serving: 12 g carb, 50 cal, 0 g fat, 0 g sat fat, 0 mg chol, 0 g fib, 1 g pro, 26 mg sod • Carb Choices: 1; Exchanges: 1 fruit

Cucumber-Mint Cooler

makes 8 servings

If you're lucky enough to have a patch of mint in your garden, use about ½ cup of fresh mint leaves instead of the mint tea bags. Garnish the drink with a mint sprig and a slice of lime and you'll feel like you're at a luxury spa.

8 cups cold water, divided
4 mint tea bags
1 hothouse (English) cucumber, peeled and chopped
8 thin lime or lemon slices

1 Bring 2 cups of the water to a boil in a small saucepan over high heat. Remove from the heat, add the tea bags, and let stand 5 minutes.

2 Place the cucumber and 1 cup of the remaining water in a food processor and process until smooth. Set a fine wire mesh strainer over a 2-quart pitcher. Pour the cucumber puree through the strainer. Discard the solids.

3 Remove and discard the tea bags and add the tea to the cucumber liquid. Stir in the remaining 5 cups water. Refrigerate until chilled, at least 2 hours and up to 1 day. Serve over ice and garnish each serving with a lime slice.

Each serving: 1 g carb, 4 cal, 0 g fat, 0 g sat fat, 0 mg chol, 0 g fib, 0 g pro, 1 mg sod • Carb Choices: 0

Grapefruit-Hibiscus Cooler

makes 8 servings

This pretty pink drink is a healthful beverage to serve at a party. If you have trouble finding hibiscus tea, try the recipe with Red Zinger tea.

4 cups water, divided
6 hibiscus tea bags
½ cup loosely packed fresh mint leaves
2 cups pink grapefruit juice
2 cups unsweetened apple juice
Mint sprigs

1 Bring 2 cups of the water to a boil in a small saucepan over high heat. Remove from the heat, add the tea bags and mint, and let stand 10 minutes.

2 Set a fine wire mesh strainer over a 2-quart pitcher. Pour the tea mixture through the strainer. Discard the solids. Stir in the remaining 2 cups water, the grapefruit juice, and apple juice. Refrigerate until chilled, at least 2 hours and up to 4 days. Serve over ice and garnish each serving with a mint sprig.

Each serving: 13 g carb, 53 cal, 0 g fat, 0 g sat fat, 0 mg chol, 0 g fib, 0 g pro, 2 mg sod • Carb Choices: 1; Exchanges: 1 fruit

Fresh Spicy Tomato Juice

makes 6 servings

When life gives you tomatoes, make tomato juice! This is an easy and delicious drink to make when you have a lot of tomatoes in late summer. It makes the best Bloody Marys you've ever had. If you want a plain version of tomato juice, just puree the tomatoes and salt together, omitting all the other ingredients, and then strain.

6 large beefsteak tomatoes, chopped
3 tablespoons lime juice
2 scallions, chopped
1 jalapeño, seeded and chopped
1 garlic clove, chopped
½ cup loosely packed fresh cilantro leaves
½ teaspoon kosher salt

Combine all the ingredients in a blender in batches and process until smooth. Set a medium wire mesh strainer over a pitcher. Pour the tomato puree mixture through the strainer. Discard the solids. Refrigerate until chilled, at least 2 hours and up to 4 days.

Each serving: 9 g carb, 38 cal, 0 g fat, 0 g sat fat, 0 mg chol, 0 g fib, 2 g pro, 104 mg sod • Carb Choices: ½; Exchanges: 2 veg

Watermelon Agua Fresca QUICK

makes 4 servings

Agua fresca is Spanish for "fresh water." Instead of watermelon, try cantaloupe, honeydew, or strawberries.

4 cups ¾-inch cubes seedless watermelon
1 cup cold water
1½ tablespoons lime juice

Combine all the ingredients in a blender in batches and process until smooth. Transfer to a pitcher. Serve over ice.

Each serving: 14 g carb, 41 cal, 0 g fat, 0 g sat fat, 0 mg chol, 1 g fib, 1 g pro, 5 mg sod • Carb Choices: 1; Exchanges: 1 fruit

Vegetable Water

makes 6 servings

A small amount of pureed vegetable gives water an amazing amount of flavor. They're really pretty, too—the cucumber and celery are pale green and the tomato is pink. Set out a selection of them in clear glass pitchers at a party for a thirst-quenching conversation starter.

6 cups cold water, divided
2 inner stalks celery with leaves attached, thinly sliced, or ½ cucumber, peeled and sliced, or 1 plum tomato, quartered, or 1 cup chopped fennel

1 Combine 1 cup of the water and the vegetable of your choice in a blender and process until smooth.

2 Set a fine wire mesh strainer over a 2-quart pitcher. Pour the vegetable mixture through the strainer. Discard the solids. Add the remaining 5 cups water to the pitcher and refrigerate until chilled, at least 2 hours and up to 2 days.

Each serving: 0 g carb, 2 cal, 0 g fat, 0 g sat fat, 0 mg chol, 0 g fib, 0 g pro, 18 mg sod • Carb Choices: 0

Herb Water

makes 8 servings

8 cups cold water, divided
¼ cup loosely packed fresh basil, dill, mint, or cilantro leaves or 2 tablespoons fresh tarragon leaves or a combination
8 thin lemon slices

1 Place 1 cup of the water and the herb of your choice in a blender and process until smooth.

2 Set a fine wire mesh strainer over a 2-quart pitcher. Pour the herb mixture through the strainer. Discard the solids. Add the remaining 7 cups water to the pitcher and refrigerate until chilled, at least 2 hours and up to 2 days.

Each serving: 0 g carb, 0 cal, 0 g fat, 0 g sat fat, 0 mg chol, 0 g fib, 0 g pro, 10 mg sod • Carb Choices: 0

Berry Water

makes 6 servings

With a handful of berries, you can turn ordinary water into a flavorful drink. Keep a clear pitcher of this water in the refrigerator and every time you open the door, there will be something delicious and calorie-free for you to enjoy. Garnish each glass with berries or a slice of citrus if you wish.

6 cups cold water, divided
1 cup fresh strawberries or frozen unsweetened strawberries, or ½ cup fresh raspberries or blueberries or frozen unsweetened raspberries or blueberries

1 Place 1 cup of the water and the berries of your choice in a blender and process until smooth.

2 Set a fine wire mesh strainer over a 2-quart pitcher. Pour the berry mixture through the strainer. Discard the solids. Add the remaining 5 cups of water to the pitcher and refrigerate until chilled, at least 2 hours and up to 2 days. Serve over ice.

Each serving: 2 g carb, 8 cal, 0 g fat, 0 g sat fat, 0 mg chol, 0 g fib, 0 g pro, 10 mg sod • Carb Choices: 0

Resources

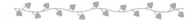

General Information

American Diabetes Association

www.diabetes.org

The American Diabetes Association website is a clearinghouse for information on all topics related to diabetes. The site includes information on healthy eating, exercise, and medications, as well as a bookstore, links to blogs and discussion groups for people with diabetes, and the latest research findings.

National Diabetes Education Program

www.ndep.nih.gov

Sponsored by the National Institutes of Health, the National Diabetes Education Program is a resource for information about managing diabetes, controlling risk factors, and making healthful lifestyle and behavior changes.

Joslin Diabetes Center

www.joslin.org

The Joslin Diabetes Center is a teaching and research affiliate of Harvard Medical School and is dedicated to diabetes research and education. The website offers free classes and newsletters, discussion boards, and extensive information on managing diabetes.

Juvenile Diabetes Research Foundation

www.jdrf.org

The Juvenile Diabetes Research Foundation International website will lead you to information on living with type 1 diabetes at any age and participating in clinical trials, and to numerous articles on everything from insurance coverage to insulin pumps.

American Association of Diabetes Educators

www.diabeteseducator.org

Find a health care professional in your area who is certified by the American Association of Diabetes Educators on this site.

www.diatraibe.com

An e-newsletter for staying informed about the latest research in diabetes management, drugs, devices, and treatments.

www.dlife .com

A comprehensive resource for information and support for living with diabetes. Check the site for local air times of *dLife TV*, a weekly television program that inspires and informs people with diabetes.

www.diabeteshealth.com

A resource for continuously updated diabetes news and diabetes blogs as well as information on new products and treatments. The site also has comprehensive information on glucose monitoring and diabetes medications.

www.fit4D.com

Offers personalized individual coaching to help meet goals for glucose control, weight loss, and fitness.

Weight Control

American Dietetic Association

www.eatright.org

The website of the American Dietetic Association is a resource for finding a registered dietitian who specializes in diabetes. The site also offers information on weight loss, shopping for healthy foods, and making healthy restaurant choices.

Weight Control Information Network

www.win.niddk.nih.gov

The Weight Control Information Network is a service of the National Institute of Diabetes and Digestive and Kidney Diseases (NIDDK). The website offers information on nutrition and fitness for all ages with tips on making healthy lifestyle changes.

Weight Watchers

www.weightwatchers.com

Offers education and support for weight management through weekly meetings and online groups.

Healthy Eating and Meal Planning

Complete Guide to Carbohydrate Counting by Hope S. Warshaw and Karmeen Kulkarni

A comprehensive manual for using the carb counting method of meal planning.

Choose Your Foods: Exchange Lists for Weight Management

An invaluable booklet on choosing foods and portions if you are following the exchange system. It is available from the American Diabetes Association website, www. diabetes.org.

My Food Advisor

www.diabetes.org/food-and-fitness/food/my-food-advisor

The My Food Advisor tool on the American Diabetes Association website is a system that allows you to track your daily food intake and calculates Exchanges for you.

www.diabetes.org/myfoodadvisor, www.calorieking.com, www.nal.usda.gov/fnic/foodcomp/search

Free online sources for carbohydrate and other nutrient content of foods.

The Ultimate Calorie, Carb, and Fat Gram Counter by Lea Ann Holzmeister and The Diabetes Carbohydrate and Calorie Counter by Annette Natow and Jo-Ann Heslin

Handy paperback books that give nutrient content of foods.

INDEX

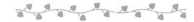

624 INDEX